PRINCIPLES AND APPLICATIONS IN ENGINEERING SERIES

Tissue Engineering

PRINCIPLES AND APPLICATIONS IN ENGINEERING SERIES

Tissue Engineering

Edited by

BERNHARD PALSSON
JEFFREY A. HUBBELL
ROBERT PLONSEY
JOSEPH D. BRONZINO

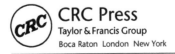

CRC Press
Taylor & Francis Group
Boca Raton London New York

CRC Press is an imprint of the
Taylor & Francis Group, an **informa** business

This material was originally published in Vol. II of *The Biomedical Engineering Handbook, Second Edition*, Joseph D. Bronzino, Ed., CRC Press, Boca Raton, FL, 2000.

CRC Press
Taylor & Francis Group
6000 Broken Sound Parkway NW, Suite 300
Boca Raton, FL 33487-2742

© 2003 by Taylor & Francis Group, LLC
CRC Press is an imprint of Taylor & Francis Group, an Informa business

First issued in paperback 2019

No claim to original U.S. Government works

ISBN 13: 978-0-367-44675-8 (pbk)
ISBN 13: 978-0-8493-1812-2 (hbk)

Visit the Taylor & Francis Web site at
http://www.taylorandfrancis.com

and the CRC Press Web site at
http://www.crcpress.com

Library of Congress Card Number 2003040913

Library of Congress Cataloging-in-Publication Data

Tissue engineering / edited by Bernhard Palsson ... [et al.].
    p. cm. — (Principles and applications in engineering ; 12)
    Includes bibliographical references and index.
    ISBN 0-8493-1812-2 (alk. paper)
    1. Biomedical engineering—Handbooks, manuals, etc. 2. Tissues—Handbooks, manuals, etc. I. Palsson, Bernhard. II. Series.

    R856.T57 2003
    610'.28—dc21

                                                          2003040913

Preface

Tissue engineering — a rapidly growing new field within biomedical engineering — represents a marriage of the rapid developments in cellular and molecular biology on the one hand, and materials, chemical, and mechanical engineering on the other. The ability to manipulate and reconstitute tissue function has tremendous clinical implications and is likely to play a major role in cell and gene therapies in the future as well as expanding the tissue supply for transplantation therapies.

Since tissue function is a rather complex topic and involves an intricate interplay of biologic and physiochemical rate processes, it is important for individuals in this field to have an understanding of physiologic systems. *Tissue Engineering* takes the most relevant sections regarding this important topic from the second edition of *The Biomedical Engineering Handbook* published by CRC Press in 2000. It begins with a section on physiologic systems, edited by Robert Plonsey, that provides an excellent overview of the human systems to set the stage for how topics related to tissue engineering can affect these important physiologic systems. The systems covered include the cardiovascular, nervous, vision, auditory, gastrointestinal, endocrine, and respiratory.

Drs. Bernhard Palsson, Jeffrey Hubbell, Robert Plonsey, and Joseph Bronzino, the editors of *Tissue Engineering*, considered three major goals: (1) to cover some of the generic engineering issues, (2) to cover generic cell biologic issues, and (3) to review the status of tissue engineering of specific organs. To accomplish these goals, topics covered include biomolecular properties of surface, engineering of scaffolds, and templates on which cells are grown for transplantation purposes, stem cell biology, cell motility, and the role of stroma in tissue engineering.

In addition, progress with the engineering of specific tissues is described. Six tissues where much progress has been made are emphasized: bone marrow, liver, the nervous system, skeletal muscle, cartilage, and kidney. These chapters provide a concise review of the accomplishments of advances in tissue engineering to date and the likely clinical implications of these developments in the future.

Advisory Board

Contributors

Patrick Aebischer
Lausanne University Medical
School
Lausanne, Switzerland

Berj L. Bardakjian
University of Toronto
Toronto, Canada

Ravi Bellamkonda
Lausanne University Medical
School
Lausanne, Switzerland

François Berthiaume
Surgical Services, Massachusetts
General Hospital, Harvard
Medical School, and the Shriners
Hospital for Children
Cambridge, Massachusetts

Joseph D. Bronzino
Trinity College/The Biomedical
Engineering Alliance and
Consortium (BEACON)
Hartford, Connecticut

Susan V. Brooks
University of Michigan
Ann Arbor, Michigan

Ewart R. Carson
City University
London, United Kingdom

Joseph A. Chinn
Sulzer Carbomedics
Austin, Texas

Ben M. Clopton
University of Washington
Seattle, Washington

Derek G. Cramp
City University
London, United Kingdom

Paul D. Drumheller
Gore Hybrid Technologies, Inc.
Flagstaff, Arizona

Karen A. Duca
University of Wisconsin
Madison, Wisconsin

Graham A. Dunn
King's College
London, United Kingdom

John A. Faulkner
University of Michigan
Ann Arbor, Michigan

L.E. Freed
Harvard University
Cambridge, Massachusetts

Jeffrey A. Hubbell
California Institute of Technology
Pasadena, California

H. David Humes
University of Michigan
Ann Arbor, Michigan

Arthur T. Johnson
University of Maryland
College Park, Maryland

Craig T. Jordan
Somatix Therapy Corp.
Alameda, California

Tao Ho Kim
Harvard University and Boston
Children's Hospital
Boston, Massachusetts

Manfred R. Koller
Oncosis
San Diego, California

Robert S. Langer
Massachusetts Institute of
Technology
Cambridge, Massachusetts

Christopher G. Lausted
University of Maryland
College Park, Maryland

Edwin N. Lightfoot
University of Wisconsin
Madison, Wisconsin

Michael W. Long
University of Michigan
Ann Arbor, Michigan

Larry V. McIntire
Rice University
Houston, Texas

**Evangelia Micheli-
Tzanakou**
Rutgers University
Piscataway, New Jersey

David J. Mooney
Massachusetts Institute of
Technology
Cambridge, Massachusetts

Brian A. Naughton
Advanced Tissue Sciences, Inc.
La Jolla, California

Bernhard Ø. Palsson
University of Michigan
Ann Arbor, Michigan

Charles W. Patrick, Jr.
Rice University
Houston, Texas

Robert Plonsey
Duke University
Durham, North Carolina

Rangarajan Sampath
Rice University
Houston, Texas

Daniel J. Schneck
Virginia Polytechnic Institute and
  State University
Blacksburg, Virginia

Steven M. Slack
The University of Memphis
Memphis, Tennessee

Francis A. Spelman
University of Washington
Seattle, Washington

George Stetten
Duke University
Durham, North Carolina

Joseph P. Vacanti
Harvard University and Boston
  Children's Hospital
Boston, Massachusetts

Gary Van Zant
University of Kentucky Medical
  Center
Lexington, Kentucky

G. Vunjak-Novakovic
Massachusetts Institute of
  Technology
Cambridge, Massachusetts

Ioannis V. Yannas
Massachusetts Institute of
  Technology
Cambridge, Massachusetts

Martin L. Yarmush
Massachusetts General Hospital,
  Harvard Medical School, and the
  Shriners Burns Hospital
Cambridge, Massachusetts

Contents

I

Physiologic Systems

Robert Plonsey
Duke University

THE CONTENT OF THIS book is devoted to the subject of *tissue engineering*. We understand biomedical engineering to involve the application of engineering science and technology to problems arising in medicine and biology. In principle, the intersection of each engineering discipline (i.e., electrical, mechanical, chemical, etc.) with each discipline in medicine (i.e., cardiology, pathology, neurology, etc.) or biology (i.e., biochemistry, pharmacology, molecular biology, cell biology, etc.) is a potential area of biomedical engineering application. As such, the discipline of biomedical engineering is potentially very extensive. However, at least to date, only a few of the aforementioned "intersections" contain active areas of research and/or development. The most significant of these are described in this book.

While the application of engineering expertise to the life sciences requires an obvious knowledge of contemporary technical theory and its applications, it also demands an adequate knowledge and under-standing of relevant medicine and biology. It has been argued that the most challenging part of finding engineering solutions to problems lies in the formulation of the solution in engineering terms. In biomedical engineering, this usually demands a full understanding of the life science substrates as well as the quantitative methodologies.

This section is devoted to an overview of the major physiologic systems of current interest to biomedical engineers, on which their work is based. The overview may contain useful definitions, tables of basic physiologic data, and an introduction to the literature. Obviously these chapters must be extremely brief. However, our goal is an introduction that may enable the reader to clarify some item of interest or to indicate a way to pursue further information. Possibly the reader will find the greatest value in the references to more extensive literature.

This section contains seven chapters, and these describe each of the major organ systems of the human body. Thus we have chapters describing the cardiovascular, endocrine, nervous, visual, auditory, gas-trointestinal, and respiratory systems. While each author is writing at an introductory and tutorial level, the audience is assumed to have some technical expertise, and consequently mathematical descriptions are not avoided. All authors are recognized as experts on the system which they describe, but all are also biomedical engineers.

The authors in this section noted that they would have liked more space but recognized that the main focus of this book is on "engineering." The hope is that readers will find this introductory section helpful to their understanding of later chapters of this book and, as noted above, that this section will at least provide a starting point for further investigation into the life sciences.

1

An Outline of Cardiovascular Structure and Function

Daniel J. Schneck
Virginia Polytechnic Institute and State University

Because not every cell in the human body is near enough to the environment to easily exchange with it mass (including nutrients, oxygen, carbon dioxide, and the waste products of metabolism), energy (including heat), and momentum, the physiologic system is endowed with a major highway network—organized to make available thousands of miles of access tubing for the transport to and from a different neighborhood (on the order of 10 μm or less) of any given cell whatever it needs to sustain life. This highway network, called the *cardiovascular system,* includes a pumping station, the heart; a working fluid, blood; a complex branching configuration of distributing and collecting pipes and channels, blood vessels; and a sophisticated means for both intrinsic (inherent) and extrinsic (autonomic and endocrine) control.

1.1   The Working Fluid: Blood

Accounting for about $8 \pm 1\%$ of total body weight, averaging 5200 ml, blood is a complex, heterogeneous suspension of formed elements—the *blood cells,* or *hematocytes*—suspended in a continuous, straw-colored fluid called *plasma.* Nominally, the composite fluid has a mass density of 1.057 ± 0.007 g/cm^3, and it is three to six times as viscous as water. The hematocytes (Table 1.1) include three basic types of cells: red blood cells (erythrocytes, totaling nearly 95% of the formed elements), white blood cells (leukocytes, averaging <0.15% of all hematocytes), and platelets (thrombocytes, on the order of 5% of all blood cells). Hematocytes are all derived in the active ("red") bone marrow (about 1500 g) of adults from undifferentiated stem cells called *hemocytoblasts,* and all reach ultimate maturity via a process called *hematocytopoiesis.*

The primary function of erythrocytes is to aid in the transport of blood gases—about 30 to 34% (by weight) of each cell consisting of the oxygen- and carbon dioxide–carrying protein hemoglobin (64,000 $\leq$ MW $\leq$ 68,000) and a small portion of the cell containing the enzyme carbonic anhydrase, which catalyzes the reversible formation of carbonic acid from carbon dioxide and water. The primary function of leukocytes is to endow the human body with the ability to identify and dispose of foreign substances (such as infectious organisms) that do not belong there—agranulocytes (lymphocytes and monocytes)

TABLE 1.1   Hematocytes

Cell Type	Number Cells per mm³ Blood*	Corpuscular Diameter (μm)*	Corpuscular Surface Area (μm²)*	Corpuscular Volume (μm³)*	Mass Density (g/cm³)*	Percent Water*	Percent Protein*	Percent Extractives*†
Erythrocytes (red blood cells)	4.2–5.4 × 10⁶ ♀ 4.6–6.2 × 10⁶ ♂ (5 × 10⁶)	6–9 (7.5) Thickness 1.84–2.84 "Neck" 0.81–1.44	120–163 (140)	80–100 (90)	1.089–1.100 (1.098)	64–68 (66)	29–35 (32)	1.6–2.8 (2)
Leukocytes (white blood cells)	4000–11000 (7500)	6–10	300–625	160–450	1.055–1.085	52–60 (56)	30–36 (33)	4–18 (11)
Granulocytes								
Neutrophils: 55–70% WBC (65%)	2–6 × 10³ (4875)	8–8.6 (8.3)	422–511 (467)	268–333 (300)	1.075–1.085 (1.080)	—	—	—
Eosinophils: 1–4% WBC (3%)	45–480 (225)	8–9 (8.5)	422–560 (491)	268–382 (321)	1.075–1.085 (1.080)	—	—	—
Basophils: 0–1.5% WBC (1%)	0–113 (75)	7.7–8.5 (8.1)	391–500 (445)	239–321 (278)	1.075–1.085 (1.080)	—	—	—
Agranulocytes								
Lymphocytes: 20–35% WBC (25%)	1000–4800 (1875)	6.75–7.34 (7.06)	300–372 (336)	161–207 (184)	1.055–1.070 (1.063)	—	—	—
Monocytes: 3–8% WBC (6%)	100–800 (450)	9–9.5 (9.25)	534–624 (579)	382–449 (414)	1.055–1.070 (1.063)	—	—	—
Thrombocytes (platelets)	(1.4 ♂), 2.14 (♀)–5 × 10⁵ (2.675 × 10⁵)	2–4 (3) Thickness 0.9–1.3	16–35 (25)	5–10 (7.5)	1.04–1.06 (1.05)	60–68 (64)	32–40 (36)	Neg.

*Normal physiologic range, with "typical" value in parentheses.
†Extractives include mostly minerals (ash), carbohydrates, and fats (lipids).

essentially doing the "identifying" and granulocytes (neutrophils, basophils, and eosinophils) essentially doing the "disposing." The primary function of platelets is to participate in the blood clotting process.

Removal of all hematocytes from blood centrifugation or other separating techniques leaves behind the aqueous (91% water by weight, 94.8% water by volume), saline (0.15 N) suspending medium called *plasma*—which has an average mass density of 1.035 ± 0.005 g/cm³ and a viscosity 1½ to 2 times that of water. Some 6.5 to 8% by weight of plasma consists of the plasma proteins, of which there are three major types—albumin, the globulins, and fibrinogen—and several of lesser prominence (Table 1.2).

TABLE 1.2 Plasma

Constituent	Concentration Range (mg/dl plasma)	Typical Plasma Value (mg/dl)	Molecular Weight Range	Typical Value	Typical size (nm)
Total protein, 7% by weight	6400–8300	7245	21,000–1,200,000	—	—
Albumin (56% TP)	2800–5600	4057	66,500–69,000	69,000	15 × 4
α_1-*Globulin* (5.5% TP)	300–600	400	21,000–435,000	60,000	5–12
α_2-*Globulin* (7.5% TP)	400–900	542	100,000–725,000	200,000	50–500
β-*Globulin* (13% TP)	500–1230	942	90,000–1,200,000	100,000	18–50
γ-*Globulin* (12% TP)	500–1800	869	150,000–196,000	150,000	23 × 4
Fibrinogen (4% TP)	150–470	290	330,000–450,000	390,000	(50–60) × (3–8)
Other (2% TP)	70–210	145	70,000–1,000,000	200,000	(15–25) × (2–6)
Inorganic ash, 0.95% by weight	930–1140	983	20–100	—	— (Radius)
Sodium	300–340	325	—	22.98977	0.102 (Na^+)
Potassium	13–21	17	—	39.09800	0.138 (K^+)
Calcium	8.4–11.0	10	—	40.08000	0.099 (Ca^{2+})
Magnesium	1.5–3.0	2	—	24,30500	0.072 (Mg^{2+})
Chloride	336–390	369	—	35.45300	0.181 (Cl^-)
Bicarbonate	110–240	175	—	61.01710	0.163 (HCO_3^-)
Phosphate	2.7–4.5	3.6	—	95.97926	0.210 (HPO_4^{2-})
Sulfate	0.5–1.5	1.0	—	96.05760	0.230 (SO_4^{2-})
Other	0–100	80.4	20–100	—	0.1–0.3
Lipids (fats), 0.80% by weight	541–1000	828	44,000–3,200,000	= Lipoproteins	Up to 200 or more
Cholesterol (34% TL)	12–105 "free" 72–259 esterified, 84–364 "total"	59 224 283	386.67	Contained mostly in intermediate to LDL β-lipoproteins; higher in women	
Phospholipid (35% TL)	150–331	292	690–1010	Contained mainly in HDL to VHDL α_1-lipoproteins	
Triglyceride (26% TL)	65–240	215	400–1370	Contained mainly in VLDL α_2-lipoproteins and chylomicrons	
Other (5% TL)	0–80	38	280–1500	Fat-soluble vitamins, prostaglandins, fatty acids	
Extractives, 0.25% by weight	200–500	259	—	—	—
Glucose	60–120, fasting	90	—	180.1572	0.86 D
Urea	20–30	25	—	60.0554	0.36 D
Carbohydrate	60–105	83	180.16–342.3	—	0.74–0.108 D
Other	11–111	61	—	—	—

The primary functions of albumin are to help maintain the osmotic (oncotic) transmural pressure differential that ensures proper mass exchange between blood and interstitial fluid at the capillary level and to serve as a transport carrier molecule for several hormones and other small biochemical constituents (such as some metal ions). The primary function of the globulin class of proteins is to act as transport carrier molecules (mostly of the α and β class) for large biochemical substances, such as fats (lipoproteins) and certain carbohydrates (muco- and glycoproteins) and heavy metals (mineraloproteins), and to work together with leukocytes in the body's immune system. The latter function is primarily the responsibility of the γ class of immunoglobulins, which have antibody activity. The primary function of fibrinogen is to work with thrombocytes in the formation of a blood clot—a process also aided by one of the most abundant of the lesser proteins, prothrombin (MW ≃ 62,000).

Of the remaining 2% or so (by weight) of plasma, just under half (0.95%, or 983 mg/dl plasma) consists of minerals (inorganic ash), trace elements, and electrolytes, mostly the cations sodium, potassium, calcium, and magnesium and the anions chlorine, bicarbonate, phosphate, and sulfate—the latter three helping as buffers to maintain the fluid at a slightly alkaline pH between 7.35 and 7.45 (average 7.4). What is left, about 1087 mg of material per deciliter of plasma, includes (1) mainly (0.8% by weight) three major types of fat, i.e., cholesterol (in a free and esterified form), phospholipid (a major ingredient of cell membranes), and triglyceride, with lesser amounts of the fat-soluble vitamins (A, D, E, and K), free fatty acids, and other lipids, and (2) "extractives" (0.25% by weight), of which about two-thirds includes glucose and other forms of carbohydrate, the remainder consisting of the water-soluble vitamins (B-complex and C), certain enzymes, nonnitrogenous and nitrogenous waste products of metabolism (including urea, creatine, and creatinine), and many smaller amounts of other biochemical constituents—the list seeming virtually endless.

Removal from blood of all hematocytes and the protein fibrinogen (by allowing the fluid to completely clot before centrifuging) leaves behind a clear fluid called *serum*, which has a density of about 1.018 ± 0.003 g/cm³ and a viscosity up to 1½ times that of water. A glimpse of Tables 1.1 and 1.2, together with the very brief summary presented above, nevertheless gives the reader an immediate appreciation for why blood is often referred to as the "river of life." This river is made to flow through the vascular piping network by two central pumping stations arranged in series: the left and right sides of the human heart.

1.2   The Pumping Station: The Heart

Barely the size of the clenched fist of the individual in whom it resides—an inverted, conically shaped, hollow muscular organ measuring 12 to 13 cm from base (top) to apex (bottom) and 7 to 8 cm at its widest point and weighing just under 0.75 lb (about 0.474% of the individual's body weight, or some 325 g)—the human heart occupies a small region between the third and sixth ribs in the central portion of the thoracic cavity of the body. It rests on the diaphragm, between the lower part of the two lungs, its base-to-apex axis leaning mostly toward the left side of the body and slightly forward. The heart is divided by a tough muscular wall—the interatrial-interventricular septum—into a somewhat crescent-shaped right side and cylindrically shaped left side (Fig. 1.1), each being one self-contained pumping station, but the two being connected in series. The left side of the heart drives oxygen-rich blood through the aortic semilunar outlet valve into the *systemic circulation,* which carries the fluid to within a differential neighborhood of each cell in the body—from which it returns to the right side of the heart low in oxygen and rich in carbon dioxide. The right side of the heart then drives this oxygen-poor blood through the pulmonary semilunar (pulmonic) outlet valve into the *pulmonary circulation,* which carries the fluid to the lungs—where its oxygen supply is replenished and its carbon dioxide content is purged before it returns to the left side of the heart to begin the cycle all over again. Because of the anatomic proximity of the heart to the lungs, the right side of the heart does not have to work very hard to drive blood through the pulmonary circulation, so it functions as a low-pressure ($P \leq 40$ mmHg gauge) pump compared with the left side of the heart, which does most of its work at a high pressure (up to 140 mmHg gauge or more) to drive blood through the entire systemic circulation to the furthest extremes of the organism.

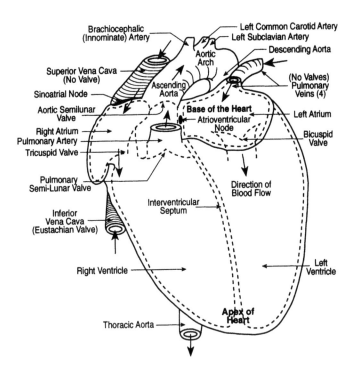

FIGURE 1.1 Anterior view of the human heart showing the four chambers, the inlet and outlet valves, the inlet and outlet major blood vessels, the wall separating the right side from the left side, and the two cardiac pacing centers—the sinoatrial node and the atrioventricular node. Boldface arrows show the direction of flow through the heart chambers, the valves, and the major vessels.

Each cardiac (heart) pump is further divided into two chambers: a small upper receiving chamber, or atrium (auricle), separated by a one-way valve from a lower discharging chamber, or ventricle, which is about twice the size of its corresponding atrium. In order of size, the somewhat spherically shaped left atrium is the smallest chamber—holding about 45 ml of blood (at rest), operating at pressures on the order of 0 to 25 mmHg gauge, and having a wall thickness of about 3 mm. The pouch-shaped right atrium is next (63 ml of blood, 0 to 10 mmHg gauge of pressure, 2-mm wall thickness), followed by the conical/cylindrically shaped left ventricle (100 ml of blood, up to 140 mmHg gauge of pressure, variable wall thickness up to 12 mm) and the crescent-shaped right ventricle (about 130 ml of blood, up to 40 mmHg gauge of pressure, and a wall thickness on the order of one-third that of the left ventricle, up to about 4 mm). All together, then, the heart chambers collectively have a capacity of some 325 to 350 ml, or about 6.5% of the total blood volume in a "typical" individual—but these values are nominal, since the organ alternately fills and expands, contracts, and then empties as it generates a *cardiac output*.

During the 480-ms or so filling phase—diastole—of the average 750-ms cardiac cycle, the inlet valves of the two ventricles (3.8-cm-diameter tricuspid valve from right atrium to right ventricle; 3.1-cm-diameter bicuspid or mitral valve from left atrium to left ventricle) are open, and the outlet valves (2.4-cm-diameter pulmonary valve and 2.25-cm-diameter aortic semilunar valve, respectively) are closed—the heart ultimately expanding to its end diastolic volume (EDV), which is on the order of 140 ml of blood for the left ventricle. During the 270-ms emptying phase—systole—electrically induced vigorous contraction of cardiac muscle drives the intraventricular pressure up, forcing the one-way inlet valves closed and the unidirectional outlet valves open as the heart contracts to its end systolic volume (ESV), which is typically on the order of 70 ml of blood for the left ventricle. Thus the ventricles normally empty about half their contained volume with each heart beat, the remainder being termed the *cardiac reserve volume*. More generally, the difference between the *actual* EDV and the *actual* ESV, called the *stroke volume* (SV), is the volume of blood expelled from the heart during each systolic interval, and the ratio of SV to EDV is called the *cardiac ejection fraction,* or *ejection ratio* (0.5 to 0.75 is normal, 0.4 to 0.5 signifies mild cardiac damage, 0.25 to 0.40 implies moderate heart damage, and <0.25 warns of severe damage to the heart's pumping ability). If the stroke volume is multiplied by the number of systolic intervals per minute, or heart rate (HR), one obtains the total cardiac output (CO):

$$CO = HR \times \left(EDV - ESV\right) \tag{1.1}$$

Dawson [1991] has suggested that the cardiac output (in milliliters per minute) is proportional to the weight W (in kilograms) of an individual according to the equation

$$CO - 224W^{3/4} \tag{1.2}$$

and that "normal" heart rate obeys very closely the relation

$$HR = 229W^{-1/4} \tag{1.3}$$

For a "typical" 68.7-kg individual (blood volume = 5200 ml), Eqs. (1.1), (1.2), and (1.3) yield CO = 5345 ml/min, HR = 80 beats/min (cardiac cycle period = 754 ms) and SV = CO/HR = $224W^{3/4}/229W^{-1/4}$ = $0.978W$ = 67.2 ml/beat, which are very reasonable values. Furthermore, assuming this individual lives about 75 years, his or her heart will have cycled over 3.1536 billion times, pumping a total of 0.2107 billion liters of blood (55.665 million gallons, or 8134 quarts per day)—all of it emptying into the circulatory pathways that constitute the vascular system.

1.3   The Piping Network: Blood Vessels

The vascular system is divided by a microscopic capillary network into an upstream, high-pressure, efferent arterial side (Table 1.3)—consisting of relatively thick-walled, viscoelastic tubes that carry blood away from the heart—and a downstream, low-pressure, afferent venous side (Table 1.4)—consisting of correspondingly thinner (but having a larger caliber) elastic conduits that return blood to the heart. Except for their differences in thickness, the walls of the largest arteries and veins consist of the same three distinct, well-defined, and well-developed layers. From innermost to outermost, these layers are (1) the thinnest *tunica intima,* a continuous lining (the vascular endothelium) consisting of a single layer of simple squamous (thin, sheetlike) endothelial cells "glued" together by a polysaccharide (sugar) intercellular matrix, surrounded by a thin layer of subendothelial connective tissue interlaced with a number of circularly arranged elastic fibers to form the subendothelium, and separated from the next adjacent wall layer by a thick elastic band called the *internal elastic lamina*; (2) the thickest *tunica media,* composed of numerous circularly arranged elastic fibers, especially prevalent in the largest blood vessels on the arterial side (allowing them to expand during systole and to recoil passively during diastole), a significant amount of smooth muscle cells arranged in spiraling layers around the vessel wall, especially prevalent in medium-sized arteries and arterioles (allowing them to function as control points for blood distribution), and some interlacing collagenous connective tissue, elastic fibers, and intercellular muco-polysaccharide substance (extractives), all separated from the next adjacent wall layer by another thick elastic band called the *external elastic lamina*; and (3) the medium-sized *tunica adventitia,* an outer vascular sheath consisting entirely of connective tissue.

The largest blood vessels, such as the aorta, the pulmonary artery, the pulmonary veins, and others, have such thick walls that they require a separate network of tiny blood vessels—the vasa vasorum—just to service the vascular tissue itself. As one moves toward the capillaries from the arterial side (see Table 1.3), the vascular wall keeps thinning, as if it were shedding 15-μm-thick, onion-peel-like concentric layers, and while the percentage of water in the vessel wall stays relatively constant at 70% (by weight),

TABLE 1.3 Arterial System*

Blood Vessel Type	(Systemic) Typical Number	Internal Diameter Range	Length Range†	Wall Thickness	Systemic Volume	(Pulmonary) Typical Number	Pulmonary Volume
Aorta	1	1.0–3.0 cm	30–65 cm	2–3 mm	156 ml	—	—
Pulmonary artery	—	2.5–3.1 cm	6–9 cm	2–3 cm	—	1	52 ml

Wall morphology: Complete tunica adventitia, external elastic lamina, tunica media, internal elastic lamina, tunica intima, subendothelium, endothelium, and vasa vasorum vascular supply

Blood Vessel Type	(Systemic) Typical Number	Internal Diameter Range	Length Range†	Wall Thickness	Systemic Volume	(Pulmonary) Typical Number	Pulmonary Volume
Main branches	32	5 mm–2.25 cm	3.3–6 cm	≃2 mm	83.2 ml	6	41.6 ml

(Along with the aorta and pulmonary artery, the largest, most well-developed of all blood vessels)

Blood Vessel Type	(Systemic) Typical Number	Internal Diameter Range	Length Range†	Wall Thickness	Systemic Volume	(Pulmonary) Typical Number	Pulmonary Volume
Large arteries	288	4.0–5.0 mm	1.4–2.8 cm	≃1 mm	104 ml	64	23.5 ml

(A well-developed tunica adventitia and vasa vasorum, although wall layers are gradually thinning)

Blood Vessel Type	(Systemic) Typical Number	Internal Diameter Range	Length Range†	Wall Thickness	Systemic Volume	(Pulmonary) Typical Number	Pulmonary Volume
Medium arteries	1152	2.5–4.0 mm	1.0–2.2 cm	≃0.75 mm	117 ml	144	7.3 ml
Small arteries	3456	1.0–2.5 mm	0.6–1.7 cm	≃0.50 mm	104 ml	432	5.7 ml
Tributaries	20,736	0.5–1.0 mm	0.3–1.3 cm	≃0.25 mm	91 ml	5184	7.3 ml

(Well-developed tunica media and external elastic lamina, but tunica adventitia virtually nonexistent)

Blood Vessel Type	(Systemic) Typical Number	Internal Diameter Range	Length Range†	Wall Thickness	Systemic Volume	(Pulmonary) Typical Number	Pulmonary Volume
Small rami	82,944	250–500 μm	0.2–0.8 cm	≃125 μm	57.2 ml	11,664	2.3 ml
Terminal branches	497,664	100–250 μm	1.0–6.0 mm	≃60 μm	52 ml	139,968	3.0 ml

(A well-developed endothelium, subendothelium, and internal elastic lamina, plus about two to three 15-μm-thick concentric layers forming just a very thin tunica media; no external elastic lamina)

Blood Vessel Type	(Systemic) Typical Number	Internal Diameter Range	Length Range†	Wall Thickness	Systemic Volume	(Pulmonary) Typical Number	Pulmonary Volume
Arterioles	18,579,456	25–100 μm	0.2–3.8 mm	≃20–30 μm	52 ml	4,094,064	2.3 ml

Wall morphology: More than one smooth muscle layer (with nerve association in the outermost muscle layer), a well-developed internal elastic lamina; gradually thinning in 25- to 50-μm vessels to a single layer of smooth muscle tissue, connective tissue, and scant supporting tissue.

Blood Vessel Type	(Systemic) Typical Number	Internal Diameter Range	Length Range†	Wall Thickness	Systemic Volume	(Pulmonary) Typical Number	Pulmonary Volume
Metarterioles	238,878,720	10–25 μm	0.1–1.8 mm	≃5–15 μm	41.6 ml	157,306,536	4.0 ml

(Well-developed subendothelium; discontinuous contractile muscle elements; one layer of connective tissue)

Blood Vessel Type	(Systemic) Typical Number	Internal Diameter Range	Length Range†	Wall Thickness	Systemic Volume	(Pulmonary) Typical Number	Pulmonary Volume
Capillaries	16,124,431,360	3.5–10 μm	0.5–1.1 mm	≃0.5–1 μm	260 ml	3,218,406,696	104 ml

(Simple endothelial tubes devoid of smooth muscle tissue; one-cell-layer-thick walls)

*Values are approximate for a 68.7-kg individual having a total blood volume of 5200 ml.

†Average uninterrupted distance between branch origins (except aorta and pulmonary artery, which are total length).

TABLE 1.4 Venous System

Blood Vessel Type	(Systemic) Typical Number	Internal Diameter Range	Length Range	Wall Thickness	Systemic Volume	(Pulmonary) Typical Number	Pulmonary Volume
Postcapillary venules	4,408,161,734	8–30 μm	0.1–0.6 mm	1.0–5.0 μm	166.7 ml	306,110,016	10.4 ml
(Wall consists of thin endothelium exhibiting occasional pericytes (pericapillary connective tissue cells) which increase in number as the vessel lumen gradually increases)							
Collecting venules	160,444,500	30–50 μm	0.1–0.8 mm	5.0–10 μm	161.3 ml	8,503,056	1.2 ml
(One complete layer of pericytes, one complete layer of veil cells (veil-like cells forming a thin membrane), occasional primitive smooth muscle tissue fibers that increase in number with vessel size)							
Muscular venules	32,088,900	50–100 μm	0.2–1.0 mm	10–25 μm	141.8 ml	3,779,136	3.7 ml
(Relatively thick wall of smooth muscle tissue)							
Small collecting veins	10,241,508	100–200 μm	0.5–3.2 mm	≈30 μm	329.6 ml	419,904	6.7 ml
(Prominent tunica media of continuous layers of smooth muscle cells)							
Terminal branches	496,900	200–600 μm	1.0–6.0 mm	30–150 μm	206.6 ml	34,992	5.2 ml
(A well-developed endothelium, subendothelium, and internal elastic lamina; well-developed tunica media but fewer elastic fibers than corresponding arteries and much thinner walls)							
Small veins	19,968	600 μm–1.1 mm	2.0–9.0 mm	≈0.25 mm	63.5 ml	17,280	44.9 ml
Medium veins	512	1–5 mm	1–2 cm	≈0.50 mm	67.0 ml	144	22.0 ml
Large veins	256	5–9 mm	1.4–3.7 cm	≈0.75 mm	476.1 ml	48	29.5 ml
(Well-developed wall layers comparable to large arteries but about 25% thinner)							
Main branches	224	9.0 mm–2.0 cm	2.0–10 cm	≈1.00 mm	1538.1 ml	16	39.4 ml
(Along with the vena cava and pulmonary veins, the largest, most well-developed of all blood vessels)							
Vena cava	1	2.0–3.5 cm	20–50 cm	≈1.50 mm	125.3 ml	—	—
Pulmonary veins	—	1.7–2.5 cm	5–8 cm	≈1.50 mm	—	4	52 ml

Wall morphology: Essentially the same as comparable major arteries but a much thinner tunica intima, a much thinner tunica media, and a somewhat thicker tunica adventitia; contains a vasa vasorum

Total systemic blood volume: 4394 ml—84.5% of total blood volume; 19.5% in arteries (~3:2 large:small), 5.9% in capillaries, 74.6% in veins (~3:1 large:small); 63% of volume is in vessels greater than 1 mm internal diameter

Total pulmonary blood volume: 468 ml—9.0% of total blood volume; 31.8% in arteries, 22.2% in capillaries, 46% in veins; 58.3% of volume is in vessels greater than 1 mm internal diameter; remainder of blood in heart, about 338 ml (6.5% of total blood volume)

the ratio of elastin to collagen decreases (actually reverses)—from 3:2 in large arteries (9% elastin, 6% collagen, by weight) to 1:2 in small tributaries (5% elastin, 10% collagen)—and the amount of smooth muscle tissue increases from 7.5% by weight of large arteries (the remaining 7.5% consisting of various extractives) to 15% in small tributaries. By the time one reaches the capillaries, one encounters single-cell-thick endothelial tubes—devoid of any smooth muscle tissue, elastin, or collagen—downstream of which the vascular wall gradually "reassembles itself," layer-by-layer, as it directs blood back to the heart through the venous system (Table 1.4).

Blood vessel structure is directly related to function. The thick-walled large arteries and main *distributing branches* are designed to withstand the pulsating 80 to 130 mmHg blood pressures that they must endure. The smaller elastic *conducting vessels* need only operate under steadier blood pressures in the range 70 to 90 mmHg, but they must be thin enough to penetrate and course through organs without unduly disturbing the anatomic integrity of the mass involved. Controlling arterioles operate at blood pressures between 45 and 70 mmHg but are heavily endowed with smooth muscle tissue (hence their being referred to as *muscular vessels*) so that they may be actively shut down when flow to the capillary bed they service is to be restricted (for whatever reason), and the smallest capillary *resistance vessels* (which operate at blood pressures on the order of 10 to 45 mmHg) are designed to optimize conditions for transport to occur between blood and the surrounding interstitial fluid. Traveling back up the venous side, one encounters relatively steady blood pressures continuously decreasing from around 30 mmHg all the way down to near zero, so these vessels can be thin-walled without disease consequence. However, the low blood pressure, slower, steady (time-dependent) flow, thin walls, and larger caliber that characterize the venous system cause blood to tend to "pool" in veins, allowing them to act somewhat like reservoirs. It is not surprising, then, that at any given instant, one normally finds about two-thirds of the total human blood volume residing in the venous system, the remaining one-third being divided among the heart (6.5%), the microcirculation (7% in systemic and pulmonary capillaries), and the arterial system (19.5 to 20%).

In a global sense, then, one can think of the human cardiovascular system—using an electrical analogy—as a voltage source (the heart), two capacitors (a large venous system and a smaller arterial system), and a resistor (the microcirculation taken as a whole). Blood flow and the dynamics of the system represent electrical inductance (inertia), and useful engineering approximations can be derived from such a simple model. The cardiovascular system is designed to bring blood to within a capillary size of each and every one of the more than 10^{14} cells of the body—but *which* cells receive blood at any given time, *how much* blood they get, the *composition* of the fluid coursing by them, and related physiologic considerations are all matters that are not left to chance.

1.4 Cardiovascular Control

Blood flows through organs and tissues either to nourish and sanitize them or to be itself processed in some sense—e.g., to be oxygenated (pulmonary circulation), stocked with nutrients (splanchnic circulation), dialyzed (renal circulation), cooled (cutaneous circulation), filtered of dilapidated red blood cells (splenic circulation), and so on. Thus any given vascular network normally receives blood according to the metabolic needs of the region it perfuses and/or the function of that region as a blood treatment plant and/or thermoregulatory pathway. However, it is not feasible to expect that our physiologic transport system can be "all things to all cells all of the time"—especially when resources are scarce and/or time is a factor. Thus the distribution of blood is further prioritized according to three basic criteria: (1) how essential the perfused region is to the maintenance of life itself (e.g., we can survive without an arm, a leg, a stomach, or even a large portion of our small intestine but not without a brain, a heart, and at least one functioning kidney and lung, (2) how essential the perfused region is in allowing the organism to respond to a life-threatening situation (e.g., digesting a meal is among the least of the body's concerns in a "fight or flight" circumstance), and (3) how well the perfused region can function and survive on a decreased supply of blood (e.g., some tissues—like striated skeletal and smooth muscle—have significant anaerobic capability; others—like several forms of connective tissue—can function quite effectively at a significantly decreased metabolic rate when necessary; some organs—like the liver—are larger than they really need to be; and some anatomic structures—like the eyes, ears, and limbs—have duplicates, giving them a built-in redundancy).

Within this generalized prioritization scheme, control of cardiovascular function is accomplished by mechanisms that are based either on the inherent physicochemical attributes of the tissues and organs themselves—so-called intrinsic control—or on responses that can be attributed to the effects on cardio-vascular tissues of other organ systems in the body (most notably the autonomic nervous system and the endocrine system)—so-called extrinsic control. For example, the accumulation of wastes and deple-tion of oxygen and nutrients that accompany the increased rate of metabolism in an active tissue both lead to an *intrinsic* relaxation of local precapillary sphincters (rings of muscle)—with a consequent widening of corresponding capillary entrances—which reduces the local resistance to flow and thereby allows more blood to perfuse the active region. On the other hand, the *extrinsic* innervation by the autonomic nervous system of smooth muscle tissues in the walls of arterioles allows the central nervous system to completely shut down the flow to entire vascular beds (such as the cutaneous circulation) when this becomes necessary (such as during exposure to extremely cold environments).

In addition to prioritizing and controlling the *distribution* of blood, physiologic regulation of cardio-vascular function is directed mainly at four other variables: cardiac output, blood pressure, blood volume, and blood composition. From Eq. (1.1) we see that cardiac output can be increased by increasing the heart rate (a chronotropic effect), increasing the EDV (allowing the heart to fill longer by delaying the onset of systole), decreasing the ESV (an inotropic effect), or doing all three things at once. Indeed, under the extrinsic influence of the sympathetic nervous system and the adrenal glands, heart rate can triple—to some 240 beats/min if necessary—EDV can increase by as much as 50%—to around 200 ml or more of blood—and ESV can decrease a comparable amount (the cardiac reserve)—to about 30 to 35 ml or less. The combined result of all three effects can lead to over a sevenfold increase in cardiac output—from the normal 5 to 5.5 liters/min to as much as 40 to 41 liters/min or more for very brief periods of strenuous exertion.

The control of blood pressure is accomplished mainly by adjusting at the arteriolar level the down-stream resistance to flow—an increased resistance leading to a rise in arterial backpressure, and vice versa. This effect is conveniently quantified by a fluid-dynamic analogue to Ohm's famous $E = IR$ law in electromagnetic theory, voltage drop E being equated to fluid pressure drop ΔP, electric current I corre-sponding to flow—cardiac output (CO)—and electric resistance R being associated with an analogous vascular "peripheral resistance" (PR). Thus one may write

$$\Delta P = \left(\text{CO}\right)\left(\text{PR}\right) \tag{1.4}$$

Normally, the total systemic peripheral resistance is 15 to 20 mmHg/liter/min of flow but can increase significantly under the influence of the vasomotor center located in the medulla of the brain, which controls arteriolar muscle tone.

The control of blood volume is accomplished mainly through the excretory function of the kidney. For example, antidiuretic hormone (ADH) secreted by the pituitary gland acts to prevent renal fluid loss (excretion via urination) and thus increases plasma volume, whereas perceived extracellular fluid over-loads such as those that result from the peripheral vasoconstriction response to cold stress lead to a sympathetic/adrenergic receptor-induced renal diuresis (urination) that tends to decrease plasma vol-ume—if not checked, to sometimes dangerously low dehydration levels. Blood composition, too, is maintained primarily through the activity of endocrine hormones and enzymes that enhance or repress specific biochemical pathways. Since these pathways are too numerous to itemize here, suffice it to say that in the body's quest for homeostasis and stability, virtually nothing is left to chance, and every biochemical end can be arrived at through a number of alternative means. In a broader sense, as the organism strives to maintain life, it coordinates a wide variety of different functions, and central to its ability to do just that is the role played by the cardiovascular system in transporting mass, energy, and momentum.

Defining Terms

Atrioventricular (AV) node: A highly specialized cluster of neuromuscular cells at the lower portion of the right atrium leading to the interventricular septum; the AV node delays sinoatrial (SA) node–generated electrical impulses momentarily (allowing the atria to contract first) and then conducts the depolarization wave to the bundle of His and its bundle branches.

Autonomic nervous system: The functional division of the nervous system that innervates most glands, the heart, and smooth muscle tissue in order to maintain the internal environment of the body.

Cardiac muscle: Involuntary muscle possessing much of the anatomic attributes of skeletal voluntary muscle and some of the physiologic attributes of involuntary smooth muscle tissue; SA node–induced contraction of its interconnected network of fibers allows the heart to expel blood during systole.

Chronotropic: Affecting the periodicity of a recurring action, such as the slowing (bradycardia) or speeding up (tachycardia) of the heartbeat that results from extrinsic control of the SA node.

Endocrine system: The system of ductless glands and organs secreting substances directly into the blood to produce a specific response from another "target" organ or body part.

Endothelium: Flat cells that line the innermost surfaces of blood and lymphatic vessels and the heart.

Homeostasis: A tendency to uniformity or stability in an organism by maintaining within narrow limits certain variables that are critical to life.

Inotropic: Affecting the contractility of muscular tissue, such as the increase in cardiac *power* that results from extrinsic control of the myocardial musculature.

Precapillary sphincters: Rings of smooth muscle surrounding the entrance to capillaries where they branch off from upstream metarterioles. Contraction and relaxation of these sphincters close and open the access to downstream blood vessels, thus controlling the irrigation of different capillary networks.

Sinoatrial (SA) node: Neuromuscular tissue in the right atrium near where the superior vena cava joins the posterior right atrium (the sinus venarum); the SA node generates electrical impulses that initiate the heartbeat, hence its nickname the cardiac "pacemaker."

Stem cell: A generalized parent cell spawning descendants that become individually specialized.

Acknowledgments

The author gratefully acknowledges the assistance of Professor Robert Hochmuth in the preparation of Table 1.1 and the Radford Community Hospital for its support of the Biomedical Engineering Program at Virginia Tech.

References

Bhagavan NV. 1992. Medical Biochemistry. Boston, Jones and Bartlett.

Beall HPT, Needham D, Hochmuth RM. 1993. Volume and osmotic properties of human neutrophils. Blood 81(10):2774–2780.

Caro CG, Pedley TJ, Schroter RC, Seed WA. 1978. The Mechanics of the Circulation. New York, Oxford University Press.

Chandran KB. 1992. Cardiovascular Biomechanics. New York, New York University Press.

Frausto da Silva JJR, Williams RJP. 1993. The Biological Chemistry of the Elements. New York, Oxford University Press/Clarendon.

Dawson TH. 1991. Engineering Design of the Cardiovascular System of Mammals. Englewood Cliffs, NJ, Prentice-Hall.

Duck FA. 1990. Physical Properties of Tissue. San Diego, Academic Press.

Kaley G, Altura BM (Eds). Microcirculation, vol I (1977), vol II (1978), vol III (1980). Baltimore, University Park Press.

Kessel RG, Kardon RH. 1979. Tissue and Organs—A Text-Atlas of Scanning Electron Microscopy. San Francisco, WH Freeman.

Lentner C (Ed). Geigy Scientific Tables, vol 3: Physical Chemistry, Composition of Blood, Hematology and Somatometric Data, 8th ed. 1984. New Jersey, Ciba-Geigy.

————Vol 5: Heart and Circulation, 8th ed. 1990. New Jersey, Ciba-Geigy.

Schneck DJ. 1990. Engineering Principles of Physiologic Function. New York, New York University Press.

Tortora GJ, Grabowski SR. 1993. Principles of Anatomy and Physiology, 7th ed. New York, HarperCollins.

2
Endocrine System

The body, if it is to achieve optimal performance, must possess mechanisms for sensing and responding appropriately to numerous biologic cues and signals in order to control and maintain its internal environment. This complex role is effected by the integrative action of the endocrine and neural systems. The endocrine contribution is achieved through a highly sophisticated set of communication and control systems involving signal generation, propagation, recognition, transduction, and response. The signal entities are chemical messengers or hormones that are distributed through the body by the blood circulatory system to their respective target organs to modify their activity in some fashion.

Endocrinology has a comparatively long history, but real advances in the understanding of endocrine physiology and mechanisms of regulation and control began only in the late 1960s with the introduction of sensitive and relatively specific analytical methods; these enabled low concentrations of circulating hormones to be measured reliably, simply, and at relatively low cost. The breakthrough came with the development and widespread adoption of competitive protein binding and radioimmunoassays that superseded existing cumbersome bioassay methods. Since then, knowledge of the physiology of individual endocrine glands and of the neural control of the pituitary gland and the overall feedback control of the endocrine system has progressed and is growing rapidly. Much of this has been accomplished by applying to endocrinological research the methods developed in cellular and molecular biology and recombinant DNA technology. At the same time, theoretical and quantitative approaches using mathematical modeling complemented experimental studies have been of value in gaining a greater understanding of endocrine dynamics.

2.1 Endocrine System: Hormones, Signals, and Communication between Cells and Tissues

Hormones are synthesized and secreted by specialized endocrine glands to act locally or at a distance, having been carried in the bloodstream (classic endocrine activity) or secreted into the gut lumen (lumocrine activity) to act on target cells that are distributed elsewhere in the body. Hormones are chemically diverse, physiologically potent molecules that are the primary vehicle for intercellular communication with the

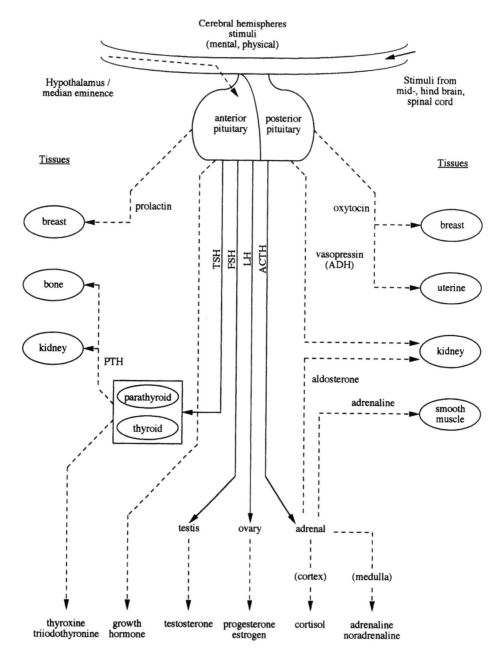

FIGURE 2.1 Representation of the forward pathways of pituitary and target gland hormone release and action: —— tropic hormones; – – – tissue-affecting hormones.

capacity to override the intrinsic mechanisms of normal cellular control. They can be classified broadly into three groups according to their physicochemical characteristics: (1) steroid hormones produced by chemical modification of cholesterol, (2) peptide and protein hormones, and (3) those derived from the aromatic amino acid tyrosine. The peptide and protein hormones are essentially hydrophilic and are therefore able to circulate in the blood in the free state; however, the more hydrophobic lipid-derived molecules have to be carried in the circulation bound to specific transport proteins. Figure 2.1 and Table 2.1 show, in schematic and descriptive form, respectively, details of the major endocrine glands of the body and the endocrine pathways.

TABLE 2.1 Main Endocrine Glands and the Hormones They Produce and Release

Gland	Hormone	Chemical Characteristics
Hypothalamus/median eminence	Thyrotropin-releasing hormone (TRH)	Peptides
	Somatostatin	
	Gonadotropin-releasing hormone	Amine
	Growth hormone-releasing hormone	
	Corticotropin-releasing hormone	
	Prolactin inhibitor factor	
Anterior pituitary	Thyrotropin (TSH)	Glycoproteins
	Luteinizing hormone	
	Follicle-stimulating hormone (FSH)	Proteins
	Growth hormone	
	Prolactin	
	Adrenocorticotropin (ACTH)	
Posterior pituitary	Vasopressin (antidiuretic hormone, ADH)	
	Oxytocin	Peptides
Thyroid	Triidothyronine (T3)	Tyrosine derivatives
	Thyroxine (T4)	
Parathyroid	Parathyroid hormone (PTH)	Peptide
Adrenal cortex	Cortisol	Steroids
	Aldosterone	
Adrenal medulla	Epinephrine	Catecholamines
	Norepinephrine	
Pancreas	Insulin	Proteins
	Glucagon	
	Somatostatin	
Gonads: Testes	Testosterone	Steroids
Ovaries	Estrogen	
	Progesterone	

The endocrine and nervous system are physically and functionally linked by a specific region of the brain called the *hypothalamus*, which lies immediately above the pituitary gland, to which it is connected by an extension called the *pituitary stalk*. The integrating function of the hypothalamus is mediated by cells that possess the properties of both nerve and processes that carry electrical impulses and on stimulation can release their signal molecules into the blood. Each of the hypothalamic neurosecretory cells can be stimulated by other nerve cells in higher regions of the brain to secrete specific peptide hormones or release factors into the adenohypophyseal portal vasculature. These hormones can then specifically stimulate or suppress the secretion of a second hormone from the anterior pituitary.

The pituitary hormones in the circulation interact with their target tissues, which, if endocrine glands, are stimulated to secrete further (third) hormones that feed back to inhibit the release of the pituitary hormones. It will be seen from Fig. 2.1 and Table 2.1 that the main targets of the pituitary are the adrenal cortex, the thyroid, and the gonads. These axes provide good examples of the control of pituitary hormone release by negative-feedback inhibition; e.g., adrenocorticotropin (ACTH), luteinizing hormone (LH), and follicle-stimulating hormone (FSH) are selectively inhibited by different steroid hormones, as is thyrotropin (TSH) release by the thyroid hormones.

In the case of growth hormone (GH) and prolactin, the target tissue is not an endocrine gland and thus does not produce a hormone; then the feedback control is mediated by inhibitors. Prolactin is under dopamine inhibitory control, whereas hypothalamic releasing and inhibitory factors control GH release. The two posterior pituitary (neurohypophyseal) hormones, oxytocin and vasopressin, are synthesized in the supraoptic and paraventricular nuclei and are stored in granules at the end of the nerve fibers in the posterior pituitary. Oxytocin is subsequently secreted in response to peripheral stimuli from the cervical stretch receptors or the suckling receptors of the breast. In a like manner, antidiuretic hormone (ADH, vasopressin) release is stimulated by the altered activity of hypothalamic osmoreceptors responding to changes in plasma solute concentrations.

It will be noted that the whole system is composed of several endocrine axes with the hypothalamus, pituitary, and other endocrine glands together forming a complex hierarchical regulatory system. There is no doubt that the anterior pituitary occupies a central position in the control of hormone secretion and, because of its important role, was often called the "conductor of the endocrine orchestra." However, the release of pituitary hormones is mediated by complex feedback control, so the pituitary should be regarded as having a permissive role rather than having the overall control of the endocrine system.

2.2 Hormone Action at the Cell Level: Signal Recognition, Signal Transduction, and Effecting a Physiological Response

The ability of target glands or tissues to respond to hormonal signals depends on the ability of the cells to recognize the signal. This function is mediated by specialized proteins or glycoproteins in or on the cell plasma membrane that are specific for a particular hormone, able to recognize it, bind it with high affinity, and react when very low concentrations are present. Recognition of the hormonal signal and activation of the cell surface receptors initiates a flow of information to the cell interior which triggers a chain of intracellular events in a pre-programmed fashion that produces a characteristic response. It is useful to classify the site of such action of hormones into two groups: those which act at the cell surface without, generally, traversing the cell membrane and those which actually enter the cell before effecting a response. In the study of this multi-step sequence, two important events can be readily studied, namely, the binding of the hormone to its receptor and activation of cytoplasmic effects. However, it is some of the steps between these events, such as receptor activation and signal generation, that are still relatively poorly defined. One method employed in an attempt to elucidate the intermediate steps has been to use ineffective mutant receptors, which when assayed are either defective in their hormone binding capabilities or in effector activation and thus unable to transduce a meaningful signal to the cell. But the difficulty with these studies has been to distinguish receptor-activation and signal-generation defects from hormone binding and effector activation defects.

Hormones Acting at the Cell Surface

Most peptide and protein hormones are hydrophilic and thus unable to traverse the lipid-containing cell membrane and must therefore act through activation of receptor proteins on the cell surface. When these receptors are activated by the binding of an extracellular signal ligand, the ligand-receptor complex initiates a series of protein interactions within or adjacent to the inner surface of the plasma membrane, which in turn brings about changes in intracellular activity. This can happen in one of two ways. The first involves the so-called second messenger, by altering the activity of a plasma membrane-bound enzyme, which in turn increases (or sometimes decreases) the concentration of an intracellular mediator. The second involves activation of other types of cell surface receptors, which leads to changes in the plasma membrane electrical potential and the membrane permeability, resulting in altered transmembrane transport of ions or metabolites. If the hormone is thought of as the "first messenger," cyclic adenosine monophosphate (cAMP) can be regarded as the "second messenger," capable of triggering a cascade of intracellular biochemical events that can lead either to a rapid secondary response such as altered ion transport, enhanced metabolic pathway flux, steroidogenesis or to a slower response such as DNA, RNA, and protein synthesis resulting in cell growth or cell division.

The peptide and protein hormones circulate at very low concentrations relative to other proteins in the blood plasma. These low concentrations are reflected in the very high affinity and specificity of the receptor sites, which permits recognition of the relevant hormones amid the profusion of protein molecules in the circulation. Adaptation to a high concentration of a signal ligand in a time-dependent reversible manner enables cells to respond to changes in the concentration of a ligand instead of to its absolute concentration. The number of receptors in a cell is not constant; synthesis of receptors may be induced or repressed by other hormones or even by their own hormones. Adaptation can occur in several ways. Ligand binding can inactivate a cell surface receptor either by inducing its internalization and degradation or by causing the receptor to adopt an inactive conformation. Alternatively, it may result from the changes in one of the non-receptor proteins involved in signal transduction following receptor activation. Downregulation is the name given to the process whereby a cell decreases the number of receptors in response to intense or frequent stimulation and can occur by degradation or more temporarily by phosphorylation and sequestration. Upregulation is the process of increasing receptor expression either by other hormones or in response to altered stimulation.

The cell surface receptors for peptide hormones are linked functionally to a cell membrane-bound enzyme that acts as the catalytic unit. This receptor complex consists of three components: (1) the receptor itself which recognizes the hormone, (2) a regulatory protein called a G-protein that binds guanine nucleotides and is located on the cytosolic face of the membrane, and (3) adenylate cyclase which catalyzes the conversion of ATP to cAMP. As the hormone binds at the receptor site, it is coupled through a regulatory protein, which acts as a transducer, to the enzyme adenyl cyclase, which catalyzes the formation of cAMP from adenosine triphosphate (ATP). The G-protein consists of three subunits, which in the unstimulated state form a heterotrimer to which a molecule of GDP is bound. Binding of the hormone to the receptor causes the subunit to exchange its GDP for a molecule of GTP (guanine triphosphate) which then dissociates from the subunits. This in turn decreases the affinity of the receptor for the hormone and leads to its dissociation. The GTP subunit not only activates adenylate cyclase, but also has intrinsic GTPase activity and slowly converts GTP back to GDP, thus allowing the subunits to reassociate and so regain their initial resting state. There are hormones, such as somatostatin, that possess the ability to inhibit AMP formation but still have similarly structured receptor complexes. The G-protein of inhibitory complexes consists of an inhibitory subunit complexed with a subunit thought to be identical to the subunits of the stimulatory G-protein. However, it appears that a single adenylate cyclase molecule can be simultaneously regulated by more than one G-protein enabling the system to integrate opposing inputs.

The adenylate cyclase reaction is rapid, and the increased concentration of intracellular cAMP is short-lived, since it is rapidly hydrolyzed and destroyed by the enzyme cAMP phosphodiesterase which terminates the hormonal response. The continual and rapid removal of cAMP and free calcium ions from the cytosol makes for both the rapid increase and decrease of these intracellular mediators when the cells respond to signals. Rising cAMP concentrations affect cells by stimulating cAMP-dependent protein kinases to phosphorylate specific target proteins. Phosphorylation of proteins leads to conformational changes that enhance their catalytic activity, thus providing a signal amplification pathway from hormone to effector. These effects are reversible because phosphorylated proteins are rapidly dephosphorylated by protein phosphatases when the concentration of cAMP falls. A similar system involving cyclic GMP, although less common and less well studied, plays an analogous role to that of cAMP. The action of thyrotropin-releasing hormone (TRH), parathyroid hormone (PTH), and epinephrine is catalyzed by adenyl cyclase, and this can be regarded as the classic reaction.

However, there are variant mechanisms. In the phosphatidylinositol-diacylglycerol (DAG)/inositol triphosphate (IP3) system, some surface receptors are coupled through another G-protein to the enzyme phospholipase C which cleaves the membrane phospholipid to form DAG and IP3 or phospholipase D which cleaves phosphatidyl choline to DAG via phosphatidic acid. DAG causes the calcium, phospholipid-dependent protein kinase C to translocate to the cell membrane from the cytosolic cell compartment becoming 20 times more active in the process. IP3 mobilizes calcium from storage sites associated with the plasma and intracellular membranes thereby contributing to the activation of protein kinase C as well as other calcium-dependent processes. DAG is cleared from the cell either by conversion to phosphatidic acid which may be recycled to phospholipid or it may be broken down to fatty acids and glycerol. The DAG derived from phosphatidylinositol usually contains arachidonic acid esterified to the middle carbon of glycerol. Arachidonic acid is the precursor of the prostaglandins and leukotrienes which are biologically active eicosanoids.

Thyrotropin and vasopressin modulate an activity of phospholipase C that catalyzes the conversion of phosphatidylinositol to diacylglycerol and inositol, 1,4,5-triphosphate, which act as the second messengers. They mobilize bound intracellular calcium and activate a protein kinase, which in turn alters the activity of other calcium-dependent enzymes within the cell.

Increased concentrations of free calcium ions affect cellular events by binding to and altering the molecular conformation of calmodulin; the resulting calcium ion-calmodulin complex can activate many different target proteins, including calcium ion-dependent protein kinases. Each cell type has a characteristic set of target proteins that are so regulated by cAMP-dependent kinases and/or calmodulin that it will respond in a specific way to an alteration in cAMP or calcium ion concentrations. In this way, cAMP or calcium ions act as second messengers in such a way as to allow the extracellular signal not only to be greatly amplified but, just as importantly, also to be made specific for each cell type.

The action of the important hormone insulin that regulates glucose metabolism depends on the activation of the enzyme tyrosine kinase catalyzing the phosphorylation of tyrosyl residues of proteins. This effects changes in the activity of calcium-sensitive enzymes, leading to enhanced movement of glucose and fatty acids across the cell membrane and modulating their intracellular metabolism. The binding of insulin to its receptor site has been studied extensively; the receptor complex has been isolated and characterized. It was such work that highlighted the interesting aspect of feedback control at the cell level, downregulation: the ability of peptide hormones to regulate the concentration of cell surface receptors. After activation, the receptor population becomes desensitized, or "downregulated," leading to a decreased availability of receptors and thus a modulation of transmembrane events.

Hormones Acting within the Cell

Steroid hormones are small hydrophobic molecules derived from cholesterol that are solubilized by binding reversibly to specify carrier proteins in the blood plasma. Once released from their carrier proteins, they readily pass through the plasma membrane of the target cell and bind, again reversibly, to steroid hormone receptor proteins in the cytosol. This is a relatively slow process when compared to protein hormones. The latter second messenger–mediated phosphorylation-dephosphorylation reactions modify enzymatic processes rapidly with the physiologic consequences becoming apparent in seconds or minutes and are as rapidly reversed. Nuclear-mediated responses, on the other hand, lead to transcription/translation-dependent changes that are slow in onset and tend to persist since reversal is dependent on degradation of the induced proteins. The protein component of the steroid hormone-receptor complex has an affinity for DNA in the cell nucleus, where it binds to nuclear chromatin and initiates the transcription of a small number of genes. These gene products may, in turn, activate other genes and produce a secondary response, thereby amplifying the initial effect of the hormone. Each steroid hormone is recognized by a separate receptor protein, but this same receptor protein has the capacity to regulate several different genes in different target cells. This, of course, suggests that the nuclear chromatin of each cell type is organized so that only the appropriate genes are made available for regulation by the hormone-receptor complex. The thyroid hormone triiodothyronine (T3) also acts, though by a different mechanism than the steroids, at the cell nucleus level to initiate genomic transcription. The hormonal activities of GH and prolactin influence cellular gene transcription and translation of messenger RNA by complex mechanisms.

2.3 Endocrine System: Some Other Aspects of Regulation and Control

From the foregoing sections it is clear that the endocrine system exhibits complex molecular and metabolic dynamics which involve many levels of control and regulation. Hormones are chemical signals released from a hierarchy of endocrine glands and propagated through the circulation to a hierarchy of cell types. The integration of this system depends on a series of what systems engineers call "feedback

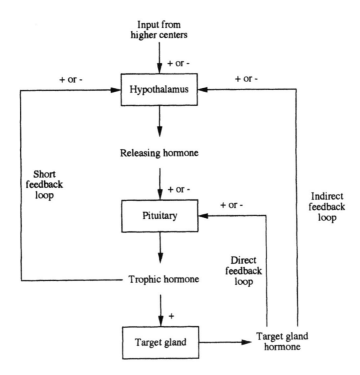

FIGURE 2.2 Illustration of the complexity of hormonal feedback control (+ indicates a positive or augmenting effect; – indicates a negative or inhibiting effect).

loops"; feedback is a reflection of mutual dependence of the system variables: variable x affects variable y, and y affects x. Further, it is essentially a closed-loop system in which the feedback of information from the system output to the input has the capacity to maintain homeostasis. A diagrammatic representation of the ways in which hormone action is controlled is shown in Fig. 2.2. One example of this control structure arises in the context of the thyroid hormones. In this case, TRH, secreted by the hypothalamus, triggers the anterior pituitary into the production of TSH. The target gland is the thyroid, which produces T3 and thyroxine (T4). The complexity of control includes both direct and indirect feedback of T3 and T4, as outlined in Fig. 2.2, together with TSH feedback on to the hypothalamus.

Negative Feedback

If an increase in y causes a change in x which in turn tends to decrease y, feedback is said to be *negative;* in other words, the signal output induces a response that feeds back to the signal generator to decrease its output. This is the most common form of control in physiologic systems, and examples are many. For instance, as mentioned earlier, the anterior pituitary releases trophic or stimulating hormones that act on peripheral endocrine glands such as the adrenals or thyroid or on gonads to produce hormones that act back on the pituitary to decrease the secretion of the trophic hormones. These are examples of what is called *long-loop feedback* (see Fig. 2.2). (**Note:** The adjectives *long* and *short* reflect the spatial distance or proximity of effector and target sites.) The trophic hormones of the pituitary are also regulated by feedback action at the level of their releasing factors. *Ultrashort-loop feedback* is also described. There are numerous examples of *short-loop feedback* as well, the best being the reciprocal relation between insulin and blood glucose concentrations, as depicted in Fig. 2.3. In this case, elevated glucose concentration (and positive rate of change, implying not only proportional but also derivative control) has a positive effect on the pancreas, which secretes insulin in response. This has an inhibiting effect on glucose metabolism, resulting in a reduction of blood glucose toward a normal concentration; in other words, classic negative-feedback control.

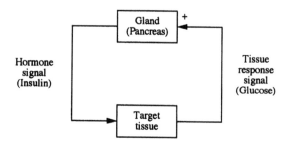

FIGURE 2.3   The interaction of insulin as an illustration of negative feedback within a hormonal control system.

Positive Feedback

If increase in *y* causes a change in *x* which tends to increase *y*, feedback is said to be *positive*; in other words, a further signal output is evoked by the response it induces or provokes. This is intrinsically an unstable system, but there are physiologic situations where such control is valuable. In the positive feedback situation, the signal output will continue until no further response is required. Suckling provides an example; stimulation of nipple receptors by the suckling child provokes an increased oxytocin release from the posterior pituitary with a corresponding increase in milk flow. Removal of the stimulus causes cessation of oxytocin release.

Rhythmic Endocrine Control

Many hormone functions exhibit rhythmically in the form of pulsatile release of hormones. The most common is the approximately 24-h cycle (circadian or diurnal rhythm). For instance, blood sampling at frequent intervals has shown that ACTH is secreted episodically, each secretory burst being followed 5 to 10 min later by cortisol secretion. These episodes are most frequent in the early morning, with plasma cortisol concentrations highest around 7 to 8 AM and lowest around midnight. ACTH and cortisol secretion vary inversely, and the parallel circadian rhythm is probably due to a cyclic change in the sensitivity of the hypothalamic feedback center to circulating cortisol. Longer cycles are also known, e.g., the infradian menstrual cycle.

It is clear that such inherent rhythms are important in endocrine communication and control, suggesting that its physiologic organization is based not only on the structural components of the system but also on the dynamics of their interactions. The rhythmic, pulsatile nature of release of many hormones is a means whereby time-varying signals can be encoded, thus allowing large quantities of information to be transmitted and exchanged rapidly in a way that small, continuous changes in threshold levels would not allow.

References

Inevitably, our brief exposition has been able to touch upon an enormous subject only by describing some of the salient features of this fascinating domain, but it is hoped that it may nevertheless stimulate a further interest. However, not surprisingly the endocrinology literature is massive and it is suggested that anyone wishing to read further turn initially to one of the many excellent textbooks and go on from there. Those we have found useful include:

Goodman HM. 1994. *Basic Medical Endocrinology*, New York, Raven Press. 2nd ed.

Greenspan FS, Strewler GJ (Eds.). 1997. *Basic and Clinical Endocrinology*, Norwalk, CT, Appleton & Lange. 5th ed.

O'Malley BW, Birnbaumer L, Hunter T (Eds.). 1998. *Hormones and Signaling*. Vol. 1. New York, Academic Press.

Wilson JD, Foster DW, Kronenberg HM (Eds.). 1998. *Williams Textbook of Endocrinology*, Philadelphia, WB Saunders. 9th ed.

3

Nervous System

Evangelia
Micheli-Tzanakou
Rutgers University

The nervous system, unlike other organ systems, is concerned primarily with signals, information encoding and processing, and control rather than manipulation of energy. It acts like a communication device whose components use substances and energy in processing signals and in reorganizing them, choosing, and commanding, as well as in developing and learning. A central question that is often asked is how nervous systems work and what are the principles of their operation. In an attempt to answer this question, we will, at the same time, ignore other fundamental questions, such as those relating to anatomic or neurochemical and molecular aspects. We will concentrate rather on relations and transactions between neurons and their assemblages in the nervous system. We will deal with neural signals (encoding and decoding), the evaluation and weighting of incoming signals, and the formulation of outputs. A major part of this chapter is devoted to higher aspects of the nervous system, such as memory and learning, rather than individual systems, such as vision and audition, which are treated extensively elsewhere in this book.

3.1 Definitions

Nervous systems can be defined as organized assemblies of nerve cells as well as nonnervous cells. Nerve cells, or *neurons*, are specialized in the generation, integration, and conduction of incoming signals from the outside world or from other neurons and deliver them to other excitable cells or to *effectors* such as muscle cells. Nervous systems are easily recognized in higher animals but not in the lower species, since the defining criteria are difficult to apply.

A central nervous system (CNS) can be distinguished easily from a peripheral nervous system (PNS), since it contains most of the motor and nucleated parts of neurons that innervate muscles and other effectors. The PNS contains all the sensory nerve cell bodies, with some exceptions, plus local *plexuses*, local *ganglia*, and peripheral axons that make up the *nerves*. Most sensory axons go all the way into the CNS, while the remaining sensory axons relay in peripheral plexuses. Motor axons originating in the CNS innervate effector cells.

The nervous system has two major roles: (1) to regulate, acting homeostatically in restoring some conditions of the organism after some external stimulus, and (2) to act to alter a preexisting condition by replacing it or modifying it. In both cases — regulation or initiation of a process — learning can be superimposed. In most species, learning is a more or less adaptive mechanism, combining and timing species-characteristic acts with a large degree of evolution toward perfection.

The nervous system is a complex structure for which realistic assumptions have led to irrelevant oversimplifications. One can break the nervous system down into four components: sensory transducers, neurons, axons, and muscle fibers. Each of these components gathers, processes, and transmits information impinging on it from the outside world, usually in the form of complex stimuli. The processing is carried out by exitable tissues — neurons, axons, sensory receptors, and muscle fibers. Neurons are the basic elements of the nervous system. If put in small assemblies or clusters, they form neuronal assemblies or neuronal networks communicating with each other either chemically via *synaptic junctions* or electrically via *tight* junctions. The main characteristics of a cell are the *cell body*, or *soma*, which contains the *nucleus*, and a number of processes originating from the cell body, called the *dendrites*, which reach out to surroundings to make contacts with other cells. These contacts serve as the incoming information to the cell, while the outgoing information follows a conduction path, the axon. The incoming information is integrated in the cell body and generates its action potential at the *axon hillock*. There are two types of outputs that can be generated and therefore two types of neurons: those which generate *graded* potentials that attenuate with distance and those which generate *action* potentials. The latter travel through the axon, a thin, long process that passively passes the action potential or rather a train of action potentials without any attenuation (*all-or-none effect*). A number of action potentials is often called a *spike train*. A threshold built into the hillock, depending on its level, allows or stops the generation of the spike train. Axons usually terminate on other neurons by means of *synaptic terminals* or *boutons* and have properties similar to those of an electric cable with varying diameters and speeds of signal transmission. Axons can be of two types: *myelinated* or *unmyelinated*. In the former case, the axon is surrounded by a thick fatty material, the myelin sheath, which is interrupted at regular intervals by gaps called the *nodes of Ranvier*. These nodes provide for the *saltatory* conduction of the signal along the axon. The axon makes functional connections with other neurons at synapses on the cell body, or the dendrites, or the axons. There exist two kinds of synapses: *excitatory* and *inhibitory*, and as the names imply, they either increase the *firing* frequency of the postsynaptic neurons or decrease it, respectively.

Sensory receptors are specialized cells that, in response to an incoming stimulus, generate a corresponding electrical signal, a graded receptor potential. Although the mechanisms by which the sensory receptors generate receptor potentials are not known exactly, the most plausible scenario is that an external stimulus alters the membrane permeabilities. The receptor potential, then, is the change in intracellular potential relative to the *resting* potential.

It is important to notice here that the term *receptor* is used in physiology to refer not only to sensory receptors but also, in a different sense, to proteins that bind neurotransmitters, hormones, and other substances with great affinity and specificity as a first step in starting up physiologic responses. This receptor is often associated with nonneural cells that surround it and form a *sense organ*. The forms of energy converted by the receptors include mechanical, thermal, electromagnetic, and chemical energy. The particular form of energy to which a receptor is most sensitive is called its *adequate stimulus*. The problem of how receptors convert energy into action potentials in the sensory nerves has been the subject of intensive study. In the complex sense organs, such as those concerned with hearing and vision, there exist separate receptor cells and synaptic junctions between receptors and afferent nerves. In other cases, such as the cutaneous sense organs, the receptors are specialized. Where a stimulus of constant strength is applied to a receptor repeatedly, the frequency of the action potentials in its sensory nerve declines over a period of time. This phenomenon is known as *adaptation*. If the adaptation is very rapid, then the receptors are called *phasic*; otherwise, they are called *tonic*.

Another important issue is the *coding* of sensory information. Action potentials are similar in all nerves, although there are variations in their speed of conduction and other characteristics. However, if the action potentials were the same in most cells, then what makes the visual cells sensitive to light and not to sound and the touch receptors sensitive to touch and not to smell? And how can we tell if these sensations are strong or not? These sensations depend on what is called the *doctrine of specific nerve energies*, which has been questioned over time by several researchers. No matter where a particular sensory pathway is stimulated along its course to the brain, the sensation produced is referred to the location of the receptor. This is the *law of projections*. An example of this law is the "phantom limb," in which an amputee complains about an itching sensation in the amputated limb.

3.2 Functions of the Nervous System

The basic unit of integrated activity is the *reflex arc*. This arc consists of a sense organ, afferent neuron, one or more synapses in a central integrating station (or sympathetic ganglion), an efferent neuron, and an effector. The simplest reflex arc is the *monosynaptic* one, which has only one synapse between the afferent and efferent neurons. With more than one synapse, the reflex arc is called *polysynaptic*. In each of these cases, activity is modified by both spatial and temporal facilitation, occlusion, and other effects.

In mammals, the concentration between afferent and efferent somatic neurons is found either in the brain or in the spinal cord. The Bell-Magendie law dictates that in the spinal cord the dorsal roots are sensory, while the ventral roots are motor. The action potential message that is carried by an axon is eventually fed to a muscle, to a secretory cell, or to the dendrite of another neuron. If an axon is carrying a graded potential, its output is too weak to stimulate a muscle, but it can terminate on a secretory cell or dendrite. The latter can have as many as 10,000 inputs. If the endpoint is a motor neuron, which has been found experimentally in the case of fibers from the primary endings, then there is a lag between the time when the stimulus was applied and when the response is obtained from the muscle. This time interval is called the *reaction time* and in humans is approximately 20 ms for a stretch reflex. The distance from the spinal cord can be measured, and since the conduction velocities of both the efferent and afferent fibers are known, another important quality can be calculated: the *central delay*. This delay is the portion of the reaction time that was spent for conduction to and from the spinal cord. It has been found that muscle spindles also make connections that cause muscle contraction via polysynaptic pathways, while the afferents from secondary endings make connections that excite extensor muscles. When a motor neuron sends a burst of action potentials to its skeletal muscle, the amount of contraction depends largely on the discharge frequency but also on many other factors, such as the history of the load on the muscle and the load itself. The *stretch error* can be calculated from the desired motion minus the actual stretch. If this error is then fed back to the motor neuron, its discharge frequency is modified appropriately. This corresponds to one of the three feedback loops that are available locally. Another loop corrects for overstretching beyond the point that the muscle or tendon may tear. Since a muscle can only contract, it must be paired with another muscle (*antagonist*) in order to effect the return motion. Generally speaking, a flexor muscle is paired with an extensor muscle that cannot be activated simultaneously. This means that the motor neurons that affect each one of these are not activated at the same time. Instead, when one set of motor neurons is activated, the other is inhibited, and vice versa. When movement involves two or more muscles that normally cooperate by contracting simultaneously, the excitation of one causes facilitation of the other *synergistic* members via cross-connections. All these networks form feedback loops. An engineer's interpretation of how these loops work would be to assume dynamic conditions, as is the case in all parts of the nervous system. This has little value in dealing with stationary conditions, but it provides for an ability to adjust to changing conditions.

The nervous system, as mentioned earlier, is a control system of processes that adjust both internal and external operations. As humans, we have experiences that change our perceptions of events in our environment. The same is true for higher animals, which, besides having an internal environment the status of which is of major importance, also share an external environment of utmost richness and variety. Objects and conditions that have direct contact with the surface of an animal directly affect the future of the animal. Information about changes at some point provides a prediction of possible future status. The amount of information required to represent changing conditions increases as the required temporal resolution of detail increases. This creates a vast amount of data to be processed by any finite system. Considering that the information reaching sensory receptors is too extensive and redundant, as well as modified by external interference (noise), the nervous system has a tremendously difficult task to accomplish. Enhanced responsiveness to a particular stimulus can be produced by structures that either increase the energy converging on a receptor or increase the effectiveness of coupling of a specific type of stimulus with its receptor. Different species have sensory systems that respond to stimuli that are important to them for survival. Often one nervous system responds to conditions that are not sensed by another nervous system. The transduction, processing, and transmission of signals in any nervous system produce a survival mechanism for an organism but only after these signals have been further modified by effector organs. Although the nerve impulses that drive a muscle, as explained earlier, are discrete events, a muscle twitch takes much longer to happen, a fact that allows for their responses to overlap and produce a much smoother output. Neural control of motor activity of skeletal muscle is accomplished entirely by the modification of muscle excitation, which involves changes in velocity, length, stiffness, and heat production. The importance of accurate timing of inputs and the maintenance of this timing across several synapses is obvious in sensory pathways of the nervous system. Cells are located next to other cells that have overlapping or adjacent receptor or motor fields. The dendrites provide important and complicated sites of interactions as well as channels of variable effectiveness for excitatory inputs, depending on their position relative to the cell body. Among the best examples are the cells of the medial superior olive in the auditory pathway. These cells have two major dendritic trees extending from opposite poles of the cell body. One receives synaptic inhibitory input from the ipsilateral cochlear nucleus, the other from the contralateral nucleus that normally is an excitatory input. These cells deal with the determination of the azimuth of a sound. When a sound is present on the contralateral side, most cells are excited, while ipsilateral sounds cause inhibition. It has been shown that the cells can go from complete excitation to full inhibition with a difference of only a few hundred milliseconds in arrival time of the two inputs.

The question then arises: How does the nervous system put together the signals available to it so that a determination of output can take place? To arrive at an understanding of how the nervous system intergrates incoming information at a given moment of time, we must understand that the processes that take place depend both on cellular forms and a topologic architecture and on the physiologic properties that relate input to output. That is, we have to know the *transfer* functions or *coupling* functions. Integration depends on the weighting of inputs. One of the important factors determining weighting is the area of synaptic contact. The extensive dendrites are the primary integrating structures. Electronic spread is the means of mixing, smoothing, attenuating, delaying, and summing postsynaptic potentials. The spatial distribution of input is often not random but systematically restricted. Also, the wide variety of characteristic geometries of synapses is no doubt important not only for the weighting of different combinations of inputs. When repeated stimuli are presented at various intervals at different junctions, increasing synaptic potentials are generated if the intervals between them are not too short or too long. This increase is due to a phenomenon called *facilitation*. If the response lasts longer than the interval between impulses, such that the second response rises from the residue of the first, then it is temporal summation. If, in addition, the response increment due to the second stimulus is larger than the preceding one, then it is facilitation. Facilitation is an important function of the nervous system and is found in quite different forms and durations ranging from a few milliseconds to tenths of seconds. Facilitation may grade from forms of sensitization to learning, especially at long intervals. A special case is the so-called *posttetanic potentiation* that is the result of high-frequency stimulation for long periods of time (about 10 s). This is an interesting case, since no effects can be seen during stimulation, but afterwards, any test stimulus at various intervals creates a marked increase in response up to many times more than the "tetanic" stimulus. *Antifacilitation* is the phenomenon where a decrease of response from the neuron is observed at certain junctions due to successive impulses. Its mechanism is less understood than facilitation. Both facilitation and antifacilitation may be observed on the same neuron but in different functions of it.

3.3 Representation of Information in the Nervous System

Whenever information is transferred between different parts of the nervous system, some communication paths have to be established, and some parameters of impulse firing relevant to communication must be set up. Since what is communicated is nothing more than impulses — spike trains — the only basic variables in a train of events are the number and intervals between spikes. With respect to this, the nervous system acts like a pulse-coded analog device, since the intervals are continuously graded. There exists a distribution of interval lengths between individual spikes, which in any sample can be expressed by the shape of the interval histogram. If one examines different examples, their distributions differ markedly. Some histograms look like Poisson distributions; some others exhibit Gaussian or bimodal shapes. The coefficient of variation — expressed as the standard deviation over the mean — in some cases is constant, while in others it varies. Some other properties depend on the sequence of longer and shorter intervals than the mean. Some neurons show no linear dependence; some others show positive or negative correlations of successive intervals. If a stimulus is delivered and a discharge from the neuron is observed, a *poststimulus time histogram* can be used, employing the onset of the stimulus as a reference point and averaging many responses in order to reveal certain consistent features of temporal patterns. Coding of information can then be based on the average frequency, which can represent relevant gradations of the input. Mean frequency is the code in most cases, although no definition of it has been given with respect to measured quantities, such as averaging time, weighting functions, and forgetting functions. Characteristic transfer functions have been found, which suggests that there are several distinct coding principles in addition to the mean frequency. Each theoretically possible code becomes a candidate code as long as there exists some evidence that is readable by the system under investigation. Therefore, one has to first test for the availability of the code by imposing a stimulus that is considered "normal." After a response has been observed, the code is considered to be available. If the input is then changed to different levels of one parameter and changes are observed at the postsynaptic level, the code is called *readable.* However, only if both are formed in the same preparation and no other parameter is available and readable can the code be said to be the *actual* code employed. Some such parameters follow:

1. Time of firing
2. Temporal pattern
3. Number of spikes in the train
4. Variance of interspike intervals
5. Spike delays or latencies
6. Constellation code

The last is a very important parameter, especially when used in conjunction with the concept of *receptive fields* of units in the different sensory pathways. The unit receptors do not need to have highly specialized abilities to permit encoding of a large number of distinct stimuli. Receptive fields are topographic and overlap extensively. Any given stimulus will excite a certain constellation of receptors and is therefore encoded in the particular set that is activated. A large degree of uncertainty prevails and requires the brain to operate probabilistically. In the nervous system there exists a large amount of *redundancy,* although neurons might have different thresholds. It is questionable, however, if these units are entirely equivalent, although they share parts of their receptive fields. The nonoverlapping parts might be of importance and critical to sensory function. On the other hand, redundancy does not necessarily mean unspecified or random connectivity. Rather, it allows for greater sensitivity and resolution, improvement of signal-to-noise ratio, while at the same time it provides stability of performance.

Integration of large numbers of converging inputs to give a single output can be considered as an averaging or probabilistic operation. The "decisions" made by a unit depend on its inputs, or some intrinsic states, and reaching a certain threshold. This way every unit in the nervous system can make a decision when it changes from one state to a different one. A theoretical possibility also exists that a mass of randomly connected neurons may constitute a trigger unit and that activity with a sharp threshold can spread through such a mass redundancy. Each part of the nervous system, and in particular the receiving side, can be thought of as a filter. Higher-order neurons do not merely pass their information on, but instead they use convergence from different channels, as well as divergence of the same channels and other processes, in order to modify incoming signals. Depending on the structure and coupling functions of the network, what gets through is determined. Similar networks exist at the output side.

They also act as filters, but since they formulate decisions and commands with precise *spatiotemporal* properties, they can be thought of as *pattern generators.*

3.4   Lateral Inhibition

This discussion would be incomplete without a description of a very important phenomenon in the nervous system. This phenomenon, called *lateral inhibition,* is used by the nervous system to improve spatial resolution and contrast. The effectiveness of this type of inhibition decreases with distance. In the retina, for example, lateral inhibition is used extensively in order to improve contrast. As the stimulus approaches a certain unit, it first excites neighbors of the recorded cell. Since these neighbors inhibit that unit, it responds by a decrease in firing frequency. If the stimulus is exactly over the recorded unit, this unit is excited and fires above its normal rate, and as the stimulus moves out again, the neighbors are excited, while the unit under consideration fires less. If we now examine the output of all the units as a whole, and while half the considered array is stimulated and the other half is not, we will notice that at the point of discontinuity of the stimulus going from stimulation to nonstimulation, the firing frequencies of the two halves have been differentiated to the extreme at the stimulus edge, which has been enhanced. The neuronal circuits responsible for lateral shifts are relatively simple. Lateral inhibition can be considered to give the negative of the second spatial derivative of the input stimulus. A second layer of neurons could be constructed to perform this spatial differentiation on the input signal to detect the edge only. It is probably lateral inhibition that explains the psychophysical illusion known as *Mach bands.* It is probably the same principle that operates widely in the nervous system to enhance the sensitivity to contrast in the visual system in particular and in all other modalities in general. Through the years, different models have been developed to describe lateral inhibition mathematically, and various methods of analysis have been employed. Such methods include:

Functional notations
Graphic solutions
Tabular solution
Taylor's series expansions
Artificial neural network modeling

These models include both one-dimensional examination of the phenomenon and two-dimensional treatment, where a two-dimensional array is used as a stimulus. This two-dimensional treatment is justified because most of the sensory receptors of the body form two-dimensional maps (receptive fields). In principle, if a one-dimensional lateral inhibition system is linear, one can extend the analysis to two dimensions by means of superposition. The two-dimensional array can be thought of as a function $f(x, y)$, and the lateral inhibition network itself is embodied in a separate $N \times N$ array, the central square of which has a positive value and can be thought of as a direct input from an incoming axon. The surrounding squares have negative values that are higher than the corner values, which are also negative. The method consists of multiplying the input signal values $f(x, y)$ and their contiguous values by the lateral inhibitory network's weighting factors to get a corresponding $g(x, y)$. Figure 3.1 presents an example of such a process. The technique illustrated here is used in the contrast enhancement of photographs. The objective is the same as that of the nervous system: to improve image sharpness without introducing too much distortion. This technique requires storage of each picture element and lateral "inhibitory" interactions between adjacent elements. Since a picture may contain millions of elements, high-speed computers with large-scale memories are required.

At a higher level, similar algorithms can be used to evaluate decision-making mechanisms. In this case, many inputs from different sensory systems are competing for attention. The brain evaluates each one of the inputs as a function of the remaining ones. One can picture a decision-making mechanism resembling a "locator" of stimulus peaks. The final output depends on what weights are used at the inputs of a push-pull mechanism. Thus a decision can be made depending on the weights as an individual's

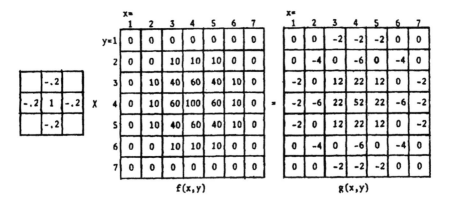

FIGURE 3.1 An example of two-dimensional lateral inhibition. On the left, the 3 × 3 array corresponds to the values of the synaptic junctions weighting coefficients. For simplicity, the corner weights are assumed to be zero. $g(x, y)$ represents the output matrix after lateral inhibition has been applied to the input matrix.

brain is applying to the incoming information about a situation under consideration. The most important information is heavily weighted, while the rest is either totally masked or weighted very lightly.

3.5 Higher Functions of the Nervous System

Pattern Recognition

One way of understanding human perception is to study the mechanism of information processing in the brain. The recognition of patterns of sensory input is one of the functions of the brain, a task accomplished by neuronal circuits, the *feature extractors*. Although such neuronal information is more likely to be processed globally by a large number of neurons, in animals, single-unit recording is one of the most powerful tools in the hands of the physiologist. Most often, the concept of the *receptive field* is used as a method of understanding sensory information processing. In the case of the visual system, one could call the receptive field a well-defined region of the visual field which, when stimulated, will change the firing rate of a neuron in the visual pathway. The response of that neuron will usually depend on the distribution of light in the receptive field. Therefore, the information collected by the brain from the outside world is transformed into spatial as well as temporal patterns of neuronal activity.

The question often asked is how do we perceive and recognize faces, objects, and scenes. Even in those cases where only noisy representations exist, we are still able to make some inference as to what the pattern represents. Unfortunately, in humans, single-unit recording, as mentioned above, is impossible. As a result, one has to use other kinds of measurements, such as *evoked potentials* (EPs). Although physiologic in nature, EPs are still far from giving us information at the neuronal level. Yet EPs have been used extensively as a way of probing human (and animal) brains because of their noninvasive character. EPs can be considered to be the result of integrations of the neuronal activity of many neurons some place in the brain. This gross potential can then be used as a measure of the response of the brain to sensory input.

The question then becomes: Can we somehow use this response to influence the brain in producing patterns of activity that we want? None of the efforts of the past closed this loop. How do we explain then the phenomenon of selective attention by which we selectively direct our attention to something of interest and discard the rest? And what happens with the evolution of certain species that change appearance according to their everyday needs? All these questions tend to lead to the fact that somewhere in the brain there is a loop where previous knowledge or experience is used as a feedback to the brain itself. This feedback then modifies the ability of the brain to respond in a different way to the same stimulus the next time it is presented. In a way, then, the brain creates mental "images" independent of the stimulus which tend to modify the representation of the stimulus in the brain.

This section describes some efforts in which different methods have been used in trying to address the difficult task of feedback loops in the brain. However, no attempt will be made to explain or even postulate where these feedback loops might be located. If one considers the brain as a huge set of neural nets, then one question has been debated for many years: What is the role of the individual neuron in the net, and what is the role of each network in the holistic process of the brain? More specifically, does the neuron act as an analyzer or a detector of specific features, or does it merely reflect the characteristic response of a population of cells of which it happens to be a member? What invariant relationships exist between sensory input and the response of a single neuron, and how much can be "read" about the stimulus parameters from the record of a single EP? In turn, then, how much feedback can one use from a single EP in order to influence the stimulus, and how successful can that influence be? Many physiologists express doubts that simultaneous observations of large numbers of individual neuronal activities can be readily interpreted. The main question we are asking is: Can a feedback process influence and modulate the stimuli patterns so that they appear optimal? If this is proved to be true, it would mean that we can reverse the pattern-recognition process, and instead of recognizing a pattern, we would be able to create a pattern from a vast variety of possible patterns. It would be like creating a link between our brain and a computer; equivalent to a brain-computer system network. Figure 3.2 is a schematic representation of such a process involved in what we call the *feedback loop* of the system. The pattern-recognition device (PRD) is connected to an ALOPEX system (a computer algorithm and an image processor in this case) and faces a display monitor where different-intensity patterns can be shown. Thin arrows representing response information and heavy arrows representing detailed pattern information are generated by the computer and relayed by the ALOPEX system to the monitor. ALOPEX is a set of algorithms described in detail elsewhere in this book. If this kind of arrangement is used for the determination of visual receptive fields of neurons, then the PRD is nothing more than the brain of an experimental animal. This way the neuron under investigation does its own selection of the best stimulus or trigger feature and reverses the role of the neuron from being a feature extractor to becoming a feature generator, as mentioned earlier. The idea is to find the response of the neuron to a stimulus and use this response as a positive feedback in the directed evaluation of the initially random pattern. Thus the cell involved filters out the key trigger features from the stimulus and reinforces them with the feedback.

As a generalization of this process, one might consider that a neuron N receives a visual input from a pattern P which is transmitted in a modified form P' to an analyzer neuron AN (or even a complex of

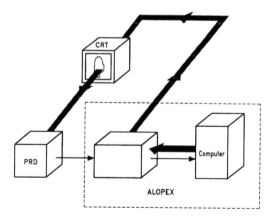

FIGURE 3.2 An ALOPEX system. The stimulus is presented on the CRT. The observer or any pattern-recognition device (PRD) faces the CRT; the subject's response is sent to the ALOPEX interface unit, where it is recorded and integrated, and the final response is sent to the computer. The computer calculates the values of the new pattern to be presented on the CRT according to the ALOPEX algorithm, and the process continues until the desired pattern appears on the CRT. At this point, the response is considered to be optimal and the process stops.

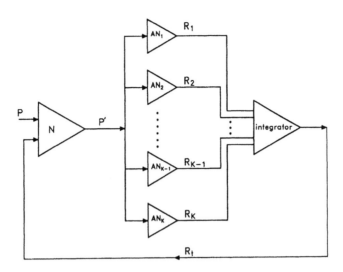

FIGURE 3.3 Diagrammatic representation of the ALOPEX "inverse" pattern-recognition scheme. Each neuron represents a feature analyzer that responds to the stimulus with a scalar quantity R called the *response*. R is then fed back to the system, and the pattern is modified accordingly. This process continues until there is a close correlation between the desired output and the original pattern.

neurons), as shown in Fig. 3.3. The analyzer responds with a scalar variable R that is then fed back to the system, and the pattern is modified accordingly. The process continues in small steps until there is an almost perfect correlation between the original pattern (template) and the one that neuron N indirectly created. This integrator sends the response back to the original modifier. The integrator need not be a linear summator. It could take any nonlinear form, a fact that is a more realistic representation of the visual cortex. One can envision the input patterns as templates preexisting in the memory of the system, a situation that might come about with visual experience. For a "naive" system, any initial pattern will do. As experience is gained, the patterns become less random. If one starts with a pattern that has some resemblance to one of the preexisting patterns, evolution will take its course. In nature, there might exist a mechanism similar to that of ALOPEX. By filtering the characteristics most important for the survival of the species, changes would be triggered. Perception, therefore, could be considered to be an interaction between sensory inputs and past experience in the form of templates stored in the memory of the perceiver and specific to the perceiver's needs. These templates are modifiable with time and adjusted accordingly to the input stimuli. With this approach, the neural nets and ensembles of nets under observation generate patterns that describe their thinking and memory properties. The normal flow of information is reversed and controls the afferent systems.

The perception processes as well as feature extraction or suppression of images or objects can be ascribed to specific neural mechanisms due to some sensory input or even due to some "wishful thinking" of the PRD. If it is true that the association cortex is affecting the sensitivity of the sensory cortex, then an ALOPEX mechanism is what one needs to close the loop for memory and learning.

Memory and Learning

If we try to define what memory is, we will face the fact that memory is not a single mental faculty but is rather composed of multiple abilities mediated by separate and distinct brain systems. Memory for a recent event can be expressed *explicitly* as a conscious recollection or *implicitly* as a facilitation of test performance without conscious recollection. The major distinction between these two memories is that explicit or *declarative* memory depends on limbic and diencephalic structures and provides the basis for recollection of events, while implicit or *nondeclarative* memory supports skills and habit learning, single conditioning, and the well-researched phenomenon of *priming*.

Declarative memory refers to memory of recent events and is usually assessed by tests of recall or recognition for specific single items. When the list of items becomes longer, a subject not only learns about each item on the list but also makes associations about what all these items have in common; i.e., the subject learns about the category that the items belong to. Learning leads to changes that increase or decrease the effectiveness of impulses arriving at the junctions between neurons, and the cumulative effect of these changes constitutes memory. Very often a particular pattern of neural activity leads to a result that occurs some time after the activity has ended. Learning then requires some means of relating the activity that is to be changed to the evaluation that can be made only by the delayed consequence. This phenomenon in physics is called *hysteresis* and refers to any modifications of future actions due to past actions. *Learning* then could be defined as change in any neuronal response resulting from previous experiences due to an external stimulus. Memory, in turn, would be the maintenance of these changes over time. The collection of neural changes representing memory is commonly known as the *engram,* and a major part of recent work has been to identify and locate engrams in the brain, since specific parts of the nervous system are capable of specific types of learning. The view of memory that has recently emerged is that information storage is tied to specific processing areas that are engaged during learning. The brain is organized so that separate regions of neocortex simultaneously carry out computations on specific features or characteristics of the external stimulus, no matter how complex that stimulus might be. If the brain learns specific properties or features of the stimulus, then we talk about the *nonassociative memory.* Associated with this type of learning is the phenomenon of *habituation,* in which if the same stimulus is presented repeatedly, the neurons respond less and less, while the introduction of a new stimulus increases the sensitization of the neuron. If the learning includes two related stimuli, then we talk about associative learning. This type of learning includes two types: *classic conditioning* and *operant conditioning.* The first deals with relationships among stimuli, while the latter deals with the relationship of the stimulus to the animal's own behavior. In humans, there exist two types of memory: *short-term* and *long-term memories.* The best way to study any physiologic process in humans, and especially memory, is to study its pathology. The study of amnesia has provided strong evidence distinguishing between these types of memory. Amnesic patients can keep a short list of numbers in mind for several minutes if they pay attention to the task. The difficulty comes when the list becomes longer, especially if the amount to be learned exceeds the brain capacity of what can be held in immediate memory. It could be that this happens because more systems have to be involved and that temporary information storage may occur within each brain area where stable changes in synaptic efficacy can eventually develop. *Plasticity* within existing pathways can account for most of the observations, and short-term memory occurs too quickly for it to require any major modifications of neuronal pathways. The capacity of long-term memory requires the integrity of the medial temporal and diencephalic regions in conjunction with neurons for storage of information. Within the domain of long-term memory, amnesic patients demonstrate intact learning and retention of certain motor, perceptual, and cognitive skills and intact priming effects. These patients do not exhibit any learning deficits but have no conscious awareness of prior study sessions or recognition of previously presented stimuli.

Priming effects can be tested by presenting words and then providing either the first few letters of the word or the last part of the word for recognition by the patient. Normal subjects, as expected, perform better than amnesic subjects. However, if these patients are instructed to "read" the incomplete word instead of memorizing it, then they perform as well as the normal individuals. Also, these amnesic patients perform well if words are cued by category names. Thus priming effects seem to be independent of the processes of recall and recognition memory, which is also observed in normal subjects. All this evidence supports the notion that the brain has organized its memory functions around fundamentally different information storage systems. In perceiving a word, a preexisting array of neurons is activated that have concurrent activities that produce perception, and priming is one of these functions.

Memory is not fixed immediately after learning but continues to grow toward stabilization over a period of time. This stabilization is called *consolidation of memory.* Memory consolidation is a *dynamic* feature of long-term memory, especially the declarative memory, but it is neither an automatic process with fixed lifetime nor is it determined at the time of learning. It is rather a process of reorganization of stored information. As time passes, some not yet consolidated memories fade out by remodeling the neural circuitry that is responsible for the original representation or by establishing new representations, since the original one can be forgotten.

The problems of learning and memory are studied continuously and with increased interest these days, especially because artificial systems such as neural networks can be used to mimic functions of the nervous system.

References

Cowan WM, Cuenod M (Eds). 1975. Use of Axonal Transport for Studies of Neuronal Connectivity. New York, Elsevier.

Deutsch S, Micheli-Tzanakou E. 1987. Neuroelectric Systems. New York, New York University Press.

Ganong WF. 1989. Review of Medical Physiology, 14th ed. Norwalk, CT, Appleton & Lange.

Hartzell HC. 1981. Mechanisms of slow postsynaptic potentials. Nature 291:593.

McMahon TA. 1984. Muscles, Reflexes and Locomotion. Princeton, NJ, Princeton University Press.

Partridge LD, Partridge DL. 1993. The Nervous System: Its Function and Interaction with the World. Cambridge, MA, MIT Press.

Shepherd GM. 1978. Microcircuits in the nervous system. Sci Am 238(2):92–103.

4

Vision System

George Stetten
Duke University

David Marr, an early pioneer in computer vision, defined *vision* as extracting "from images of the external world, a description that is useful for the viewer and not cluttered with irrelevant information" [Marr, 1982]. Advances in computers and video technology in the past decades have created the expectation that artificial vision should be realizable. The nontriviality of the task is evidenced by the continuing proliferation of new and different approaches to computer vision without any observable application in our everyday lives. Actually, computer vision is already offering practical solutions in industrial assembly and inspection, as well as for military and medical applications, so it seems we are beginning to master some of the fundamentals. However, we have a long way to go to match the vision capabilities of a 4-year-old child. In this chapter we will explore what is known about how nature has succeeded at this formidable task — that of interpreting the visual world.

4.1 Fundamentals of Vision Research

Research into biologic vision systems has followed several distinct approaches. The oldest is psychophysics, in which human and animal subjects are presented with visual stimuli and their responses recorded. Important early insights also were garnered by correlating clinical observations of visual defects with known neuroanatomic injury. In the past 50 years, a more detailed approach to understanding the mechanisms of vision has been undertaken by inserting small electrodes deep within the living brain to monitor the electrical activity of individual neurons and by using dyes and biochemical markers to track the anatomic course of nerve tracts. This research has led to a detailed and coherent, if not complete, theory of a visual system capable of explaining the discrimination of form, color, motion, and depth. This theory has been confirmed by noninvasive radiologic techniques that have been used recently to study the physiologic responses of the visual system, including positron emission tomography [Zeki et al., 1991] and functional magnetic resonance imaging [Belliveau et al., 1992; Cohen and Bookheimer, 1994], although these noninvasive techniques provide far less spatial resolution and thus can only show general regions of activity in the brain.

4.2 A Modular View of the Vision System

The Eyes

Movement of the eyes is essential to vision, not only allowing rapid location and tracking of objects but also preventing stationary images on the retina, which are essentially invisible. Continual movement of the image on the retina is essential to the visual system.

0-8493-1812-2/03/$0.00+$1.50

The eyeball is spherical and therefore free to turn in both the horizontal and vertical directions. Each eye is rotated by three pairs of mutually opposing muscles, innervated by the oculomotor nuclei in the brainstem. The eyes are coordinated as a pair in two useful ways: turning together to find and follow objects and turning inward to allow adjustment for parallax as objects become closer. The latter is called *convergence.*

The optical portion of the eye, which puts an image on the retina, is closely analogous to a photographic or television camera. Light enters the eye, passing through a series of transparent layers — the cornea, the aqueous humor, the lens, and the vitreous body — to eventually project on the retina.

The *cornea*, the protective outer layer of the eye, is heavily innervated with sensory neurons, triggering the blink reflex and tear duct secretion in response to irritation. The cornea is also an essential optical element, supplying two-thirds of the total refraction in the eye. Behind the cornea is a clear fluid, the *aqueous humor,* in which the central aperture of the iris, the pupil, is free to constrict or dilate. The two actions are accomplished by opposing sets of muscles.

The *lens,* a flexible transparent object behind the iris, provides the remainder of refraction necessary to focus an image on the retina. The ciliary muscles surrounding the lens can increase the lens' curvature, thereby decreasing its focal length and bringing nearer objects into focus. This is called *accommodation.* When the ciliary muscles are at rest, distant objects are in focus. There are no contradictory muscles to flatten the lens. This depends simply on the elasticity of the lens, which decreases with age. Behind the lens is the *vitreous humor,* consisting of a semigelatinous material filling the volume between the lens and the retina.

The Retina

The retina coats the back of the eye and is therefore spherical, not flat, making optical magnification constant at 3.5° of scan angle per millimeter. The retina is the neuronal front end of the visual system, the image sensor. In addition, it accomplishes the first steps in edge detection and color analysis before sending the processed information along the optic nerve to the brain. The retina contains five major classes of cells, roughly organized into layers. The dendrites of these cells each occupy no more than 1 to 2 mm^2 in the retina, limiting the extent of spatial integration from one layer of the retina to the next.

First come the *receptors,* which number approximately 125 million in each eye and contain the light-sensitive pigments responsible for converting photons into chemical energy. Receptor cells are of two general varieties: *rods* and *cones.* The cones are responsible for the perception of color, and they function only in bright light. When the light is dim, only rods are sensitive enough to respond. Exposure to a single photon may result in a measurable increase in the membrane potential of a rod. This sensitivity is the result of a chemical cascade, similar in operation to the photo multiplier tube, in which a single photon generates a cascade of electrons. All rods use the same pigment, whereas three different pigments are found in three separate kinds of cones.

Examination of the retina with an otoscope reveals its gross topography. The yellow circular area occupying the central 5° of the retina is called the *macula lutea,* within which a small circular pit called the *fovea* may be seen. Detailed vision occurs only in the fovea, where a dense concentration of cones provides visual activity to the central 1° of the visual field.

On the inner layer of the retina one finds a layer of *ganglion cells,* whose axons make up the optic nerve, the output of the retina. They number approximately 1 million, or less than 1% of the number of receptor cells. Clearly, some data compression has occurred in the space between the receptors and the ganglion cells. Traversing this space are the *bipolar cells,* which run from the receptors through the retina to the ganglion cells. Bipolar cells exhibit the first level of information processing in the visual system; namely, their response to light on the retina demonstrates "center/surround" receptive fields. By this I mean that a small dot on the retina elicits a response, while the area surrounding the spot elicits the opposite response. If both the center and the surround are illuminated, the net result is no response.

Thus bipolar cells respond only at the border between dark and light areas. Bipolar cells come in two varieties, on-center and off-center, with the center brighter or darker, respectively, than the surround.

The center response of bipolar cells results from direct contact with the receptors. The surround response is supplied by the *horizontal cells,* which run parallel to the surface of the retina between the receptor layer and the bipolar layer, allowing the surrounding area to oppose the influence of the center. The *amacrine cells,* a final cell type, also run parallel to the surface but in a different layer, between the bipolar cells and the ganglion cells, and are possibly involved in the detection of motion.

Ganglion cells, since they are triggered by bipolar cells, also have center/surround receptive fields and come in two types, on-center and off-center. On-center ganglion cells have a receptive field in which illumination of the center increases the firing rate and a surround where it decreases the rate. Off-center ganglion cells display the opposite behavior. Both types of ganglion cells produce little or no change in firing rate when the entire receptive field is illuminated, because the center and surround cancel each other. As in many other areas of the nervous system, the fibers of the optic nerve use frequency encoding to represent a scalar quantity.

Multiple ganglion cells may receive output from the same receptor, since many receptive fields overlap. However, this does not limit overall spatial resolution, which is maximum in the fovea, where two points separated by 0.5 min of arc may be discriminated. This separation corresponds to a distance on the retina of 2.5 μm, which is approximately the center-to-center spacing between cones. Spatial resolution falls off as one moves away from the fovea into the peripheral vision, where resolution is as low as 1° of arc.

Several aspects of this natural design deserve consideration. Why do we have center/surround receptive fields? The ganglion cells, whose axons make up the optic nerve, do not fire unless there is meaningful information, i.e., a border, falling within the receptive field. It is the edge of a shape we see rather than its interior. This represents a form of data compression. Center/surround receptive fields also allow for relative rather than absolute measurements of color and brightness. This is essential for analyzing the image independent of lighting conditions. Why do we have both on-center and off-center cells? Evidently, both light and dark are considered information. The same shape is detected whether it is lighter or darker than the background.

Optic Chiasm

The two optic nerves, from the left and right eyes, join at the optic chiasm, forming a *hemidecussation,* meaning that half the axons cross while the rest proceed uncrossed. The resulting two bundles of axons leaving the chiasm are called the *optic tracts.* The left optic tract contains only axons from the left half of each retina. Since the images are reversed by the lens, this represents light from the right side of the visual field. The division between the right and left optic tracts splits the retina down the middle, bisecting the fovea. The segregation of sensory information into the contralateral hemispheres corresponds to the general organization of sensory and motor centers in the brain.

Each optic tract has two major destinations on its side of the brain: (1) the superior colliculus and (2) the lateral geniculate nucleus (LGN). Although topographic mapping from the retina is scrambled within the optic tract, it is reestablished in both major destinations so that right, left, up, and down in the image correspond to specific directions within those anatomic structures.

Superior Colliculus

The *superior colliculus* is a small pair of bumps on the dorsal surface of the midbrain. Another pair, the *inferior colliculus,* is found just below it. Stimulation of the superior colliculus results in contralateral eye movement. Anatomically, output tracts from the superior colliculus run to areas that control eye and neck movement. Both the inferior and superior colliculi are apparently involved in locating sound. In the bat, the inferior colliculus is enormous, crucial to that animal's remarkable echolocation abilities.

The superior colliculus processes information from the inferior colliculus, as well as from the retina, allowing the eyes to quickly find and follow targets based on visual and auditory cues.

Different types of eye movements have been classified. The *saccade* (French, for "jolt") is a quick motion of the eyes over a significant distance. The saccade is how the eyes explore an image, jumping from landmark to landmark, rarely stopping in featureless areas. *Nystagmus* is the smooth pursuit of a moving image, usually with periodic backward saccades to lock onto subsequent points as the image moves by. *Microsaccades* are small movements, several times per second, over 1 to 2 min of arc in a seemingly random direction. Microsaccades are necessary for sight; their stabilization leads to effective blindness.

LGN

The thalamus is often called "the gateway to the cortex" because it processes much of the sensory information reaching the brain. Within the thalamus, we find the *lateral geniculate nucleus* (LGN), a peanut-sized structure that contains a single synaptic stage in the major pathway of visual information to higher centers. The LGN also receives information back from the cortex, so-called reentrant connections, as well as from the nuclei in the brainstem that control attention and arousal.

The cells in the LGN are organized into three pairs of layers. Each pair contains two layers, one from each eye. The upper two pairs consist of parvocellular cells (*P cells*) that respond with preference to different colors. The remaining lower pair consists of magnocellular cells (*M cells*) with no color preference (Fig. 4.1). The topographic mapping is identical for all six layers; i.e., passing through the layers at a given point yields synapses responding to a single area of the retina. Axons from the LGN proceed to the primary visual cortex in broad bands, the *optic radiations*, preserving this topographic mapping and displaying the same center/surround response as the ganglion cells.

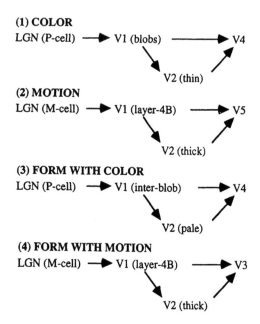

FIGURE 4.1 Visual pathways to cortical areas showing the separation of information by type. The lateral geniculate nucleus (LGN) and areas V1 and V2 act as gateways to more specialized higher areas.

Area V1

The LGN contains approximately 1.5 million cells. By comparison, the *primary visual cortex,* or *striate cortex,* which receives the visual information from the LGN, contains 200 million cells. It consists of a thin (2-mm) layer of gray matter (neuronal cell bodies) over a thicker collection of white matter (myelinated axons) and occupies a few square inches of the occipital lobes. The primary visual cortex has been called *area 17* from the days when the cortical areas were first differentiated by their cytoarchitectonics (the microscopic architecture of their layered neurons). In modern terminology, the primary visual cortex is often called *visual area 1,* or simply *V1.*

Destroying any small piece of V1 eliminates a small area in the visual field, resulting in *scotoma,* a local blind spot. Clinical evidence has long been available that a scotoma may result from injury, stroke, or tumor in a local part of V1. Between neighboring cells in V1's gray matter, horizontal connections are at most 2 to 5 mm in length. Thus, at any given time, the image from the retina is analyzed piecemeal in V1. Topographic mapping from the retina is preserved in great detail. Such mapping is seen elsewhere in the brain, such as in the somatosensory cortex [Mountcastle, 1957]. Like all cortical surfaces, V1 is a highly convoluted sheet, with much of its area hidden within its folds. If unfolded, V1 would be roughly pear shaped, with the top of the pear processing information from the fovea and the bottom of the pear processing the peripheral vision. Circling the pear at a given latitude would correspond roughly to circling the fovea at a fixed radius.

The primary visual cortex contains six layers, numbered 1 through 6. Distinct functional and anatomic types of cells are found in each layer. Layer 4 contains neurons that receive information from the LGN. Beyond the initial synapses, cells demonstrate progressively more complex responses. The outputs of V1 project to an area known as *visual area 2* (*V2*), which surrounds V1, and to higher visual areas in the occipital, temporal, and parietal lobes as well as to the superior colliculus. V1 also sends reentrant projections back to the LGN. Reentrant projections are present at almost every level of the visual system [Felleman and Essen, 1991; Edelman, 1978].

Cells in V1 have been studied extensively in animals by inserting small electrodes into the living brain (with surprisingly little damage) and monitoring the individual responses of neurons to visual stimuli. Various subpopulations of cortical cells have thus been identified. Some, termed *simple cells,* respond to illuminated edges or bars at specific locations and at specific angular orientations in the visual field. The angular orientation must be correct within 10° to 20° for the particular cell to respond. All orientations are equally represented. Moving the electrode parallel to the surface yields a smooth rotation in the orientation of cell responses by about 10° for each 50 μm that the electrode is advanced. This rotation is subject to reversals in direction, as well as "fractures," or sudden jumps in orientation.

Other cells, more common than simple cells, are termed *complex cells.* Complex cells respond to a set of closely spaced parallel edges within a particular receptive field. They may respond specifically to movement perpendicular to the orientation of the edge. Some prefer one direction of movement to the other. Some complex and simple cells are *end-stopped,* meaning they fire only if the illuminated bar or edge does not extend too far. Presumably, these cells detect corners, curves, or discontinuities in borders and lines. End-stopping takes place in layers 2 and 3 of the primary visual cortex. From the LGN through the simple cells and complex cells, there appears to be a sequential processing of the image. It is probable that simple cells combine the responses of adjacent LGN cells and that complex cells combine the responses of adjacent simple cells.

A remarkable feature in the organization of V1 is binocular convergence, in which a single neuron responds to identical receptive fields in both eyes, including location, orientation, and directional sensitivity to motion. It does not occur in the LGN, where axons from the left and right eyes are still segregated into different layers. Surprisingly, binocular connections to neurons are present in V1 at birth. Some binocular neurons are equally weighted in terms of responsiveness to both eyes, while others are more sensitive to one eye than to the other. One finds columns containing the latter type of cells in which one eye dominates, called *ocular dominance columns,* in uniform bands approximately 0.5 mm wide everywhere in V1. Ocular dominance columns occur in adjacent pairs, one for each eye, and are prominent in animals with forward-facing eyes, such as cats, chimpanzees, and humans. They are nearly absent in rodents and other animals whose eyes face outward.

The topography of orientation-specific cells and of ocular dominance columns is remarkably uniform throughout V1, which is surprising because the receptive fields near the fovea are 10 to 30 times smaller than those at the periphery. This phenomenon is called magnification. The fovea maps to a greater relative distance on the surface of V1 than does the peripheral retina, by as much as 36-fold [Daniel and Whitteridge, 1961]. In fact, the majority of V1 processes only the central 10° of the visual field. Both simple and complex cells in the foveal portion can resolve bars as narrow as 2 min of arc. Toward the periphery, the resolution falls off to 1° of arc.

As an electrode is passed down through the cortex *perpendicular* to the surface, each layer demonstrates receptive fields of characteristic size, the smallest being at layer 4, the input layer. Receptive fields are larger in other layers due to lateral integration of information. Passing the electrode *parallel* to the surface of the cortex reveals another important uniformity to V1. For example, in layer 3, which sends output fibers to higher cortical centers, one must move the electrode approximately 2 mm to pass from one collection of receptive fields to another that does not overlap. An area approximately 2 mm across thus represents the smallest unit piece of V1, i.e., that which can completely process the visual information.

Indeed, it is just the right size to contain a complete set of orientations and more than enough to contain information from both eyes. It receives a few tens of thousands of fibers from the LGN, produces perhaps 50,000 output fibers, and is fairly constant in cytoarchitectonics whether at the center of vision, where it processes approximately 30 min of arc, or at the far periphery, where it processes 7° to 8° of arc.

The topographic mapping of the visual field onto the cortex suffers an abrupt discontinuity between the left and right hemispheres, and yet our perception of the visual scene suffers no obvious rift in the midline. This is due to the *corpus collousum,* an enormous tract containing at least 200 million axons, that connects the two hemispheres. The posterior portion of the corpus collousum connects the two halves of V1, linking cells that have similar orientations and whose receptive fields overlap in the vertical midline. Thus a perceptually seamless merging of left and right visual fields is achieved. Higher levels of the visual system are likewise connected across the corpus collousum. This is demonstrated, for example, by the clinical observation that cutting the corpus collousum prevents a subject from verbally describing objects in the left field of view (the right hemisphere). Speech, which normally involves the left hemisphere, cannot process visual objects from the right hemisphere without the corpus collousum.

By merging the information from both eyes, V1 is capable of analyzing the distance to an object. Many cues for depth are available to the visual system, including occlusion, parallax (detected by the convergence of the eyes), optical focusing of the lens, rotation of objects, expected size of objects, shape based on perspective, and shadow casting. Stereopsis, which uses the slight difference between images due to the parallax between the two eyes, was first enunciated in 1838 by Sir Charles Wheatstone and it is probably the most important cue [Wheatstone, 1838]. Fixating on an object causes it to fall on the two foveas. Other objects that are nearer become outwardly displaced on the two retinas, while objects that are farther away become inwardly displaced. About 2° of horizontal disparity is tolerated, with fusion by the visual system into a single object. Greater horizontal disparity results in double vision. Almost no vertical displacement (a few minutes of arc) is tolerated. Physiologic experiments have revealed a particular class of complex cells in V1 which are *disparity tuned.* They fall into three general classes. One class fires only when the object is at the fixation distance, another only when the object is nearer, and a third only when it is farther away [Poggio and Talbot, 1981]. Severing the corpus collousum leads to a loss of stereopsis in the vertical midline of the visual field.

When the inputs to the two retinas cannot be combined, one or the other image is rejected. This phenomenon is known as *retinal rivalry* and can occur in a piecewise manner or can even lead to blindness in one eye. The general term *amblyopia* refers to the partial or complete loss of eyesight not caused by abnormalities in the eye. The most common form of amblyopia is caused by *strabismus,* in which the eyes are not aimed in a parallel direction but rather are turned inward (cross-eyed) or outward (wall-eyed). This condition leads to habitual suppression of vision from one of the eyes and sometimes to blindness in that eye or to *alternation,* in which the subject maintains vision in both eyes by using only one eye at a time. Cutting selected ocular muscles in kittens causes strabismus, and the kittens respond by alternation, preserving functional vision in both eyes. However, the number of cells in the cortex displaying binocular responses is greatly reduced. In humans with long-standing alternating strabismus, surgical repair making the eyes parallel again does not bring back a sense of depth. Permanent damage has been caused by the subtle condition of the images on the two retinas not coinciding. This may be explained by the Hebb model for associative learning, in which temporal association between inputs strengthens synaptic connections [Hebb, 1961].

Further evidence that successful development of the visual system depends on proper input comes from clinical experience with children who have *cataracts* at birth. Cataracts constitute a clouding of the lens, permitting light, but not images, to reach the retina. If surgery to remove the cataracts is delayed until the child is several years old, the child remains blind even though images are restored to the retina. Kittens and monkeys whose eyelids are sewn shut during a critical period of early development stay blind even when the eyes are opened. Physiologic studies in these animals show very few cells responding in the visual cortex. Other experiments depriving more specific elements of an image, such as certain orientations or motion in a certain direction, yield a cortex without the corresponding cell type.

Color

Cones, which dominate the fovea, can detect wavelengths between 400 and 700 nm. The population of cones in the retina can be divided into three categories, each containing a different pigment. This was established by direct microscopic illumination of the retina [Wald, 1974; Marks et al., 1964]. The pigments have a bandwidth on the order of 100 nm, with significant overlap, and with peak sensitivities at 560 nm (yellow-green), 530 nm (blue-green), and 430 nm (violet). These three cases are commonly known as red, green, and blue. Compared with the auditory system, whose array of cochlear sensors can discriminate thousands of different sonic frequencies, the visual system is relatively impoverished with only three frequency parameters. Instead, the retina expends most of its resolution on spatial information. Color vision is absent in many species, including cats, dogs, and some primates, as well as in most nocturnal animals, since cones are useless in low light.

By having three types of cones at a given locality on the retina, a simplified spectrum can be sensed and represented by three independent variables, a concept known as *trichromacy*. This model was developed by Thomas Young and Hermann von Helmholtz in the 19th century before neurobiology existed and does quite well at explaining the retina [Young, 1802; Helmholtz, 1889]. The model is also the underlying basis for red-green-blue (RGB) video monitors and color television [Ennes, 1981]. Rods do not help in discriminating color, even though the pigment in rods does add a fourth independent sensitivity peak.

Psychophysical experimentation yields a complex, redundant map between spectrum and perceived color, or *hue*, including not only the standard red, orange, yellow, green, and blue but hues such as pink, purple, brown, and olive green that are not themselves in the rainbow. Some of these may be achieved by introducing two more variables: *saturation*, which allows for mixing with white light, and *intensity*, which controls the level of color. Thus three variables are still involved: hue, saturation, and intensity.

Another model for color vision was put forth in the 19th century by Ewald Hering [Hering, 1864]. This theory also adheres to the concept of trichromacy, espousing three independent variables. However, unlike the Young-Helmholtz model, these variables are signed; they can be positive, negative, or zero. The resulting three axes are *red-green, yellow-blue,* and *black-white.* The Hering model is supported by the physiologic evidence for the center/surround response, which allows for positive as well as negative information. In fact, two populations of cells, activated and suppressed along the red-green and yellow-blue axes, have been found in monkey LGN. Yellow is apparently detected by a combination of red and green cones.

The Hering model explains, for example, the perception of the color brown, which results only when orange or yellow is surrounded by a brighter color. It also accounts for the phenomenon of color constancy, in which the perceived color of an object remains unchanged under differing ambient light conditions provided background colors are available for comparison. Research into color constancy was pioneered in the laboratory of Edwin Land [Land and McCann, 1971]. As David Hubel says, "We require color borders for color, just as we require luminance borders for black and white" [Hubel, 1988, p. 178]. As one might expect, when the corpus collousum is surgically severed, color constancy is absent across the midline.

Color processing in V1 is confined to small circular areas, known as *blobs*, in which *double-opponent cells* are found. They display a center/surround behavior based on the red-green and yellow-blue axes but lack orientation selectivity. The V1 blobs were first identified by their uptake of certain enzymes, and only later was their role in color vision discovered [Livingstone and Hubel, 1984]. The blobs are especially prominent in layers 2 and 3, which receive input from the P cells of the LGN.

Higher Cortical Centers

How are the primitive elements of image processing so far discussed united into an understanding of the image? Beyond V1 are many higher cortical centers for visual processing, at least 12 in the occipital lobe and others in the temporal and parietal lobes. Areas V2 receives axons from both the blob and interblob areas of V1 and performs analytic functions such as filling in the missing segments of an edge. V2 contains three areas categorized by different kinds of stripes: *thick stripes* which process relative horizontal position and stereopsis, *thin stripes* which process color without orientations, and *pale stripes* which extend the process of end-stopped orientation cells.

Beyond V2, higher centers have been labeled V3, V4, V5, etc. Four parallel systems have been delineated [Zeki, 1992], each system responsible for a different attribute of vision, as shown in Fig. 4.1. This is obviously an oversimplification of a tremendously complex system.

Corroborative clinical evidence supports this model. For example, lesions in V4 lead to *achromatopsia*, in which a patient can only see gray and cannot even recall colors. Conversely, a form of poisoning, *carbon monoxide chromatopsia*, results when the V1 blobs and V2 thin stripes selectively survive exposure to carbon monoxide thanks to their rich vasculature, leaving the patient with a sense of color but not of shape. A lesion in V5 leads to *akinetopsia*, in which objects disappear.

As depicted in Fig. 4.1, all visual information is processed through V1 and V2, although discrete channels within these areas keep different types of information separate. A total lesion of V1 results in the perception of total blindness. However, not all channels are shown in Fig. 4.1, and such a "totally blind" patient may perform better than randomly when forced to guess between colors or between motion in different directions. The patient with this condition, called *blindsight*, will deny being able to see anything [Weiskrantz, 1990].

Area V1 preserves retinal topographic mapping and shows receptive fields, suggesting a piecewise analysis of the image, although a given area of V1 receives sequential information from disparate areas of the visual environment as the eyes move. V2 and higher visual centers show progressively larger receptive fields and less defined topographic mapping but more specialized responses. In the extreme of specialization, neurobiologists joke about the "grandmother cell," which would respond only to a particular face. No such cell has yet been found. However, cortical regions that respond to faces in general have been found in the temporal lobe. Rather than a "grandmother cell," it seems that face-selective neurons are members of ensembles for coding facts [Gross and Sergen, 1992].

Defining Terms

Binocular convergence: The response of a single neuron to the same location in the visual field of each eye.

Color constancy: The perception that the color of an object remains constant under different lighting conditions. Even though the spectrum reaching the eye from that object can be vastly different, other objects in the field of view are used to compare.

Cytoarchitectonics: The organization of neuron types into layers as seen by various staining techniques under the microscope. Electrophysiologic responses of individual cells can be correlated with their individual layer.

Magnification: The variation in amount of retinal area represented per unit area of V1 from the fovea to the peripheral vision. Even though the fovea takes up an inordinate percentage of V1 compared with the rest of the visual field, the scale of the cellular organization remains constant. Thus the image from the fovea is, in effect, magnified before processing.

Receptive field: The area in the visual field that evokes a response in a neuron. Receptive fields may respond to specific stimuli such as illuminated bars or edges with particular directions of motion, etc.

Stereopsis: The determination of distance to objects based on relative displacement on the two retinas because of parallax.

Topographic mapping: The one-to-one correspondence between location on the retina and location within a structure in the brain. Topographic mapping further implies that contiguous areas on the retina map to contiguous areas in the particular brain structure.

References

Belliveau JH, Kwong KK, et al. 1992. Magnetic resonance imaging mapping of brain function: Human visual cortex. Invest Radiol 27(suppl 2):S59.

Cohen MS, Bookheimer SY. 1994. Localization of brain function using magnetic resonance imaging. Trends Neurosci 17(7):268.

Daniel PM, Whitteridge D. 1961. The representation of the visual field on the cerebral cortex in monkeys. J Physiol 159:203.

Edelman GM. 1978. Group selection and phasic reentrant signalling: A theory of higher brain function. In GM Edelman and VB Mountcastle (eds), The Mindful Brain, pp 51–100, Cambridge, MA, MIT Press.

Ennes HE. 1981. NTSC color fundamentals. In Television Broadcasting: Equipment, Systems, and Operating Fundamentals. Indianapolis, Howard W. Sams & Co.

Felleman DJ, V Essen DC. 1991. Distributed hierarchical processing in the primate cerebral cortex. Cerebral Cortex 1(1):1.

Gross CG, Sergen J. 1992. Face recognition. Curr Opin Neurobiol 2(2):156.

Hebb DO. 1961. The Organization of Behavior. New York, Wiley.

Helmholtz H. 1889, Popular Scientific Lectures. London, Longmans.

Hering E. 1864. Outlines of a Theory of Light Sense. Cambridge, MA, Harvard University Press.

Hubel DH. 1995. Eye, Brain, and Vision. New York, Scientific American Library.

Land EH, McCann JJ. 1971. Lightness and retinex theory. J Opt Soc Am 61:1.

Livingstone MS, Hubel DH. 1984. Anatomy and physiology of a color system in the primate visual cortex. J Neurosci 4:309.

Marks WB, Dobelle WH, MacNichol EF. 1964. Visual pigments of single primate cones. Science 143:1181.

Marr D. 1982. Vision. San Francisco, WH Freeman.

Mountcastle VB. 1957. Modality and topographic properties of single neurons of cat's somatic sensory cortex. J Neurophysiol 20(3):408.

Poggio GF, Talbot WH. 1981. Mechanisms of static and dynamic stereopsis in foveal cortex of the rhesus monkey. J Physiol 315:469.

Wald G. 1974. Proceedings: Visual pigments and photoreceptors — Review and outlook. Exp Eye Res 18(3):333.

Weiskrantz L. 1990. The Ferrier Lecture: Outlooks for blindsight: Explicit methodologies for implicit processors. Proc R Soc Lond B239:247.

Wheatstone SC. 1838. Contribution to the physiology of vision. Philos Trans R Soc Lond.

Young T. 1802. The Bakerian Lecture: On the theory of lights and colours. Philos Trans R Soc Lond 92:12.

Zeki S. 1992. The visual image in mind and brain. Sci Am, Sept., p. 69.

Zeki S, Watson JD, Lueck CJ, et al. 1991. A direct demonstration of functional specialization in human visual cortex. J Neurosci 11(3):641.

Further Reading

An excellent introductory text about the visual system is *Eye, Brain, and Vision,* by Nobel laureate, David H. Hubel (1995, Scientific American Library, New York). A more recent general text with a thorough treatment of color vision, as well as the higher cortical centers, is *A Vision of the Brain,* by Semir Zeki (1993, Blackwell Scientific Publications, Oxford).

Other useful texts with greater detail about the nervous system are *From Neuron to Brain,* by Nicholls, Martin, Wallace, and Kuffler (3rd ed., 1992, Sinauer Assoc., Sunderand, MA), *The Synaptic Organization of the Brain,* by Shepherd (4th ed., 1998, Oxford University Press, New York), and *Fundamental Neuroanatomy,* by Nauta and Feirtag (1986, WH Freeman, New York).

A classic text that laid the foundation of computer vision is *Vision,* by David Marr (1982, WH Freeman, New York). Other texts dealing with the mathematics of image processing and image analysis are *Digital Image Processing,* by Pratt (1991, Wiley, New York), and *Digital Imaging Processing and Computer Vision,* by Schalkoff (1989, Wiley, New York).

5

Auditory System

Ben M. Clopton
University of Washington

Francis A. Spelman
University of Washington

The auditory system can be divided into two large subsystems, peripheral and central. The peripheral auditory system converts the condensations and rarefactions that produce sound into neural codes that are interpreted by the central auditory system as specific sound tokens that may affect behavior.

The peripheral auditory system is subdivided into the external ear, the middle ear, and the inner ear (Fig. 5.1). The external ear collects sound energy as pressure waves, which are converted to mechanical motion at the *eardrum*. This motion is transformed across the *middle ear* and transferred to the *inner ear*, where it is frequency analyzed and converted into neural codes that are carried by the eighth cranial nerve, or *auditory nerve*, to the central auditory system.

Sound information, encoded as discharges in an array of thousands of auditory nerve fibers, is processed in nuclei that make up the central auditory system. The major centers include the *cochlear nuclei* (CN), the *superior olivary complex* (SOC), the *nuclei of the lateral lemniscus* (NLL), the *inferior colliculi* (IC), the *medial geniculate body* (MGB) of the thalamus, and the *auditory cortex* (AC). The CN, SOC, and NLL are brainstem nuclei; the IC is at the midbrain level; and the MGB and AC constitute the auditory thalamocortical system.

While interesting data have been collected from groups other than mammals, this chapter will emphasize the mammalian auditory system. This chapter ignores the structure and function of the vestibular system. While a few specific references are included, most are general in order to provide a more introductory entry into topics.

5.1 Physical and Psychological Variables

Acoustics

Sound is produced by time-varying motion of the particles in air. The motions can be defined by their pressure variations or by their volume velocities. *Volume velocity* is defined as the average particle velocity produced across a cross-sectional area and is the acoustic analogue of electric current. *Pressure* is the acoustic analogue of voltage. *Acoustic intensity* is the average rate of the flow of energy through a unit

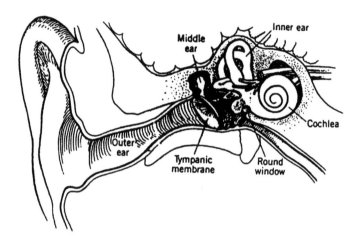

FIGURE 5.1   The peripheral auditory system showing the ear canal, tympanic membrane, middle ear and ossicles, and the inner ear consisting of the cochlea and semicircular canals of the vestibular system. Nerves communicating with the brain are also shown.

area normal to the direction of the propagation of the sound wave. It is the product of the acoustic pressure and the volume velocity and is analogous to electric power. *Acoustic impedance,* the analogue of electrical impedance, is the complex ratio of acoustic pressure and volume velocity. Sound is often described in terms of either acoustic pressure or acoustic intensity [Kinsler and Frey, 1962].

The auditory system has a wide dynamic range; i.e., it responds to several decades of change in the magnitude of sound pressure. Because of this wide dynamic range, it is useful to describe the independent variables in terms of decibels, where acoustic intensity is described by $dB = 10 \log(I/I_0)$, where I_0 is the reference intensity, or equivalently for acoustic pressure, $dB = 20 \log(P/P_0)$, where P_0 is the reference pressure.

Psychoacoustics

Physical variables, such as *frequency* and *intensity,* may have correlated psychological variables, such as *pitch* and *loudness.* Relationships between acoustic and psychological variables, the subject of the field of *psychoacoustics,* are generally not linear and may be very complex, but measurements of human detection and discrimination can be made reliably. Humans without hearing loss detect tonal frequencies from 20 Hz to 20 kHz. At 2 to 4 kHz their *dynamic range,* the span between threshold and pain, is approximately 120 dB. The minimum threshold for sound occurs between 2 and 5 kHz and is about 20 µPa. At the low end of the auditory spectrum, threshold is 80 dB higher, while at the high end, it is 70 dB higher. Intensity differences of 1 dB can be detected, while frequency differences of 2 to 3 Hz can be detected at frequencies below about 3 kHz [Fay, 1988].

5.2   The Peripheral Auditory System

The External Ear

Ambient sounds are collected by the *pinna,* the visible portion of the external ear, and guided to the middle ear by the *external auditory meatus,* or ear canal. The pinna acquires sounds selectively due to its geometry and the sound shadowing effect produced by the head. In those species whose ears can be moved voluntarily through large angles, selective scanning of the auditory environment is possible.

The ear canal serves as an acoustic waveguide that is open at one end and closed at the other. The open end at the pinna approximates a short circuit (large volume velocity and small pressure variation), while that at the closed end is terminated by the *tympanic membrane* (eardrum). The tympanic membrane has a relatively high acoustic impedance compared with the characteristic impedance of the meatus and looks like an open circuit. Thus the ear canal can resonate at those frequencies for which its length is an odd number of quarter wavelengths. The first such frequency is at about 3 kHz in the human. The meatus is antiresonant for those frequencies for which its length is an integer number of half wavelengths. For a discussion of resonance and antiresonance in an acoustic waveguide, see a text on basic acoustics, e.g., Kinsler and Frey [1962].

The acoustic properties of the external ear produce differences between the sound pressure produced at the tympanic membrane and that at the opening of the ear canal. These differences are functions of frequency, with larger differences found at frequencies between 2 and 6 kHz than those below 2 kHz. These variations have an effect on the frequency selectivity of the overall auditory system.

The Middle Ear

Anatomy

Tracing the acoustic signal, the boundaries of the middle ear include the tympanic membrane at the input and the oval window at the output. The middle ear bones, the ossicles, lie between. Pressure relief for the tympanic membrane is provided by the eustachian tube. The middle ear is an air-filled cavity.

The Ossicles

The three bones that transfer sound from the tympanic membrane to the *oval window* are called the *malleus* (hammer), *incus* (anvil), and *stapes* (stirrup). The acoustic impedance of the atmospheric source is much less than that of the aqueous medium of the load. The ratio is 3700 in an open medium, or 36 dB [Kinsler and Frey, 1962]. The ossicles comprise an impedance transformer for sound, producing a mechanical advantage that allows the acoustic signal at the tympanic membrane to be transferred with low loss to the round window of the cochlea (inner ear). The air-based sound source produces an acoustic signal of low-pressure and high-volume velocity, while the mechanical properties of the inner ear demand a signal of high-pressure and low-volume velocity.

The impedance transformation is produced in two ways: The area of the tympanic membrane is greater than that of the footplate of the stapes, and the lengths of the malleus and incus produce a lever whose length is greater on the side of the tympanic membrane than it is on the side of the oval window. In the human, the mechanical advantage is about 22:1 [Dobie and Rubel, 1989] and the impedance ratio of the transformer is 480, 27 dB, changing the mismatch from 3700:1 to about 8:1.

This simplified discussion of the function of the ossicles holds at low frequencies, those below 2 kHz. First, the tympanic membrane does not behave as a piston at higher frequencies but can support modes of vibration. Second, the mass of the ossicles becomes significant. Third, the connections between the ossicles is not lossless, nor can the stiffness of these connections be ignored. Fourth, pressure variations in the middle ear cavity can change the stiffness of the tympanic membrane. Fifth, the cavity of the middle ear produces resonances at acoustic frequencies.

Pressure Relief

The eustachian tube is a bony channel that is lined with soft tissue. It extends from the middle ear to the nasopharynx and provides a means by which pressure can be equalized across the tympanic membrane. The function is clearly observed with changes in altitude or barometric pressure. A second function of the eustachian tube is to aerate the tissues of the middle ear.

The Inner Ear

The mammalian inner ear is a spiral structure, the *cochlea* (snail), consisting of three fluid-filled chambers, or scalae, the *scala vestibuli*, the *scala media*, and the *scala tympani* (Fig. 5.2). The stapes footplate introduces mechanical displacements into the scala vestibuli through the oval window at the *base* of the

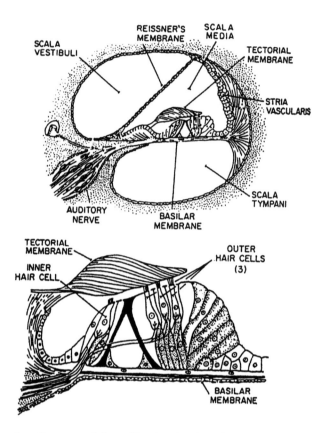

FIGURE 5.2 Cross section of one turn of the cochlea showing the scala vestibuli, scala media, and scala tympani. Reissner's membrane separates the SM and SV, while the basilar membrane and organ of Corti separate the SM and ST.

cochlea. At the other end of the spiral, the *apex* of the cochlea, the scala vestibuli and the scala tympani communicate by an opening, the *helicotrema*. Both are filled with an aqueous medium, the *perilymph*. The scala media spirals between them and is filled with *endolymph*, a medium that is high in K^+ and low in Na^+. The scala media is separated from the scala vestibuli by *Reissner's membrane*, which is impermeable to ions, and the scala media is separated from the scala tympani by the *basilar membrane* (BM) and *organ of Corti*. The organ of Corti contains the hair cells that transduce acoustic signals into neural signals, the cells that support the hair cells, and the tectorial membrane to which the outer hair cells are attached. The BM provides the primary filter function of the inner ear and is permeable so that the cell bodies of the hair cells are bathed in perilymph.

Fluid and tissue displacements travel from the footplate of the stapes along the cochlear spiral from base to apex. Pressure relief is provided for the incompressible fluids of the inner ear by the round window membrane; e.g., if a transient pressure increase at the stapes displaces its footplate inward, there will be a compensatory outward displacement of the round window membrane.

The Basilar Membrane

Physiology

The BM supports the hair cells and their supporting cells (see Fig. 5.2). Sound decomposition into its frequency components is a major code of the BM. A transient sound, such as a click, initiates a *traveling wave* of displacement in the BM, and this motion has frequency-dependent characteristics which arise from properties of the membrane and its surrounding structures [Bekesy, 1960]. The membrane's width varies as it traverses the cochlear duct: It is narrower at its basal end than at its apical end. It is stiffer at the base than at the apex, with stiffness varying by about two orders of magnitude [Dobie and Rubel, 1989]. The membrane is a distributed structure, which acts as a delay line, as suggested by the nature of the traveling wave [Lyon and Mead, 1989]. The combination of mechanical properties of the BM produces a structure that demonstrates a distance-dependent displacement when the ear is excited sinusoidally. The distance from the apex to the maximum displacement is logarithmically related to the frequency of a sinusoidal tone [LePage, 1991].

Tuning is quite sharp for sinusoidal signals. The slope of the tuning curve is much greater at the high-frequency edge than at the low-frequency edge, with slopes of more than 100 dB per octave at the high edge and about half that at the low edge [Lyon and Mead, 1989]. The filter is sharp, with a 10-dB bandwidth of 10 to 25% of the center frequency.

The auditory system includes both passive and active properties. The outer hair cells (see below) receive efferent output from the brain and actively modify the characteristics of the auditory system. The result is to produce a "cochlear amplifier," which sharpens the tuning of the BM [Lyon and Mead, 1989], as well as adding nonlinear properties to the system [Geisler, 1992; Cooper and Rhode, 1992], along with otoacoustic emissions [LePage, 1991].

The Organ of Corti

The organ of Corti is attached to the BM on the side of the aqueous fluid of the scala media. It is comprised of the supporting cells for the hair cells, the hair cells themselves, and the *tectorial membrane*. The cilia of the *inner hair cells* (IHCs) do not contact the tectorial membrane, while those of the *outer hair cells* (OHCs) do. Both IHCs and OHCs have precise patterns of stereocilia at one end which are held within the tectorial plate next to the overlying tectorial membrane. The IHCs synapse with *spiral ganglion cells*, the afferent neurons, while the OHCs synapse with efferent neurons. Both IHCs and OHCs are found along the length of the organ of Corti. The IHCs are found in a single line, numbering between about 3000 and 4000 in human. There are three lines of OHCs, numbering about 12,000 in human [Nadol, 1988].

Inner Hair Cells

The stereocilia of the IHCs are of graded, decreasing length from one side of the cell where a kinocilium is positioned early in ontogeny. If the cilia are deflected in a direction toward this position, membrane channels are further opened to allow potassium to enter and depolarize the cell [Hudspeth, 1987]. Displacement in the other direction reduces channel opening and produces a relative hyperpolarization [Hudspeth and Corey, 1977]. These changes in intracellular potential modulate transmitter release at the base of the IHCs.

The IHCs are not attached to the tectorial membrane, so their response to motion of the membrane is proportional to the velocity of displacement rather than to displacement itself, since the cilia of the hair cells are bathed in endolymph. When the membrane vibrates selectively in response to a pure tone, the stereocilia are bent atop a small number of hair cells, which depolarize in response to the mechanical event. Thus, the *tonotopic organization* of the BM is transferred to the hair cells and to the rest of the auditory system. The auditory system is organized tonotopically, i.e., in order of frequency, because the frequency ordering of the cochlea is mapped through successive levels of the system. While this organization is preserved throughout the system, it is much more complex than a huge set of finely tuned filters.

Hair cells in some species exhibit frequency tuning when isolated [Crawford and Fettiplace, 1985], but mammalian hair cells exhibit no tuning characteristics. The tuning of the mammalian auditory system depends on the mechanical characteristics of the BM as modified by the activity of the OHCs.

Outer Hair Cells

The OHCs have cilia that are attached to the tectorial membrane. Since their innervation is overwhelmingly efferent, they do not transfer information to the brain but are modulated in their mechanical action by the brain. There are several lines of evidence that lead to the conclusion that the OHCs play an active role in the processes of the inner ear. First, OHCs change their length in response to neurotransmitters

[Dobie and Rubel, 1989]. Second, observation of the Henson's cells, passive cells that are intimately connected to OHCs, shows that spontaneous vibrations are produced by the Henson's cells in mammals and likely in the OHCs as well. These vibrations exhibit spectral peaks that are appropriate in frequency to their locations on the BM [Khanna et al., 1993]. Third, action of the OHCs as amplifiers leads to spontaneous otoacoustic emissions [Kim, 1984; Lyon and Mead, 1989] and to changes in the response of the auditory system [Lyon and Mead, 1989; Geisler, 1992]. Fourth, AC excitation of the OHCs of mammals produces changes in length [Cooke, 1993].

The OHCs appear to affect the response of the auditory system in several ways. They enhance the tuning characteristics of the system to sinusoidal stimuli, decreasing thresholds and narrowing the filter's bandwidth [Dobie and Rubel, 1989]. They likely influence the damping of the BM dynamically by actively changing its stiffness.

Spiral Ganglion Cells and the Auditory Nerve

Anatomy

The auditory nerve of the human contains about 30,000 fibers consisting of myelinated proximal processes of spiral ganglion cells (SGCs). The somas of spiral ganglion cells (SGCs) lie in *Rosenthal's canal,* which spirals medial to the three scalae of the cochlea. Most (93%) are large, heavily myelinated, *type I* SGCs whose distal processes synapse on IHCs. The rest are smaller *type II* SGCs, which are more lightly myelinated. Each IHC has, on average, a number of fibers that synapse with it, 8 in the human and 18 in the cat, although some fibers contact more than one IHC. In contrast, each type II SGC contacts OHCs at a rate of about 10 to 60 cells per fiber.

The auditory nerve collects in the center of the cochlea, its *modiolus,* as SGC fibers join it. Low-frequency fibers from the apex join first, and successively higher frequency fibers come to lie concentrically on the outer layers of the nerve in a spiraling fashion before it exits the modiolus to enter the internal auditory meatus of the temporal bone. A precise tonotopic organization is retained in the concentrically wrapped fibers.

Physiology

Discharge spike patterns from neurons can be recorded extracellularly while repeating tone bursts are presented. A *threshold level* can be identified from the resulting *rate-level function* (RLF). In the absence of sound and at lower, subthreshold levels, a *spontaneous rate* of discharge is measured. In the nerve this ranges from 50 spikes per second to fewer than 10. As intensity is raised, the *threshold level* is encountered, where the evoked discharge rate significantly exceeds the spontaneous discharge rate. The plot of threshold levels as a function of frequency is the neuron's *threshold tuning curve.* The tuning curves for axons in the auditory nerve show a minimal threshold (maximum sensitivity) at a *characteristic frequency* (CF) with a narrow frequency range of responding for slightly more intense sounds. At high intensities, a large range of frequencies elicits spike discharges. RLFs for nerve fibers are *monotonic* (i.e., spike rate increases with stimulus intensity), and although a saturation rate is usually approached at high levels, the spike rate does not decline. Mechanical tuning curves for the BM and neural threshold tuning curves are highly similar (Fig. 5.3). Mechanical frequency analysis in the cochlea and the orderly projection of fibers through the nerve lead to correspondingly orderly maps for CFs in the nerve and the nuclei of the central pathways.

Sachs and Young [1979] found that the frequency content of lower intensity vowel sounds is represented as corresponding tonotopic rate peaks in nerve activity, but for higher intensities this rate code is lost as fibers tend toward equal discharge rates. At high intensities spike synchrony to frequencies near CF continue to signal the relative spectral content of vowels, a temporal code. These results hold for *high-spontaneous-rate fibers* (over 15 spikes per second), which are numerous. Less common, *low-spontaneous-rate fibers* (less than 15 spikes per second) appear to maintain the rate code at higher intensities, suggesting different coding roles for these two fiber populations.

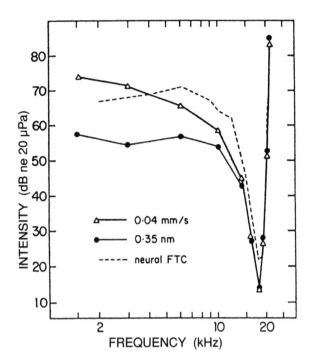

FIGURE 5.3 Mechanical and neural turning curves from the BM and auditory nerve, respectively. The two mechanical curves show the intensity and frequency combinations for tones required to obtain a criterion displacement or velocity, while the neural curve shows the combinations needed to increase neural discharge rates a small amount over spontaneous rate.

5.3 The Central Auditory System

Overview

In ascending paths, obligatory synapses occur at the CN, IC, MGB, and AC, but a large number of alternative paths exist with ascending and descending internuclear paths and the shorter intranuclear connections between neighboring neurons and subdivisions within a major nuclear group. Each of the centers listed contains subpopulations of neurons that differ in aspects of their morphologies, discharge patterns to sounds, segregation in the nucleus, biochemistry, and synaptic connectivities. The arrangement of the major ascending auditory pathways is schematically illustrated in Fig. 5.4. For references, see Altschuler et al. [1991].

Neural Bases of Processing

The Cochlear Nuclei

Anatomy of the Cochlear Nuclei. The CN can be subdivided into at least three distinct regions, the *anteroventral CN* (AVCN), the *posteroventral CN* (PVCN), and the *dorsal CN* (DCN). Each subdivision has one or more distinctive neuron types and unique intra- and internuclear connections. The axon from each type I SGC in the nerve branches to reach each of the three divisions in an orderly manner so that tonotopic organization is maintained. Neurons with common morphologic classifications are found in all three divisions, especially *granule cells,* which tend to receive connections from type II spiral ganglion cells.

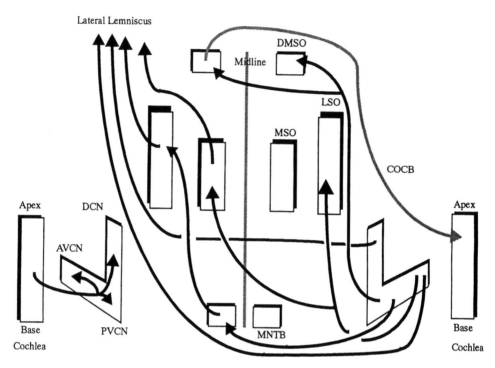

FIGURE 5.4 A schematic of major connections in the auditory brainstem discussed in the text. All structures and connections are bilaterally symmetrical, but connections have been shown on one side only for clarity. No cell types are indicated, but the subdivisions of origin are suggested in the CN. Note that the LSO and MSO receive inputs from both CN.

Morphologic classification of neurons based on the shapes of their dendritic trees and somas show that the anterior part of the AVCN contains many *spherical bushy cells,* while in its posterior part both *globular bushy cells* and spherical bushy cells are found. Spherical bushy cells receive input from one type I ganglion cell through a large synapse formation containing end bulbs of Held, while the globular cells may receive inputs from a few afferent fibers. These endings cover a large part of the soma surface and parts of the proximal dendrite, especially in spherical bushy cells, and they have rounded vesicles pre-synaptically, indicating excitatory input to the bushy cells, while other synaptic endings of noncochlear origins tend to have flattened vesicles associated with inhibitory inputs. *Stellate cells* are found throughout the AVCN, as well as in the lower layers of the DCN. The AVCN is tonotopically organized, and neurons having similar CFs have been observed to lie in layers or laminae [Bourk et al., 1981]. *Isofrequency laminae* also have been indicated in other auditory nuclei.

The predominant neuron in the PVCN is the *octopus cell,* a label arising from its distinctive shape with asymmetrically placed dendrites. Octopus cells receive cochlear input from type I SGCs on their somas and proximal dendrites. Their dendrites cross the incoming array of cochlear fibers, and these often branch to follow the dendrite toward the soma.

The DCN is structurally the most intricate of the CN. In many species, four or five layers are noticeable, giving it a "cortical" structure, and its local circuitry has been compared with that of the cerebellum. *Fusiform cells* are the most common morphologic type. Their somas lie in the deeper layers of the DCN, and their dendrites extend toward the surface of the nucleus and receive primarily noncochlear inputs. Cochlear fibers pass deeply in the DCN and turn toward the surface to innervate fusiform and *giant cells* that lie in the deepest layer of the DCN. The axons of fusiform and giant cells project out of the DCN to the contralateral IC.

Intracellular recording in slice preparation is beginning to identify the membrane characteristics of neuronal types in the CN. The diversity of neuronal morphologic types, their participation in local

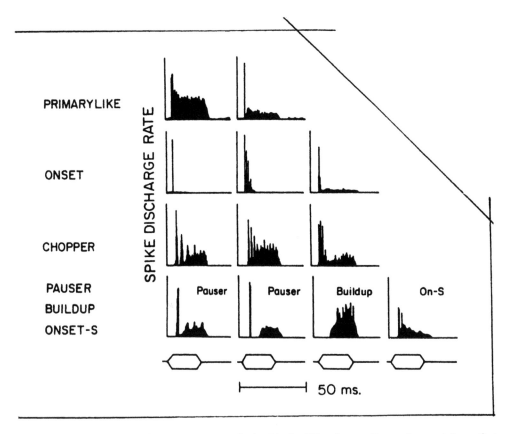

FIGURE 5.5 Peristimulus time histogram patterns obtained in the CN and nerve. Repeated presentations of a tone burst at CF are used to obtain these estimates of discharge rate during the stimulus. (Adapted from Young, 1984.)

circuits, and the emerging knowledge of their membrane biophysics are motivating detailed compartmental modeling [Arle and Kim, 1991].

Spike Discharge Patterns. Auditory nerve fibers and neurons in central nuclei may discharge only a few times during a brief tone burst, but if a histogram of spike events is synchronized to the onset of the tone burst, a *peristimulus time histogram* (PSTH) is obtained that is more representative of the neuron's response than any single one. The PSTH may be expressed in terms of spike counts, spike probability, or spike rate as a function of time, but all these retain the underlying temporal pattern of the response. PSTHs taken at the CF for a tone burst intensity roughly 40 dB above threshold have shapes that are distinctive to different nuclear subdivisions and even different morphologic types. They have been used for functionally classifying auditory neurons.

Figure 5.5 illustrates some of the major pattern types obtained from the auditory nerve and CN. Auditory nerve fibers and spherical bushy cells in AVCN have *primary-like* patterns in their PSTHs, an elevated spike rate after tone onset, falling to a slowly adapting level until the tone burst ends. Globular bushy cells may have primary-like, *pri-notch* (primary-like with a brief notch after onset), or chopper patterns. Stellate cells have non-primary-like patterns. *Onset* response patterns, one or a few brief peaks of discharge at onset with little or no discharges afterward, are observed in the PVCN from octopus cells. *Chopper, pauser,* and *buildup* patterns are observed in many cells of the DCN. For most neurons of the CN, these patterns are not necessarily stable over different stimulus intensities; a primary-like pattern may change to a pauser pattern and then to a chopper pattern as intensity is raised [Young, 1984].

Functional classification also has been based on the *response map,* a plot of a neuron's spike discharge rate as a function of tonal frequency and intensity. Fibers and neurons with primary-like PSTHs generally have response maps with only an *excitatory region* of elevated rate. The lower edges of this region approximate the threshold tuning curve. Octopus cells often have very broad tuning curves and extended response maps, as suggested by their frequency-spanning dendritic trees. More complex response maps are observed for some neurons, such as those in the DCN. Inhibitory regions alone, a frequency-intensity area of suppressed spontaneous discharge rates, or combinations of excitatory regions and inhibitory regions have been observed. Some neurons are excited only within islands of frequency-intensity combinations, demonstrating a CF but having no response to high-intensity sounds. In these cases, an RLF at CF would be *nonmonotonic;* i.e., spike rate decreases as the level is raised. Response maps in the DCN containing both excitatory and inhibitory regions have been shown to arise from a convergence of inputs from neurons with only excitatory or inhibitory regions in their maps [Young and Voigt, 1981].

Superior Olivary Complex (SOC)

The SOC contains 10 or more subdivisions in some species. It is the first site at which connections from the two ears converge and is therefore a center for binaural processing that underlies sound localization. There are large differences in the subdivisions between mammalian groups such as bats, primates, cetaceans, and burrowing rodents that utilize vastly different binaural cues. Binaural cues to the locus of sounds include *interaural level differences* (ILDs), *interaural time differences* (ITDs), and detailed spectral differences for multispectral sounds due to head and pinna filtering characteristics.

Neurons in the *medial superior olive* (MSO) and *lateral superior olive* (LSO) tend to process ITDs and ILDs, respectively. A neuron in the MSO receives projections from spherical bushy cells of the CN from both sides and thereby the precise timing and tuning cues of nerve fibers passed through the large synapses mentioned. The time accuracy of the pathways and the comparison precision of MSO neurons permit the discrimination of changes in ITD of a few tens of microseconds. MSO neurons project to the ipsilateral IC through the lateral lemniscus. Globular bushy cells of the CN project to the medial nucleus of the trapezoid body (MNTB) on the contralateral side, where they synapse on one and only one neuron in a large, excitatory synapse, the calyx of Held. MNTB neurons send inhibitory projections to neurons of the LSO on the same side, which also receives excitatory input from spherical bushy cells from the AVCN on the same side. Sounds reaching the ipsilateral side will excite discharges from an LSO neuron, while those reaching the contralateral side will inhibit its discharge. The relative balance of excitation and inhibition is a function of ILD over part of its physiological range, leading to this cue being encoded in discharge rate.

One of the subdivisions of the SOC, the *dorsomedial periolivary nucleus* (DMPO), is a source of efferent fibers that reach the contralateral cochlea in the *crossed olivocochlear bundle* (COCB). Neurons of the DMPO receive inputs from collaterals of globular bushy cell axons of the contralateral ACVN that project to the MNTB and from octopus cells on both sides. The functional role of the feedback from the DMPO to the cochlea is not well understood.

Nuclei of the Lateral Lemniscus (NLL)

The lateral lemniscus consists of ascending axons from the CN and LSO. The NLL lie within this tract, and some, such as the dorsal nucleus (DNLL), are known to process binaural information, but less is known about these nuclei as a group than others, partially due to their relative inaccessibility.

Inferior Colliculi (IC)

The IC are paired structures lying on the dorsal surface of the rostral brainstem. Each colliculus has a large *central nucleus* (ICC), a surface cortex, and paracentral nuclei. Each colliculus receives afferents from a number of lower brainstem nuclei, projects to the MGB through the *brachium,* and communicates with the other colliculus through a *commissure.* The ICC is the major division and has distinctive laminae in much of its volume. The laminae are formed from *disk-shaped cells* and afferent fibers. The disk-shaped cells, which make up about 80% of the ICC neuronal population, have flattened dendritic fields that lie in the laminar plane. The terminal endings of afferents form fibrous layers between laminae. The remaining neurons in the ICC are *stellate cells* that have dendritic trees spanning laminae. Axons from these two cell types make up much of the ascending ICC output.

Tonotropic organization is preserved in the ICC laminae, each corresponding to an *isofrequency lamina.* Both monaural and binaural information converges at the IC through direct projections from the CN and from the SOC and NLL. Crossed CN inputs and those from the ipsilateral MSO are excitatory. Inhibitory synapses in the ICC arise from the DNLL, mediated by gamma-aminobutyric acid (GABA), and from the ipsilateral LSO, mediated by glycine.

These connections provide an extensive base for identifying sound direction at this midbrain level, but due to their convergence, it is difficult to determine what binaural processing occurs at the IC as opposed to being passed from the SOC and NLL. Many neurons in the IC respond differently depending on binaural parameters. Varying ILDs for clicks or high-frequency tones often indicates that contralateral sound is excitatory. Ipsilateral sound may have no effect on responses to contralateral sound, classifying the cell as E0, or it may inhibit responses, in which case the neuron is classified as EI, or maximal excitation may occur for sound at both ears, classifying the neuron as EE. Neurons responding to lower frequencies are influenced by ITDs, specifically the phase difference between sinusoids at the ears. Spatial receptive fields for sounds are not well documented in the mammalian IC, but barn owls, who use the sounds of prey for hunting at night, have sound-based spatial maps in the homologous structure. The superior colliculus, situated just rostral to the IC, has spatial auditory receptive field maps for mammals and owl.

Auditory Thalamocortical System

Medial Geniculate Body (MGB).   The MGB and AC form the auditory thalamocortical system. As with other sensory systems, extensive projections to and from the cortical region exist in this system. The MGB has three divisions, the *ventral, dorsal,* and *medial.* The ventral division is the largest and has the most precise tonotopic organization. Almost all its input is from the ipsilateral ICC through the brachium of the IC. Its large *bushy cells* have dendrites oriented so as to lie in isofrequency layers, and the axons of these neurons project to the AC, terminating in layers III and IV.

Auditory Cortex.   The auditory cortex (AC) consists of areas of the cerebral cortex that respond to sounds. In mammals, the AC is bilateral and has a primary area with surrounding secondary areas. In nonprimates, the AC is on the lateral surface of the cortex, but in most primates, it lies within the lateral fissure on the superior surface of the temporal lobe. Figure 5.6 reveals the area of the temporal lobe involved with auditory function in humans. Tonotopic mapping is usually evident in these areas as isofrequency surface lines. The primary AC responds most strongly and quickly to sounds. In echo-locating bats, the cortex has a large tonotopic area devoted to the frequency region of its emitted cries and cues related to its frequency modulation and returned Doppler shift [Aitkin, 1990].

The cytoarchitecture of the primary AC shows layers I (surface) through VI (next to white matter), with the largest neurons in layers V and VI. Columns with widths of 50 to 75 μm are evident from dendritic organization in layers III and IV, with fibers lying between the columns. A description of cell types is beyond this treatment.

Discharge patterns in the AC for sound stimuli are mainly of the onset type. Continuous stimuli often evoke later spikes, after the onset discharge, in unanesthetized animals. About half the neurons in the primary AC have monotonic RLFs, but the proportion of nonmonotonic RLFs in secondary areas is much higher. A number of studies have used complex sounds to study cortical responses. Neural responses to species-specific cries, speech, and other important sounds have proved to be labile and to a great extent dependent on the arousal level and behavioral set of the animal.

Cortical lesions in humans rarely produce deafness, although deficits in speech comprehension and generation may exist. Audiometric tests will generally indicate that sensitivity to tonal stimuli is retained. It has been known for some time that left-hemisphere lesions in the temporal region can disrupt comprehension (Wernicke's area) and in the region anterior to the precentral gyrus (Broca's area) can interfere with speech production. It is difficult to separate the effects of these areas because speech comprehension provides vital feedback for producing correct speech.

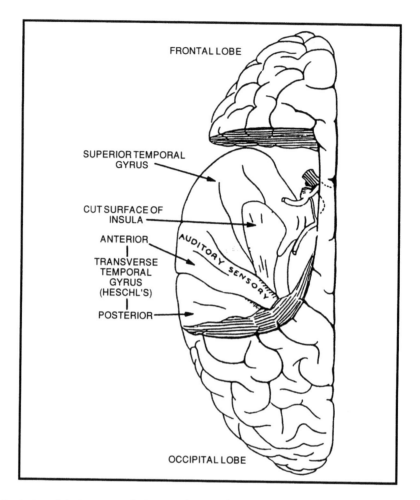

FIGURE 5.6 A view of the human cerebral cortex showing the auditory cortex on the superior surface of the left temporal lobe after removal of the overlying parietal cortex.

5.4 Pathologies

Hearing loss results from conductive and neural deficits. Conductive hearing loss due to attenuation in the outer or middle ear often can be alleviated by amplification provided by hearing aids and may be subject to surgical correction. Sensorineural loss due to the absence of IHCs results from genetic deficits, biochemical insult, exposure to intense sound, or aging (*presbycusis*). For some cases of sensorineural loss, partial hearing function can be restored with the cochlear prosthesis, electrical stimulation of remaining SGCs using small arrays of electrodes inserted into the scala tympani [Miller and Spelman, 1990]. In a few patients having no auditory nerve, direct electrical stimulation of the CN has been used experimentally to provide auditory sensation. Lesions of the nerve and central structures occur due to trauma, tumor growth, and vascular accidents. These may be subject to surgical intervention to prevent further damage and promote functional recovery.

5.5 Models of Auditory Function

Hearing mechanisms have been modeled for many years at a phenomenologic level using psychophysical data. As physiologic and anatomic observations have provided detailed parameters for peripheral and central processing, models of auditory encoding and processing have become more quantitative and physically based. Compartmental models of single neurons, especially SGCs and neurons in the CN, having accurate morphometric geometries, electrical properties, membrane biophysics, and local circuitry are seeing increasing use.

References

Aitkin L. 1990. The Auditory Cortex: Structural and Functional Bases of Auditory Perception. London, Chapman & Hall.

Altschuler RA, Bobbin RP, Clopton BM, Hoffman DW (Eds). 1991. Neurobiology of Hearing: The Central Auditory System. New York, Raven Press.

Arle JE, Kim DO. 1991. Neural modeling of intrinsic and spike-discharge properties of cochlear nucleus neurons. Biol Cybern 64:273.

Bekesy G. von. 1960. Experiments in Hearing. New York, McGraw-Hill.

Bourk TR, Mielcarz JP, Norris BE. 1981. Tonotopic organization of the anteroventral cochlear nucleus of the cat. Hear Res 4:215.

Cooke M. 1993. Modelling Auditory Processing and Organisation. Cambridge, England, Cambridge University Press.

Cooper NP, Rhode WS. 1992. Basilar membrane mechanics in the hook region of cat and guinea-pig cochleae: Sharp tuning and nonlinearity in the absence of baseline position shifts. Hear Res 63:163.

Crawford AC, Fettiplace R. 1985. The mechanical properties of ciliary bundles of turtle cochlear hair cells. J Physiol 364:359.

Dobie RA, Rubel EW. 1989. The auditory system: Acoustics, psychoacoustics, and the periphery. In HD Patton et al. (Eds), Textbook of Physiology, vol 1: Excitable Cells and Neurophysiology, 21st ed. Philadelphia, Saunders.

Fay RR. 1988. Hearing in Vertebrates: A Psychophysics Databook. Winnetka, Hill-Fay Associates.

Geisler CD. 1992. Two-tone suppression by a saturating feedback model of the cochlear partition. Hear Res 63:203.

Hudspeth AJ. 1987. Mechanoelectrical transduction by hair cells in the acousticolateralis sensory system. Annu Rev Neurosci 6:187.

Hudspeth AJ, Corey DP. 1977. Sensitivity, polarity, and conductance change in the response of vertebrate hair cells to controlled mechanical stimuli. Proc Natl Acad Sci USA 74:2407.

Khanna SM, Keilson SE, Ulfendahl M, Teich MC. 1993. Spontaneous cellular vibrations in the guinea-pig temporal-bone preparation. Br J Audiol 27:79.

Kim DO. 1984. Functional roles of the inner- and outer-hair-cell subsystems in the cochlea and brainstem. In CI Berlin (Ed), Hearing Science: Recent Advances. San Diego, College-Hill Press.

Kinsler LE, Frey AR. 1962. Fundamentals of Acoustics. New York, Wiley.

LePage EL. 1991. Helmholtz revisited: Direct mechanical data suggest a physical model for dynamic control of mapping frequency to place along the cochlear partition. In Lecture Notes in Biomechanics. New York, Springer-Verlag.

Lyon RF, Mead C. 1989. Electronic cochlea. In C Mead (Ed), Analog VLSI and Neural Systems. Reading, MA, Addison-Wesley.

Miller JM, Spelman FA (Eds). 1990. Cochlear Implants: Models of the Electrically Stimulated Ear. New York, Springer-Verlag.

Nadol JB Jr. 1988. Comparative anatomy of the cochlea and auditory nerve in mammals. Hear Res 34:253.

Sachs MB, Young ED. 1979. Encoding of steady-state vowels in the auditory nerve: Representation in terms of discharge rate. J Acoust Soc Am 66:470.

Young ED, Voigt HF. 1981. The internal organization of the dorsal cochlear nucleus. In J Syka and L Aitkin (Eds), Neuronal Mechanisms in Hearing, pp 127–133. New York, Plenum Press.

Young ED. 1984. Response characteristics of neurons of the cochlear nuclei. In CI Berlin (Ed), Hearing Science: Recent Advances. San Diego, College-Hill Press.

6

Gastrointestinal System

Berj L. Bardakjian
University of Toronto

6.1   Introduction

The primary function of the gastrointestinal system (Fig. 6.1) is to supply the body with nutrients and water. The ingested food is moved along the alimentary canal at an appropriate rate for digestion, absorption, storage, and expulsion. To fulfill the various requirements of the system, each organ has adapted one or more functions. The esophagus acts as a conduit for the passage of food into the stomach for trituration and mixing. The ingested food is then emptied into the small intestine, which plays a major role in the digestion and absorption processes. The chyme is mixed thoroughly with secretions and it is propelled distally (1) to allow further gastric emptying, (2) to allow for uniform exposure to the absorptive mucosal surface of the small intestine, and (3) to empty into the colon. The vigor of mixing and the rate of propulsion depend on the required contact time of chyme with enzymes and the mucosal surface for efficient performance of digestion and absorption. The colon absorbs water and electrolytes from the chyme, concentrating and collecting waste products that are expelled from the system at appropriate times. All of these motor functions are performed by contractions of the muscle layers in the gastrointestinal wall.

6.2   Gastrointestinal Electrical Oscillations

Gastrointestinal motility is governed by myogenic, neural, and chemical control systems (Fig. 6.2). The myogenic control system is manifest by periodic depolarizations of the smooth muscle cells, which constitute autonomous electrical oscillations called the electrical control activity (ECA) or slow waves [Daniel and Chapman, 1963]. The properties of this myogenic system and its electrical oscillations dictate to a large extent the contraction patterns in the stomach, small intestine, and colon [Szurszewski, 1987].

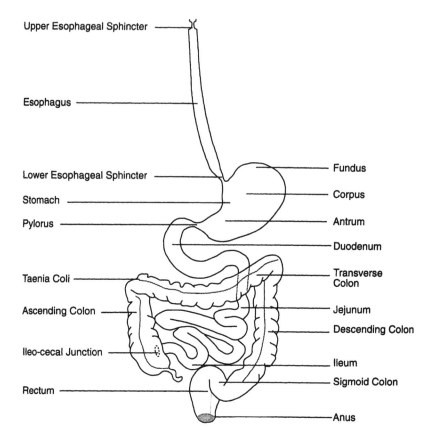

FIGURE 6.1   The gastrointestinal tract.

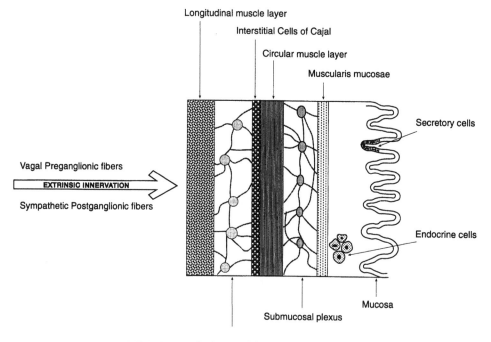

FIGURE 6.2   The layers of the gastrointestinal wall.

The ECA controls the contractile excitability of smooth muscle cells since the cells may contract only when depolarization of the membrane voltage exceeds an excitation threshold. The normal spontaneous amplitude of ECA depolarization does not exceed this excitation threshold except when neural or chemical excitation is present. The myogenic system affects the frequency, direction, and velocity of the contractions. It also affects the coordination or lack of coordination between adjacent segments of the gut wall. Hence, the electrical activities in the gut wall provide an electrical basis for gastrointestinal motility.

In the distal stomach, small intestine, and colon, there are intermittent bursts of rapid electrical oscillations, called the electrical response activity (ERA) or spike bursts. The ERA occurs during the depolarization plateaus of the ECA if a cholinergic stimulus is present, and it is associated with muscular contractions (Fig. 6.3). Thus, neural and chemical control systems determine whether contractions will occur or not, but when contractions are occurring, the myogenic control system (Fig. 6.4) determines the spatial and temporal patterns of contractions.

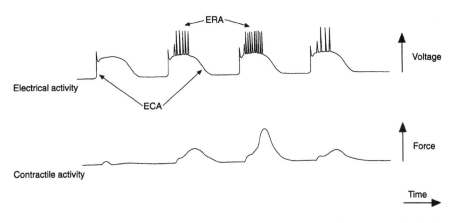

FIGURE 6.3 The relationships between ECA, ERA and muscular contractions. The ERA occurs in the depolarized phase of the ECA. Muscular contractions are associated with the ERA, and their amplitude depends on the frequency of response potentials within an ERA burst.

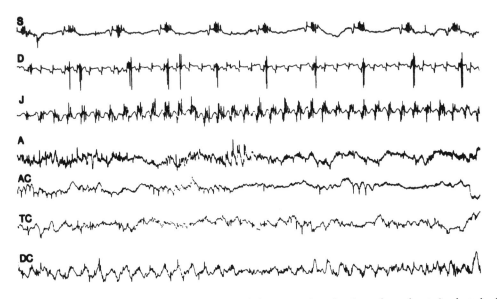

FIGURE 6.4 The gastrointestinal ECA and ERA, recorded in a conscious dog from electrode sets implanted subserosally on stomach (S), duodenum (D), jejunum (J), proximal ascending colon (A), distal ascending colon (AC), transverse colon (TC), and descending colon (DC), respectively. Each trace is of 2 min duration.

There is also a cyclical pattern of of distally propagating ERA that appears in the small intestine during the fasted state [Szurszewski, 1969], called the migrating motility complex (MMC). This pattern consists of four phases [Code and Marlett, 1975]: Phase I has little or no ERA, phase II consists of irregular ERA bursts, phase III consists of intense repetitive ERA bursts where there is an ERA burst on each ECA cycle, and phase IV consists of irregular ERA bursts but is usually much shorter than phase II and may not be always present. The initiation and propagation of the MMC is controlled by enteric cholinergic neurons in the intestinal wall (Fig. 6.2). The propagation of the MMC may be modulated by inputs from extrinsic nerves or circulating hormones [Sarna et al., 1981]. The MMC keeps the small intestine clean of residual food, debris, and desquamated cells.

6.3   A Historical Perspective

Minute Rhythms

Alvarez and Mahoney [1922] reported the presence of a rhythmic electrical activity (which they called "action currents") in the smooth muscle layers of the stomach, small intestine, and colon. Their data were acquired from cat (stomach, small intestine), dog (stomach, small intestine, colon), and rabbit (small intestine, colon). They also demonstrated the existence of frequency gradients in excised stomach and bowel. Puestow [1933] confirmed the presence of a rhythmic electrical activity (which he called "waves of altered electrical potential") and a frequency gradient in isolated canine small intestinal segments. He also demonstrated the presence of an electrical spiking activity (associated with muscular contractions) superimposed on the rhythmic electrical activity. He implied that the rhythmic electrical activity persisted at all times, whereas the electrical spike activity was of an intermittent nature. Bozler [1938, 1939, 1941] confirmed the occurrence of an electrical spiking activity associated with muscular contractions both *in vitro* in isolated longitudinal muscle strips from guinea pig (colon, small intestine) and rabbit (small intestine), and *in situ* in exposed loops of small intestine of anesthetized cat, dog, and rabbit as well as in cat stomach. He also suggested that the strength of a spontaneous muscular contraction is proportional to the frequency and duration of the spikes associated with it.

The presence of two types of electrical activity in the smooth muscle layers of the gastrointestinal tract in several species has been established [Milton and Smith, 1956; Bulbring et al., 1958; Burnstock et al., 1963; Daniel and Chapman, 1963; Bass, 1965; Gillespie, 1962; Duthie, 1974; Christensen, 1975; Daniel, 1975; Sarna, 1975a]. The autonomous electrical rhythmic activity is an omnipresent myogenic activity [Burnstock et al., 1963] whose function is to control the appearance *in time and space* of the electrical spiking activity (an intermittent activity associated with muscular contractions) when neural and chemical factors are appropriate [Daniel and Chapman, 1963]. Neural and chemical factors determine whether or not contractions will occur, but when contractions are occurring, the myogenic control system determines the *spatial and temporal* patterns of contractions.

Isolation of a distal segment of canine small intestine from a proximal segment (using surgical transection or clamping) has been reported to produce a decrease in the frequency of both the rhythmic muscular contractions [Douglas, 1949; Milton and Smith, 1956] and the electrical rhythmic activity [Milton and Smith, 1956] of the distal segment, suggesting frequency entrainment or pulling of the distal segment by the proximal one. It was demonstrated [Milton and Smith, 1956] that the repetition of the electrical spiking activity changed in the same manner as that of the electrical rhythmic activity, thus confirming a one-to-one temporal relationship between the frequency of the electrical rhythmic activity, the repetition rate of the electrical spiking activity, and the frequency of the muscular contractions (when all are present at any one site). Nelson and Becker [1968] suggested that the electrical rhythmic activity of the small intestine behaves like a system of coupled relaxation oscillators. They used two forward coupled relaxation oscillators, having different intrinsic frequencies, to demonstrate frequency entrainment of the two coupled oscillators. Uncoupling of the two oscillators caused a decrease in the frequency of the distal oscillator simulating the effect of transection of the canine small intestine.

The electrical rhythmic activity in canine stomach [Sarna et al., 1972], canine small intestine [Nelson and Becker, 1968; Diamant et al., 1970; Sarna et al., 1971], human small intestine [Robertson-Dunn and Linkens, 1974], human colon [Bardakjian and Sarna, 1980], and human rectosigmoid [Linkens et al., 1976] has been modeled by populations of coupled nonlinear oscillators. The interaction between coupled nonlinear oscillators is governed by both intrinsic oscillator properties and coupling mechanisms.

Hour Rhythms

The existence of periodic gastric activity in the fasted state in both dog [Morat, 1882] and man [Morat, 1893] has been reported. The occurrence of a periodic pattern of motor activity, comprising bursts of contractions alternating with "intervals of repose," in the gastrointestinal tracts of fasted animals was noted early in the 20th century by Boldireff [1905]. He observed that (1) the bursts recurred with a periodicity of about 1.5 to 2.5 h, (2) the amplitude of the gastric contractions during the bursts were larger than those seen postprandially, (3) the small bowel was also involved, and (4) with longer fasting periods, the bursts occurred less frequently and had a shorter duration. Periodic bursts of activity were also observed in (1) the lower esphageal sphincter [Cannon and Washburn, 1912] and (2) the pylorus [Wheelon and Thomas, 1921]. Further investigation of the fasting contractile activity in the upper small intestine was undertaken in the early 1920s with particular emphasis on the coordination between the stomach and duodenum [Wheelon and Thomas, 1922; Alvarez and Mahoney, 1923]. More recently, evidence was obtained [Itoh et al., 1978] that the cyclical activity in the lower esophageal sphincter noted by Cannon and Washburn [1912] was also coordinated with that of the stomach and small intestine.

With the use of implanted strain gauges, it was possible to observe contractile activity over long periods of time and it was demonstrated that the cyclical fasting pattern in the duodenum was altered by feeding [Jacoby et al., 1963]. The types of contractions observed during fasting and feeding were divided into four groups [Reinke et al., 1967; Carlson et al., 1972]. Three types of contractile patterns were observed in fasted animals: (1) quiescent interval, (2) a shorter interval of increasing activity, and (3) an interval of maximal activity. The fourth type was in fed animals and it consisted of randomly occurring contractions of varying amplitudes. With the use of implanted electrodes in the small intestine of fasted dogs, Szurszewski [1969] demonstrated that the cyclical appearance of electrical spiking activity at each electrode site was due to the migration of the cyclical pattern of quiescence, increasing activity and maximal electrical activity down the small intestine from the duodenum to the terminal ileum. He called this electrical pattern the *migrating myoelectric complex* (MMC). Grivel and Ruckebusch [1972] demonstrated that the mechanical correlate of this electrical pattern, which they called the *migrating motor complex*, occurs in other species such as sheep and rabbits. They also observed that the velocity of propagation of the maximal contractile activity was proportional to the length of the small intestine. Code and Marlett [1975] observed the electrical correlate of the cyclical activity in dog stomach that was reported by Morat [1882, 1893], and they demonstrated that the stomach MMC was coordinated with the duodenal MMC.

The MMC pattern has been demonstrated in other mammalian species [Ruckebusch and Fioramonti, 1975; Ruckebusch and Bueno, 1976], including humans. Bursts of distally propagating contractions has been noted in the gastrointestinal tract of man [Beck et al., 1965], and their cyclical nature was reported by Stanciu and Bennet [1975]. The MMC has been described in both normal volunteers [Vantrappen et al., 1977; Fleckenstein, 1978; Thompson et al., 1980; Kerlin and Phillips, 1982; Rees et al., 1982] and in patients [Vantrappen et al., 1977; Thompson et al., 1982; Summers et al., 1982].

Terminology

A nomenclature to describe the gastrointestinal electrical activities has been proposed to describe the minute rhythm [Sarna, 1975b] and the hour rhythm [Carlson et al., 1972; Code and Marlett, 1975].

Control cycle is one depolarization and repolarization of the transmembrane voltage. *Control wave (or slow wave)* is the continuing rhythmic electrical activity recorded at any one site. It was assumed to be generated by the smooth muscle cells behaving like a relaxation oscillator at that site. However, recent evidence [Hara et al., 1986; Suzuki et al., 1986; Barajas-Lopez et al., 1989; Serio et al., 1991] indicates that it is generated by a system of interstitial cells of Cajal (ICC) and smooth muscle cells at that site. *Electrical Control Activity* (ECA) is the totality of the control waves recorded at one or several sites. *Response Potentials* (or *spikes*) are the rapid oscillations of transmembrane voltage in the depolarized state of smooth muscle cells. They are associated with muscular contraction and their occurrence is assumed to be in response to a control cycle when acetylcholine is present. *Electrical Response Activity* (ERA) is the totality of the groups of response potentials at one or several sites.

Migrating Motility Complex (MMC) is the entire cycle which is composed of four phases. Initially, the electrical and mechanical patterns were referred to as the migrating myoelectric complex and the migrating motor complex, respectively. *Phase I* is the interval during which fewer than 5% of ECA have associated ERA, and no or very few contractions are present. *Phase II* is the interval when 5 to 95% of the ECA has associated ERA, and intermittent contractions are present. *Phase III* is the interval when more than 95% of ECA have associated ERA, and large cyclical contractions are present. *Phase IV* is a short and waning interval of intermittent ERA and contractions. Phases II and IV are not always present and are difficult to characterize, whereas phases I and III are always present. *MMC Cycle Time* is the interval from the end of one phase III to the end of a subsequent phase III at any one site. *Migration Time* is the time taken for the MMC to migrate from the upper duodenum to the terminal ileum.

6.4   The Stomach

Anatomical Features

The stomach is somewhat pyriform in shape with its large end directed upward at the lower esophageal sphincter and its small end bent to the right at the pylorus. It has two curvatures, the greater curvature which is four to five times as long as the lesser curvature, and it consists of three regions: the fundus, corpus (or body), and antrum. It has three smooth muscle layers. The outermost layer is the longitudinal muscle layer, the middle is the circular muscle layer, and the innermost is the oblique muscle layer. These layers thicken gradually in the distal stomach toward the pylorus, which is consistent with stomach function since trituration occurs in the distal antrum. The size of the stomach varies considerably among subjects. In an adult male, its greatest length when distended is about 25 to 30 cm and its widest diameter is about 10 to 12 cm [Pick and Howden, 1977].

The structural relationships of nerve, muscle, and interstitial cells of Cajal in the canine corpus indicated a high density of gap junctions indicating very tight coupling between cells. Nerves in the corpus are not located close to circular muscle cells but are found exterior to the muscle bundles, whereas ICCs have gap junction contact with smooth muscle cells and are closely innervated [Daniel and Sakai, 1984].

Gastric ECA

In the canine stomach, the fundus does not usually exhibit spontaneous electrical oscillations, but the corpus and antrum do exhibit such oscillations. In the intact stomach, the ECA is entrained to a frequency of about 5 cpm (about 3 cpm in humans) throughout the electrically active region with phase lags in both the longitudinal and circumferential directions [Sarna et al., 1972]. The phase lags decrease distally from corpus to antrum.

There is a marked intrinsic frequency gradient along the axis of the stomach and a slight intrinsic frequency gradient along the circumference. The intrinsic frequency of gastric ECA in isolated circular muscle of the orad and mid corpus is the highest (about 5 cpm) compared to about 3.5 cpm in the rest of the corpus, and about 0.5 cpm in the antrum. Also, there is an orad to aborad intrinsic gradient in resting membrane potential, with the terminal antrum having the most negative resting membrane potential, about 30 mV more negative than the fundal regions [Szurszewski, 1987]. The relatively depolarized state of the fundal muscle may explain its electrical inactivity since the voltage-sensitive ionic channels may be kept in a state of inactivation. Hyperpolarization of the fundus to a transmembrane voltage of −60 mV produces fundal control waves similar to those recorded from mid and orad corpus.

The ECA in canine stomach was modeled [Sarna et al., 1972] using an array of 13 bidirectionally coupled relaxation oscillators. The model featured (1) an intrinsic frequency decline from corpus to the pylorus and from greater curvature to the lesser curvature, (2) entrainment of all coupled oscillators at a frequency close to the highest intrinsic frequency, and (3) distally decreasing phase lags between the entrained oscillators. A simulated circumferential transection caused the formation of another frequency plateau aboral to the transection. The frequency of the orad plateau remained unaffected while that of the aborad plateau was decreased. This is consistent with the observed experimental data.

The Electrogastrogram

In a similar manner to other electrophysiological measures such as the electrocardiogram (EKG) and the electroencephalogram (EEG), the electrogastrogram (EGG) was identified [Stern and Koch, 1985; Chen and McCallum, 1994]. The EGG is the signal obtained from cutaneous recording of the gastric myoelectrical activity by using surface electrodes placed on the abdomen over the stomach. Although the first EGG was recorded in the early 1920s [Alvarez, 1922], progress *vis-à-vis* clinical applications has been relatively slow, in particular when compared to the progress made in EKG, which also started in the early 1920s. Despite many attempts made over the decades, visual inspection of the EGG signal has not led to the identification of waveform characteristics that would help the clinician to diagnose functional or organic diseases of the stomach. Even the development of techniques such as time-frequency analysis [Qiao et al., 1998] and artificial neural network-based feature extraction [Liang et al., 1997; Wang et al., 1999] for computer analysis of the EGG did not provide *clinically relevant* information about gastric motility disorders. It has been demonstrated that increased EGG frequencies (1) were seen in perfectly healthy subjects [Pffafenbach et al., 1995], and (2) did not always correspond to serosally recorded tachygastria in dogs [Mintchev and Bowes, 1997]. As yet, there is no effective method of detecting a change in the direction or velocity of propagation of gastric ECA from the EGG.

6.5 The Small Intestine

Anatomical Features

The small intestine is a long hollow organ which consists of the duodenum, jejunum, and ileum. Its length is about 650 cm in humans and 300 cm in dogs. The duodenum extends from the pylorus to the ligament of Treitz (about 30 cm in humans and dogs). In humans, the duodenum forms a C-shaped pattern, with the ligament of Treitz near the corpus of the stomach. In dogs, the duodenum lies along the right side of the peritoneal cavity, with the ligament of Treitz in the pelvis. The duodenum receives pancreatic exocrine secretions and bile. In both humans and dogs, the jejunum consists of the next one-third whereas the ileum consists of the remaining two-thirds of the intestine. The major differences between the jejunum and ileum are functional in nature, relating to their absorption characteristics and motor control. The majority of sugars, amino acids, lipids, electrolytes, and water are absorbed in the jejunum and proximal ileum, whereas bile acids and vitamin B12 are absorbed in the terminal ileum.

Small Intestinal ECA

In the canine small intestine, the ECA is not entrained throughout the entire length [Diamant and Bortoff, 1969a; Sarna et al., 1971]. However, the ECA exhibits a plateau of constant frequency in the proximal region whereby there is a distal increase in phase lag. The frequency plateau (of about 20 cpm) extends over the entire duodenum and part of the jejunum. There is a marked intrinsic frequency gradient in the longitudinal direction with the highest intrinsic frequency being less than the plateau frequency. When the small intestine was transected *in vivo* into small segments (15 cm long), the intrinsic frequency of the ECA in adjacent segments tended to decrease aborally in an exponential manner [Sarna et al.,

1971]. A single transection of the duodenum caused the formation of another frequency plateau aboral to the transection. The ECA frequency in the orad plateau was generally unaffected, while that in the aborad plateau was decreased [Diamant and Bortoff, 1969b; Sarna et al., 1971]. The frequency of the aborad plateau was either higher than or equal to the highest intrinsic frequency distal to the transection, depending on whether the transection of the duodenum was either above or below the region of the bile duct [Diamant and Bortoff, 1969b].

The ECA in canine small intestine was modeled using a chain of 16 bidirectionally coupled relaxation oscillators [Sarna et al., 1971]. Coupling was not uniform along the chain, since the proximal oscillators were strongly coupled and the distal oscillators were weakly coupled. The model featured (1) an exponential intrinsic frequency decline along the chain, (2) a frequency plateau which is higher than the highest intrinsic frequency, and (3) a temporal variation of the frequencies distal to the frequency plateau region. A simulated transection in the frequency plateau region caused the formation of another frequency plateau aboral to the transection, such that the frequency of the orad plateau was unchanged whereas the frequency of the aborad plateau decreased.

The ECA in human small intestine was modeled using a chain of 100 bidirectionally coupled relaxation oscillators [Robertson-Dunn and Linkens, 1976]. Coupling was nonuniform and asymmetrical. The model featured (1) a piecewise linear decline in intrinsic frequency along the chain, (2) a piecewise linear decline in coupling similar to that of the intrinsic frequency, (3) forward coupling which is stronger than backward coupling, and (4) a frequency plateau in the proximal region which is higher than the highest intrinsic frequency in the region.

Small Intestinal MMC

The MMCs in canine small intestine have been observed in intrinsically isolated segments [Sarna et al., 1981, 1983], even after the isolated segment has been stripped of all extrinsic innervation [Sarr and Kelly, 1981] or removed in continuity with the remaining gut as a Thiry Vella loop [Itoh et al., 1981]. This intrinsic mechanism is able to function independently of extrinsic innervation since vagotomy [Weisbrodt et al., 1975; Ruckebusch and Bueno, 1977] does not hinder the initiation of the MMC. The initiation of the small intestinal MMC is controlled by integrative networks within the intrinsic plexuses utilizing nicotinic and muscarinic cholinergic receptors [Ormsbee et al., 1979; El-Sharkawy et al., 1982].

When the canine small intestine was transected into four equal strips [Sarna et al., 1981, 1983], it was found that each strip was capable of generating an independent MMC that would appear to propagate from the proximal to the distal part of each segment. This suggested that the MMC can be modeled by a chain of coupled relaxation oscillators. The average intrinsic periods of the MMC for the four segments were reported to be 106.2, 66.8, 83.1, and 94.8 min, respectively. The segment containing the duodenum had the longest period, while the subsequent segment containing the jejunum had the shortest period. However, in the intact small intestine, the MMC starts in the duodenum and not the jejunum. Bardakjian et al. [1981, 1984] have demonstrated that both the intrinsic frequency gradients and resting level gradients have major roles in the entrainment of a chain of coupled oscillators. In modeling the small intestinal MMC with a chain of four coupled oscillators, it was necessary to include a gradient in the intrinsic resting levels of the MMC oscillators (with the proximal oscillator having the lowest resting level) in order to entrain the oscillators and allow the proximal oscillator to behave as the leading oscillator [Bardakjian and Ahmed, 1992].

6.6   The Colon

Anatomical Features

In humans, the colon is about 100 cm in length. The ileum joins the colon approximately 5 cm from its end, forming the cecum which has a worm-like appendage, the appendix. The colon is sacculated, and the longitudinal smooth muscle is concentrated in three bands (the taeniae). It lies in front of the small intestine against the abdominal wall and it consists of the ascending (on the right side), transverse (across the lower stomach), and descending (on the left side) colon. The descending colon becomes the sigmoid colon in the pelvis as it runs down and forward to the rectum. Major functions of the colon are (1) to absorb water, certain electrolytes, short chain fatty acids, and bacterial metabolites; (2) to slowly propel its luminal contents in the caudad direction; (3) to store the residual matter in the distal region; and (4) to rapidly move its contents in the caudad direction during mass movements [Sarna, 1991]. In dogs, the colon is about 45 cm in length and the cecum has no appendage. The colon is not sacculated, and the longitudinal smooth muscle coat is continuous around the circumference [Miller et al., 1968]. It lies posterior to the small intestine and it consists mainly of ascending and descending segments with a small transverse segment. However, functionally it is assumed to consist of three regions, each of about 15 cm in length, representing the ascending, transverse, and descending colon, respectively.

Colonic ECA

In the human colon, the ECA is almost completely phase-unlocked between adjacent sites as close as 1 to 2 cm apart, and its frequency (about 3 to 15 cpm) and amplitude at each site vary with time [Sarna et al., 1980]. This results in short duration contractions that are also disorganized in time and space. The disorganization of ECA and its associated contractions is consistent with the colonic function of extensive mixing, kneading, and slow net distal propulsion [Sarna, 1991]. In the canine colon, the reports about the intrinsic frequency gradient were conflicting [Vanasin et al., 1974; Shearin et al., 1978; El-Sharkawy, 1983].

The human colonic ECA was modeled [Bardakjian and Sarna, 1980] using a tubular structure of 99 bidirectionally coupled nonlinear oscillators arranged in 33 parallel rings where each ring contained three oscillators. Coupling was nonuniform and it increased in the longitudinal direction. The model featured (1) no phase-locking in the longitudinal or circumferential directions, (2) temporal and spatial variation of the frequency profile with large variations in the proximal and distal regions and small variations in the middle region, and (3) waxing and waning of the amplitudes of the ECA which was more pronounced in the proximal and distal regions. The model demonstrated that the "silent periods" occurred because of the interaction between oscillators and they did not occur when the oscillators were uncoupled. The model was further refined [Bardakjian et al., 1990] such that when the ECA amplitude exceeded an excitation threshold, a burst of ERA was exhibited. The ERA bursts occurred in a seemingly random manner in adjacent sites because (1) the ECA was not phase-locked and (2) the ECA amplitudes and waveshapes varied in a seemingly random manner.

6.7 Epilogue

The ECA in stomach, small intestine, and colon behaves like the outputs of a population of coupled nonlinear oscillators. The populations in the stomach and the proximal small intestine are entrained, whereas those in the distal small intestine and colon are not entrained. There are distinct intrinsic frequency gradients in the stomach and small intestine but their profile in the colon is ambiguous.

The applicability of modeling of gastrointestinal ECA by coupled nonlinear oscillators has been reconfirmed [Daniel et al., 1994], and a novel nonlinear oscillator, the mapped clock oscillator, was proposed [Bardakjian and Diamant, 1994] for modeling the cellular ECA. The oscillator consists of two coupled components: a clock which represents the interstitial cells of Cajal, and a transformer which represents the smooth muscle transmembrane ionic transport mechanisms [Skinner and Bardakjian, 1991]. Such a model accounts for the mounting evidence supporting the role of the interstitial cells of Cajal as a pacemaker for the smooth muscle transmembrane voltage oscillations [Hara et al., 1986; Suzuki et al., 1986; Barajas-Lopez et al., 1989; Serio et al., 1991; Sanders, 1996].

Modeling of the gastrointestinal ECA by populations of coupled nonlinear oscillators [Bardakjian, 1987] suggests that gastrointestinal motility disorders associated with abnormal ECA can be effectively treated by (1) electronic pacemakers to coordinate the oscillators, (2) surgical interventions to remove regional ectopic foci, and (3) pharmacotherapy to stimulate the oscillators. Electronic pacing has been demonstrated in canine stomach [Kelly and LaForce, 1972; Sarna and Daniel, 1973; Bellahsene et al., 1992] and small intestine [Sarna and Daniel, 1975c; Becker et al., 1983]. Also, pharmacotherapy with prokinetic drugs such as Domperidone and Cisapride has demonstrated improvements in the coordination of the gastric oscillators.

Acknowledgments

The author would like to thank his colleagues Dr. Sharon Chung and Dr. Karen Hall for providing biological insight.

References

Alvarez, W.C. and Mahoney, L.J. 1922. Action current in stomach and intestine. *Am. J. Physiol.*, 58:476-493.

Alvarez, W.C. 1922. The electrogastrogram and what it shows. *J. Am. Med. Assoc.*, 78:1116-1119.

Alvarez, W.C. and Mahoney, L.J. 1923. The relations between gastric and duodenal peristalsis. *Am. J. Physiol.*, 64:371-386.

Barajas-Lopez, C., Berezin, I., Daniel, E.E., and Huizinga, J.D. 1989. Pacemaker activity recorded in interstitial cells of Cajal of the gastrointestinal tract. *Am. J. Physiol.*, 257:C830-C835.

Bardakjian, B.L. and Sarna, S.K. 1980. A computer model of human colonic electrical control activity (ECA). *IEEE Trans. Biomed. Eng.*, 27:193-202.

Bardakjian, B.L. and Sarna, S.K. 1981. Mathematical investigation of populations of coupled synthesized relaxation oscillators representing biological rhythms. *IEEE Trans. Biomed. Eng.*, 28:10-15.

Bardakjian, B.L., El-Sharkawy, T.Y., and Diamant, N.E. 1984. Interaction of coupled nonlinear oscillators having different intrinsic resting levels. *J. Theor. Biol.*, 106:9-23.

Bardakjian, B.L. 1987. Computer models of gastrointestinal myoelectric activity. *Automedica*, 7:261-276.

Bardakjian, B.L., Sarna, S.K., and Diamant, N.E. 1990. Composite synthesized relaxation oscillators: Application to modeling of colonic ECA and ERA. *Gastrointest. J. Motil.*, 2:109-116.

Bardakjian, B.L. and Ahmed, K. 1992. Is a peripheral pattern generator sufficient to produce both fasting and postprandial patterns of the migrating myoelectric complex (MMC)? *Dig. Dis. Sci.*, 37:986.

Bardakjian, B.L. and Diamant, N.E. 1994. A mapped clock oscillator model for transmembrane electrical rhythmic activity in excitable cells. *J. Theor. Biol.*, 166:225-235.

Bass, P. 1965. Electric activity of smooth muscle of the gastrointestinal tract. *Gastroenterology*, 49:391-394.

Beck, I.T., McKenna, R.D., Peterfy, G., Sidorov, J., and Strawczynski, H. 1965. Pressure studies in the normal human jejunum. *Am. J. Dig. Dis.*, 10:437-448.

Becker, J.M., Sava, P., Kelly, K.A., and Shturman, L. 1983. Intestinal pacing for canine postgastrectomy dumping. *Gastroenterology*, 84:383-387.

Bellahsene, B.E., Lind, C.D., Schirmer, B.D., et al. 1992. Acceleration of gastric emptying with electrical stimulation in a canine model of gastroparesis. *Am. J. Physiol.*, 262:G826-G834.

Boldireff, W.N. 1905. Le travail periodique de l'appareil digestif en dehors de la digestion. *Arch. Des. Sci. Biol.*, 11:1-157.

Bozler, E. 1938. Action potentials of visceral smooth muscle. *Am. J. Physiol.*, 124:502-510.

Bozler, E. 1939. Electrophysiological studies on the motility of the gastrointestinal tract. *Am. J. Physiol.*, 127:301-307.

Bozler, E. 1941. Action potentials and conduction of excitation in muscle. *Biol. Symp.*, 3:95-110.

Bulbring, E., Burnstock G., and Holman, M.E. 1958. Excitation and conduction in the smooth muscle of the isolated taenia coli of the guinea pig. *J. Physiol.*, 142:420-437.

Burnstock, G., Holman, M.E., and Prosser, C.L. 1963. Electrophysiology of smooth muscle. *Physiol. Rev.*, 43:482-527.

Cannon, W.B. and Washburn, A.L. 1912. An explanation of hunger. *Am. J. Physiol.*, 29:441-454.

Carlson, G.M., Bedi, B.S., and Code, C.F. 1972. Mechanism of propagation of intestinal interdigestive myoelectric complex. *Am. J. Physiol.*, 222:1027-1030.

Chen, J.Z. and McCallum, R.W. 1994. *Electrogastrography: Principles and Applications*. Raven Press, New York.

Christensen, J. 1975. Myoelectric control of the colon. *Gastroenterology*, 68:601-609.

Code, C.F. and Marlett, J.A. 1975. The interdigestive myoelectric complex of the stomach and small bowel of dogs. *J. Physiol.*, 246:289-309.

Daniel, E.E. and Chapman, K.M. 1963. Electrical activity of the gastrointestinal tract as an indication of mechanical activity. *Am. J. Dig. Dis.*, 8:54-102.

Daniel, E.E. 1975. Electrophysiology of the colon. *Gut*, 16:298-329.

Daniel, E.E. and Sakai, Y. 1984. Structural basis for function of circular muscle of canine corpus. *Can. J. Physiol. Pharmacol.*, 62:1304-1314.

Daniel, E.E., Bardakjian, B.L., Huizinga, J.D., and Diamant, N.E. 1994. Relaxation oscillators and core conductor models are needed for understanding of GI electrical activities. *Am. J. Physiol.*, 266:G339-G349.

Diamant, N.E. and Bortoff, A. 1969a. Nature of the intestinal slow wave frequency gradient. *Am. J. Physiol.*, 216:301-307.

Diamant, N.E. and Bortoff, A. 1969b. Effects of transection on the intestinal slow wave frequency gradient. *Am. J. Physiol.*, 216:734-743.

Douglas, D.M. 1949. The decrease in frequency of contraction of the jejunum after transplantation to the ileum. *J. Physiol.*, 110:66-75.

Duthie, H.L. 1974. Electrical activity of gastrointestinal smooth muscle. *Gut*, 15:669-681.

El-Sharkawy, T.Y., Markus, H., and Diamant, N.E. 1982. Neural control of the intestinal migrating myoelectric complex: A pharmacological analysis. *Can. J. Physiol. Pharm.*, 60:794-804.

El-Sharkawy, T.Y. 1983. Electrical activity of the muscle layers of the canine colon. *J. Physiol.*, 342:67-83.

Fleckenstein, P. 1978. Migrating electrical spike activity in the fasting human small intestine. *Dig. Dis. Sci.*, 23:769-775.

Gillespie, J.S. 1962. The electrical and mechanical responses of intestinal smooth muscle cells to stimulation of their extrinsic parasympathetic nerves. *J. Physiol.*, 162:76-92.

Grivel, M.L. and Ruckebusch, Y. 1972. The propagation of segmental contractions along the small intestine. *J. Physiol.*, 277:611-625.

Hara, Y.M., Kubota, M., and Szurszewski, J.H. 1986. Electrophysiology of smooth muscle of the small intestine of some mammals. *J. Physiol.*, 372:501-520.

Itoh, Z., Honda, R., Aizawa, I., Takeuchi, S., Hiwatashi, K., and Couch, E.F. 1978. Interdigestive motor activity of the lower esophageal sphincter in the conscious dog. *Dig. Dis. Sci.*, 23:239-247.

Itoh, Z., Aizawa, I., and Takeuchi, S. 1981. Neural regulation of interdigestive motor activity in canine jejunum. *Am. J. Physiol.*, 240:G324-G330.

Jacoby, H.I., Bass, P., and Bennett, D.R. 1963. *In vivo* extraluminal contractile force transducer for gastrointestinal muscle. *J. Appl. Physiol.*, 18:658-665.

Kelly, K.A. and LaForce, R.C. 1972. Pacing the canine stomach with electric stimulation. *Am. J. Physiol.*, 222:588-594.

Kerlin, P. and Phillips, S. 1982. The variability of motility of the ileum and jejunum in healthy humans. *Gastroenterology*, 82:694-700.

Liang, J., Cheung, J.Y., and Chen, J.D.Z. 1997. Detection and deletion of motion artifacts in electrogastrogram using feature analysis and neural networks. *Ann. Biomed. Eng.*, 25:850-857.

Linkens, D.A., Taylor, I., and Duthie, H.L. 1976. Mathematical modeling of the colorectal myoelectrical activity in humans. *IEEE Trans. Biomed. Eng.*, 23:101-110.

Milton, G.W. and Smith, A.W.M. 1956. The pacemaking area of the duodenum. *J. Physiol.*, 132:100-114.

Miller, M.E., Christensen, G.C., and Evans, H.E. 1968. *Anatomy of the Dog*, Saunders, Philadelphia.

Mintchev, M.P. and Bowes, K.L. 1997. Do increased electrogastrographic frequencies always correspond to internal tachygastria? *Ann. Biomed. Eng.*, 25:1052-1058.

Morat, J.P. 1882. Sur l'innervation motrice de l'estomac. *Lyon. Med.,* 40:289-296.

Morat, J.P. 1893. Sur quelques particularites de l'innervation motrice de l'estomac et de l'intestin. *Arch. Physiol. Norm. Path.,* 5:142-153.

Nelson, T.S. and Becker, J.C. 1968. Simulation of the electrical and mechanical gradient of the small intestine. *Am. J. Physiol.,* 214:749-757.

Ormsbee, H.S., Telford, G.L., and Mason, G.R. 1979. Required neural involvement in control of canine migrating motor complex. *Am. J. Physiol.,* 237:E451-E456.

Pffafenbach, B., Adamek, R.J., Kuhn, K., and Wegener, M. 1995. Electrogastrography in healthy subjects. Evaluation of normal values: influence of age and gender. *Dig. Dis. Sci.,* 40:1445-1450.

Pick, T.P. and Howden, R. 1977. *Gray's Anatomy,* Bounty Books, New York.

Puestow, C.B. 1933. Studies on the origins of the automaticity of the intestine: the action of certain drugs on isolated intestinal transplants. *Am. J. Physiol.,* 106:682-688.

Qiao, W., Sun, H.H., Chey, W.Y., and Lee, K.Y. 1998. Continuous wavelet analysis as an aid in the representation and interpretation of electrogastrographic signals. *Ann. Biomed. Eng.,* 26:1072-1081.

Rees, W.D.W., Malagelada, J.R., Miller, L.J., and Go, V.L.W. 1982. Human interdigestive and postprandial gastrointestinal motor and gastrointestinal hormone patterns. *Dig. Dis. Sci.,* 27:321-329.

Reinke, D.A., Rosenbaum, A.H., and Bennett, D.R. 1967. Patterns of dog gastrointestinal contractile activity monitored *in vivo* with extraluminal force transducers. *Am. J. Dig. Dis.,* 12:113-141.

Robertson-Dunn, B. and Linkens, D.A. 1974. A mathematical model of the slow wave electrical activity of the human small intestine. *Med. Biol. Eng.,* 12:750-758.

Ruckebusch, Y. and Fioramonti, S. 1975. Electrical spiking activity and propulsion in small intestine in fed and fasted states. *Gastroenterology,* 68:1500-1508.

Ruckebusch, Y. and Bueno, L. 1976. The effects of feeding on the motility of the stomach and small intestine in the pig. *Br. J. Nutr.,* 35:397-405.

Ruckebusch, Y. and Bueno, L. 1977. Migrating myoelectrical complex of the small intestine. *Gastroenterology,* 73:1309-1314.

Sanders, K.M. 1996. A case for interstitial cells of Cajal as pacemakers and mediators of neurotransmission in the gastrointestinal tract. *Gastroenterology,* 111(2):492-515.

Sarna, S.K., Daniel, E.E., and Kingma, Y.J. 1971. Simulation of slow wave electrical activity of small intestine. *Am. J. Physiol.,* 221:166-175.

Sarna, S.K., Daniel, E.E., and Kingma, Y.J. 1972. Simulation of the electrical control activity of the stomach by an array of relaxation oscillators. *Am. J. Dig. Dis.,* 17:299-310.

Sarna, S.K. and Daniel, E.E. 1973. Electrical stimulation of gastric electrical control activity. *Am. J. Physiol.,* 225:125-131.

Sarna, S.K. 1975a. Models of smooth muscle electrical activity. In *Methods in Pharmacology,* E.E. Daniel and D.M. Paton, Eds., Plenum Press, New York, 519-540.

Sarna, S.K. 1975b. Gastrointestinal electrical activity: terminology. *Gastroenterology,* 68:1631-1635.

Sarna, S.K. and Daniel, E.E. 1975c. Electrical stimulation of small intestinal electrical control activity. *Gastroenterology,* 69:660-667.

Sarna, S.K., Bardakjian, B.L., Waterfall, W.E., and Lind, J.F. 1980. Human colonic electrical control activity (ECA). *Gastroenterology,* 78:1526-1536.

Sarna, S.K., Stoddard, C., Belbeck, L., and McWade, D. 1981. Intrinsic nervous control of migrating myoelectric complexes. *Am. J. Physiol.,* 241:G16-G23.

Sarna, S., Condon, R.E., and Cowles, V. 1983. Enteric mechanisms of initiation of migrating myoelectric complexes in dogs. *Gastroenterology,* 84:814-822.

Sarna, S.K. 1991. Physiology and pathophysiology of colonic motor activity. *Dig. Dis. Sci.,* 6:827-862.

Sarr M.G. and Kelly, K.A. 1981. Myoelectric activity of the autotransplanted canine jejunoileum. *Gastroenterology,* 81:303-310.

Serio, R., Barajas-Lopez, C., Daniel, E.E., Berezin, I., and Huizinga, J.D. 1991. Pacemaker activity in the colon: Role of interstitial cells of Cajal and smooth muscle cells. *Am. J. Physiol.,* 260:G636-G645.

Shearin, N.L., Bowes, K.L. and Kingma, Y.J. 1978. *In vitro* electrical activity in canine colon. *Gut,* 20:780-786.

Stanciu, C. and Bennett, J.R. 1975. The general pattern of gastroduodenal motility: 24 hour recordings in normal subjects. *Rev. Med. Chir. Soc. Med. Nat. Iasi.,* 79:31-36.

Skinner, F.K. and Bardakjian, B.L. 1991. A barrier kinetic mapping unit. Application to ionic transport in gastric smooth muscle. *Gastrointest. J. Motil.,* 3:213-224.

Stern, R.M. and Koch, K.L. 1985. *Electrogastrography: Methodology, Validation, and Applications.* Praeger, New York.

Summers, R.W., Anuras, S., and Green, J. 1982. Jejunal motility patterns in normal subjects and symptomatic patients with partial mechanical obstruction or pseudo-obstruction. In *Motility of the Digestive Tract,* M. Weinbeck, Ed., Raven Press, New York, 467-470.

Suzuki, N., Prosser, C.L., and Dahms, V., 1986. Boundary cells between longitudinal and circular layers: Essential for electrical slow waves in cat intestine. *Am. J. Physiol.,* 280:G287-G294.

Szurszewski, J.H. 1969. A migrating electric complex of the canine small intestine. *Am. J. Physiol.,* 217:1757-1763.

Szurszewski, J.H. 1987. Electrical basis for gastrointestinal motility. In *Physiology of the Gastrointestinal Tract,* L.R. Johnson, Ed., Raven Press, New York, chap. 12.

Thompson, D.G., Wingate, D.L., Archer, L., Benson, M.J., Green, W.J., and Hardy, R.J. 1980. Normal patterns of human upper small bowel motor activity recorded by prolonged radiotelemetry. *Gut,* 21:500-506.

Vanasin, B., Ustach, T.J., and Schuster, M.M. 1974. Electrical and motor activity of human and dog colon in vitro. *Johns Hopkins Med. J.,* 134:201-210.

Vantrappen, G., Janssens, J.J., Hellemans, J., and Ghoos, Y. 1977. The interdigestive motor complex of normal subjects and patients with bacterial overgrowth of the small intestine. *J. Clin. Invest.,* 59:1158-1166.

Wang, Z., He, Z., and Chen, J.D.Z. 1999. Filter banks and neural network-based feature extraction and automatic classification of electrogastrogram. *Ann. Biomed. Eng.,* 27:88-95.

Weisbrodt, N.W., Copeland, E.M., Moore, E.P., Kearly, K.W., and Johnson, L.R. 1975. Effect of vagotomy on electrical activity of the small intestine of the dog. *Am. J. Physiol.,* 228:650-654.

Wheelon, H. and Thomas, J.E. 1921. Rhythmicity of the pyloric sphincter. *Am. J. Physiol.,* 54:460-473.

Wheelon, H. and Thomas, J.E. 1922. Observations on the motility of the duodenum and the relation of duodenal activity to that of the pars pylorica. *Am. J. Physiol.,* 59:72-96.

7

Respiratory System

Arthur T. Johnson
University of Maryland

Christopher G. Lausted
University of Maryland

Joseph D. Bronzino
Trinity College/The Biomedical Engineering Alliance and Consortium (BEACON)

As functioning units, the lung and heart are usually considered a single complex organ, but because these organs contain essentially two compartments — one for blood and one for air — they are usually separated in terms of the tests conducted to evaluate heart or pulmonary function. This chapter focuses on some of the physiologic concepts responsible for normal function and specific measures of the lung's ability to supply tissue cells with enough oxygen while removing excess carbon dioxide.

7.1 Respiration Anatomy

The respiratory system consists of the lungs, conducting airways, pulmonary vasculature, respiratory muscles, and surrounding tissues and structures (Fig. 7.1). Each plays an important role in influencing respiratory responses.

Lungs

There are two lungs in the human chest; the right lung is composed of three incomplete divisions called *lobes,* and the left lung has two, leaving room for the heart. The right lung accounts for 55% of total gas volume and the left lung for 45%. Lung tissue is spongy because of the very small (200 to 300 × 10⁻⁶ m diameter in normal lungs at rest) gas-filled cavities called *alveoli,* which are the ultimate structures for gas exchange. There are 250 million to 350 million alveoli in the adult lung, with a total alveolar surface area of 50 to 100 m² depending on the degree of lung inflation [Johnson, 1991].

Conducting Airways

Air is transported from the atmosphere to the alveoli beginning with the oral and nasal cavities, through the pharynx (in the throat), past the glottal opening, and into the trachea or windpipe. Conduction of air begins at the larynx, or voice box, at the entrance to the trachea, which is a fibromuscular tube 10 to 12 cm in length and 1.4 to 2.0 cm in diameter [Kline, 1976]. At a location called the *carina,* the trachea

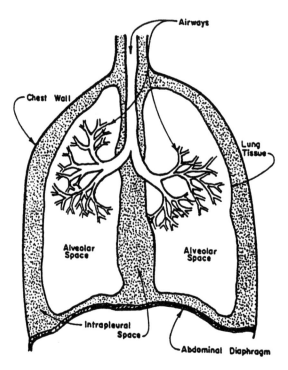

FIGURE 7.1   Schematic representation of the respiratory system.

terminates and divides into the left and right bronchi. Each bronchus has a discontinuous cartilaginous support in its wall. Muscle fibers capable of controlling airway diameter are incorporated into the walls of the bronchi, as well as in those of air passages closer to the alveoli. Smooth muscle is present throughout the respiratory bronchiolus and alveolar ducts but is absent in the last alveolar duct, which terminates in one to several alveoli. The alveolar walls are shared by other alveoli and are composed of highly pliable and collapsible squamous epithelium cells.

The bronchi subdivide into subbronchi, which further subdivide into bronchioli, which further subdivide, and so on, until finally reaching the alveolar level. Table 7.1 provides a description and dimensions of the airways of adult humans. A model of the geometric arrangement of these air passages is presented in Fig. 7.2. It will be noted that each airway is considered to branch into two subairways. In the adult human there are considered to be 23 such branchings, or generations, beginning at the trachea and ending in the alveoli.

Movement of gases in the respiratory airways occurs mainly by bulk flow (convection) throughout the region from the mouth to the nose to the 15th generation. Beyond the 15th generation, gas diffusion is relatively more important. With the low gas velocities that occur in diffusion, dimensions of the space over which diffusion occurs (alveolar space) must be small for adequate oxygen delivery into the walls; smaller alveoli are more efficient in the transfer of gas than are larger ones. Thus animals with high levels of oxygen consumption are found to have smaller-diameter alveoli compared with animals with low levels of oxygen consumption.

Alveoli

Alveoli are the structures through which gases diffuse to and from the body. To ensure gas exchange occurs efficiently, alveolar walls are extremely thin. For example, the total tissue thickness between the inside of the alveolus to pulmonary capillary blood plasma is only about 0.4×10^{-6} m. Consequently, the principal barrier to diffusion occurs at the plasma and red blood cell level, not at the alveolar membrane [Ruch and Patton, 1966].

TABLE 7.1 Classification and Approximate Dimensions of Airways of Adult Human Lung (inflated to about 3/4 of total lung capacity)*

Common Name	Numerical Order of Generation	Number of Each	Diameter, mm	Length, mm	Total Cross-Sectional Area, cm²	Description and Comment
Trachea	0	1	18	120	2.5	Main cartilaginous airway; partly in thorax
Main bronchus	1	2	12	47.6	2.3	First branching of airway; one to each lung; in lung root; cartilage
Lobar bronchus	2	4	8	19.0	2.1	Named for each lobe; cartilage
Segmental bronchus	3	8	6	7.6	2.0	Named for radiographical and surgical anatomy; cartilage
Subsegmental bronchus	4	16	4	12.7	2.4	Last generally named bronchi; may be referred to as medium-sized bronchi; cartilage
Small bronchi	5–10	1,024†	1.3†	4.6†	13.4†	Not generally named; contain decreasing amounts of cartilage; beyond this level airways enter the lobules as defined by a strong elastic lobular limiting membrane
Bronchioles	11–13	8,192†	0.8†	2.7†	44.5†	Not named; contain no cartilage, mucus-secreting elements, or cilia; tightly embedded in lung tissue
Terminal bronchioles	14–15	32,768†	0.7†	2.0†	113.0†	Generally 2 or 3 orders so designated; morphology not significantly different from orders 11–13
Respiratory bronchioles	16–18	262,144†	0.5†	1.2†	534.0†	Definite class; bronchiolar cuboidal epithelium present, but scattered alveoli are present giving these airways a gas exchange function; order 16 often called first-order respiratory bronchiole; 17, second-order; 18, third-order
Alveolar ducts	19–22	4,194,304†	0.4†	0.8†	5,880.0†	No bronchial epithelium; have no surface except connective tissue framework; open into alveoli
Alveolar sacs	23	8,388,608	0.4	0.6	11,800.0	No reason to assign a special name; are really short alveolar ducts
Alveoli	24	300,000,000	0.2			Pulmonary capillaries are in the septae that form the alveoli

* The number of airways in each generation is based on regular dichotomous branching.

† Numbers refer to last generation in each group.

Source: Used with permission from Staub [1963] and Weibel [1963]; adapted by Comroe [1965].

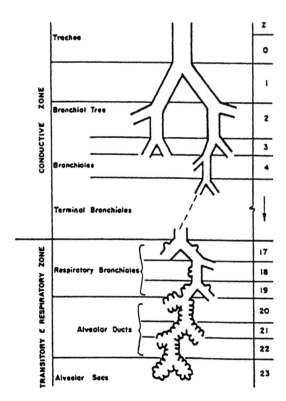

FIGURE 7.2   General architecture of conductive and transitory airways. (Used with permission from Weibel, 1963.) In the conductive zone air is conducted to and from the lungs while in the respiration zone, gas exchange occurs.

Molecular diffusion within the alveolar volume is responsible for mixing of the enclosed gas. Due to small alveolar dimensions, complete mixing probably occurs in less than 10 ms, fast enough that alveolar mixing time does not limit gaseous diffusion to or from the blood [Astrand and Rodahl, 1970].

Of particular importance to proper alveolar operation is a thin surface coating of surfactant. Without this material, large alveoli would tend to enlarge and small alveoli would collapse. It is the present view that surfactant acts like a detergent, changing the stress-strain relationship of the alveolar wall and thereby stabilizing the lung [Johnson, 1991].

Pulmonary Circulation

There is no true pulmonary analogue to the systemic arterioles, since the pulmonary circulation occurs under relatively low pressure [West, 1977]. Pulmonary blood vessels, especially capillaries and venules, are very thin walled and flexible. Unlike systemic capillaries, pulmonary capillaries increase in diameter, and pulmonary capillaries within alveolar walls separate adjacent alveoli with increases in blood pressure or decreases in alveolar pressure. Flow, therefore, is significantly influenced by elastic deformation. Although pulmonary circulation is largely unaffected by neural and chemical control, it does respond promptly to hypoxia.

There is also a high-pressure systemic blood delivery system to the bronchi that is completely independent of the pulmonary low-pressure ($\sim$3330 N/m^2) circulation in healthy individuals. In diseased states, however, bronchial arteries are reported to enlarge when pulmonary blood flow is reduced, and some arteriovenous shunts become prominent [West, 1977].

Total pulmonary blood volume is approximately 300 to 500 cm^3 in normal adults, with about 60 to 100 cm^3 in the pulmonary capillaries [Astrand and Rodahl, 1970]. This value, however, is quite variable, depending on such things as posture, position, disease, and chemical composition of the blood [Kline, 1976].

Since pulmonary arterial blood is oxygen poor and carbon dioxide rich, it exchanges excess carbon dioxide for oxygen in the pulmonary capillaries, which are in close contact with alveolar walls. At rest, the transit time for blood in the pulmonary capillaries is computed as

$$t = V_c / \dot{V}_c$$

where t = blood transmit time, s
V_c = capillary blood volume, m^3
$\dot{V}_c$ = total capillary blood flow = cardiac output, m^3/s

and is somewhat less than 1 s, while during exercise it may be only 500 ms or even less.

Respiratory Muscles

The lungs fill because of a rhythmic expansion of the chest wall. The action is indirect in that no muscle acts directly on the lung. The diaphragm, the muscular mass accounting for 75% of the expansion of the chest cavity, is attached around the bottom of the thoracic cage, arches over the liver, and moves downward like a piston when it contracts. The external intercostal muscles are positioned between the ribs and aid inspiration by moving the ribs up and forward. This, then, increases the volume of the thorax. Other muscles are important in the maintenance of thoracic shape during breathing. (For details, see Ruch and Patton [1966] and Johnson [1991]).

Quiet expiration is usually considered to be passive; i.e., pressure to force air from the lungs comes from elastic expansion of the lungs and chest wall. During moderate to severe exercise, the abdominal and internal intercostal muscles are very important in forcing air from the lungs much more quickly than would otherwise occur. Inspiration requires intimate contact between lung tissues, pleural tissues (the pleura is the membrane surrounding the lungs), and chest wall and diaphragm. This is accomplished by reduced intrathoracic pressure (which tends toward negative values) during inspiration.

Viewing the lungs as an entire unit, one can consider the lungs to be elastic sacs within an airtight barrel — the thorax — which is bounded by the ribs and the diaphragm. Any movement of these two boundaries alters the volume of the lungs. The normal breathing cycle in humans is accomplished by the active contraction of the inspiratory muscles, which enlarges the thorax. This enlargement lowers intrathoracic and interpleural pressure even further, pulls on the lungs, and enlarges the alveoli, alveolar ducts, and bronchioli, expanding the alveolar gas and decreasing its pressure below atmospheric. As a result, air at atmospheric pressure flows easily into the nose, mouth, and trachea.

7.2   Lung Volumes and Gas Exchange

Of primary importance to lung functioning is the movement and mixing of gases within the respiratory system. Depending on the anatomic level under consideration, gas movement is determined mainly by diffusion or convection.

Without the thoracic musculature and rib cage, as mentioned above, the barely inflated lungs would occupy a much smaller space than they occupy *in situ*. However, the thoracic cage holds them open. Conversely, the lungs exert an influence on the thorax, holding it smaller than should be the case without the lungs. Because the lungs and thorax are connected by tissue, the volume occupied by both together is between the extremes represented by relaxed lungs alone and thoracic cavity alone. The resting volume V_R, then, is that volume occupied by the lungs with glottis open and muscles relaxed.

Lung volumes greater than resting volume are achieved during inspiration. Maximum inspiration is represented by *inspiratory reserve volume* (IRV). IRV is the maximum additional volume that can be

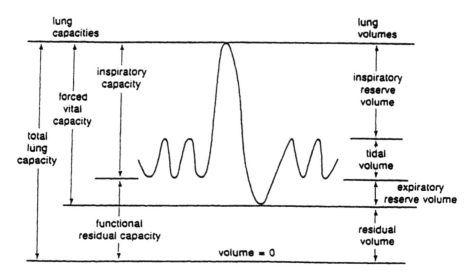

FIGURE 7.3   Lung capacities and lung volumes.

accommodated by the lung at the end of inspiration. Lung volumes less than resting volume do not normally occur at rest but do occur during exhalation while exercising (when exhalation is active). Maximum additional expiration, as measured from lung volume at the end of expiration, is called *expiratory reserve volume* (ERV). *Residual volume* is the amount of gas remaining in the lungs at the end of maximal expiration.

Tidal volume V_T is normally considered to be the volume of air entering the nose and mouth with each breath. Alveolar ventilation volume, the volume of fresh air that enters the alveoli during each breath, is always less than tidal volume. The extent of this difference in volume depends primarily on the *anatomic dead space*, the 150- to 160-ml internal volume of the conducting airway passages. The term *dead* is quite appropriate, since it represents wasted respiratory effort; i.e., no significant gas exchange occurs across the thick walls of the trachea, bronchi, and bronchiolus. Since normal tidal volume at rest is usually about 500 ml of air per breath, one can easily calculate that because of the presence of this dead space, about 340 to 350 ml of fresh air actually penetrates the alveoli and becomes involved in the gas exchange process. An additional 150 to 160 ml of stale air exhaled during the previous breath is also drawn into the alveoli.

The term *volume* is used for elemental differences of lung volume, whereas the term *capacity* is used for combination of lung volumes. Figure 7.3 illustrates the interrelationship between each of the following lung volumes and capacities:

1. *Total lung capacity* (TLC): The amount of gas contained in the lung at the end of maximal inspiration.
2. *Forced vital capacity* (FVC): The maximal volume of gas that can be forcefully expelled after maximal inspiration.
3. *Inspiratory capacity* (IC): The maximal volume of gas that can be inspired from the resting expiratory level.
4. *Functional residual capacity* (FRC): The volume of gas remaining after normal expiration. It will be noted that functional residual capacity (FRC) is the same as the resting volume. There is a small difference, however, between resting volume and FRC because FRC is measured while the patient breathes, whereas resting volume is measured with no breathing. FRC is properly defined only at end-expiration at rest and not during exercise.

TABLE 7.2 Typical Lung Volumes for Normal, Healthy Males

Lung Volume	Normal Values	
Total lung capacity (TLC)	6.0×10^{-3} m^3	(6,000 cm^3)
Residual volume (RV)	1.2×10^{-3} m^3	(1,200 cm^3)
Vital capacity (VC)	4.8×10^{-3} m^3	(4,800 cm^3)
Inspiratory reserve volume (IRV)	3.6×10^{-3} m^3	(3,600 cm^3)
Expiratory reserve volume (ERV)	1.2×10^{-3} m^3	(1,200 cm^3)
Functional residual capacity (FRC)	2.4×10^{-3} m^3	(2,400 cm^3)
Anatomic dead volume (V_D)	1.5×10^{-4} m^3	(150 cm^3)
Upper airways volume	8.0×10^{-5} m^3	(80 cm^3)
Lower airways volume	7.0×10^{-5} m^3	(70 cm^3)
Physiologic dead volume (V_D)	1.8×10^{-4} m^3	(180 cm^3)
Minute volume ($\dot{V}_e$) at rest	1.0×10^{-4} m^3/s	(6,000 cm^3/min)
Respiratory period (T) at rest	4s	
Tidal volume (V_T) at rest	4.0×10^{-4} m^3	(400 cm^3)
Alveolar ventilation volume (V_A) at rest	2.5×10^{-4} m^3	(250 cm^3)
Minute volume during heavy exercise	1.7×10^{-3} m^3/s	(10,000 cm^3/min)
Respiratory period during heavy exercise	1.2 s	
Tidal volume during heavy exercise	2.0×10^{-3} m^3	(2,000 cm^3)
Alveolar ventilation volume during exercise	1.8×10^{-3} m^3	(1,820 cm^3)

Source: Adapted and used with permission from Forster et al. [1986].

These volumes and specific capacities, represented in Fig. 7.3, have led to the development of specific tests (that will be discussed below) to quantify the status of the pulmonary system. Typical values for these volumes and capacities are provided in Table 7.2.

7.3 Perfusion of the Lung

For gas exchange to occur properly in the lung, air must be delivered to the alveoli via the conducting airways, gas must diffuse from the alveoli to the capillaries through extremely thin walls, and the same gas must be removed to the cardiac atrium by blood flow. This three-step process involves (1) alveolar ventilation, (2) the process of diffusion, and (3) ventilatory perfusion, which involves pulmonary blood flow. Obviously, an alveolus that is ventilated but not perfused cannot exchange gas. Similarly, a perfused alveolus that is not properly ventilated cannot exchange gas. The most efficient gas exchange occurs when ventilation and perfusion are matched.

There is a wide range of ventilation-to-perfusion ratios that naturally occur in various regions of the lung [Johnson, 1991]. Blood flow is somewhat affected by posture because of the effects of gravity. In the upright position, there is a general reduction in the volume of blood in the thorax, allowing for larger lung volume. Gravity also influences the distribution of blood, such that the perfusion of equal lung volumes is about five times greater at the base compared with the top of the lung [Astrand and Rodahl, 1970]. There is no corresponding distribution of ventilation; hence the ventilation-to-perfusion ratio is nearly five times smaller at the top of the lung (Table 7.3). A more uniform ventilation-to-perfusion ratio is found in the supine position and during exercise [Jones, 1984b].

Blood flow through the capillaries is not steady. Rather, blood flows in a halting manner and may even be stopped if intraalveolar pressure exceeds intracapillary blood pressure during diastole. Mean blood flow is not affected by heart rate [West, 1977], but the highly distensible pulmonary blood vessels admit more blood when blood pressure and cardiac output increase. During exercise, higher pulmonary blood pressures allow more blood to flow through the capillaries. Even mild exercise favors more uniform perfusion of the lungs [Astrand and Rodahl, 1970]. Pulmonary artery systolic pressures increases from 2670 N/m^2 (20 mmHg) at rest to 4670 N/m^2 (35 mmHg) during moderate exercise to 6670 N/m^2 (50 mmHg) at maximal work [Astrand and Rodahl, 1970].

TABLE 7.3   Ventilation-to-Perfusion Ratios from the Top to Bottom
of the Lung of Normal Man in the Sitting Position

Percent Lung Volume, %	Alveolar Ventilation Rate, cm³/s	Perfusion Rate, cm³/s	Ventilation-to-Perfusion Ratio
		Top	
7	4.0	1.2	3.3
8	5.5	3.2	1.8
10	7.0	5.5	1.3
11	8.7	8.3	1.0
12	9.8	11.0	0.90
13	11.2	13.8	0.80
13	12.0	16.3	0.73
13	13.0	19.2	0.68
		Bottom	
13	13.7	21.5	0.63
100	84.9	100.0	

Source: Used with permission from West [1962].

7.4   Gas Partial Pressures

The primary purpose of the respiratory system is gas exchange. In the gas-exchange process, gas must diffuse through the alveolar space, across tissue, and through plasma into the red blood cell, where it finally chemically joins to hemoglobin. A similar process occurs for carbon dioxide elimination.

As long as intermolecular interactions are small, most gases of physiologic significance can be considered to obey the ideal gas law:

$$pV = nRT$$

where p = pressure, N/m²
V = volume of gas, m³
n = number of moles, mol
R = gas constant, (N × m)/(mol × K)
T = absolute temperature, K

The ideal gas law can be applied without error up to atmospheric pressure; it can be applied to a mixture of gases, such as air, or to its constituents, such as oxygen or nitrogen. All individual gases in a mixture are considered to fill the total volume and have the same temperature but reduced pressures. The pressure exerted by each individual gas is called the *partial pressure* of the gas.

Dalton's law states that the total pressure is the sum of the partial pressures of the constituents of a mixture:

$$p = \sum_{i=1}^{N} p_i$$

where p_i = partial pressure of the ith constituent, N/m²
N = total number of constituents

Dividing the ideal gas law for a constituent by that for the mixture gives

$$\frac{P_i V}{PV} = \frac{n_i R_i T}{nRT}$$

so that

$$\frac{p_i}{p} = \frac{n_i R_i}{nR}$$

which states that the partial pressure of a gas may be found if the total pressure, mole fraction, and ratio of gas constants are known. For most respiratory calculations, p will be considered to be the pressure of 1 atmosphere, 101 kN/m². Avogadro's principle states that different gases at the same temperature and pressure contain equal numbers of molecules:

$$\frac{V_1}{V_2} = \frac{nR_1}{nR_2} = \frac{R_1}{R_2}$$

Thus

$$\frac{p_i}{p} = \frac{V_i}{V}$$

where V_i/V is the volume fraction of a constituent in air and is therefore dimensionless. Table 7.4 provides individual gas constants, as well as volume fractions, of constituent gases of air.

Gas pressures and volumes can be measured for many different temperature and humidity conditions. Three of these are body temperature and pressure, saturated (BTPS); ambient temperature and pressure (ATP); and standard temperature and pressure, dry (STPD). To calculate constituent partial pressures at STPD, total pressure is taken as barometric pressure minus vapor pressure of water in the atmosphere:

$$p_i = \left(V_i/V\right)\left(p - pH_2O\right)$$

where p = total pressure, kN/m²
        pH_2O = vapor pressure of water in atmosphere, kN/m²

and V_i/V as a ratio does not change in the conversion process.

TABLE 7.4   Molecular Masses, Gas Constants, and Volume Fractions for Air and Constituents

Constituent	Molecular Mass kg/mol	Gas Constant, N·m/(mol·K)	Volume Fraction in Air, m³/m³
Air	29.0	286.7	1.0000
Ammonia	17.0	489.1	0.0000
Argon	39.9	208.4	0.0093
Carbon dioxide	44.0	189.0	0.0003
Carbon monoxide	28.0	296.9	0.0000
Helium	4.0	2078.6	0.0000
Hydrogen	2.0	4157.2	0.0000
Nitrogen	28.0	296.9	0.7808
Oxygen	32.0	259.8	0.2095

Note: Universal gas constant is 8314.43 N·m/kg·mol·K.

TABLE 7.5 Gas Partial Pressures (kN/m^2) throughout the Respiratory and Circulatory Systems

Gas	Inspired Air*	Alveolar Air	Expired Air	Mixed Venous Blood	Arterial Blood	Muscle Tissue
H_2O	—	6.3	6.3	6.3	6.3	6.3
CO_2	0.04	5.3	4.2	6.1	5.3	6.7
O_2	21.2	14.0	15.5	5.3	13.3	4.0
N_2†	80.1	75.7	75.3	76.4	76.4	76.4
Total	101.3	101.3	101.3	94.1	101.3	93.4

*Inspired air considered dry for convenience.
†Includes all other inert components.
Source: Used with permission from Astrand and Rodahl [1970].

Gas volume at STPD is converted from ambient condition volume as

$$V_i = V_{amb}\left[273/(273+\Theta)\right]\left[(p - pH_2O)/101.3\right]$$

where V_i = volume of gas i corrected to STPD, m^3
V_{amb} = volume of gas i at ambient temperature and pressure, m^3
Θ = ambient temperature, °C
p = ambient total pressure, kN/m^2
pH_2O = vapor pressure of water in the air, kN/m^2

Partial pressures and gas volumes may be expressed in BTPS conditions. In this case, gas partial pressures are usually known from other measurements. Gas volumes are converted from ambient conditions by

$$V_i = V_{amb}\left[310/(273+\Theta)\right]\left[(p - pH_2O)/p - 6.28\right]$$

Table 7.5 provides gas partial pressure throughout the respiratory and circulatory systems.

7.5 Pulmonary Mechanics

The respiratory system exhibits properties of resistance, compliance, and inertance analogous to the electrical properties of resistance, capacitance, and inductance. Of these, inertance is generally considered to be of less importance than the other two properties.

Resistance is the ratio of pressure to flow:

$$R = p/V$$

where R = resistance, $N \times s/m^5$
P = pressure, N/m^2
V = volume flow rate, m^3/s

Resistance can be found in the conducting airways, in the lung tissue, and in the tissues of the chest wall. Airways exhalation resistance is usually higher than airways inhalation resistance because the surrounding lung tissue pulls the smaller, more distensible airways open when the lung is being inflated. Thus airways inhalation resistance is somewhat dependent on lung volume, and airways exhalation resistance can be very lung volume dependent [Johnson, 1991]. Respiratory tissue resistance varies with frequency, lung volume, and volume history. Tissue resistance is relatively small at high frequencies but increases greatly at low frequencies, nearly proportional to $1/f$. Tissue resistance often exceeds airway resistance below 2 Hz. Lung tissue resistance also increases with decreasing volume amplitude [Stamenovic et al., 1990].

Compliance is the ratio of lung volume to lung pressure:

$$C = V/p$$

where C = compliance, m^5/N
  V = lung volume/m^3
  P = pressure, N/m^2

As the lung is stretched, it acts as an expanded balloon that tends to push air out and return to its normal size. The static pressure-volume relationship is nonlinear, exhibiting decreased static compliance at the extremes of lung volume [Johnson, 1991]. As with tissue resistance, dynamic tissue compliance does not remain constant during breathing. Dynamic compliance tends to increase with increasing volume and decrease with increasing frequency [Stamenovic et al., 1990].

Two separate approaches can be used to model lung tissue mechanics. The traditional approach places a linear viscoelastic system in parallel with a plastoelastic system. A linear viscoelastic system consists of ideal resistive and compliant elements and can exhibit the frequency dependence of respiratory tissue. A plastoelastic system consists of dry-friction elements and compliant elements and can exhibit the volume dependence of respiratory tissue [Hildebrandt, 1970]. An alternate approach is to utilize a nonlinear viscoelastic system that can characterize both the frequency dependence and the volume dependence of respiratory tissue [Suki and Bates, 1991].

Lung tissue hysteresivity relates resistance and compliance:

$$wR = \eta/C_{dyn}$$

where ω = frequency, radians/s
  R = resistance, $N \times s/m^5$
  η = hysteresivity, unitless
  C_{dyn} = dynamic compliance, m^5/n

Hysteresivity, analogous to the structural damping coefficient used in solid mechanics, is an empirical parameter arising from the assumption that resistance and compliance are related at the microstructural level. Hysteresivity is independent of frequency and volume. Typical values range from 0.1 to 0.3 [Fredberg and Stamenovic, 1989].

7.6 Respiratory Control

Control of respiration occurs in many different cerebral structures [Johnson, 1991] and regulates many things [Hornbein, 1981]. Respiration must be controlled to produce the respiratory rhythm, ensure adequate gas exchange, protect against inhalation of poisonous substances, assist in maintenance of body pH, remove irritations, and minimize energy cost. Respiratory control is more complex than cardiac control for at least three reasons:

1. Airway airflow occurs in both directions.
2. The respiratory system interfaces directly with the environment outside the body.
3. Parts of the respiratory system are used for other functions, such as swallowing and speaking.

As a result, respiratory muscular action must be exquisitely coordinated; it must be prepared to protect itself against environmental onslaught, and breathing must be temporarily suspended on demand.

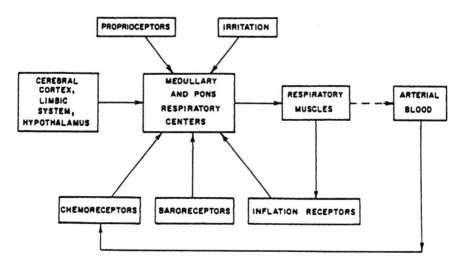

FIGURE 7.4   General scheme of respiratory control.

All control systems require sensors, controllers, and effectors. Figure 7.4 presents the general scheme for respiratory control. There are mechanoreceptors throughout the respiratory system. For example, nasal receptors are important in sneezing, apnea (cessation of breathing), bronchodilation, bronchoconstriction, and the secretion of mucus. Laryngeal receptors are important in coughing, apnea, swallowing, bronchoconstriction, airway mucus secretion, and laryngeal constriction. Tracheobronchial receptors are important in coughing, pulmonary hypertension, bronchoconstriction, laryngeal constriction, and mucus production. Other mechanoreceptors are important in the generation of the respiratory pattern and are involved with respiratory sensation.

Respiratory chemoreceptors exist peripherally in the aortic arch and carotic bodies and centrally in the ventral medulla oblongata of the brain. These receptors are sensitive to partial pressures of CO_2 and O_2 and to blood pH.

The respiratory controller is located in several places in the brain. Each location appears to have its own function. Unlike the heart, the basic respiratory rhythm is not generated within the lungs but rather in the brain and is transmitted to the respiratory muscles by the phrenic nerve.

Effector organs are mainly the respiratory muscles, as described previously. Other effectors are muscles located in the airways and tissues for mucus secretion. Control of respiration appears to be based on two criteria: (1) removal of excess CO_2 and (2) minimization of energy expenditure. It is not the lack of oxygen that stimulates respiration but increased CO_2 partial pressure that acts as a powerful respiratory stimulus. Because of the buffering action of blood bicarbonate, blood pH usually falls as more CO_2 is produced in the working muscles. Lower blood pH also stimulates respiration.

A number of respiratory adjustments are made to reduce energy expenditure during exercise: Respiration rate increases, the ratio of inhalation time to exhalation time decreases, respiratory flow waveshapes become more trapezoidal, and expiratory reserve volume decreases. Other adjustments to reduce energy expenditure have been theorized but not proved [Johnson, 1991].

7.7   The Pulmonary Function Laboratory

The purpose of a pulmonary function laboratory is to obtain clinically useful data from patients with respiratory dysfunction. The pulmonary function tests (PFTs) within this laboratory fulfill a variety of functions. They permit (1) quantification of a patient's breathing deficiency, (2) diagnosis of different types of pulmonary diseases, (3) evaluation of a patient's response to therapy, and (4) preoperative screening to determine whether the presence of lung disease increases the risk of surgery.

Although PFTs can provide important information about a patient's condition, the limitations of these tests must be considered. First, they are nonspecific in that they cannot determine which portion of the lungs is diseased, only that the disease is present. Second, PFTs must be considered along with the medical history, physical examination, x-ray examination, and other diagnostic procedures to permit a complete evaluation. Finally, the major drawback to *some* PFTs is that they require a full patient cooperation and for this reason cannot be conducted on critically ill patients. Consider some of the most widely used PFTs: spirometry, body plethysmography, and diffusing capacity.

Spirometry

The simplest PFT is the spirometry maneuver. In this test, the patient inhales to total lung capacity (TLC) and exhales forcefully to residual volume. The patient exhales into a displacement bell chamber that sits on a water seal. As the bell rises, a pen coupled to the bell chamber inscribes a tracing on a rotating drum. The spirometer offers very little resistance to breathing; therefore, the shape of the spirometry curve (Fig. 7.5) is purely a function of the patient's lung compliance, chest compliance, and airway resistance. At high lung volumes, a rise in intrapleural pressure results in greater expiratory flows. However, at intermediate and low lung volumes, the expiratory flow is independent of effort after a certain intrapleural pressure is reached.

Measurements made from the spirometry curve can determine the degree of a patient's ventilatory obstruction. Forced vital capacity (FVC), forced expiratory volumes (FEV), and forced expiratory flows (FEF) can be determined. The FEV indicates the volume that has been exhaled from TLC for a particular time interval. For example, $FEV_{0.5}$ is the volume exhaled during the first half-second of expiration, and $FEV_{1.0}$ is the volume exhaled during the first second of expiration; these are graphically represented in Fig. 7.5. Note that the more severe the ventilatory obstruction, the lower are the timed volumes ($FEV_{0.5}$ and $FEV_{1.0}$). The FEF is a measure of the average flow (volume/time) over specified portions of the spirometry curve and is represented by the slope of a straight line drawn between volume levels. The average flow over the first quarter of the forced expiration is the $FEF_{0-25\%}$, whereas the average flow over the middle 50% of the FVC is the $FEF_{25-75\%}$. These values are obtained directly from the spirometry curves. The less steep curves of obstructed patients would result in lower values of $FEF_{0-25\%}$ and $FEF_{25-75\%}$ compared with normal values, which are predicted on the basis of the patient's sex, age, and height.

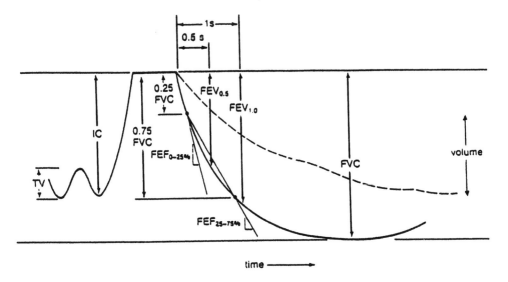

FIGURE 7.5 Typical spirometry tracing obtained during testing; inspiratory capacity (IC), tidal volume (TV), forced vital capacity (FVC), forced expiratory volume (FEV), and forced expiratory flows. Dashed line represents a patient with obstructive lung disease; solid line represents a normal, healthy individual.

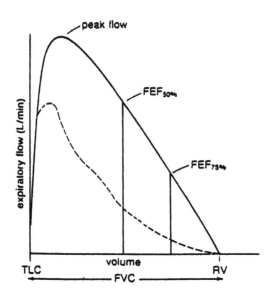

FIGURE 7.6   Flow-volume curve obtained from a spirometry maneuver. Solid line is a normal curve; dashed line represents a patient with obstructive lung disease.

Equations for normal values are available from statistical analysis of data obtained from a normal population. Test results are then interpreted as a percentage of normal.

Another way of presenting a spirometry curve is as a flow-volume curve. Figure 7.6 represents a typical flow-volume curve. The expiratory flow is plotted against the exhaled volume, indicating the maximum flow that may be reached at each degree of lung inflation. Since there is no time axis, a time must mark the $FEV_{0.5}$ and $FEV_{1.0}$ on the tracing. To obtain these flow-volume curves in the laboratory, the patient usually exhales through a *pneumotach*. The most widely used pneumotach measures a pressure drop across a flow-resistive element. The resistance to flow is constant over the measuring range of the device; therefore, the pressure drop is proportional to the flow through the tube. This signal, which is indicative of flow, is then integrated to determine the volume of gas that has passed through the tube.

Another type of pneumotach is the heated-element type. In this device, a small heated mass responds to airflow by cooling. As the element cools, a greater current is necessary to maintain a constant temperature. This current is proportional to the airflow through the tube. Again, to determine the volume that has passed through the tube, the flow signal is integrated.

The flow-volume loop in Fig. 7.7 is a dramatic representation displaying inspiratory and expiratory curves for both normal breathing and maximal breathing. The result is a graphic representation of the patient's reserve capacity in relation to normal breathing. For example, the normal patient's tidal breathing loop is small compared with the patient's maximum breathing loop. During these times of stress, this tidal breathing loop can be increased to the boundaries of the outer ventilatory loop. This increase in ventilation provides the greater gas exchange needed during the stressful situation. Compare this condition with that of the patient with obstructive lung disease. Not only is the tidal breathing loop larger than normal, but the maximal breathing loop is smaller than normal. The result is a decreased ventilatory reserve, limiting the individual's ability to move air in and out of the lungs. As the disease progresses, the outer loop becomes smaller, and the inner loop becomes larger.

The primary use of spirometry is in detection of obstructive lung disease that results from increased resistance to flow through the airways. This can occur in several ways:

1. Deterioration of the structure of the smaller airways that results in early airways closure.
2. Decreased airway diameters caused by bronchospasm or the presence of secretions increases the airway's resistance to airflow.
3. Partial blockage of a large airway by a tumor decreases airway diameter and causes turbulent flow.

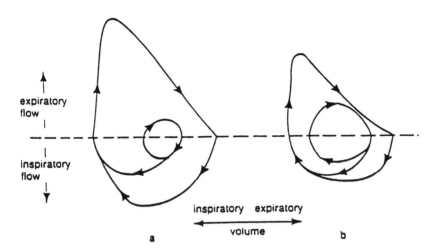

FIGURE 7.7 Typical flow-volume loops. (a) Normal flow-volume loop. (b) Flow-volume loop of patient with obstructive lung disease.

Spirometry has its limitations, however. It can measure only ventilated volumes. It cannot measure lung capacities that contain the residual volume. Measurements of TLC, FRC, and RV have diagnostic value in defining lung overdistension or restrictive pulmonary disease; the body plethysmograph can determine these absolute lung volumes.

Body Plethysmography

In a typical plethysmograph, the patient is put in an airtight enclosure and breathes through a pneumotach. The flow signal through the pneumotach is integrated and recorded as tidal breathing. At the end of a normal expiration (at FRC), an electronically operated shutter occludes the tube through which the patient is breathing. At this time the patient pants lightly against the occluded airway. Since there is no flow, pressure measured at the mouth must equal alveolar pressure. But movements of the chest that compress gas in the lung simultaneously rarify the air in the plethysmograph, and vice versa. The pressure change in the plethysmograph can be used to calculate the volume change in the plethysmograph, which is the same as the volume change in the chest. This leads directly to determination of FRC.

At the same time, alveolar pressure can be correlated to plethysmographic pressure. Therefore, when the shutter is again opened and flow rate is measured, airway resistance can be obtained as the ratio of alveolar pressure (obtainable from plethysmographic pressure) to flow rate [Carr and Brown, 1993]. Airway resistance is usually measured during panting, at a nominal lung volume of FRC and flow rate of ±1 liter/s.

Airway resistance during inspiration is increased in patients with asthma, bronchitis, and upper respiratory tract infections. Expiratory resistance is elevated in patients with emphysema, since the causes of increased expiratory airway resistance are decreased driving pressures and the airway collapse. Airway resistance also may be used to determine the response of obstructed patients to bronchodilator medications.

Diffusing Capacity

So far the mechanical components of airflow through the lungs have been discussed. Another important parameter is the diffusing capacity of the lung, the rate at which oxygen or carbon dioxide travel from the alveoli to the blood (or vice versa for carbon dioxide) in the pulmonary capillaries. Diffusion of gas across a barrier is directly related to the surface area of the barrier and inversely related to the thickness. Also, diffusion is directly proportional to the solubility of the gas in the barrier material and inversely related to the molecular weight of the gas.

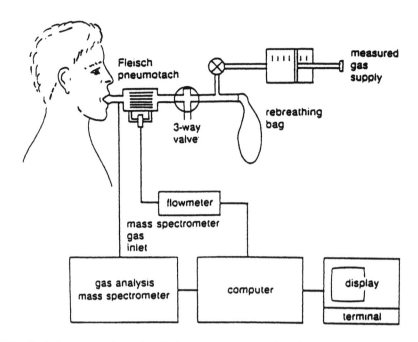

FIGURE 7.8   Typical system configuration for the measurement of rebreathing pulmonary diffusing capacity.

Lung diffusing capacity (D_L) is usually determined for carbon monoxide but can be related to oxygen diffusion. The popular method of measuring carbon monoxide diffusion utilizes a rebreathing technique in which the patient rebreathes rapidly in and out of a bag for approximately 30 s. Figure 7.8 illustrates the test apparatus. The patient begins breathing from a bag containing a known volume of gas consisting of 0.3 to 0.5% carbon monoxide made with heavy oxygen, 0.3 to 0.5% acetylene, 5% helium, 21% oxygen, and a balance of nitrogen. As the patient rebreathes the gas mixture in the bag, a modified mass spectrometer continuously analyzes it during both inspiration and expiration. During this rebreathing procedure, the carbon monoxide disappears from the patient-bag system; the rate at which this occurs is a function of the lung diffusing capacity.

The helium is inert and insoluble in lung tissue and blood and equilibrates quickly in unobstructed patients, indicating the dilution level of the test gas. Acetylene, on the other hand, is soluble in blood and is used to determine the blood flow through the pulmonary capillaries. Carbon monoxide is bound very tightly to hemoglobin and is used to obtain diffusing capacity at a constant pressure gradient across the alveolar-capillary membrane.

Decreased lung diffusing capacity can occur from the thickening of the alveolar membrane or the capillary membrane as well as the presence of interstitial fluid from edema. All these abnormalities increase the barrier thickness and cause a decrease in diffusing capacity. In addition, a characteristic of specific lung diseases is impaired lung diffusing capacity. For example, fibrotic lung tissue exhibits a decreased permeability to gas transfer, whereas pulmonary emphysema results in the loss of diffusion surface area.

Defining Terms

Alveoli: Respiratory airway terminals where most gas exchange with the pulmonary circulation takes place.

BTPS: Body temperature (37°C) and standard pressure (1 atm), saturated (6.28 kN/m²).

Chemoreceptors: Neural receptors sensitive to chemicals such as gas partial pressures.

Dead space: The portion of the respiratory system that does not take part in gas exchange with the blood.

Diffusion: The process whereby a material moves from a region of higher concentration to a region of lower concentration.

Expiration: The breathing process whereby air is expelled from the mouth and nose. Also called *exhalation*.

Functional residual capacity: The lung volume at rest without breathing.

Inspiration: The breathing process whereby air is taken into the mouth and noise. Also called *inhalation*.

Mass spectrometer: A device that identifies relative concentrations of gases by means of mass-to-charge ratios of gas ions.

Mechanoreceptors: Neural receptors sensitive to mechanical inputs such as stretch, pressure, irritants, etc.

Partial pressure: The pressure that a gas would exert if it were the only constituent.

Perfusion: Blood flow to the lungs.

Plethysmography: Any measuring technique that depends on a volume change.

Pleura: The membrane surrounding the lung.

Pneumotach: A measuring device for airflow.

Pulmonary circulation: Blood flow from the right cardiac ventricle that perfuses the lung and is in intimate contact with alveolar membranes for effective gas exchange.

STPD: Standard temperature (0°C) and pressure (1 atm), dry (moisture removed).

Ventilation: Airflow to the lungs.

References

Astrand PO, Rodahl K. 1970. Textbook of Work Physiology. New York, McGraw-Hill.

Carr JJ, Brown JM. 1993. Introduction to Biomedical Equipment Technology. Englewood Cliffs, NJ, Prentice-Hall.

Fredberg JJ, Stamenovic D. 1989. On the imperfect elasticity of lung tissue. J Appl Physiol 67(6):2408–2419.

Hildebrandt J. 1970. Pressure-volume data of cat lung interpreted by plastoelastic, linear viscoelastic model. J Appl Physiol 28(3):365–372.

Hornbein TF (ed). 1981. Regulation of Breathing. New York, Marcel Dekker.

Johnson AT. 1991. Biomechanics and Exercise Physiology. New York, Wiley.

Jones NL. 1984. Normal values for pulmonary gas exchange during exercise. Am Rev Respir Dis 129:544–546.

Kline J. (ed). 1976. Biologic Foundations of Biomedical Engineering. Boston, Little, Brown.

Parker JF Jr, West VR. (eds). 1973. Bioastronautics Data Book. Washington, NASA.

Ruch TC, Patton HD. (eds). 1966. Physiology Biophysics. Philadelphia, Saunders.

Stamenovic D, Glass GM, Barnas GM, Fredberg JJ. 1990. Viscoplasticity of respiratory tissues. J Appl Physiol 69(3):973–988.

Suki B, Bates JHT. 1991. A nonlinear viscoelastic model of lung tissue mechanics. J Appl Physiol 71(3):826–833.

Weibel ER. 1963. Morphometry of the Human Lung. New York, Academic Press.

West J. 1962. Regional differences in gas exchange in the lung of erect man. J Appl Physiol 17:893–898.

West JB. (ed). 1977. Bioengineering Aspects of the Lung. New York, Marcel Dekker.

Additional References

Fredberg JJ, Jones KA, Nathan A, Raboudi S, Prakash YS, Shore SA, Butler JP, Sieck GC. 1996. Friction in airway smooth muscle: Mechanism, latch, and implications in asthma. J Appl Physiol 81(6):2703–2712.

Hantos Z, Daroczy B, Csendes T, Suki B, Nagy S. 1990. Modeling of low-frequency pulmonary impedance in dogs. J Appl Physiol 68(3):849–860.

Hantos Z, Daroczy B, Suki B, Nagy S. 1990. Low-frequency respiratory mechanical impedance in rats. J Appl Physiol 63(1):36–43.

Hantos Z, Petak F, Adamicza A, Asztalos T, Tolnai J, Fredberg JJ. 1997. Mechanical impedance of the lung periphery. J Appl Physiol 83(5):1595–1601.

Maksym GN, Bates JHT. 1997. A distributed nonlinear model of lung tissue elasticity. J Appl Physiol 82(1):32–41.

Petak F, Hall GL, Sly PD. 1998. Repeated measurements of airway and parenchymal mechanics in rats by using low frequency oscillations. J Appl Physiol 84(5):1680–1686.

Thorpe CW, Bates JHT. 1997. Effect of stochastic heterogeneity on lung impedance during acute bronchoconstriction: A model analysis. J Appl Physiol 82(5):1616–1625.

Yuan H, Ingenito EP, Suki B. 1997. Dynamic properties of lung parenchyma: Mechanical contributions of fiber network and interstitial cells. J Appl Physiol 83(5):1420–1431.

II

Tissue Engineering

Bernhard Ø. Palsson
University of Michigan

Jeffrey A. Hubbell
California Institute of Technology

T ISSUE ENGINEERING IS A NEW field that is rapidly growing in both scope and importance within biomedical engineering. It represents a marriage of the rapid developments in cellular and molecular biology on the one hand and materials, chemical, and mechanical engineering on the other. The ability to manipulate and reconstitute tissue function has tremendous clinical implications and is likely to play a major role in cell and gene therapies during the next few years in addition to expanding the tissue supply for transplantation therapies.

Tissue function is complex and involves an intricate interplay of biologic and physicochemical rate processes. A major difficulty with selecting topics for this section was to define its scope. After careful consideration we focused on three goals: first, to cover some of the generic engineering issues; second, to cover generic cell biologic issues; and third, to review the status of tissue engineering of specific organs.

In the first category we have two common engineering themes of material properties and development and the analysis of physical rate processes. The role of materials is treated in terms of two length scales—the molecular and the cellular size scales. On the smaller size scale, Chapter 9 deals with engineering the biomolecular properties of a surface, and Chapter 10 deals with protein adsorption onto surfaces to which cells will be exposed. Chapters 11 and 12 deal with the engineering of scaffolds and templates on which cells are grown for transplantation purposes. The effects of physical rate processes are treated in Chapter 13 and 14. Both fluid mechanical forces and mass transfer rates influence important attributes of tissue function and relate to the physical constraints under which tissues operate. The issues associated with materials and the physical rate process represent important engineering challenges that need to be met to further the development of tissue engineering.

In the second category we have common cell biologic themes: stem cell biology, cell motion, the tissue microenvironment, and the role of stroma in tissue function. It is now believed that many tissues contain stem cells from which the tissue is generated. Chapter 15 describes the basic concepts of stem cell biology. Cell motion is an important process in tissue function and tissue development. Basic concepts of cell motility are covered in Chapter 16, and the manipulation of this process is likely to become an essential part of tissue engineering. It is well established that the cellular microenvironment *in vivo* is critical to tissue function. This complex set of tissues is treated in Chapter 17. The specific interaction between cells performing a tissue-specific function and the accessory cells (or stroma) found in tissues has proved to be a key to reconstituting tissue function *ex vivo*. The important role of the stroma in tissue engineering is described in Chapter 18. The understanding and mastery of these cell biologic issues are essential for the future tissue engineer.

Chapters in the third and last category describe progress with the engineering of specific tissues. Six tissues where much progress has been made were selected: bone marrow, liver, the nervous system, skeletal muscle, cartilage, and kidney. These chapters provide a concise review of the accomplishments to date and the likely clinical implications of these developments.

By focusing on these three categories we hope that the reader will acquire a good understanding of the engineering and cell biological fundamentals of tissue engineering and of the progress that has been made and will develop ideas for further development of this emerging and important field.

8

Fundamentals of Tissue Engineering

François Berthiaume
Surgical Services, Massachusetts General Hospital, Department of Surgery, Harvard Medical School, and the Shriners Hospital for Children

Martin L. Yarmush
Surgical Services, Massachusetts General Hospital, Department of Surgery, Harvard Medical School, and the Shriners Hospital for Children

8.1 Introduction

Tissue engineering can be defined as the application of scientific principles to the design, construction, modification, growth, and maintenance of living tissues. Tissue engineering can be divided into two broad categories: (1) *in vitro* construction of bioartificial tissues from cells isolated by enzymatic dissociation of donor tissue, and (2) *in vivo* alteration of cell growth and function. The first category of applications includes bioartificial tissues (i.e., tissues which are composed of natural and synthetic substances) to be used as an alternative to organ transplantation. Besides their potential clinical use, reconstructed organs may also be used as tools to study complex tissue functions and morphogenesis *in vitro*. For tissue engineering *in vivo*, the objective is to alter the growth and function of cells *in situ*, an example being the use of implanted polymeric tubes to promote the growth and reconnection of damaged nerves. Some representative examples of applications of tissue engineering currently being pursued are listed in Table 8.1.

Conceptually, bioartificial tissues involve three-dimensional structures with cell masses that are orders of magnitude greater than that used in traditional two-dimensional cell culture techniques. In addition, bioartificial organ technology often involves highly differentiated somatic and parenchymal cells isolated from normal tissues. In this chapter, we will provide an overview on tissue reconstruction *in vitro* with particular emphasis on the techniques used to control cell function and organization and to scale up bioartificial tissues. Other equally important issues in tissue engineering, such as cell isolation and biomaterial fabrication will not be presented here. A chapter on cell preservation is presented later within this section.

8.2 Basic Principles and Considerations

Cell Type and Source

In tissue engineering, differentiated cells offer some advantages over tumor cell lines: (1) tumor cells often do not express the full spectrum of functions at the same level as the somatic cell lines they originated

TABLE 8.1   Representative Applications of Tissue Engineering

Application	Examples
Implantable device	Endothelialized vascular grafts
Extracorporeal device	Bone and cartilage implants
Cell production	Bioartificial skin
In situ tissue growth and repair	Bioartificial pancreatic islets
	Neurotransmitter-secreting cells
	Bioartificial liver
	Hematopoiesis *in vitro*
	Nerve regeneration
	Artificial skin

from, (2) tumor cell growth can be very rapid and uncontrollable which can cause design problems (e.g., clogging of microchannels), (3) there is a potential risk of seeding tumor cells in the patient. Notwithstanding these limitations, appropriate selection procedures can be used to derive tumor cell lines which are easily propagated, are contact inhibited, and maintain most of the parent somatic cell features.

Certain human cell types can be easily propagated using standard culture techniques, such as human keratinocytes [Parenteau, 1991]. Conversely, other cell types, such as adult hepatocytes or pancreatic islet cells, do not replicate to any appreciable extent *in vitro*. Because there is currently a shortage of human organs, animal sources are also considered. Success in using xenogeneic cells will largely depend on our ability to control the immunological response of the host to these cells as well as the proteins that they produce. Genetic engineering offers the possibility of creating new cells (i.e., cells which perform a new function) which are easy to grow (e.g., fibroblasts); however, care must be taken to verify that these cells also exhibit the necessary control mechanisms for responding appropriately to the host's metabolic changes.

Control of Cell Function by the Extracellular Matrix

Since the vast majority of mammalian cells are anchorage dependent, they must attach and spread on a substrate to proliferate and function normally. Cell adhesion is generally mediated by certain extracellular matrix proteins such as fibronectin, vitronectin, laminin, and collagen as well as various glycosaminoglycans. Adsorption of these proteins to surfaces and the conformation of the adsorbed proteins appear to be important factors influencing cell attachment and growth on synthetic substrates [Grinnell, 1981]. Small sequences of the cell binding region of these proteins (RGDS in fibronectin and vitronectin, YIGSR in laminin) can also be covalently attached to surfaces to promote cell-substrate adhesion [Massia, 1990].

In general, seeding density is important for normal cell function, especially if cell-cell communications must be established, either by direct cell-cell contacts or via the secretion of trophic factors by the cells. Efficient cell seeding will mainly depend on (1) the affinity of certain cell surface proteins for extracellular matrix components, (2) the density of cell-substrate binding sites on the material surface, (3) the presence or absence of certain nutritional factors. While the first two factors can be controlled independently of the number of cells placed on the surface, the last issue can be problematic because attempts at seeding large numbers of cells can significantly deplete nutrients, with the result that less cells than expected will attach. This point is discussed below in the section on "metabolic requirements of cells."

After seeding, the cells spread on the surface and reach a stable shape. The final morphology of the cells depends on three factors: (1) adherence of the substrate for the cells, which is a function of the affinity and number of the adhesion sites, (2) rigidity of the substrate (i.e., ability to resist cell-generated tractional forces, (3) cell-cell adherence. The effect of substrate adherence and compliance on cell shape and function has been studied on hepatocytes. Increased adherence by increasing the amount of fibronectin adsorbed on a surface leads to increased cell spreading, increased DNA synthesis, and reduced expression of liver-specific functions [Mooney, 1992]. Conversely, reduced adherence or the use of a compliant substrate where little spreading is observed helps maintain liver-specific function but reduces

TABLE 8.2   Effect of Extracellular Matrix (ECM) on Cell Shape and Function

ECM Characteristics		Hepatocytes[a]		Capillary Endothelial
Surface Chemistry	Geometry	Cell shape[b]	Liver-Specific Function	Cell Shape[c]
1 ng/cm^2 Fibronectin on polystyrene	Single surface	Round (1.2)	+	
1000 ng/cm^2 Fibronectin on polystyrene	Single surface	Spread, flat (5)	—	
0.1% w/v Collagen gel	Single surface sandwich	Spread, flat (3.5) Cuboidal, flat (1.5)	— +	Cobblestone, flat capillary network
Heat denatured collagen	Single surface	Round, cell aggregates	+	
Basement membrane extract	Single surface	Round, cell aggregates	+	Capillary network

  [a] Data from [Mooney, 1992; Lindblad, 1990; Ezzell, 1993].
  [b] The number between brackets indicates the projected surface area relative to that of isolated hepatocytes (~1200 μm^2).
  [c] Data from [Montesano, 1983; Madri, 1983].

DNA synthesis [Lindblad, 1991]. The quantitative difference between cell-substrate and cell-cell adhesion strength on a rigid substrate is also a potential factor which may dramatically affect the organization of cells on the substrate. A thermodynamic view of the problem suggests that the overall system (consisting of the cells and the extracellular support) ultimately reaches an equilibrium state when the surface free energy is minimized [Martz, 1974]. According to this hypothesis, the existence of large cell-substrate adhesion forces relative to cell-cell adhesion forces may be a sufficient condition to prevent cell-cell overlapping. In contrast, the opposite situation would lead to cell clumping or multilayered growth on the substrate. This prediction is in agreement with the observation of cellular aggregate formation when hepatocytes are plated on a nonadherent surface as opposed to a highly adherent surface such as type I collagen [Koide, 1990].

One of the most striking features of endothelial and epithelial cells (as opposed to connective tissue cells such as fibroblasts) is the organization of the membrane, which exhibits distinct basal and apical domains, where different proteins and receptors are found. Most epithelial cells can be cultured on a single surface of plastic or extracellular matrix materials which allows the basal surface to be in contact with the substrate and the apical surface to be exposed to the liquid medium. Changing the extracellular matrix configuration can induce these cells to adopt different morphologies. For example, capillary endothelial cells grown on a single collagen gel reorganize into branching capillary-like structures when overlaid with a second layer of collagen [Montesano, 1983]. Unlike most epithelial cells, which exhibit only two distinct membrane domains (one apical and one basal), hepatocytes possess two basolateral surfaces separated by a belt of apical membrane. To express and maintain this particular phenotype, these cells have been cultured between two layers of extracellular matrix, thereby creating a "sandwich" configuration which closely mimics the *in vivo* geometry. Examples of the effect of the extracellular matrix on cell shape and function are summarized in Table 8.2.

Control of Tissue Organization

New ways of controlling cell distribution and shape on surfaces are being developed. These methods provide finer control of cell distribution and creation of microstructures (e.g., microchannels) at a scale that rivals that of natural organs.

The current approach to control cell distribution at size scales down to cell size (10 μm) involves micropatterning techniques. A micropatterning technique based on the utilization of photoreactive cross-linking of hydrophobic or hydrophilic compounds to a polymeric surface has recently been described. Cells attach and grow along the less hydrophilic micropatterned domains. Micropatterned surfaces produced with this technique have been used to produce two-dimensional neuronal networks with neuroblastoma cells [Matsuda, 1992]. Small micropatterned adherent squares of different sizes have been used to control the extent of spreading of hepatocytes [Bhatia, 1994; Singhvi, 1994].

The control of cell orientation may be important when nonisotropic connective tissues are desired. For example, cells can be mixed with a chilled solution of collagen in physiologic buffer, followed by exposure to 37°C to induce the gelation of the collagen. The result is a loose gel comprised of small collagen fibrils where cells and fluid are entrapped. Fibroblasts embedded in a collagen gel cause the contraction of the gel [Bell, 1979]. The contraction process can be controlled to a certain extent by mechanically restricting the motion along certain directions; this also induces a preferential alignment of the collagen fibers as well as the cells within it. A mathematical description of the effect of cell tractional forces on the deformation of collagen-cell lattices and the resulting alignment of the collagen fibers has been presented by Tranquillo [1994]. Other strategies to align cells have been reported: (1) alignment of fibroblasts in collagen gels where collagen fibrils were aligned by a magnetic field during gelation [Guido, 1993], (2) repetitive stretching of endothelial cells cultured on an extensible surface [Banes, 1993], and (3) flow-induced alignment of endothelial cells [Girard, 1993].

Heterotypic cell systems or "co-culture" systems have been used for the production of skin grafts, in long-term cultures of hepatocytes, and in long-term cultures of mixed bone marrow cells. These systems take advantage of the trophic factors (for the most part unknown) secreted by "feeder" cells. Greater use of different cell types used in co-culture will enable engineered cell systems to closely mimic *in vivo* organization, with potential benefits including increased cell function and viability, and greater range of functions expressed by the bioartificial tissue. The organization of multicellular three-dimensional structures may not be obvious. Provided that the adherence of homotypic and heterotypic interactions is known, a thermodynamic analysis similar to that used to describe the morphology of a pure cell culture on a surface can be used to predict how cells will organize in these systems [Wiseman, 1972]. The process of cell-cell sorting in multicellular systems may be altered by changing the composition of the medium or altering the expression of proteins mediating cell-cell adhesion via genetic engineering [Kuhlenschmidt, 1982; Nose, 1988]. Furthermore, micropatterned surfaces can be used to control the initial interface between two cell types in co-culture systems [Bhatia et al., 1998].

Metabolic Requirements of Cells

Oxygen is very often the limiting nutrient in reconstructed tissues. The oxygen requirements vary largely with cell type. Among cells commonly used in bioartificial systems, hepatocytes and pancreatic islet cells are particularly sensitive to the availability of oxygen. Oxygen is required for efficient cell attachment and spreading to planar surfaces as well as microcarriers [Foy, 1993; Rotem, 1994].

Based on a simple mathematical model, we can estimate the critical distance at which the oxygen concentration at the cell surface becomes limiting (this concentration is arbitrarily set equal to K_m) if an unstirred aqueous layer is placed between the gas phase (air) and a confluent monolayer of cells [Yarmush, 1992]. In the case of a confluent monolayer of hepatocytes (2×10^5 cells/cm^2), this distance is 0.95 mm. Thus, in a first approximation, a successful bioartificial liver system containing hepatocytes will have to keep the diffusional distance between the oxygen-carrying medium and the cells to below 1 mm (assuming a confluent cell monolayer on the surface).

Figure 8.1 can be used to estimate the maximum half thickness of a cell mass surrounded by a membrane or external diffusion barrier before the nutrient concentration in the center falls below the Michaelis-Menten constant for nutrient uptake, a sign of nutrient limitation at the cellular level. Oxygen uptake rate parameters for different cell types are given by Fleischaker [1981]. Values for hepatocytes and pancreatic islets can be found in Yarmush [1992], Rotem [1992], and Dionne [1989]. For illustrative purposes, we will use cylindrical hepatocyte aggregates, as an example. We assumed the following: no external diffusion barrier (R_1/R_0) = 1; medium saturated with air at 37°C at the aggregate surface (160 mmHg = 190 nmol/cm^3); diffusivity of oxygen in aggregates (D_0) similar to that in water (2×10^{-5} cm^2/s); a packed cell mass (given a cell diameter of approximately 20 μm, this corresponds to 1.25×10^8 cells/cm^3). The oxygen uptake parameters for hepatocytes were μ_{max} = 0.4 nmol/10^{6}cells/s (thus 50 nmol/cm^3/s for the above cell concentration) and K_m = 0.5 mmHg (e.g., 0.6 nmol/cm^3). We obtain $C_1/K_m = C_0/K_m = 320$, ($\mu_{max} R^2$)/($D_0 K_m$) = 724, 1370, and 2010 for the slab, cylindrical, and spherical

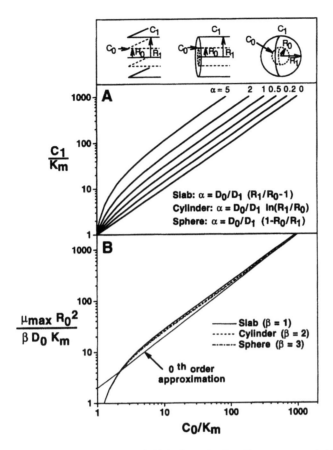

FIGURE 8.1 Correlation to predict the maximum half-thickness R of a cell mass surrounded by a shell of thickness R_1-R_0 without nutrient limitation, assuming that diffusion is the only transport mechanism involved. A: The nutrient concentration at the surface of the cell mass normalized to the Michaelis-Menten constant for the nutrient uptake by the cells (C_0/K_m) is obtained from the normalized bulk nutrient concentration (C_1/K_m), and the aspect ratio of the system (R_1/R_0). D_0, D_1 are the diffusivities for the nutrient within the cell mass and the external diffusion barrier, respectively. The partition coefficient between the cell mass and the surrounding shell is assumed to be equal to 1. B: The half thickness R for which $C/K_m = 1$ in the center ($R = 0$) is obtained from the value of the y-axis corresponding to C_0/K_m, knowing, in addition to the parameters listed above, the maximum nutrient uptake rate by the cells (μ_{max}). If K_m is unknown, a zero order approximation may be used, in which case K_m is set arbitrarily so that C_1/K_m falls in the linear portion of the curve in A. In B, R_0 is obtained using the line labeled "0th order approximation," and corresponds to the half thickness R for which $C = 0$ at the center ($R = 0$).

geometries, respectively, and thus the corresponding maximum half thicknesses obtained are $R = 132$, 181, and 220 μm, respectively. We now consider the case where there is a 100 μm thick membrane around a cylindrical cell aggregate assuming that the diffusivity of oxygen in the membrane (D_1) is the same as in the cell mass. An aspect ratio (α) must be assumed and the values of C_0/K_m, $(\mu_{max} R^2)/(D_0 K_m)$, and R_0 are calculated. R_1 is then obtained from the assumed aspect ratio. Calculations must be performed with several aspect ratios until the difference $R_1 - R_0$ equates the membrane thickness. Here, we found that $\alpha = 0.6$ generates $C_0/K_m = 141$, $(\mu_{max} R^2)/(D_0 K_m) = 622$, $R_0 = 122$ μm. For a cylinder, $\alpha = D_0/D_1$ $\ln(R_1/R_0)$, and thus in this case $R_1 = 222$ μm. Thus, the maximum half-thickness of the cell mass is 122 μm, as compared to 181 μm in the absence of the membrane. These estimates can be used as first guidelines to design a bioartificial liver, and they clearly suggest that the thickness of the cell mass must be limited to a few hundred microns to prevent the formation of an anoxic core.

TABLE 8.3   Maximum Oxygen Uptake Rates of Cells Used in Tissue Reconstruction

Cell Type	μ_{max} (nmol/10^6cells/s)	$K_{0.5}{}^a$ (mmHg)	Reference
$S_p2/0$-derived mouse hybridoma	0.053	0.28	[Miller, 1987]
Hepatocytes	0.38 (day 1, single gel)	5.6	Oxyvice paper
	0.25 (day 3, single gel)	3.3	
Pancreatic islet cells	25.9 nmol/cm^3/s (100 mg/dl glucose)	0.44	[Dionne, 1989]
	46.1 nmol/cm^3/s (300 mg/dl glucose)		

^{a} Oxygen tension for which the oxygen uptake rate equals half of the maximum.

Tissue assembled *in vitro* may have different metabolic requirements than their *in vivo* counterparts, so that exposure of bioartificial tissues to biological fluids and the *in vivo* environment may lead to unexpected alterations in function that may impact on their clinical effectiveness. For example, stable cultures of hepatocytes suddenly exposed to heparinized plasma accumulate fat droplets and exhibit a progressive deterioration of hepatospecific functions [Stefanovich et al., 1996]. Thus, it is important to consider the response of cultured cells and bioartificial tissues to biological fluids when evaluating their performance after implantation.

8.3   Reconstruction of Connective Tissues

The simplest method to create connective tissue *in vitro* is to incorporate connective tissue cells within a loose network of extracellular matrix components. A dermal equivalent has been produced by embedding fibroblasts in collagen gels [Bell et al., 1979]. When fibroblasts (2.5×10^4/ml) were seeded in collagen, the collagen lattice contracted 30- to 50-fold after 4 days of culture. The result is a dense cell-collagen matrix which can be used to support a cultured epidermis. Another example is the production of a bioartificial vascular media by seeding smooth muscle cells in collagen tubes [Weinberg, 1986]. In the latter case, orientation of the cells along the circumference of the tube may be necessary in order to eventually obtain a tissue with contractile properties similar to that exhibited by native blood vessels. More recently, L'Heureux et al. [1998] showed that smooth muscle cells and fibroblasts cultured in the presence of ascorbic acid produce large amounts of extracellular matrix and generate cell-extracellular matrix composite membranes which can be harvested from the substrate. Vascular grafts generated by wrapping around these membranes had a higher burst strength than human saphenous veins commonly used for arterial reconstructions.

When reconstructing connective tissue, it may be advantageous to use a relatively low seeding density with the expectation that cell replication together with the migration of blood vessels from the host's surrounding tissue would occur after implantation. This approach may not be appropriate for tissues that grow slowly and that are subjected to high stresses after implantation. This is the case of bioartificial cartilage, which would be best implanted once its mechanical properties are similar to that of the authentic tissue. Chondrocytes seeded at high density (10^7 cells/cm^3) in agarose gels and in serum-free medium retain their phenotype and remain viable for up to 6 months [Bruckner, 1989]. In this system, the deposition of type II collagen and highly charged proteoglycans can be observed over a period of 43 days [Buschmann, 1992]. The cartilage obtained in the latter studies had a stiffness of approximately 1/3 that of the cartilage explants used to isolate the cells. It should be recognized that in these experiments, the cell density was considerably lower than that found in the native cartilage explants (7.5×10^7 cells/cm^3). Higher chondrocyte seeding density in the initial gel could potentially yield a material with mechanical properties closer to that of native cartilage.

Meshes made of slowly biodegradable polymers may be particularly suitable for dense connective tissue synthesis, such as bone and cartilage. Loose meshes made of lactic and glycolic acid copolymer seeded with calf chondrocytes (5×10^7/ml) have been shown to harbor the production of cartilage *in vitro*

[Freed, 1993]. In the same studies, meshes seeded with cells were implanted in nude mice and recovered at different time following implantation. Implants excised at the 7-week time point consisted almost entirely of cartilage-like tissue with an overall shape similar to that of the original synthetic matrix. Histochemical analysis of the specimens revealed the presence of type II collagen and sulfated glycosaminoglycans at week 7 and later.

Angiogenesis may be necessary if there is cell growth in the reconstructed tissue after implantation. Because open matrices are mainly used to reconstruct these tissues, the host's capillaries can migrate into the implant. The presence of angiogenic factors (e.g., heparin-binding growth factor-1) may be used to improve the kinetics of implant vascularization [Thompson, 1989]. Genetically modified cells have been used to provide stable long-term release of angiogenic factors by the implant [Eming et al., 1995].

8.4 Reconstruction of Epithelial or Endothelial Surfaces

Cells Embedded in Extracellular Matrix Materials

A simple way to maintain certain epithelial cells in a three-dimensional matrix is to seed them in gels or meshes in a similar manner as connective tissues are constructed. For example, hepatocytes can be maintained in the same mesh-type matrices made of biodegradable materials used to create bioartificial cartilage [Cima, 1991]. In this configuration, hepatocytes have a tendency to aggregate; such aggregates (sometimes called organoids) are known to contain cells which have maintained their phenotypic stability [Koide, 1990]. However, this process may be somewhat limited unless the aggregate size can be controlled to prevent the formation of large aggregates with anoxic cores. Also, this method may not be used to produce continuous epithelial cell sheets.

Culture on a Single Surface

Bioartificial vascular grafts have been produced by seeding endothelial cells on the luminal surface of small diameter (6 mm or less) synthetic vascular grafts. These prostheses have given poor results because of inflammatory responses at the anastomotic sites and the poor retention of the seeded endothelium under *in vivo* conditions. A more intrinsically biocompatible approach to vascular graft production is to reproduce more closely the organization of actual blood vessels. For instance, a bioartificial media has been produced by embedding vascular smooth muscle cells in a collagen gel annulus, and the intima re-established by seeding endothelial cells on the inside surface of the gel [Weinberg, 1986].

A dermal equivalent consisting of fibroblasts embedded in collagen has been used to support a stratified layer of human keratinocytes [Parenteau, 1991]. Exposure to air induces the terminal differentiation of the keratinocytes near the air-liquid interface, which is characterized by the formation of tight cell-cell contacts and cornified envelopes. The resulting bioartificial skin has a morphological and biochemical organization very similar to that of real skin including a stratum corneum which exhibits a high resistance to chemical damage. This type of bioartificial skin has been tested successfully in animals, but acceptance of allogeneic skin grafts remains problematic in humans, which means that the production of grafts requires that both fibroblasts and keratinocytes be obtained from the patient and propagated *in vitro*.

Culture in a Sandwich Configuration

This culture technique has been successfully used to maintain hepatocyte polarity and function *in vitro*. Hepatocytes are first plated on a single gel of collagen and then a top layer of type I collagen is placed on the cells after 1 day in culture. The resulting extracellular geometry closely mimics that found *in vivo* and maintains a wide spectrum of liver-specific functions, including protein secretion (e.g., albumin, transferrin, and fibrinogen), detoxification (e.g., cytochrome P450-dependent pathways) for up to 6 to 8 weeks [Dunn, 1991].

8.5 Bioreactor Design in Tissue Engineering

A bioreactor is a system containing a large number of cells that transform an input of reactants into an output of products. Bioreactors have been designed primarily for use as bioartificial liver or pancreas, and more recently for the production of blood cells from hematopoietic tissue. These systems require the maintenance of the function of a large number of cells in a small volume. For example, a hypothetical bioartificial liver device possessing 10% of the detoxification and protein synthesis capacity of the normal human liver (a rough estimate of the minimum processing and secretory capacities that can meet a human body's demands) would contain a total of 10^{10} adult hepatocytes. Thus, to keep the total bioreactor volume within reasonable limits (1 l or less), 10^7 cells/ml or more are required. For comparison, the normal human liver contains approximately 10^8 hepatocytes/ml. Two main types of bioreactor design have been considered in tissue engineering: (1) hollow fiber systems and (2) microcarrier systems.

Hollow Fiber Systems

Hollow fiber systems consist of a shell traversed by a large number of small-diameter tubes. The cells may be placed within the fibers in the intracapillary space or on the shell side in the extracapillary space. The compartment which does not contain the cells is generally perfused with culture medium or the patient's plasma or blood. The fiber walls may provide the attaching surface for the cells and/or act as barrier against the immune system of the host. Some of these systems are essentially designed to be implanted as vascular shunts, but may also be perfused with the patient's blood or plasma extracorporeally.

For the selection of fiber dimensions, spacing, and reactor length, the reader is referred to previously published experimental and theoretical studies [Chresand, 1988; Piret, 1991]. If the pressure gradient across the fiber length is sufficiently high and relatively permeable fibers are used, the pressure difference between the inlet and outlet induces convective flow (called Starling flow) across the fiber wall and through the shell compartement [Kelsey, 1990; Pillarella, 1990]. The maintenance of Starling flow in implanted hollow fiber devices is contingent upon the prevention of a gradual decrease in fiber permeability due to protein deposition over time on the fiber walls, which may difficult to achieve with fluids containing high levels of proteins such as plasma.

There are several reports in the literature describing the use of hollow fiber systems in the development of a bioartificial pancreas [Colton, 1991; Ramírez, 1992]. Most designs place the islets on the shell side, while perfusing the fibers with the animal's plasma or blood. Recent studies using implantable devices connected to the vascular system of the patient have given some encouraging results [Sullivan, 1991], but it appears that none of the pancreatic islet devices tested to date has shown long-term function in a reproducible manner. It is interesting to note that none of the studies involving pancreatic islets encapsulated in hollow fiber systems has recognized that oxygen transport can be severely compromised within the isolated islets alone, resulting in a substantial reduction in the insulin secretion capacity of the islets in response to glucose changes [Dionne, 1993].

It may be advantageous to place cells in the lumen of small fibers because the diffusional distance between the shell (where the nutrient supply would be) and the cells is essentially equal to the fiber diameter, which is easier to control than the inter-fiber distance. In one configuration, cells have been suspended in a collagen solution and injected into the lumen of fibers where the collagen is allowed to gel. Contraction of the collagen lattice by the cells creates a void in the intraluminal space [Scholz, 1991]. Such a configuration has been described for the construction of a bioartificial liver using adult hepatocytes [Nyberg, 1993]. It has been further proposed that the lumen be perfused with culture medium containing the appropriate hormones for cell maintenance while the patient's plasma would flow on the shell side.

Microcarrier-Based Systems

Microcarriers are small beads (usually less than 500 μm in diameter) with surfaces treated to support cell attachment. The surface area available per microcarrier can be increased by using porous microcarriers, where cells can migrate and proliferate within the porous matrix as well as on the microcarrier surface. Porous ceramic beads have been used to support a rat cell line transfected with the human proinsulin gene [Park, 1993]; under certain conditions intraparticle flow significantly enhances mass transport (especially that of oxygen) to the cells in the beads [Stephanopoulos, 1989].

Maintaining a constant number of microcarriers while increasing the number of cells increases the surface coverage of the microcarriers as long as the concentration of nutrients (especially oxygen) is not limiting. With the adult rat hepatocyte-Cytodex 3 microcarrier system, we observed that sufficient supply of oxygen to the hepatocytes is required for the efficient attachment (approximately 90%) of cells to microcarriers. A simple oxygen diffusion-reaction model indicated that a cell surface oxygen partial pressure greater than 0.1 mmHg was needed [Foy, 1993].

Two bioreactor configurations using microcarriers may find potential use in tissue engineering: (1) packed or fluidized bed, and (2) microcarriers incorporated in hollow fiber cartridges. A packed bed of microcarriers consists of a column filled with microcarriers with porous plates at the inlet and outlet of the column to allow perfusion while preventing microcarrier entrainment by the flow. Total flow rate is mainly dependent on cell number and the nutrient uptake rate of the cells. Reactor volume is proportional to the microcarrier diameter. From that point of view, it is therefore advantageous to reduce the microcarrier size as much as possible. However, packed beds with small beads may be potentially more prone to clogging and the cells may have tendency to accumulate in the channels between the microcarrier surfaces. The aspect ratio of the bed (height/diameter) is adjusted so that the magnitude of fluid mechanical forces (proportional to the aspect ratio) within the bed is below damaging levels. Given a fixed flow rate and microcarrier diameter, decreasing column diameter increases fluid velocity, and therefore increases the shear stress at the surface of the microcarriers and cells, with potential mechanical damage to cells. On the other hand, low aspect ratios may be difficult to perfuse evenly. Fluidized beds differ from packed beds in that the perfusing fluid motion maintains the microcarriers in suspension [Runstadler, 1988].

Packed bed systems have been used to support high densities (5×10^8 cells/ml) of anchorage-dependent cell lines seeded on microporous microcarriers (589 to 850 µm in diameter) [Park, 1993]. In addition, packed beads (1.5 mm diameter) have been used to entrap aggregates of hepatocytes. This system was shown to maintain a relatively stable level of albumin secretion (a liver-specific product) for up to 3 weeks [Li, 1993].

Microcarriers have also been used as a way to provide an attachment surface for anchorage-dependent cells introduced in the shell side of hollow fiber devices, as in the case of a hollow fiber bioartificial liver device [Demetriou, 1986]. A flat bed device, which is in principle similar to a hollow fiber system (cells are separated from the circulating medium by a membrane), for the maintenance of cultured human bone marrow at high densities on porous microcarriers has been recently described [Palsson, 1993].

References

Banes AJ. 1993. Mechanical strain and the mammalian cell. In JA Frangos (ed), *Physical Forces and the Mammalian Cell*, pp. 81-123. San Diego, Academic Press.

Bell E, Ivarsson B, Merill C. 1979. Production of a tissue-like structure by contraction of collagen lattices by human fibroblasts of different proliferative potential *in vitro*. *Proc. Natl. Acad. Sci. U.S.A.* 76: 1274.

Bhatia SN, Toner M, Tompkins RG, Yarmush ML. 1994. Selective adhesion of hepatocytes on patterned surfaces *in vitro*. *Ann. N.Y. Acad. Sci.* 745: 187.

Bhatia SN, Balis UJ, Yarmush ML, Toner M. 1998. Microfabrication of hepatocyte/fibroblast co-cultures: Role of homotypic cell interactions. *Biotechnol. Prog.* 14: 378.

Bruckner P, Hoerler I, Mendler M, Houze Y, Winterhalter KA, Eich-Bender SG, Spycher MA. 1989. Induction and prevention of chondrocyte hypertrophy in culture. *J. Cell Biol.* 109: 2537.

Buschmann MD, Gluzband YA, Grodzinsky AJ, Kimura JH, Hunziker EB. 1992. Chondrocytes in agarose culture synthesize a mechanically functional extracellular matrix. *J. Orthop. Res.* 10: 745.

Chresand TJ, Gillies RJ, Dale BE. 1988. Optimum fiber spacing in a hollow fiber bioreactor. *Biotechnol. Bioeng.* 32: 983.

Cima LG, Vacanti JP, Vacanti C, Ingber D, Mooney D, Langer R. 1991. Tissue engineering by cell transplantation using degradable polymer substrates. *J. Biomech. Eng.* 113: 143.

Colton CK, Avgoustiniatos ES. 1991. Bioengineering in development of the hybrid artificial pancreas. *J. Biomech. Eng.* 113: 152.

Demetriou A, Chowdhury NR, Michalski S, Whiting J, Schechner R, Feldman D, Levenson SM, Chowdhury JR. 1986. New method of hepatocyte transplantation and extracorporeal liver support. *Ann. Surg.* 204: 259.

Dionne KE, Colton CK, Yarmush ML. 1993. Effect of hypoxia on insulin secretion by isolated rat and canine islets of Langherans. *Diabetes.* 42: 12.

Dunn JCY, Tompkins RG, Yarmush ML. 1991. Long-term *in vitro* function of adult hepatocytes in a collagen sandwich configuration. *Biotechnol. Prog.* 7: 237.

Eming SA, Lee J, Snow RG, Tompkins RG, Yarmush ML, Morgan JR. 1995. Genetically modified human epidermis overexpressing PDGF-A directs the development of a cellular and vascular connective tissue stroma when transplanted to athymic mice. Implications for the use of genetically modified keratinocytes to modulate dermal generation. *J. Invest. Dermatol.* 105: 756.

Ezzell RM, Toner M, Hendricks K, Dunn JCY, Tompkins RG, Yarmush ML. 1993. Effect of collagen configuration on the cytoskeleton in cultured rat hepatocytes. *Exp. Cell Res.* 208: 442.

Fleischaker RJ Jr, Sinskey AJ. 1981. Oxygen demand and supply in culture. *Eur. J. Appl. Microbiol. Biotechnol.* 12: 193.

Foy BD, Lee J, Morgan J, Toner M, Tompkins RG, Yarmush ML. 1993. Optimization of hepatocyte attachment to microcarriers: importance of oxygen. *Biotechnol. Bioeng.* 42: 579.

Freed LE, Marquis JC, Nohria A, Emmanual J, Mikos AG, Langer R. 1993. Neocartilage formation *in vitro* and *in vivo* using cells cultured on synthetic biodegradable polymers. *J. Biomed. Mater. Res.* 27: 11.

Girard PR, Helmlinger G, Nerem RM. 1993. Shear stress effects on the morphology and cytomatrix of cultured vascular endothelial cells. In JA Frangos (ed), *Physical Forces and the Mammalian Cell*, pp. 193-222. San Diego, Academic Press.

Grinnell F, Feld MK. 1981. Adsorption characteristics of plasma fibronectin in relationship to biological activity. *J. Biomed. Mater. Res.* 15: 363.

Guido S, Tranquillo RT. 1993. A methodology for the systematic and quantitative study of cell contact guidance in oriented collagen gels. *J. Cell Sci.* 105: 317.

Kelsey LJ, Pillarella MR, Zydney AL. 1990. Theoretical analysis of convective flow profiles in a hollow-fiber membrane bioreactor. *Chem. Eng. Sci.* 45: 3211.

Koide N, Sakaguchi K, Koide Y, Asano K, Kawaguchi M, Matsushima H, Takenami T, Shinji T, Mori M, Tsuji T. 1990. Formation of multicellular spheroids composed of adult rat hepatocytes in dishes with positively charged surfaces and under other nonadherent environments. *Exp. Cell Res.* 186: 227.

Kuhlenschmidt MS, Schmell E, Slife CF, Kuhlenschmidt TB, Sieber F, Lee YC, Roseman S. 1982. Studies on the intercellular adhesion of rat and chicken hepatocytes. Conditions affecting cell-cell specificity. *J. Biol. Chem.* 257: 3157.

L'Heureux N, Pâquet S, Labbé R, Germain L, Auger FA. 1998. A completely biological tissue-engineered human blood vessel. *FASEB J.* 12: 47.

Li AP, Barker G, Beck D, Colburn S, Monsell R, Pellegrin C. 1993. Culturing of primary hepatocytes as entrapped aggregates in a packed bed bioreactor: a potential bioartificial liver. *In Vitro Cell. Dev. Biol.* 29A: 249.

Lindblad WJ, Schuetz EG, Redford KS, Guzelian PS. 1991. Hepatocellular phenotype *in vitro* is influenced by biphysical features of the collagenous substratum. *Hepatology.* 13: 282.

Madri JA, Williams SK. 1983. Capillary endothelial cell cultures: phenotypic modulation by matrix components. *J. Cell Biol.* 97: 153.

Martz E, Phillips HM, Steinberg MS. 1974. Contact inhibition of overlapping and differential cell adhesion: a sufficient model for the control of certain cell culture morphologies. *J. Cell Sci.* 16: 401.

Massia SP, Hubbell JA. 1990. Covalently attached GRGD on polymer surfaces promotes biospecific adhesion of mammalian cells. *Ann. N.Y. Acad. Sci.* 589: 261.

Matsuda T, Sugawara T, Inoue K. 1992. Two-dimensional cell manipulation technology. An artificial neural circuit based on surface microphotoprocessing. *ASAIO J.* 38: M243.

Montesano R, Orci L, Vassalli P. 1983. *In vitro* rapid organization of endothelial cells into capillary-like networks is promoted by collagen matrices. *J. Cell Biol.* 97: 1648.

Mooney D, Hansen L, Vacanti J, Langer R, Farmer S, Ingber D. 1992. Switching from differentiation to growth in hepatocytes: control by extracellular matrix. *J. Cell. Physiol.* 151: 497.

Nose A, Nagafuchi A, Takeichi M. 1988. Expressed recombinant cadherins mediate cell sorting in model systems. *Cell.* 54: 993.

Nyberg SL, Shatford RA, Peshwa MV, White JG, Cerra FB, Hu W-S. 1993. Evaluation of a hepatocyte-entrapment hollow fiber bioreactor: a potential bioartificial liver. *Biotechnol. Bioeng.* 41: 194.

Palsson BO, Paek S-H, Schwartz RM, Palsson M, Lee G-M, Silver S, Emerson SG. 1993. Expansion of human bone marrow progenitor cells in a high cell density continuous perfusion system. *Bio/Technology.* 11: 368.

Parenteau NL, Nolte CM, Bilbo P, Rosenberg M, Wilkins LM, Johnson EW, Watson S, Mason VS, Bell E. 1991. Epidermis generated *in vitro*: practical considerations and applications. *J. Cell. Biochem.* 45: 245.

Park S, Stephanopoulos G. 1993. Packed bed bioreactor with porous ceramic beads for animal cell culture. *Biotechnol. Bioeng.* 41: 25.

Pillarella MR, Zydney AL. 1990. Theoretical analysis of the effect of convective flow on solute transport and insulin release in a hollow fiber bioartificial pancreas. *J. Biomech. Eng.* 112: 220.

Piret JM, Cooney CL. 1991. Model of oxygen transport limitations in hollow fiber bioreactors. *Biotechnol. Bioeng.* 37: 80.

Ramírez CA, López M, Stephens CL. 1992. *In vitro* perfusion of hybrid artificial pancreas devices at low flow rates. *ASAIO J.* 38: M443.

Rotem A, Toner M, Bhatia S, Foy BD, Tompkins RG, Yarmush ML. 1994. Oxygen is a factor determining *in vitro* tissue assembly: effects on attachment and spreading of hepatocytes. *Biotechnol. Bioeng.* 43: 654.

Runstadler PW, Cerneck SR. 1988. Large-scale fluidized-bed, immobilized cultivation of animal cells at high densities. In *Animal Cell Biotechnology*, pp. 306-320. London, Academic Press.

Scholz M, Hu WS. 1991. A two-compartment cell entrapment bioreactor with three different holding times for cells, high and low molecular weight compounds. *Cytotechnology.* 4: 127.

Singhvi R, Kumar A, Lopez GP, Stephanopoulos GN, Wang DIC, Whitesides GM, Ingber DE. 1994. Engineering cell shape and function. *Science.* 264: 696.

Stephanopoulos GN, Tsiveriotis K. 1989. The effect of intraparticle convection on nutrient transport in porous biological pellets. *Chem. Eng. Sci.* 44: 2031.

Stefanovich P, Matthew HWT, Toner M, Tompkins RG, Yarmush ML. 1996. Extracorporeal perfusion of cultured hepatocytes: Effect of intermittent perfusion on hepatocyte function and morphology. *J. Surg. Res.* 66: 57.

Sullivan SJ, Maki T, Borland KM, Mahoney MD, Solomon BA, Muller TE, Monaco AP, Chick WL. 1991. Biohybrid artificial pancreas: long-term implantation studies in diabetic, pancreatomized dogs. *Science.* 252: 718.

Thompson JA, Haudenschild CC, Anderson KD, DiPietro JM, Anderson WF, Maciag T. 1989. Heparin-binding growth factor 1 induces the formation of organoid neovascular structures in vivo. *Proc. Natl. Acad. Sci. U.S.A.* 86: 7928.

Tranquillo RT, Durrani MA, Moon AG. 1992. Tissue engineering science: consequences of cell traction force. *Cytotechnology.* 10: 225.

Weinberg CB, Bell E. 1986. A blood vessel model constructed from collagen and cultured vascular cells. _Science._ 230: 669.

Wiseman LL, Steinberg MS, Phillips HM. 1972. Experimental modulation of intercellular cohesiveness: reversal of tissue assembly patterns. _Dev. Biol._ 28: 498.

Yarmush ML, Toner M, Dunn JCY, Rotem A, Hubel A, Lee J, Tompkins RG. 1992. Hepatic tissue engineering: development of critical technologies. _Ann. N.Y. Acad. Sci._ 21: 472.

Further Information

Books, reviews and special issues of scientific and engineering journals on tissue engineering which may be of interest to the reader are listed below.

Morgan JR, Yarmush ML (eds). 1999. _Tissue Engineering Methods and Protocols._ Totowa, NJ, Humana Press.

Lanza RP, Langer RS. 1997. _Principles of Tissue Engineering._ San Diego, Academic Press.

Special issue on tissue engineering. 1996. _Biomaterials,_ 17(2-3).

Vacanti CA, Mikos AG (eds). 1995. _Tissue Engineering._ The official journal of the Tissue Engineering Society. Larchmont, NY, Mary Ann Liebert, Inc.

Silver FH. 1995. _Biomaterials, Medical Devices, and Tissue Engineering: An Integrated Approach._ London, Chapman & Hall.

Special issue on tissue engineering. 1995. _Ann. Biomed. Eng.,_ 43(7 and 8).

Special issue on tissue engineering. 1994. _Biotechnol. Bioeng.,_ 43(7 and 8).

Berthiaume F, Toner M, Tompkins RG, Yarmush ML. 1993. Tissue engineering. In _Implantation Biology: the Response of the Host,_ Boca Raton, FL, CRC Press, 363-386.

Special issue on tissue engineering. 1992. _Cytotechnology,_ 10(3).

Special issue on tissue engineering. 1991. _J. Biomech. Eng.,_ 113(2).

Special issue on tissue engineering. 1991. _J. Cell Biochem.,_ 45(4-5).

9

Surface Immobilization of Adhesion Ligands for Investigations of Cell-Substrate Interactions

Paul D. Drumheller
Gore Hybrid Technologies, Inc.

Jeffrey A. Hubbell
California Institute of Technology

The interaction between cells and surfaces plays a major biologic role in cellular behavior. Cell membrane receptors responsible for adhesion may influence cell physiology in numerous ways. Examples of these interactions are the rolling and activation of leukocytes on vascular endothelium, the spatial differentiation of embryonic basement membranes in development, the extension of neurites on adhesion proteins, the proliferation of cells induced by mitogenic factors, and the spreading and recruitment of platelets onto the vascular subendothelium. These and other cell-surface interactions influence or control many aspects of cell physiology, such as adhesion, spreading, activation, recruitment, migration, proliferation, and differentiation.

There is great interest in understanding cell-surface interactions. This understanding is paramount to the development of pharmaceutical compounds to enhance or inhibit cell-substrate interactions, such as agents to enhance cell adhesion for tissue regeneration or biomaterials integration or to reduce cell adhesion in metastasis or fibrosis. In the emerging area of tissue engineering, the adhesion of cells to a culture support is essential for many products such as biohybrid dermal dressings, synthetic articular cartilage, and hepatocyte scaffolds. Investigations of cell-surface interactions are central to many areas of biomedicine and bioengineering, including tissue engineering, biomaterials design, immunology, oncology, hematology, and developmental biology.

To examine the interactions of cells with substrates and how they may influence cell behavior, simplified models that simulate basement membranes, cell surfaces, or extracellular matrices have been developed. These models involve the immobilization of biologically active ligands of natural and synthetic origin onto various substrates to produce chemically defined bioactive surfaces. Ligands that have been immobilized include cell-membrane receptor fragments, antibiotics, adhesion peptides, enzymes, adhesive carbohydrates, lectins, membrane lipids, and glycosaminoglycan matrix components. Functionalized two-dimensional surfaces are important tools to elucidate the molecular mechanisms of cell-mediated bioadhesion.

Techniques for preparing these ligand-functionalized two-dimensional substrates for investigation of cell adhesion are similar to methods for labeling ligands, preparing immunomatrices, or immobilizing enzymes. This brief tutorial review will focus primarily on schemes for immobilizing bioactive ligands specifically for purposes of investigating cell-surface interactions. Topics that will be addressed include (1) general considerations of bioconjugation; (2) examples of surface bioconjugation; (3) preparation of surfaces for ligand immobilization; (4) examples of ligand-containing copolymers; (5) techniques for characterizing these surfaces; and (6) examples of applications of surface immobilized ligands in cell-substrate investigations.

9.1 General Considerations

Numerous reviews are available that describe the chemistry of ligand conjugation and immobilization, and the reader is encouraged to consult them for more detailed descriptions [1–12]. When immobilizing ligands for the preparation of cell-adhesive substrates, several factors must be considered to retain maximum bioactivity. Ligand surface immobilization may proceed in low yields due to sterically inaccessible reactive sites on the ligand molecule; the immobilized ligand may not have optimum cell-receptor interactions due to physical constraints imposed by the surface or by the active site being buried; or the immobilized ligand may be partially denatured upon immobilization. The inclusion of spacer arms on the surface may help relieve these limitations [13]. If the ligand has a directionality, then the cell adhesive response may vary depending upon the orientation of the immobilized ligand [14, 15] or upon the length of the spacer arm [16].

Ligands have been physicochemically absorbed onto polymeric substrates to investigate cell-surface interactions. The advantage of covalently immobilizing a ligand is that a chemical bond is present to prevent desorption. The general chemical scheme for grafting a ligand onto a surface is shown in Fig. 9.1. Activation usually is a necessary step to produce highly reactive species to enable surface immobilization under mild conditions. Typically the surface is activated, since the chemical steps are somewhat simpler than for ligand activation, but each strategy may have its own advantages and limitations.

The activation of ligands may require suitable protective schemes to prevent homopolymerization or cross-linking if these competing reactions are not desired. Ligands may also be activated at more than one site, some of which may remain unconsumed after coupling is complete and have biological activity. In contrast, the activation of surfaces usually does not require protective schemes; nonetheless, activated surfaces may contain unconsumed sites after immobilization that may require deactivation so as not to influence cell-mediated adhesive responses.

Because most ligands immobilized for cell-surface studies are biologic in origin, water is often the only choice of solvent as the coupling medium. Water is nucleophilic, and hydrolysis can be a competing reaction during activation and coupling, especially at higher pH (>9–10). To reduce hydrolysis, surfaces are commonly activated in nonaqueous solvents; ligands are then coupled using concentrated aqueous solutions (>1 mg/ml) for extended periods (>12 h). Some ligands are soluble in polar solvents such as dimethylsulfoxide (DMSO), dimethylformamide (DMF), acetone, dioxane, or ethanol, or their aqueous cosolvents, and these combinations may be used to reduce hydrolysis during coupling.

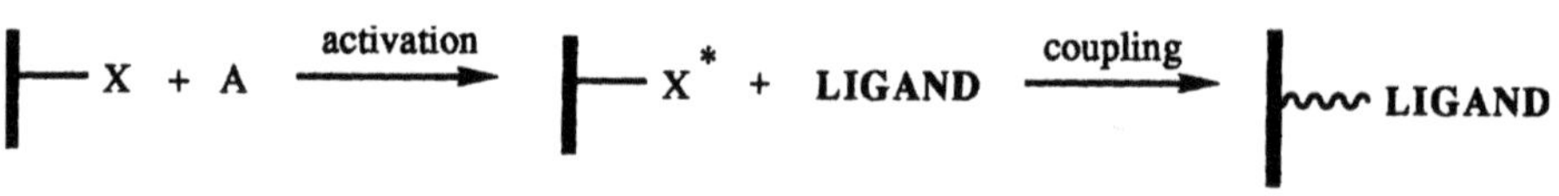

FIGURE 9.1   General chemical scheme for grafting a ligand onto a surface.

9.2   Surface Bioconjugation

The typical chemical groups involved in immobilizing ligands for cell-surface studies are hydroxyls, amines, carboxylic acids, and thiols. Other groups, such as amides, disulfides, phenols, guanidines, thioethers, indoles, and imidazoles, have also been modified, but these will not be described.

Hydroxyls and carboxylic acids are commonly activated to produce more reactive agents for ligand acylation. Elimination is a possible competing reaction for secondary and aryl alcohols. Primary amines, present on many biologic ligands from N-amino acid termini and lysine, are good nucleophiles when unprotonated ($pK_a \sim 9$); moderately basic pH (8–10) ensures their reactivity. Thiols, present on cysteine ($pK_a \sim 8.5$), are stronger nucleophiles than amines, and as such they can be selectively coupled in the presence of amines at lower pH (5–7). Sulhydryl groups often exist as their disulfide form and may be reduced to free thiols using mild agents such as dithiothreitol.

The following paragraphs review activation schemes for particular chemical groups present on the surface, giving brief coupling schemes. Due to the advantages of surface versus ligand activation, only general methods involving surface activation will be discussed.

Immobilization to Surface Alcohols

A hydroxyl-bearing surface may be activated with numerous reagents to produce more reactive species for substitution, the most common example being the cyanogen bromide activation of cellulose and agarose derivatives [2–5, 11, 17]. Due to problems with high volatility of the cyanogen bromide, sensitivity of the activated species to hydrolysis, competing reactions during activation and coupling, and the desire to use culture substrates other than polysaccharides, other activation schemes have been developed for more defined activation and coupling. These schemes have been used to modify functionalized glasses and polymers for cell-mediated adhesion studies.

Alcohols react with sulfonyl halides [18–25], carbonyldiimidazole [26, 27], succinimidyl chloroformate [28], epoxides [29, 30], isocyanates [31–33], and heterocyclic [34, 35] and alkyl halides [21]. Activation of surface alcohols with these agents can be performed in organic solvents such as acetonitrile, methylene chloride, acetone, benzene, dioxane, diethyl ether, toluene, or DMF.

Reactive Esters

Alcohols can be activated to reactive sulfonic ester leaving groups by reaction with sulfonyl halides [18–25] (Fig. 9.2) such as *p*-toluenesulfonyl chloride (tosyl chloride), trifluoroethanesulfonyl chloride (tresyl chloride), methanesulfonyl chloride (mesyl chloride), or fluorobenzenesulfonyl chloride (fosyl chloride). The resulting sulfonic esters are readily displaced in mild aqueous conditions with amines or thiols to produce amino- or thioether-bound ligands. Aryl alcohols should not be activated in this manner, since the sulfonate group may irreversibly transfer to the aromatic nucleus [36]. Sulfonic esters differ in their ease of nucleophilic substitution and resistance to hydrolysis, tosyl esters being low in coupling potential [23] and fosyl esters being high in hydrolysis resistance [24]. Activation can be performed in many organic solvents that are properly dry: trace water and other species such as ammonia will react. DMSO should not be used as a solvent, as it will react with sulfonyl halides. A tert-amino base such as pyridine, dimethylaminopyridine, triethylamine, diisopropylethyl amine, or ethylmorpholine can be added in equimolar amounts to serve as a nucleophilic catalyst and to combine with the liberated HCl. It has been suggested that hydroxyls be converted to alkoxides prior to sulfonic ester activation in the presence of ethers as they may be sensitive to the HCl generated during activation [25].

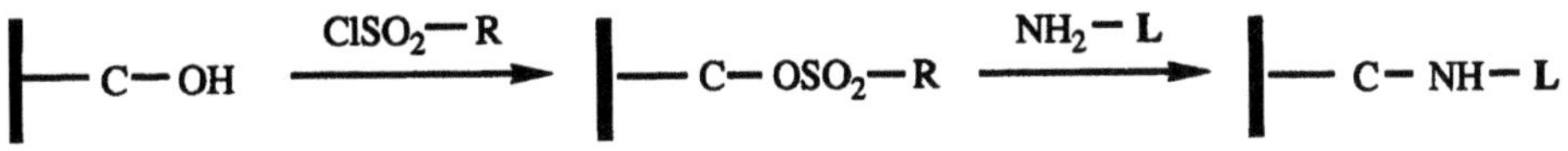

FIGURE 9.2   Alcohols can be activated with sulfonyl halides, which are readily displaced with amine- (shown) or thiol-containing (not shown) ligands.

An alcohol-containing surface is typically incubated with the sulfonyl halide for 0.5–6.0 h. Any precipitated salts can be rinsed away with 1 mM HCl. The ligand is coupled to the surface for 12–24 h in borate or carbonate buffer (pH 9–10) at a concentration of 1 mg/ml. Coupling can proceed at more mild pH (~7) with more concentrated solutions (>10 mg ligand/ml) or with thiol-bearing ligands. Excess sulfonic esters can be displaced with aqueous solutions (10–50 mM, pH = 8–9) of tris(hydroxymethyl)aminomethane, aminoethanol, glycine, or mercaptoethanol, or by hydrolysis.

Other Acylating Agents

Surface hydroxyls may be activated to groups other than sulfonic esters. Alcohols react readily with carbonyldiimidazole [26, 27] (Fig. 9.3) and succinimidyl chloroformate [28] (Fig. 9.4) to produce reactive imidazole-N-carboxylates and succinimidyl carbonates, respectively. These species acylate amines to urethane linkages. Activation typically proceeds in organic solvent for 2–6 h. Dimethylaminopyridine catalyzes formation of the succinimidyl carbonate. Amine-bearing ligands (>10 mg/ml) are coupled to the surface in borate or phosphate buffer (pH 8–9) for 12–24 h, or 4°C, 2–3 days. Thiol-bearing groups may also be immobilized onto these activated groups; however, the thiocarbamate linkage can be sensitive to hydrolysis and may not be generally applicable to preparing well-defined substrates for long-term biologic investigations.

Bifunctional Bridges

In lieu of alcohol conversion to activated reaction groups, the hydroxyl may be added to homo- or heterobifunctional bridges, wherein alcholysis consumes one terminus to produce newly functionalized surfaces (Figure 9.5). Epoxide bridges can be added to surface-bound alcohols in aqueous base (to reduce hydrolysis or polymerization of the epoxide, 10–100 mM NaOH) or in organic solvent, 12 h. Isocyanate bridges are added to surface alcohols in organic solvents with organotin catalysts (such as dibutyltin dilaurate), 12 h. Halo alkylation of surface-bound alcohols or alkoxides proceeds in organic solvents, 2–3 days, or with heat (~80°C), 12 h. The unconsumed free group (isocyanate, epoxide, or alkyl halide) is substituted with amine- or thiol-bearing ligands in buffered aqueous conditions, pH 8–10, 1–10 mg/ml, 12–24 h. Hydroxyl-bearing ligands, such as carbohydrates, can be coupled in aqueous DMSO, dioxane, or DMF, 12–24 h, 60–80°C. Hydroxyl coupling may also be performed in aqueous base (10–100 mM NaOH) for ligands that are resistant to ester or amide hydrolysis, such as mono- or polysaccharides.

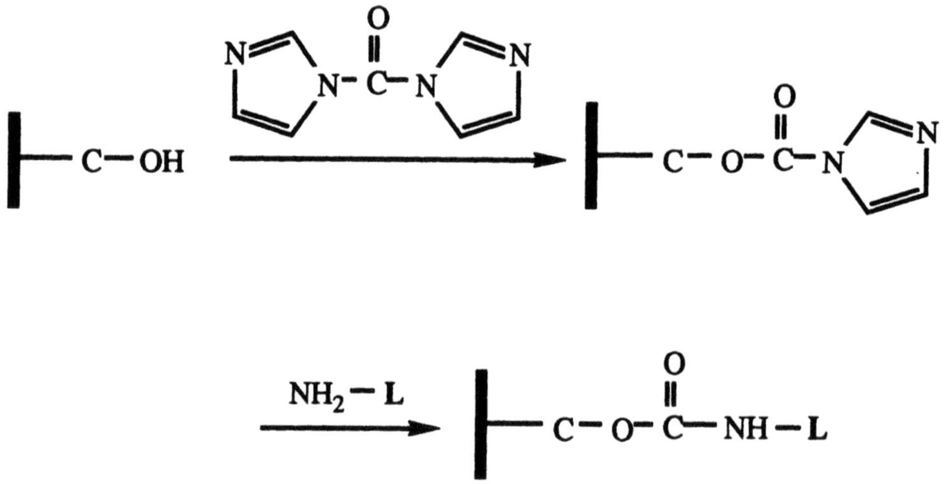

FIGURE 9.3 Alcohols react readily with carbonyldiimidazole to produce reactive imidazole-N-carboxylates for coupling to amine-containing ligands.

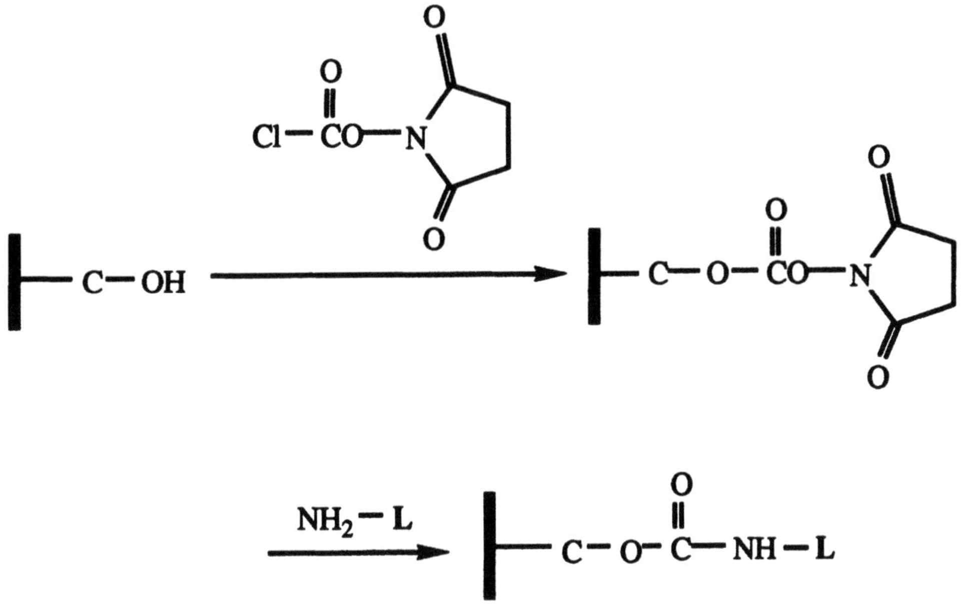

FIGURE 9.4 Alcohols react readily with succinimidyl chloroformate to produce a succinimidyl carbonate for coupling to amine-containing ligands.

Heterocyclic aryl halides, such as cyanuric chloride [34, 35], react with free hydroxyl groups in polar solvents containing sodium carbonate, 40–50°C, 30 min. Amine-bearing ligands are immobilized to the surface in borate buffer, pH 9, 1–10 mg/ml, 5–10°C, 12–24 h.

Immobilization to Surface Carboxylic Acids

Acids may be converted to activated leaving groups by reaction with carbodiimides [36]. The generated O-acylureas react with amines to produce amide linkages and can react with alcohols to produce ester linkages with acid or base catalysts. An undesirable competing reaction is urea rearrangement to nonre-active N-acylurea; this effect may be accelerated in aprotic polar solvents such as DMF but is reduced at low temperatures (0–10°C) or by the addition of agents such as hydroxybenztriazole to convert the O-acylurea to benztriazole derivatives. Acids may also be activated with carbonyldiimidizole to produce easily amino- and alcoholyzed imidazolide intermediates; however, imidazolides are highly susceptible to hydrolysis and necessitate anhydrous conditions for activation and coupling [37].

Water-soluble carbodiimides such as ethyl(dimethylaminopropyl)-carbodiimide (EDC) can be used in either aqueous or organic media for the immobilization of ligands to produce bioactive substrates [20, 38, 39]. To reduce hydrolysis of the O-acylurea, conversion to more resistant succinimidyl esters can be performed using EDC and N-hydroxysuccinimide or its water-soluble sulfonate derivative, and base catalysts (Fig. 9.6). Alternatively, the acid may be converted directly to a succinimidyl ester via reaction with tetramethyl(succinimido)uronium tetrafluoroborate [40, 41]. The activation of surface-bound carboxylic acids with EDC in organic media (ethanol, DMF, dioxane) is complete with 1–2 h at 0–10°C;

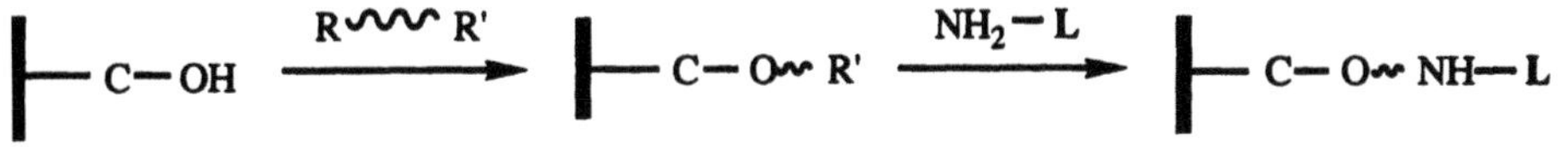

FIGURE 9.5 Bifunctional coupling agents may be used, e.g., to couple an amine-containing ligand to a hydroxyl-containing surface via a spacer.

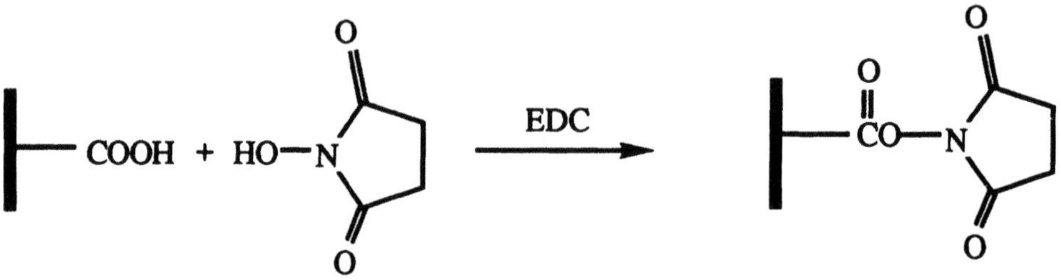

FIGURE 9.6 Carboxylated surfaces can be achieved to succinimidyl esters to subsequently couple amine-containing ligands.

in aqueous media at pH 4–6, 0–5°C, 0.5–2 h. Amine-bearing ligands may be coupled onto the surface in buffered media, pH 7.5–9, 1 mg/ml, 2–24 h. Since the reaction of carbodiimides with amines is slow compared to reaction with acids, activation and coupling may proceed simultaneously [42] by including amine-bearing ligands (1–10 mg/ml) with the EDC and allowing coupling to proceed in buffered media, pH 5–7, 0–10°C, 12–24 h, or 25–30°C, 4–6 h. Acid dehydration directly to succinimidyl esters using tetramethyl(succinimido)uronium tetrafluoroborate is performed in anhydrous conditions with equimolar tert-amino base, 2–4 h, followed by coupling in aqueous organic cosolvents (water/DMF or water/dioxane), 1–10 mg/ml ligand, pH 8–9, 12–24 h.

Immobilization to Surface Amines

Primary and secondary amine-containing surfaces may be reacted with homo- or heterobifunctional bridges (Fig. 9.7). Amines are more nucleophilic than alcohols, they generally do not require the addition of catalysts, and their addition is faster. These bridges may contain isocyanates [31, 33], isothiocyanates [43], cyclic anhydrides [44], succinimidyl esters [45–47], or epoxides [48, 49].

Isocyanates add to amines with good efficiency but are susceptible to hydrolysis; epoxides and cyclic anhydrides are somewhat less reactive yet are still sensitive to hydrolysis. Hydrolysis-resistant diisothiocyanates have been used for many years to label ligands with reporter molecules; however, the thiourea linkage may be hydrolytically labile (especially at lower pH) and may be unsuitable for investigations of cell-surface interactions. Succinimidyl esters, although not as resistant to hydrolysis as isothiocyanates, have very good reactivity to amines and form stable amide linkages. Hydrolysis is all these reagents is accelerated at higher pH (≥ 9–10).

Coupling to surface-bound amines is performed in organic conditions (DMF, DMSO, acetone) for 1–3 h. Coupling of amine-bearing ligands onto immobilized bridges is performed in buffered media, pH 8–10.5, 2–12, 1–10 mg/ml. Excess reagent can be displaced with buffered solutions of tris(hydroxymethyl)aminomethane, aminoethanol, glycine, or mercaptoethanol, or hydrolysis.

Bifunctional aldehydes, such as glutaraldehyde and formaldehyde, have been used classically as cross-linkers for purposes of immunohistochemistry and ultrastructural investigations. They have been used also to couple ligands onto amine-bearing substrates [50–52]. Hydrolysis of aldehydes is usually not a concern, since the hydrolysis product, alkyl hydrate, is reversible back to the carbonyl. Amines add to aldehydes to produce imine linkages over a wide range of pH (6–10). These Schiff bases are potentially hydrolytically labile; reductive amination can be performed with mild reducing agents such as sodium

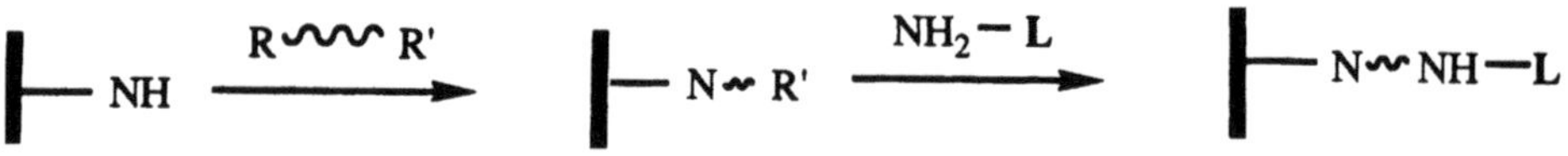

FIGURE 9.7 Primary and secondary amine-containing surfaces may be reacted with homo- or heterobifunctional bridges.

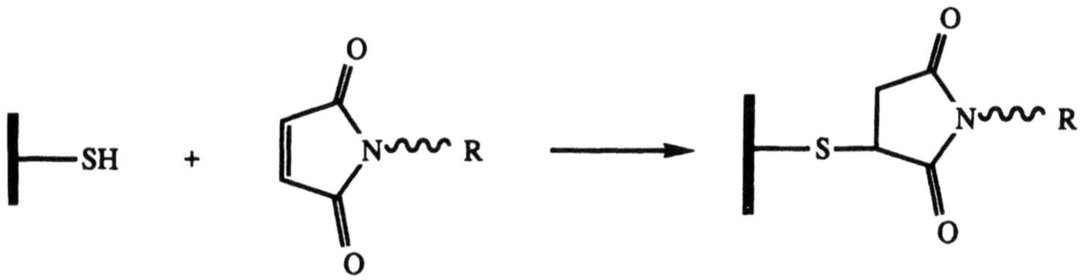

FIGURE 9.8 Thiol-containing surfaces may be coupled to malcimide activated species, either heterobifunctional linkers or ligands.

cyanoborohydride, pH 8–9, without substantial losses in ligand bioactivity [53]. Acetalization of poly-hydric alcohols may commence in the presence of Lewis acid catalysts followed by dehydrating the hemiacetal linkage, an acetal [54, 55]. The dehydration conditions (air-drying followed by 70–90°C, 2 h) may damage many biologic ligands.

Alkyl halide-bearing surfaces can be coupled to amine-bearing ligands [49, 56, 57]; their reaction is slower, but they are resistant to hydrolysis. Ligands can be immobilized in buffered medium (pH 9–10), 12–24 h, 1–10 mg/ml, or in organic medium. Heat may be used to increase yields (60–80°C).

Immobilization to Surface Thiols

Thiols are more nucleophilic than amines or alcohols and may be selectively coupled in their presence at more neutral pH. Thiols can be reacted with reagents that are not reactive toward amines, such as homo- or heterobifunctional maleimide bridges [32, 58–60]. Surface-bound thiols react with maleimides in acetone, methanol, DMF, etc., for 1–2 h, to produce a thioether linkage (Fig. 9.8). Thiol-bearing ligands can be immobilized to surface maleimides by incubating in mild buffered media, pH 5–7, 12–24 h, 1–10 mg/ml. More basic pH should be avoided as hydrolysis of the maleimide to nonreactive maleamic acid may occur.

Photoimmobilization

Surfaces can be modified using photoactivated heterobifunctional bridges in one of three schemes: (1) the bridge may be immobilized onto a functionalized surface, followed by photocoupling of the ligand onto the photoactivated group [58, 61]; (2) the reagent may be photocoupled onto the surface, followed by immobilization onto the free terminus [58, 62]; or (3) the ligand may be coupled to the reagent, followed by photoimmobilization to the surface [63, 64]. The photoactivatible group may be light-sensitive azides, benzophenones, diazinines, or acrylates; polymerization initiator-transfer agent-terminators [65] and plasma-deposited free radicals [64] have also been used. Photoactivation produces highly reactive radical intermediates that immobilize onto the surface via a nonspecific insertion of the radical into a carbon-carbon bond. Photolabile reagents may be coupled to amine- or thiol-bearing ligands using succinimidyl esters or maleimides. One utility of photoimmobilization is the ability to produce patterns of ligands on the surface by lithography.

9.3 Surface Preparation

Polymeric materials can be functionalized using plasma deposition or wet chemical methods to produce surfaces containing reactive groups for ligand bioconjugation. Plasma polymerization has been widely used to deposit numerous functional groups and alter the surface chemistry of many medically relevant polymers [66, 67]. Polyesters such as polyethyleneterephthalate can be partially saponified with aqueous base (5% NaOH, 100°C, 30 min) to produce surface-bound carboxylic acids [39], partially aminolyzed with diamines such as ethylenediamine (50% aqueous, 12 h) to produce surface-bound amines [68] or electrophilically substituted with formaldehyde (20% in 1 M acetic acid) to produce surface-bound alcohols [19].

Polyurethanes can be carboxylated via a bimolecular nucleophilic substitution [69]. Carbamate anions are prepared by abstraction of hydrogen from the urethane nitrogen at low temperatures to prevent chain cleavage (–5°C), followed by coupling of cyclic lactones such as β-propiolactone. Ligands are then immobilized onto the grafted carboxylic acids.

Polytetrafluoroethylene can be functionalized with a number of reactive groups using wet chemical or photochemical methods. Fluoropolymers are reduced with concentrated benzion dianion solutions to form carbonaceous surface layers which can then be halogenated, hydroxylated, carboxylated, or aminated [70]. Photochemical modification of fluoropolymers is possible by incubating the polymer in solutions of alkoxides or thiolate anions and exposing to UV light [71]. The patterning of surfaces is possible using this technique in conjunction with photolithography.

Glasses and oxidized polymers can be functionalized with bifunctional silanating reagents to generate surfaces containing alkyl halides, epoxides, amines, thiols, or carboxylic acids [19, 49, 59, 72]. The substrate must be thoroughly clean and free of any contaminating agents. Glass is soaked in strong acid or base for 30–60 min. Polymers are cleaned with plasma etching or with strong oxidizers such as chromic acid. Clean substrates are immersed in silane solutions (5–10% in acetone, toluene, or ethanol/water 95%/5%) for 1 h and cured 50–100°C, 2–4 h, or at 25°C, 24 h, for oxidation-sensitive silanes such as mercaptosilanes. Prepared surfaces stored under Ar are stable for several weeks.

Metals such as gold can be functionalized via the chemisorption of self-assembled monolayers of alkanethiols [73–75]. Gold substrates, prepared by evaporating gold on chromium-primed silicon substrates, are immersed in organic solutions of alkanethiol (1–10 mM) for 5–60 min. The monolayer is adsorbed via a gold-sulfur bond; competitive displacement of the alkanethiol may occur [75], and it is unclear if these surfaces are applicable for use in reducing media. Similar substrates can be prepared from the chemisorption of carboxylic acids onto alumina [76]. Prepared substrates stored under Ar are stable for several months.

Amine-bearing surfaces have been produced by the adsorption of biologically inert proteins such as albumin. Cells do not have adhesion receptors for albumin, and for this reason albumin has been used to passivate surfaces against cell adhesion. Bioactive ligands can be amino-immobilized onto the albumin-coated surfaces [45, 46, 48].

Functional polymers and copolymers containing alcohols, amines, alkyl halides, carboxylic acids, or other groups can be synthesized, coated onto a surface, and used as the substrate for immobilization of bioactive ligands [77, 78]. Examples include poly(vinyl alcohol) [31, 33], chloromethyl polystyrene [56], aminopolystyrene [79, 80], poly(acrylic acid) [20, 38], polyallylamine [80], poly(maleic acid anhydride) [12], poly(carbodiimide) [81], and poly(succinimide) [82].

9.4   Ligand/Polymer Hybrids

Hybrid copolymers may be synthesized in which one of the components is the biologically active ligand. These copolymers may then be coated onto a substrate or cross-linked into a three-dimensional network. Since the ligand is a component of the copolymer, no additional ligand immobilization may be necessary to produce bioactive substrates.

Examples are available for particular cases of hybrid copolymers (54, 55, 82–87], including gamma-irradiated cross-linked poly(peptide) [86, 88], dialdehyde cross-linked poly(vinyl alcohol)-glycosaminoglycan [54], poly(amino acid-etherurethane) [47, 87], poly(amino acid-lactic acid) [89], poly(amino acid-carbonate) [90], poly(peptide-styrene) [84], and linear [83] or cross-linked [82] poly(glycoside-acrylamide).

9.5   Determining Ligand Surface Densities

The concentration of ligands immobilized upon a surface can be measured using radiolabeling, photochrome labeling, surface analysis, or gravimetry. Since most materials can support the nonspecific adsorption of bioactive ligands, especially proteins, controls must be utilized to differentiate between covalent immobilization and physicochemical adsorption occurring during coupling. For example, ligands immobilized onto unactivated versus activated substrates give relative differences between non-specific adsorption and specific bioconjugation.

The surface immobilization of radiolabeled ligands with markers such as ^3H, ^{35}S, or ^{125}I can be followed to give information on the kinetics of coupling, the coupling capacity of the substrate, and the surface density of ligands. Densities on the order of pmol-fmol/cm^2 are detectable using radiolabeled molecules.

The coupling capacity and density of immobilized acids, amines, and thiols can be evaluated using colorimetric procedures. Substrates can be incubated in solutions of Ellman's reagent [91, 92]; the absorbances of the reaction products give the surface density. Antigens which have been immobilized can be exposed to photochrome-labeled antibodies and surface concentrations calculated using standard enzyme immunosorbent assays [49, 93].

Verification of ligand immobilization may be performed using a number of surface analysis techniques. Mass spectroscopy, x-ray photoelectron spectroscopy, and dynamic contact angle analysis can give information on the chemical composition of the substance's outermost layers. Changes in composition are indicative of modification. Ellipsometry can be used to gauge the thickness of overlapping surface layers; increases imply the presence of additional layers. Highly sensitive gravimetric balances, such as quartz crystal microbalances, can detect *in situ* changes in the mass of immobilized ligand in the nanogram range [65].

9.6 Applications of Immobilized Ligands

Extracellular matrix proteins, such as fibronectin, laminin, vitronectin and collagen, or adhesion molecules, such as ICAM-1, VCAM-1, PCAM-1, and sialyl Lewis X, interact with cell surface receptors and mediate cell adhesion. The tripeptide adhesion sequence Arg-Gly-Asp (RGD) is a ubiquitous signal present in many cell adhesion proteins. It interacts with the integrin family of cell surface adhesion receptors, and comprises the best studied ligand-receptor pair [94–96]. In lieu of immobilizing complex multifunctional proteins for purposes of cell adhesion studies, synthetic RGD sequences have instead been immobilized onto many substrates as simplified models to understand various molecular aspects of cell adhesion phenomena. The following paragraphs cite examples of RGD-grafted substrates that have been used in biomedicine and bioengineering.

The density of RGD necessary to mediate cell adhesion has been determined in a number of fashions. RGD-containing peptides and protein fragments have been physicochemically adsorbed onto tissue culture substrates [97, 98] or covalently bound to albumin-coated substrates [45, 46] to titrate the dependency of cell adhesion function upon RGD surface densities. To remove potential complications due to desorption of ligands or albumin, RGD has been covalently bound onto functionalized substrates. Immobilization also restricts the number of conformations the peptide may assume, helping to ensure that all the peptide is accessible to the cells. RGD has been immobilized onto silanated glasses by its amino [19, 99] and carboxyl [15] termini. The effects of RGD density on cell adhesion, spreading, and cytoskeletal organization was examined [99] using this well-defined system. Other peptides have been immobilized in identical fashion to determine if they influence cell physiology [100].

RGD peptides have been immobilized onto highly cell-resistant materials to ensure that the peptide is the only cell adhesion signal responsible for cell adhesion to diminish signals borne of nonspecifically adsorbed serum proteins. Hydrogels of polyacrylamide [101], poly(vinyl alcohol) [31] and poly(ethylene glycol) [85] and nonhydrogel networks of polyacrylate/poly(ethylene glycol) [102] have been grafted with RGD; these background materials were highly resistant to the adhesion of cells even in the presence of serum proteins, demonstrating that the RGD sequence was solely responsible for mediating cell adhesion.

RGD-containing peptides have been immobilized onto medically relevant polymers in an effort to enhance their biocompatibilities by containing an adhered layer of viable cells. RGD-grafted surfaces can be more efficient in supporting the number and strength of cell adhesion by the peptide facilitating cell adhesion additionally to adsorbed adhesion proteins from the biological milieu. RGD has been conjugated onto surfaces by means of photoimmobilization [103] and plasma glow discharge [64]. In an effort to promote cell adhesion onto biodegradable implants, RGD peptides have been covalently grafted onto poly(amino acid-lactic acid) copolymers [89]. In this manner, cells adherent on the degradable material can eventually obtain a completely natural environment. Self-assembled monolayers of biologic ligands have been immobilized onto gold substrates by adsorbing functionalized thiol-containing bridges followed by covalent grafting of the ligand [93] or by adsorbing alkanethiol-containing ligands [104]. It has been suggested [105] that RGD-containing peptides could be immobilized onto gold substrates in these manners to engineer highly defined surfaces for cell culture systems.

These examples only partially illustrate the utility of ligand-grafted substrates for bioengineering and biomedicine. These substrates offer simplified models of basement membranes to elucidate mechanisms and requirements of cell adhesion. They have applications in biomedicine as biocompatible, cell-adhesive biomaterials for tissue engineering or for clinical implantation.

References

1. Brinkley M. 1992. A brief survey of methods for preparing protein conjugate with dyes, haptens, and cross-linking reagents. Bioconjugate Chem 3:2.
2. Means GE, Feeney RE. 1990. Chemical modification of proteins: History and applications. Bioconjugate Chem 1:2.
3. Wong SS. 1991. Chemistry of Protein Conjugation and Cross-Linking, Boca Raton, FL, CRC Press.
4. Pharmacia Inc. 1988. Affinity chromatography principles and methods, Tech Bull, Uppsala, Sweden.
5. Trevan MD. 1980. Immobilized Enzymes: An Introduction and Applications in Biotechnology, New York, Wiley.
6. Wimalasena RL, Wilson GS. 1991. Factors affecting the specific activity of immobilized antibodies and their biologically active fragments. J Chromatogr 572:85.
7. Mason RS, Little MC. 1988. Strategy for the immobilization of monoclonal antibodies on solid-phase supports. J Chromatogr 458:67.
8. Wingard LB Jr, Katchalski-Katzir E, Goldstein L. 1976. Applied Biochemistry and Bioengineering: Immobilized Enzyme Principles, vol 1, New York, Academic Press.
9. Smalla K, Turkova J, Coupek J, et al. 1988. Influence on the covalent immobilization of proteins to modified copolymers of 2-hydroxyethyl methacrylate with ethylene dimethacrylate. Biotech Appl Biochem 10:21.
10. Schneider C, Newmanm RA, Sutherland DR, et al. 1982. A one-step purification of membrane proteins using a high efficiency immunomatrix. J Biol Chem 257:10766.
11. Scouten W. 1987. A survey of enzyme coupling techniques. Methods Enzymol 135:30.
12. Maeda H, Seymour LW, Miyamoto Y. Conjugates of anticancer agents and polymers: advantages of macromolecular therapeutics in vivo. Bioconjugate Chem 3:351.
13. Nojiri C, Okano T, Park KD, et al. 1988. Suppression mechanisms for thrombus formation on heparin-immobilized segmented polyurethane-ureas. Trans ASAIO 34:386.
14. Fassina G. 1992. Oriented immobilization of peptide ligands on solid supports. J Chromatogr 591:99.
15. Hubbell JA, Massia SP, Drumheller PD. 1992. Surface-grafted cell-binding peptides in tissue engineering of the vascular graft. Ann NY Acad Sci 665:253.
16. Beer JH, Coller BS. 1989. Immobilized Arg-Gly-Asp (RGD) peptides of varying lengths as structural probes of the platelet glycoprotein IIb/IIIa receptor. Blood 79:117.
17. Axen R, Porath J, Ernback S. Chemical coupling of peptides and proteins to polysaccharides by means of cyanogen halides. Nature 214:1302.
18. Delgado C, Patel JN, Francis GE, et al. 1990. Coupling of poly(ethylene glycol) to albumin under very mild conditions by activation with tresyl chloride: Characterization of the conjugate by partitioning in aqueous two-phase systems. Biotech Appl Biochem 12:119.

19. Massia SP, Hubbell JA. 1991. Human endothelial cell interactions with surface-coupled adhesion peptides on a nonadhesive glass substrate and two polymeric biomaterials. J Biomed Mater Res 25:223.

20. Nakajima K, Hirano Y, Iida T, et al. 1990. Adsorption of plasma proteins on Agr-Gly-Asp-Ser peptide-immobilized poly(vinyl alcohol) and ethylene-acrylic acid copolymer films. Polym J 22:985.

21. Testoff MA, Rudolph AS. 1992. Modification of dry 1,2-dipalmitoylphosatidylcholine phase behavior with synthetic membrane-bound stabilizing carbohydrates. Bioconjugate Chem 3:203.

22. Fontanel M-L, Bazin H, Teoule R. 1993. End attachment of phenololigonucleotide conjugates to diazotized cellulose. Bioconjugate Chem 4:380.

23. Nilsson K, Mosbach K. 1984. Immobilization of ligands with organic sulfonyl chlorides. Methods Enzymol 104:56.

24. Chang Y-A, Gee A, Smith A, et al. Activating hydroxyl groups of polymeric carriers using 4-fluorobenzenesulfonyl chloride. Bioconjugate Chem 3:200.

25. Harris JM, Struck EC, Case MG. 1984. Synthesis and characterization of poly(ethylene glycol) derivatives. J Polym Sci Polym Chem Edn 22:341.

26. Sawhney AS, Hubbell JA. 1992. Poly(ethylene oxide)-graft-poly(L-lysine) copolymers to enhance the biocompatibility of poly(L-lysine)-alginate microcapsule membranes. Biomaterials 13:863.

27. Hearn MTW. 1987. 1,1'-Carbonyldiimidazole-mediated immobilization of enzymes and affinity ligands. Methods Enzymol 135:102.

28. Miron T, Wilchek M. 1993. A simplified method for the preparation of succinimidyl carbonate polyethylene glycol for coupling to proteins. Bioconjugate Chem 4:568.

29. Uy R, Wold F. 1977. 1,4-Butanediol diglycidyl ether coupling of carbohydrates to sepharose: Affinity adsorbents for lectins and glycosidases. Anal Biochem 81:98.

30. Sundberg L, Porath J. 1974. Preparation of adsorbents for biospecific affinity chromatography: I. Attachment of group-containing ligands to insoluble polymers by means of bifunctional oxiranes. J Chromatogr 90:87.

31. Kondoh A, Makino K, Matsuda T. 1993. Two-dimensional artificial extracellular matrix: bioadhesive peptide-immobilized surface design. J Appl Polym Sci 47:1983.

32. Annunziato ME, Patel US, Ranade M, et al. 1993. P-Maleimidophenyl isocyanate: A novel heterobifunctional linker for hydroxyl to thiol coupling. Bioconjugate Chem 4:212.

33. Kobayashi H, Ikada Y. 1991. Covalent immobilization of proteins onto the surface of poly(vinyl alcohol) hydrogel. Biomaterials 12:747.

34. Shafer SG, Harris JM. 1986. Preparation of cyanuric-chloride activated poly(ethylene glycol). J Polym Sci Polym Chem Edn 24:375.

35. Kay G, Cook EM. 1967. Coupling of enzymes to cellulose using chloro-s-triazine. Nature (London) 216:514.

36. Bodanszky M. 1988. Peptide Chemistry, Berlin, Springer-Verlag.

37. Staab HA. 1962. Syntheses using heterocyclic amides (azolides). Agnew Chem Int Edn 7:351.

38. Hirano Y, Okuno M, Hayashi T, et al. 1993. Cell-attachment activities of surface immobilized oligopeptides RGD, RGDS, RGDT, and YIGSR toward five cell lines. J Biomater Sci Polym Edn 4:235.

39. Ozaki CK, Phaneuf MD, Hong SL, et al. 1993. Glycoconjugate mediated endothelial cell adhesion to Dacron polyester film. J Vasc Surg 18:486.

40. Barnwarth W, Schmidt D, Stallard RL, et al. 1988. Bathophenanthroline-ruthenium(II) complexes as non-radioactive labels for oligonucleotides which can be measured by time-resolved fluorescence techniques. Helv Chim Acta 71:2085.

41. Drumheller PD, Elbert DL, Hubbell JA. 1994. Multifunctional poly(ethylene glycol) semi-interpenetrating polymer networks as highly selective adhesive substrates for bioadhesive peptide grafting. Biotech Bioeng 43:772.

42. Liu SQ, Ito Y, Imanishi Y. 1993. Cell growth on immobilized cell growth factor: 9. Covalent immobilization of insulin, transferrin, and collagen to enhance growth of bovine endothelial cells. J Biomed Mater Res 27:909.

43. Wachter E, Machleidt W, Hofner H, Otto J. 1973. Aminopropyl glass and its p-phenylene diisothio-cyanate derivative, a new support in solid-phase Edman degradation of peptides and proteins. FEBS Lett 35:97.

44. Maisano F, Gozzini L, de Haen C. 1992. Coupling of DTPA to proteins: A critical analysis of the cyclic dianhydride method in the case of insulin modification. Bioconjugate Chem 3:212.

45. Streeter HB, Rees DA. 1987. Fibroblast adhesion to RGDS shows novel features compared with fibronectin. J Cell Biol 105:507.

46. Singer II, Kawka DW, Scott S, et al. 1987. The fibronectin cell attachment Arg-Gly-Asp-Ser pro-motes focal contact formation during early fibroblast attachment and spreading. J Cell Biol 104:573.

47. Nathan A, Bolikal D, Vyavahare N, et al. 1992. Hydrogels based on water-soluble poly(ether urethanes) derived from L-lysine and poly(ethylene glycol). Macromolecules 25:4476.

48. Elling L, Kula M-R. 1991. Immunoaffinity partitioning: Synthesis and use of polyethylene glycol-oxirane for coupling to bovine serum albumin and monoclonal antibodies. Biotech Appl Biochem 13:354.

49. Pope NM, Kulcinski DL, Hardwick A, et al. 1993. New applications of silane coupling agents for covalently binding antibodies to glass and cellulose solid supports. Bioconjugate Chem 4:166.

50. Werb Z, Tremble PM, Behrendtsen O, et al. 1989. Signal transduction through the fibronectin receptor induces collagenase and stromelysin gene expression. J Cell Biol 109:877.

51. Yamagata M, Suzuki S, Akiyama SK, et al. 1989. Regulation of cell-substrate adhesion by proteogly-cans immobilized on extracellular substrates. J Biol Chem 264:8012.

52. Robinson PJ, Dunnill P, Lilly MD. 1971. Porous glass as a solid support for immobilization or affinity chromatography of enzymes. Biochim Biophys Acta 242:659.

53. Harris JM, Dust JM, McGill RA, et al. 1991. New polyethylene glycols for biomedical applications. ACS Symp Ser 467:418.

54. Cholakis CH, Zingg W, Sefton MV. 1989. Effect of heparin-PVA hydrogel on platelets in a chronic arterio-venous shunt. J Biomed Mater Res 23:417.

55. Cholakis CH, Sefton MV. 1984. Chemical characterization of an immobilized heparin: heparin-PVA. In SW Shalaby, AS Hoffman, BD Ratner, et al. (eds), Polymers as Biomaterials, New York, Plenum.

56. Gutsche AT, Parsons-Wingerter P, Chand D, et al. 1994. N-Acetylglucosamine and adenosine deriva-tized surfaces for cell culture: 3T3 fibroblast and chicken hepatocyte response. Biotech Bioeng 43:801.

57. Jagendorf AT, Patchornik A, Sela M. 1963. Use of antibody bound to modified cellulose as an immunospecific adsorbent of antigen. Biochim Biophys Acta 78:516.

58. Collioud A, Clemence J-F, Sanger M, et al. 1993. Oriented and covalent immobilization of target molecules to solid supports: Synthesis and application of a light-activatible and thiol-reactive cross-linking reagent. Bioconjugate Chem 4:528.

59. Bhatia SK, Shriver-Lake LC, Prior KJ, et al. Use of thiol-terminal silanes and heterobifunctional crosslinkers for immobilization of antibodies on silica surfaces. Anal Biochem 178:408.

60. Moeschler HJ, Vaughan M. 1983. Affinity chromatography of brain cyclic nucleotide phospho-diesterase using 3-(2-pyridyldithio)proprionyl-substituted calmodulin linked to thiol-Sepharose. Biochemistry 22:826.

61. Tseng Y-C, Park K. 1992. Synthesis of photoreactive poly(ethylene glycol) and its application to the prevention of surface-induced platelet activation. J Biomed Mater Res 26:373.

62. Yan M, Cai SX, Wybourne MN, et al. 1993. Photochemical functionalization of polymer surfaces and the production of biomolecule-carrying micrometer-scale structures by deep-UV lithography using 4-substituted perfluorophenyl azides. J Am Chem Soc 115:814.

63. Guire PE. 1993. Biocompatible device with covalently bonded biocompatible agent, U.S. patent 5,263,992.

64. Ito Y, Suzuki K, Imanishi Y. 1994. Surface biolization by grafting polymerizable bioactive chemicals. ACS Symp Ser 540:66.

65. Nakayama Y, Matsuda T, Irie M. 1993. A novel surface photo-graft polymerization method for fabricated devices. ASAIO J 39:M542.

66. Ratner BD, Chilkoti A, Lopez GP. 1990. Plasma deposition and treatment for biomaterial applications. In R d'Agostino (ed), Plasma Deposition, Treatment, and Etching of Polymers, p 463, New York, Academic Press.

67. Ratner BD. 1992. Plasma deposition for biomedical applications: a brief review. J Biomater Sci Polym Edn 4:3.

68. Desai NP, Hubbell JA. 1991. Biological responses to polyethylene oxide modified polyethylene terephthalate surfaces. J Biomed Mater Res 25:829.

69. Lin H-B, Zhao Z-C, Garcia-Echeverria C, et al. 1992. Synthesis of a novel polyurethane co-polymer containing covalently attached RGD peptide. J Biomater Sci Polymer Edn 3:217.

70. Costello CA, McCarthy TJ. 1987. Surface-selective introduction of specific functionalities onto poly(tetrafluoroethylene). Macromolecules 20:2819.

71. Allmer K, Feiring AE. 1991. Photochemical modification of a fluoropolymer surface. Macromolecules 24:5487.

72. Ferguson GS, Chaudhury MK, Biebuyck HA, et al. 1993. Monolayers on disordered substrates: Self-assembly of alkyltrichlorosilanes on surface-modified polyethylene and poly(dimethylsiloxane). Macromolecules 26:5870.

73. Plant AL. 1993. Self-assembled phospholipid/alkanethiol biomimetic bilayers on gold. Langmuir 9:2764.

74. Prime KL, Whitesides GM. 1993. Adsorption of proteins onto surfaces containing end-attached oligo(ethylene oxide): A model system using self-assembled monolayers. J Am Chem Soc 115:10714.

75. Biebuyck HA, Whitesides GM. 1993. Interchange between monolayers on gold formed from unsymmetrical disulfides and solutions of thiols: Evidence for sulfur-sulfur bond cleavage by gold metal. Langmuir 9:1766.

76. Laibinis PE, Hickman JJ, Wrightson MS, et al. 1989. Orthogonal self-assembled monolayers: Alkanethiols on gold and alkane carboxylic acids on alumina. Science 245:845.

77. Veronese FM, Visco C, Massarotto S, et al. 1987. New acrylic polymers for surface modification of enzymes of therapeutic interest and for enzyme immobilization. Ann NY Acad Sci 501:444.

78. Scouten WH. 1987. A survey of enzyme coupling techniques. Methods Enzymol 135:30.

79. Mech C, Jeschkeit H, Schellenberger A. 1976. Investigation of the covalent bond structure of peptide-matrix systems by Edman degradation of support-fixed peptides. Eur J Biochem 66:133.

80. Iio K, Minoura N, Aiba S, et al. 1994. Cell growth on poly(vinyl alcohol) hydrogel membranes containing biguanido groups. J Biomed Mater Res 28:459.

81. Weinshenker NM, Shen C-M. 1972. Polymeric reagents: I. Synthesis of an insoluble polymeric carbodiimide. Tetrahedron Lett 32:3281.

82. Schnaar RL, Brandley BK, Needham LK, et al. 1989. Adhesion of eukaryotic cells to immobilized carbohydrates. Methods Enzymol 179:542.

83. Sparks MA, Williams KW, Whitesides GM. 1993. Neuraminidase-resistant hemagglutination inhibitors: Acrylamide copolymers containing a C-glycoside of N-acetylneuramic acid. J Med Chem 36:778.

84. Ozeki E, Matsuda T. 1990. Development of an artificial extracellular matrix. Solution castable polymers with cell recognizable peptidyl side chains. ASAIO Trans 36:M294.

85. Drumheller PD. 1994. Polymer Networks of Poly(Ethylene Glycol) as Biospecific Cell Adhesive Substrates, PhD dissertation, University of Texas at Austin.

86. Nicol A, Gowda DC, Parker TM, et al. 1993. Elastomeric polytetrapeptide matrices: Hydrophobicity dependence of cell attachment from adhesive $(GGIP)_n$ to nonadhesive $(GGAP)_n$ even in serum. J Biomed Mater Res 27:801.

87. Kohn J, Gean KF, Nathan A, et al. 1993. New drug conjugates: attachment of small molecules to poly(PEG-Lys). Polym Mater Sci Eng 69:515.

88. Nicol A, Gowda DC, Urry DW. 1992. Cell adhesion and growth on synthetic elastomeric matrices containing ARG-GLY-ASP-SER. J Biomed Mater Res 26:393.

89. Barrera DA, Zylstra E, Lansbury PT, et al. 1993. Synthesis and RGD peptide modification of a new biodegradable copolymer: Poly(lactic acid-colysine). J Am Chem Soc 115:11010.

90. Pulapura S, Kohn J. 1993. Tyrosine-derived polycarbonate: Backbone-modified "pseudo"-poly(amino acids) designed for biomedical applications. Biopolymers 32:411.

91. Ngo TT. Coupling capacity of solid-phase carboxyl groups. Determination by a colorimetric procedure. Appl Biochem Biotech 13:207.

92. Ngo TT. 1986. Colorimetric determination of reactive amino groups of a solid support using Traut's and Ellman's reagents. Appl Biochem Biotech 13:213.

93. Duan C, Meyerhoff ME. 1994. Separation-free sandwich enzyme immunoassays using microporous gold electrodes and self-assembled monolayer/immobilized capture antibodies. Anal Chem 66:1369.

94. Albeda SM, Buck CA. 1990. Integrins and other cell adhesion molecules. FASEB J 4:2868.

95. Ruoslahti E. 1991. Integrins. J Clin Invest 87:1.

96. Humphries MJ. 1990. The molecular basis and specificity of integrin-ligand interactions. J Cell Sci 97:585.

97. Underwood PA, Bennett FA. 1989. A comparison of the biological activities of the cell-adhesive proteins vitronectin and fibronectin. J Cell Sci 93:641.

98. Yamada KM, Kennedy DW. 1985. Amino acid sequence specificities of an adhesive recognition signal. J Cell Biochem 28:99.

99. Massia SP, Hubbell JA. 1991. An RGD spacing of 44 nm is sufficient for integrin $\alpha_v\beta_3$-mediated fibroblast spreading and 140 nm for focal contact and stress fiber formation. J Cell Biol 114:1089.

100. Hubbell JA, Massia SP, Desai NP, et al. 1992. Endothelial cell-selective materials for tissue engineering in the vascular graft via a new receptor. Bio/Technology 9:568.

101. Brandley BK, Schnaar RL. 1989. Tumor cell haptotaxis on covalently immobilized linear and exponential gradients of a cell adhesion peptide. Dev Biol 135:74.

102. Drumheller PD, Elbert DL, Hubbell JA. 1994. Multifunctional poly(ethylene glycol) semi-interpenetrating polymer networks as highly selective adhesive substrates for bioadhesive peptide grafting. Biotech Bioeng 43:772.

103. Clapper DL, Daws KM, Guire PE. 1994. Photoimmobilized ECM peptides promote cell attachment and growth on biomaterials. Trans Soc Biomater 17:345.

104. Spinke J, Liley M, Guder H-J, et al. 1993. Molecular recognition at self-assembled monolayers: The construction of multicomponent multilayers. Langmuir 9:1821.

105. Singhvi R, Kumar A, Lopez GP, et al. 1994. Engineering cell shape and function. Science 264:696.

10

Biomaterials: Protein-Surface Interactions

Joseph A. Chinn
Sulzer Carbomedics

Steven M. Slack
The University of Memphis

10.1 Introduction

A common assumption in biomaterials research is that cellular interactions with natural and artificial surfaces are mediated through adsorbed proteins. Such diverse processes as **thrombosis** and **hemostasis**, hard and soft tissue healing, infection, and inflammation are each affected by protein adsorption to surfaces *in vivo*. Many *in vitro* diagnostic analyses, chromatographic separation techniques, and genetic engineering processes also involve protein adsorption at solid-liquid interfaces.

The adsorption of fibrinogen, a prevalent blood plasma protein, has been studied extensively because of its role in blood coagulation and thrombosis, as has the adsorption of albumin, because it is thought to inhibit the adhesion of blood platelets [Young et al., 1982]. The amount of protein adsorbed to a substrate is best measured directly using radiolabeled proteins, whereas the thickness of an adsorbed protein film can be calculated from ellipsometric measurements. Further, the importance of the state of an adsorbed protein in mediating cellular interactions is now becoming evident. Molecularly sensitive indirect measurement techniques, e.g., circular dichroism (CD), differential scanning calorimetry (DSC), enzyme-linked immunosorbent assay (ELISA), Fourier transform infrared spectroscopy/attenuated total reflectance (FTIR/ATR), radio-immunoassay (RIA), or total internal reflection fluorescence (TIRF), can be used to characterize the **conformation** and **organization** of adsorbed proteins. (The amount of protein adsorbed to a substrate is best measured directly using radiolabeled proteins; the thickness of an adsorbed protein film can be calculated from ellipsometric measurements.) Highly specific monoclonal (MAb) (against specific protein **epitopes**) [Shiba et al., 1991] and polyclonal (PAb) (against multiple epitopes) [Lindon et al., 1986] antibodies provide direct probes of adsorbed protein conformation and organization. Thus, cellular responses can be compared not only with the amounts of proteins adsorbed but also the organization of the proteins on the surface of the substrate.

Whereas previous studies confirmed roles for adsorbed proteins in subsequent cell-surface interactions, much current research aims to better understand cell-protein-surface interactions on a molecular level. Recently, peptide sequences contained within the cell binding domains of adhesive proteins have been identified and characterized, synthesized, and demonstrated to bind cellular receptors known as **integrins** [Ruoslahti, 1991; Yamada, 1991]. Current and potential applications range from selective or enhanced *in vitro* cell culture to selective *in vivo* cellular responses such as endothelialization in the absence of inflammation, infection, or thrombosis [Hubbell et al., 1991].

10.2   Fundamentals of Protein Adsorption

Detailed and comprehensive reviews of protein adsorption have been published [Andrade, 1985; Andrade & Hlady, 1986; Horbett, 1982; Norde and Lyklema, 1991]. A thorough understanding of key principles will prove helpful in critically evaluating reports in literature. Particularly important concepts are protein structure and heterogeneity, factors that dramatically affect the thermodynamics and kinetics of adsorption, reversibility of adsorption, and the dynamics of multicomponent adsorption.

A protein is a complex molecule consisting of amino acid copolymer (polypeptide) chains that interact with each other to give the molecule a three-dimensional structure. Importantly, each amino acid in the polymer contributes to the chemical and physical properties of the protein. A dramatic example of this is the oxygen-carrying protein, hemoglobin, which consists of four polypeptide chains denoted $\alpha_2\beta_2$. A single amino acid substitution in the 146 amino acid β-chain results in the conversion of normal hemoglobin (HbA) to sickle-cell hemoglobin (HbS) and underlies the serious consequences of sickle-cell disease [Stryer, 1995]. Protein structure and function are relevant to protein adsorption and have been described on four different scales or orders [Andrade and Hlady, 1986]. Primary structure refers to the sequence and number of amino acids in a copolymer chain. The 20 amino acids that are polymerized to make proteins are termed **residues**. Of these, 8 have non-polar side chains, 7 have neutral polarity side chains, and 5 have charged polar side chains [Stryer, 1995]. Secondary structure results from hydrogen bonding associated with the amide linkages in the polymer chain backbone to form structures such as the α-helix and β-pleated sheet. Tertiary structure results from associations within chains, including hydrogen bonding, ionic and hydrophobic interactions, salt bridges, and disulfide bonds and dictates the three-dimensional structure adopted by protein molecules. Quaternary structure results from associations between chains. Many blood proteins contain polar, non-polar, and charged residues. In polar media such as buffered saline or blood plasma, hydrophilic residues tend to self-associate (often at the outer, water-contacting surface of the protein), as do hydrophobic residues (often "inside" the protein). This results in distinct domains (Fig. 10.1) that dictate higher order protein structure.

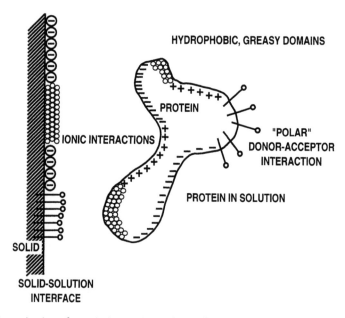

FIGURE 10.1 Schematic view of protein interacting with a well characterized surface. The protein has a number of surface domains with hydrophobic, charged, and polar character. The solid surface has a similar domain like character [Andrade and Hlady, 1986].

When a single, static protein solution contacts a surface, the rate of adsorption depends upon transport of the protein from the bulk to the surface. Andrade and Hlady [1986] identified four primary transport mechanisms, namely, diffusion, thermal convection, flow convection, and coupled convection-diffusion. In isothermal, parallel laminar flow or static systems, protein transport to the interface occurs exclusively by diffusion. In turbulent or stirred systems, each of the four transport modes can be significant.

When adsorption is reaction limited, the net rate of adsorption can sometimes be described by the classic Langmuir theory of gas adsorption [Smith, 1981]:

$$r_A = k_A * C_b * (1 - \Theta) - k_D * \Theta \qquad (10.1)$$

where r_A is the net adsorption rate, k_A is the adsorption rate constant, C_b is the bulk concentration of the protein in solution, Θ is fractional surface coverage, and k_D is the desorption rate constant. At equilibrium, the net rate of adsorption, r_A, is zero, and Θ can be calculated from Eq. (10.1) as the Langmuir adsorption isotherm,

$$\Theta = \frac{K * C_b}{1 + K * C_b} \qquad (10.2)$$

where $K = k_A/k_D$. This model assumes reversible monolayer adsorption, no conformational changes upon adsorption, and no interactions between adsorbed molecules. It is most applicable to dilute solutions and non-hydrophobic substrates. When adsorption is diffusion limited, the initial rate of adsorption is equivalent to the rate of diffusion, described mathematically as [Andrade and Hlady, 1986]

$$r_A = r_\mathcal{D} = 2 * C_\mathcal{D} * \sqrt{\frac{\mathcal{D}}{\pi t}} \qquad (10.3)$$

where $\mathcal{D}$ is the diffusivity of the protein, and t is time.

Protein adsorption to hydrophobic substrates differs from that to hydrophilic materials. The primary driving force for adsorption to hydrophilic substrates is often enthalpic, whereas that to hydrophobic substrates is entropic [Norde, 1986]. Water near a hydrophobic surface tends to hydrogen bond to neighboring water molecules, resulting in a highly ordered water structure [Andrade and Hlady, 1986]. Disruption of this structure (dehydration) by adsorption of a protein to the surface increases the entropy of the system and is therefore thermodynamically favored. As a result, adsorption to hydrophilic substrates is generally reversible, whereas that to hydrophobic substrates is not. Denaturation of the adsorbed protein by hydrophobic interactions with the substrate can also contribute to irreversible adsorption [Feng and Andrade, 1994].

The amount of a specific protein adsorbed to a substrate can be measured directly if the protein is radiolabeled. Gamma emitting isotopes are preferred because their signal is directly proportional to the amount of protein present. Radioisotopes of iodine (^{125}I, [129]I, and ^{131}I) are commonly used because iodine readily attaches to tyrosine residues [Macfarlane, 1958]. An ^{125}I monochloride radiolabeling technique has been published [Horbett, 1986] but others, such as those using chloramine-T or lactoperoxidase, can also be used.

If neither the ^{125}I-protein nor the unlabeled protein preferentially adsorbs to the substrate at the expense of the other, then the amount of that protein adsorbed to a substrate from multicomponent media such as plasma can be measured by adding a small amount of the ^{125}I-protein to the adsorption medium. Studies have shown that ^{125}I-fibrinogen generally behaves like its unlabeled analog [Horbett, 1981]. The total amount of the protein adsorbed (both unlabeled and ^{125}I-protein) is calculated by dividing the measured radioactivity by the **specific activity** of the protein in the medium. (Specific activity is determined by dividing the gamma activity in a measured aliquot of the adsorption medium by the total amount of that protein, both labeled and unlabeled, in the aliquot.) To verify that neither labeled nor unlabeled fibrinogen preferentially adsorbs to the substrates, the specific activity of the protein in a small aliquot of the plasma dilution from which adsorption was maximum should be increased ten times, and adsorption from that dilution again measured. Changes in calculated adsorption values should be attributable only to the variability in the data and differences in the signal to noise ratio, not the ratio of labeled to unlabeled fibrinogen in the plasma. Similarly, to verify that absorption into the sample materials of free ^{125}I in the buffer is not significant, adsorption from dilute plasma to which only 0.01 M unlabeled free iodide is added should be measured. Sample calculations for measuring protein adsorption using this technique are illustrated in the next section.

The use of radioisotopes for the measurement of protein adsorption to surfaces offers a significant, though underused, advantage compared with other techniques. Because the radioisotopes, e.g., ^{125}I and ^{131}I, emit unique energy spectra, i.e., their peak radiation emissions occur at distinct energies, one can simultaneously measure the adsorption of two different proteins from a protein mixture. By labeling one protein with ^{125}I and the other with ^{131}I, the adsorption behavior of both can be determined in one experiment. Modern gamma counters come with preset energy windows specific to common isotopes, making such measurements routine. In the absence of such an instrument, one can still perform dual-labeling experiments by exploiting the fact that the half-lives of the isotopes differ. For example, the half-life of ^{125}I is 60 days whereas that of ^{131}I is only 8 days. After measuring the ^{131}I emission immediately after the experiment, one can allow the radioactivity associated with it to decay to background levels (ten half-lives or 80 days for ^{131}I) and then measure the signal associated solely with ^{125}I [Dewanjee, 1992].

Indirect methods are also used to study proteins adsorbed to a substrate. ELISA and RIA analytical techniques exploit specific antibody-antigen interactions as follows. Antibodies against specific epitopes of an adsorbed protein are either conjugated to an enzyme (ELISA), or radiolabeled (RIA). Substrates are first incubated with the medium, then with a solution containing the antibody or antibody conjugate. In the case of ELISA, the substrates are subsequently incubated with substrate solution. As the substrate is converted to product, the color of the solution changes in proportion to the amount of bound antibody present and is measured spectrophotometrically. However, extensive calibration is required to quantify results. In the case of RIA, the radioactivity originating from the radiolabeled antibody (bound to the protein adsorbed to the substrate) is measured and the amount of antibody bound calculated. With both methods, the relative amount of the adsorbed protein to which the antibody has bound, rather than the total amount of protein adsorbed, is measured. Antibody binding is a function of not only the amount of protein adsorbed, but also the particular antibody used, total protein surface loading, and protein residence time. Thus, although antibody techniques provide direct probes of adsorbed protein conformation and organization, such measurements do not necessarily reflect the absolute amounts of protein adsorbed. Other indirect methods used to study adsorbed proteins include ellipsometry, electron microscopy, high performance liquid chromatography (HPLC), and staining techniques.

10.3 Example Calculations and Applications of Protein Adsorption

The following example illustrates how radiolabeled proteins are used to measure the amount of protein adsorbed to a substrate. The fibrinogen concentration in 10 ml plasma is determined to be 5.00 mg/ml by measuring the light absorbance at 280 nm of a redissolved, thrombin-induced clot [Ratnoff and Menzie, 1950]. The concentration and specific activity of a 10 μl aliquot of ^{125}I-fibrinogen are 1.00 mg/ml and 10^9 cpm/μg, respectively. Fibrinogen adsorption from dilute plasma to a series of polymer samples, each having 1.00 cm^2 total surface area (counting both sides of the sample) is to be measured. Based upon reports in literature, maximal adsorption of 250 ng/cm^2 is expected. The background signal in the gamma radiation counter is 25 cpm. To achieve a maximum signal/noise ratio of 10, the specific activity of fibrinogen in the plasma should be

$$\mathrm{sp.ac.} = \frac{(\mathrm{signal/noise})*\mathrm{noise}}{\mathrm{mass\ adsorbed}} = \frac{10*25\ \mathrm{cpm}}{25\ \mathrm{ng/cm^2}*1.00\ \mathrm{cm^2}}*\frac{10^3\ \mathrm{ng}}{\mu g} = 10^3\ \mathrm{cpm/\mu g} \qquad (10.4)$$

The volume of ^{125}I-fibrinogen solution to be added to the plasma to obtain 10^3 cpm/g specific activity (neglecting the mass of ^{125}I-fibrinogen added) is calculated as

$$\frac{10^3\ \mathrm{cpm/\mu g}*10^3\ \mu g/\mathrm{mg}*5.00\ \mathrm{mg/ml}*10\ \mathrm{ml}}{10^9\ \mathrm{cpm/mg}*1.00\ \mathrm{mg/ml}*\mathrm{ml}/10^3\ \mu l} = 50\ \mu l \qquad (10.5)$$

Addition of 50 μl ^{125}I-fibrinogen solution should increase the total fibrinogen concentration in the plasma by only a small fraction,

$$\frac{50\ \mu l*\mathrm{ml}/10^3\ \mu l*1.00\ \mathrm{mg/ml}}{10\ \mathrm{ml}*5.00\ \mathrm{mg/ml}} = 10^{-3} \qquad (10.6)$$

To determine the amount of protein adsorbed to the substrate, the radioactivity of samples incubated with plasma is measured and compared with the specific activity of the protein in the plasma. In this example, if the amount of radioactivity retained by a sample is measured to be 137 cpm, then the mass of fibrinogen adsorbed is calculated as,

$$\frac{(137\ \mathrm{cpm/sample}-25\ \mathrm{cpm\ background})*10^3\ \mathrm{ng/\mu g}}{10^3\ \mathrm{cpm/\mu g\ fibrinogen}*1.00\ \mathrm{cm^2/sample}} = 112\ \mathrm{ng/cm^2} \qquad (10.7)$$

Adsorption of proteins to polymeric substrates is measured because adsorbed proteins influence cellular processes. Adsorbed albumin is proposed to favor biocompatibility, whereas adsorbed fibrinogen is proposed to discourage biocompatibility because of its role in mediating initial adhesion of blood platelets [Young et al., 1982]. This simplified view inadequately describes biocompatibility *in vivo* for several reasons. First, the relationships between processes involved in thrombosis, hemostasis, inflammation, and healing (e.g., adhesion of platelets, fibroblasts, white blood cells, endothelial cells) and long-term biocompatibility remain mostly unknown. For example, Sakariassen and colleagues [1979] proposed that exclusively adsorbed von Willebrand factor (vWF) mediates platelet adhesion to vascular subendothelial structures, yet although some people that lack serum vWF in their blood exhibit bleeding disorders, others remain asymptomatic. Second, biological processes that do not require fibrinogen mediated cell adhesion (e.g., contact activation [Kaplan, 1978], complement activation [Chenowith, 1988]) are also related to material biocompatibility. Third, biological factors and serum proteins other than fibrinogen and albumin (e.g., vWF, fibronectin, vitronectin, laminin) significantly affect cellular processes. Fourth, the reactivity of adsorbed proteins depends upon their organization upon the substrate.

Studies of fibrinogen adsorption *in vitro* illustrate the dynamic nature of protein adsorption from plasma. Vroman and Adams [1969] reported that oxidized silicon and anodized tantalum incubated 2s with plasma bind fibrinogen anti-serum, whereas the same materials incubated 25s with plasma do not. Ellipsometric measurements indicated that the observed decrease in antibody binding was not due to loss of protein. Brash and ten Hove [1984] and Horbett [1984] reported that maximal equilibrium fibrinogen adsorption to different materials occurred from intermediate dilutions of plasma. The adsorption maximum is sometimes called a **Vroman peak**, which describes the shape of the adsorption versus log (**plasma concentration**) curve referred to as an adsorption isotherm. Both the location and the magnitude of the peak depend upon the surface chemistry of the substrate. (For this reason, it is wise to fully characterize any substrate prior to measuring protein adsorption. Electron spectroscopy for chemical analysis, ESCA [Ratner and McElroy, 1986], and secondary ion mass spectroscopy, SIMS [Andrade, 1985], are often appropriate.)

Wojciechowski and colleagues [1986] reported that at short contact times, adsorption was greatest from undiluted plasma. As contact time increased, the plasma concentration at which adsorption was greatest decreased. The unusual observed adsorption behavior occurs because fibrinogen adsorption is driven initially by mass action, i.e., a gradient between surface and bulk concentration. However, as coverage of the surface increases, bulk proteins must compete for surface binding sites. The composition of the adsorbed layer continues to change as proteins of higher surface activity displace adsorbed proteins of lower surface activity [Horbett, 1984]. Vroman and colleagues [1980] called this process conversion of the fibrinogen layer, and proposed that fibrinogen adsorbed at early time is at later time displaced by other plasma proteins, possibly high molecular weight kininogen (HMWK). Because Vroman pioneered much of this work, these phenomena are collectively referred to as the **Vroman effect** [Slack and Horbett, 1995]. This principle is most applicable to hydrophilic substrates and is commonly used in biocompatibility studies to vary the composition of the protein layer adsorbed from plasma in a controlled manner.

Slack and Horbett [1989] postulated the existence of two distinct types of adsorbed fibrinogen molecules, displaceable and non-displaceable. Protein adsorption from plasma was modeled as competitive adsorption from a binary solution of fibrinogen and a hypothetical protein H (representing all other plasma components). In this model, protein H adsorbs to unoccupied surface sites in a non-displaceable state, and fibrinogen molecules first adsorb to unoccupied surface sites in a displaceable state, then are displaced by protein H, or spread to become resistant to displacement. The latter process is referred to as fibrinogen transition. Neglecting desorption and mass transfer limitations, rate equations for surface coverage by protein H, displaceable fibrinogen, and non-displaceable fibrinogen were solved simultaneously for a surface initially free of adsorbate. The analytical solution is given by Eq. (10.8) and Eq. (10.9).

$$\Theta_1(t) = \beta\left(e^{r_1^* t} - e^{r_2^* t}\right) \tag{10.8}$$

$$\Theta_2(t) = \left(\beta * k_2 / r_1 * r_2\right) * \left[r_1\left(1 - e^{r_2^* t}\right) - r_2\left(1 - e^{r_1^* t}\right)\right] \tag{10.9}$$

where Θ_1, Θ_2, and Θ_3 are fractional coverages by displaceable fibrinogen, non-displaceable fibrinogen, and the hypothetical protein, respectively, k_1 is the fibrinogen adsorption rate constant, k_2 is the fibrinogen transition rate constant, k_3 is the hypothetical protein adsorption rate constant, k_4 is the fibrinogen displacement rate constant, C_F is the bulk concentration of fibrinogen, C_H is the bulk concentration of the hypothetical protein in solution, and β, r_1, and r_2 are constants related to rate constants and bulk concentrations. This model predicts maximal fibrinogen coverage at intermediate adsorption time (Fig. 10.2), consistent with reported experimental results. Surface exclusion and molecular mobility arguments have also been proposed to explain the Vroman effect [Willems et al., 1991].

Changes in protein conformation upon adsorption have been inferred from a variety of indirect measurements. For example, Castillo and colleagues [1984] inferred substrate, adsorption time, and residence time dependent conformational changes in human serum albumin (HSA) adsorbed to different hydrogels based upon changes in FTIR/ATR and CD spectra. Specific conformational changes, i.e., decreased α-helix and increased random coil and β-pleated sheet content upon adsorption were proposed. Similarly, Norde and colleagues [1986] reported lower α-helix content in HSA first adsorbed to, then desorbed from different substrates compared with native HSA. Castillo and colleagues [1985] also reported that lysozyme became increasingly denatured with increased adsorption time and residence time, and that denatured lysozyme adsorbed irreversibly to contact lens materials. De Baillou and colleagues [1984] proposed conformational changes in fibrinogen upon adsorption to glass based upon DSC measurements. Similarly, Feng and Andrade [1994] proposed that low temperature isotropic (LTI)

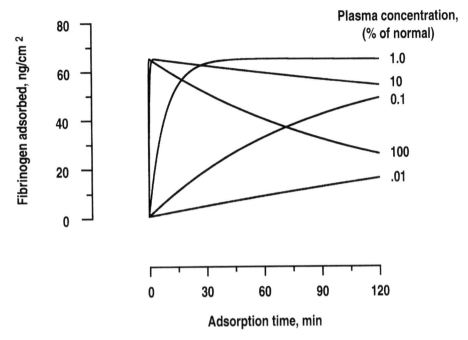

FIGURE 10.2 Time course of fibrinogen adsorption to a polymeric substrate as predicted by the model proposed by Slack and Horbett [1989].

carbon significantly denatures adsorbed proteins through hydrophobic interactions. Rainbow and colleagues [1987] proposed conformational changes in albumin upon adsorption to quartz, based upon changes in fluorescence lifetimes calculated from TIRF measurements. Finally, investigators noted that certain enzymes, following their adsorption to solid surfaces, lose a considerable amount of their enzymatic activity compared with enzymes in solution, suggesting that a surface-induced structural rearrangement had occurred [Sandwick and Schray, 1987, 1988].

Whereas indirect methods provide evidence for changes in protein organization upon adsorption, antibodies against specific protein epitopes provide direct evidence, as antibody-binding measurements directly reflect the availability of different protein epitopes. Proteins at interfaces can undergo both covalent (e.g., conversion of fibrinogen to fibrin) and non-covalent (e.g., denaturation, change in conformation, change in epitope accessibility) organizational changes. Therefore, epitopes inaccessible in solution might become available upon adsorption of the protein, and consequently, the biological activity of the adsorbed protein may differ from that of the same protein in solution. For example, receptor-induced binding site (RIBS) anti-fibrinogens bind to adsorbed but not free fibrinogen molecules [Zamarron et al., 1990]. Because an MAb binds to a single protein epitope, whereas a PAb binds to multiple epitopes on the protein, MAbs rather than PAbs should be more sensitive to such changes. Also, epitopes available at low surface loadings may become unavailable at higher loadings due to steric hindrance by proteins adsorbed to neighboring surface sites.

Horbett and Lew [1994] used the Vroman effect principle to maximize the amount of fibrinogen adsorbed from plasma to different polymers, and then measured the binding of different MAbs directed against various epitopes of fibrinogen. Binding was reported to be substrate dependent and, with some MAbs, changed with protein residence time. Thus, different fibrinogen epitopes become more or less available as the adsorbed molecule reorganizes upon the surface. Soria and colleagues [1985] demonstrated that a MAb directed against fragment D of the fibrinogen molecule, which did not bind to the molecule in solution, did bind to it following its adsorption to a surface. Although this method cannot distinguish between changes in protein conformation (higher order structure) and changes in surface orientation (e.g., rotation, steric effects), several authors reported that with increased adsorption time or residence time, adsorbed proteins became less readily displaced by plasma or surfactant eluting agents [Balasubramanian et al., in press; Bohnert and Horbett, 1986; Chinn et al., 1992; Rapoza and Horbett, 1990; Slack and Horbett, 1992]. These results suggest that **post-adsorptive transitions** in adsorbed proteins are primarily structural.

Protein organization is also a function of surface loading. Chinn and colleagues [1992] and Rapoza and Horbett [1990] used the Vroman effect principle to vary both the amounts of fibrinogen and total protein adsorbed from plasma to different polymers. Fibrinogen retention by all substrates was greater when the protein was adsorbed from more dilute than from less dilute plasma. This suggests that at higher total protein loadings, each fibrinogen molecule directly contacts the surface at fewer points (because individual molecules compete for binding sites), and a greater fraction of molecules is displaceable. Conversely, at lower total protein loadings, individual molecules compete less for binding sites and are not hindered from reorganizing on the surface. Because each molecule directly contacts the surface at more points, a greater fraction of adsorbed molecules is non-displaceable. Pettit and colleagues [1994] reported a negative correlation, independent of substrate, between anti-fibronectin binding (normalized to the amount of fibronectin adsorbed) and the amount of fibronectin adsorbed. They proposed that the conformation or orientation of the adsorbed fibronectin molecule favors exposure of the cell binding domain at lower rather than higher fibronectin surface concentrations.

Although the implications of protein transitions in long-term *in vivo* biocompatibility remain largely unknown, changes in the states of adsorbed proteins are related to cellular interactions. More platelets adhered to glass first contacted 5s with plasma than 3 min with plasma [Zucker and Vroman, 1969]. Platelet adhesion *in vitro* to polymers upon which the Vroman effect principle was used to vary the composition of adsorbed protein layer was reported related not to total fibrinogen binding, but to anti-fibrinogen binding [Lindon et al., 1986; Shiba et al., 1991], as well as the fraction of adsorbed protein that can be eluted by surfactant such as sodium dodecyl sulfate (SDS) [Chinn et al., 1991].

10.4   Summary, Conclusions, and Directions

Clearly, adsorbed proteins affect biocompatibility in ways that are not entirely understood. Fibrinogen has been extensively studied because blood platelets involved in thrombosis and hemostasis have a receptor for this protein [Phillips et al., 1988]. Adsorbed fibrinogen is often proposed to discourage biocompatibility, but this view does not consider that adsorbed proteins exist in different states, depending upon adsorption conditions, residence time, and substrate. Evidence suggests that fibrinogen adsorbed from blood to substrates upon which the protein readily denatures, e.g., LTI carbon, may in fact promote biocompatibility. Because it is the organization and not the amount of an adsorbed protein that determines its biological activity, what happens to proteins after they adsorb to the substrate must be determined to properly evaluate the biocompatibility of a material. Further, a material might be made blood compatible if protein organization can be controlled such that the cell binding epitopes become unavailable for cell binding [Horbett et al., 1994]. Much current research aims to understand the relationship between the states of adsorbed proteins and cell-protein-surface interactions.

Fundamental to better understanding of material biocompatibility is understanding the importance of protein and surface structure and heterogeneity in determining the organization of proteins at the solid-liquid interface, the dynamics of multicomponent adsorption from complex media, e.g., the Vroman effect, and the significance of post-adsorptive events and subsequent cellular interactions. MAbs against specific protein epitopes provide direct evidence of changes in the states of adsorbed proteins, and indirect methods provide corroborative evidence. Molecular imaging techniques such as atomic (AFM), lateral force (LFM), and scanning tunneling (STM) microscopies have been adapted to aqueous systems to better define the states of adsorbed proteins with limited success [Sit et al., 1998], as have surface analysis techniques such as surface-matrix assisted laser desorption ionization (MALDI) [Kingshott et al., 1998].

Identification and characterization of the cell binding domains of adhesive proteins have led to better understanding of cell adhesion at the molecular level. Pierschbacher and colleagues [1981] used monoclonal antibodies and proteolytic fragments of fibronectin to identify the location of the cell attachment site of the molecule. Subsequently, residue sequences within the cell binding domains of other adhesive proteins were identified as summarized by Yamada [1991]. The Arg-Gly-Asp (RGD) amino acid sequence first isolated from fibronectin was later found present within vitronectin, osteopontin, collagens, thrombospondin, fibrinogen, and vWF [Ruoslahti and Pierschbacher, 1987]. Different adhesive peptides exhibit cell line dependent biological activity *in vitro*, but relatively few *in vivo* studies of adhesive peptides have been reported.

Haverstick and colleagues [1985] reported that addition of RGD-containing peptides to protein-free platelet suspension inhibited thrombin induced platelet aggregation, as well as platelet adhesion *in vitro* to fibronectin, fibrinogen, and vWF coated polystyrene. These results suggest that binding of the peptide to the platelet renders the platelet's receptor for the proteins unavailable for further binding. Similarly, Hanson and Harker [1988] used MAbs against the platelet glycoprotein IIb/IIIa (fibrinogen binding) complex to prevent thrombus formation upon Dacron vascular grafts placed within a chronic baboon AV shunt. Controlled release of either MAbs or adhesive peptides at the site of medical device implant might allow localized control of thrombosis. Locally administered adhesive peptides might also be used to selectively control cell behavior; e.g., Ruoslahti [1992] used RGD containing peptides to inhibit tumor invasion *in vitro* and dissemination *in vivo*. A recently developed drug delivery system offers great promise with respect to these therapeutic interventions [Markou et al., 1996, 1998].

Alternatively, adhesive peptides can be used to promote cell proliferation. Hubbell and colleagues [1991] reported that immobilization of different adhesive peptides resulted in selective cell response *in vitro*. Whereas the immobilized RGD and YIGSR peptides both enhanced spreading of human foreskin fibroblasts, human vascular smooth muscle cells, and human vascular endothelial cells, immobilization of REDV enhanced spreading of only endothelial cells. If this concept can be applied *in vivo*, then endothelialization in the absence of inflammation, infection, or thrombosis might be achieved.

Defining Terms

Conformation: Higher order protein structure that describes the spatial relationship between the amino acid chains that a protein comprises.

Epitope: Particular regions of a protein to which an antibody or cell can bind.

Hemostasis: Mechanism by which damaged blood vessels are repaired without compromising normal blood flow.

Integrin: Cellular transmembrane protein that acts as a receptor for adhesive extracellular matrix proteins such as fibronectin. The tripeptide RGD is the sequence recognized by many integrins.

Organization: The manner in which a protein resides upon a surface, in particular, the existence, arrangement, and availability of different protein epitopes.

Plasma concentration: Not the concentration of total protein in the plasma, but rather the volume fraction of plasma in the adsorption medium when protein adsorption from different dilutions of plasma is measured.

Post-adsorptive transitions: Changes in protein conformation and organization that occur when adsorbed proteins reside upon a surface.

Residue: The individual amino acids of a peptide or protein.

Specific activity: The amount of radioactivity detected per unit mass of a specific protein.

State: The reactive state of an adsorbed protein as determined by its conformation and organization.

Thrombosis: Formation of plug comprising blood platelets and fibrin that stops blood flow through damaged blood vessels. Embolized thrombus refers to a plug that has detached from the wound site and entered the circulation.

Vroman effect: Collective term describing (1) maximal adsorption of a specific protein from multi-component medium at early time, (2) maximal equilibrium adsorption from intermediate dilution, and (3) decrease with increased adsorption time in the plasma concentration at which adsorption is maximum.

Vroman peak: The adsorption maximum in the adsorption versus log (plasma concentration) curve when protein adsorption from different dilutions of plasma is measured.

References

Andrade JD. 1985. Principles of protein adsorption. In JD Andrade (ed), *Surface and Interfacial Aspects of Biomedical Polymers: Protein Adsorption,* vol 2, pp 1–80, Plenum, New York.

Andrade JD, Hlady V. 1986. Protein adsorption and materials biocompatibility: A tutorial review and suggested hypotheses. In *Advances in Polymer Science 79.* Biopolymers/Non-Exclusion HPLC, pp 1–63, Springer-Verlag, Berlin.

Andrade JD. 1985. Polymer surface analysis: Conclusions and expectations. In JD Andrade (ed), *Surface and Interfacial Aspects of Biomedical Polymers,* vol 1, Surface Chemistry and Physics, pp. 443-460, Plenum Press, New York.

Balasubramanian V, Grusin NK, Bucher RW, et al. In Press. Residence-time dependent changes in fibrinogen adsorbed to polymeric biomaterials. *J. Biomed. Mater. Res.*

Bohnert JL, Horbett TA. 1986. Changes in adsorbed fibrinogen and albumin interactions with polymers indicated by decreases in detergent elutability. *J. Coll. Interface Sci.* 111:363.

Brash JL, ten Hove P. 1984. Effect of plasma dilution on adsorption of fibrinogen to solid surfaces. *Thromb. Haemostas.* 51:326.

Castillo EJ, Koenig JL, Anderson JM et al., 1984. Characterization of protein adsorption on soft contact lenses. I. Conformational changes of adsorbed serum albumin. *Biomaterials* 5:319.

Castillo EJ, Koenig JL, Anderson JM et al., 1985. Characterization of protein adsorption on soft contact lenses. II. Reversible and irreversible interactions between lysozyme and soft contact lens surfaces. *Biomaterials* 6:338.

Chenowith DE. 1988. Complement activation produced by biomaterials. *Artif. Organs* 12:502.

Chinn JA, Posso SE, Horbett TA et al., 1991. Post-adsorptive transitions in fibrinogen adsorbed to Biomer: Changes in baboon platelet adhesion, antibody binding, and sodium dodecyl sulfate elutability. *J. Biomed. Mater. Res.* 25:535.

Chinn JA, Posso SE, Horbett TA et al., 1992. Post-adsorptive transitions in fibrinogen adsorbed to polyurethanes: Changes in antibody binding and sodium dodecyl sulfate elutability. *J. Biomed. Mater. Res.* 26:757.

De Baillou N, Dejardin P, Schmitt A et al., 1984. Fibrinogen dimensions at an interface: Variations with bulk concentration, temperature, and pH. *J. Colloid Interface Sci.* 100:167.

Dewanjee MK. 1992. *Radioiodination: Theory, Practice, and Biomedical Application,* Kluwer Academic Press, Norwell.

Feng L, Andrade JD. 1994. Protein adsorption on low temperature isotropic carbon. I. Protein conformational change probed by differential scanning calorimetry. *J. Biomed. Mater. Res.* 28:735.

Hanson SR, Harker LA. 1988. Interruption of acute platelet-dependent thrombosis by the synthetic antithrombin D-phenylalanyl-L-prolyl-L-arginyl chloromethylketone. *Proc. Natl. Acad. Sci. U.S.A.* 85:3184.

Haverstick DM, Cowan JF, Yamada KM et al., 1985. Inhibition of platelet adhesion to fibronectin, fibrinogen, and von Willebrand factor substrates by a synthetic tetrapeptide derived from the cell-binding domain of fibronectin. *Blood* 66:946.

Horbett TA. 1981. Adsorption of proteins from plasma to a series of hydrophilic-hydrophobic copolymers. II. Compositional analysis with the prelabeled protein technique. *J. Biomed. Mater. Res.* 15:673.

Horbett TA. 1982. Protein adsorption on biomaterials. In SL Cooper, NA Peppas (eds), *Biomaterials: Interfacial Phenomena and Applications,* ACS Advances in Chemistry Series, vol 199, pp 233–244, American Chemical Society, Washington, D.C.

Horbett TA. 1984. Mass action effects on competitive adsorption of fibrinogen from hemoglobin solutions and from plasma. *Thromb. Haemostas.* 51:174.

Horbett TA. 1986. Techniques for protein adsorption studies. In DF Williams (ed), *Techniques of Biocompatibility Testing,* pp 183–214, CRC Press, Boca Raton, FL.

Horbett TA, Grunkemeier JM, Lew KR. 1994. Fibrinogen orientation of a surface coated with a GP IIb/IIIa peptide detected with monoclonal antibodies. *Trans. Soc. Biomater.* 17:335.

Horbett TA, Lew KR. 1994. Residence time effects on monoclonal antibody binding to adsorbed fibrinogen. *J. Biomater. Sci. Polym. Edn.* 6:15.

Hubbell JA, Massia SP, Desai NP et al., 1991. Endothelial cell-selective materials for tissue engineering in the vascular graft via a new receptor. *Biotechnology (NY)* 9:568.

Kaplan AP. 1978. Initiation of the intrinsic coagulation and fibrinolytic pathway of man: The role of surfaces, Hageman factor, prekallikrein, high molecular weight kininogen, and factor XI. *Prog. Hemostas. Thromb.* 4:127.

Kingshott P, St. John HAW, Vaithianathan T et al., 1998. Study of protein adsorption at monolayer and sub-monolayer levels by surface-MALDI spectroscopy. *Trans. Soc. Biomater.* 21:253.

Lindon JN, McManama G, Kushner L et al., 1986. Does the conformation of adsorbed fibrinogen dictate platelet interactions with artificial surfaces? *Blood* 68:355.

Macfarlane AS. 1958. Efficient trace-labelling of proteins with iodine. *Nature* 182:53.

Markou CP, Chronos NF, Harker LA et al., 1996. Local endovascular drug delivery for inhibition of thrombosis. *Circulation* 94:1563.

Markou CP, Lutostansky EM, Ku DN et al., 1998. A novel method for efficient drug delivery. *Ann. Biomed. Eng.* 26:502.

Norde W, MacRitchie F, Nowicka G et al. 1986. Protein adsorption at solid-liquid interfaces: reversibility and conformation aspects. *J. Colloid Interface Sci.* 112:447.

Norde W. 1986. Adsorption of proteins from solution at the solid-liquid interface. *Adv. Colloid Interface Sci.* 25:267.

Norde W, Lyklema J. 1991. Why proteins prefer interfaces. *J. Biomater. Sci. Polym. Edn.* 2:183.

Pettit DK, Hoffman AS, Horbett TA. 1994. Correlation between corneal epithelial cell outgrowth and monoclonal antibody binding to the cell domain of fibronectin. *J. Biomed. Mater. Res.* 228:685.

Phillips DR, Charo IF, Parise LV et al., 1988. The platelet membrane glycoprotein IIb-IIIa complex. *Blood* 71:831.

Pierschbacher MD, Hayman EG, Ruoslahti E. 1981. Location of the cell-attachment site in fibronectin with monoclonal antibodies and proteolytic fragments of the molecule. *Cell* 26:259.

Rainbow MR, Atherton S, Eberhart RE. 1987. Fluorescence lifetime measurements using total internal reflection fluorimetry: Evidence for a conformational change in albumin adsorbed to quartz. *J. Biomed. Mater. Res.* 21:539.

Rapoza RJ, Horbett TA. 1990. Postadsorptive transitions in fibrinogen: Influence of polymer properties. *J. Biomed. Mater. Res.* 24:1263.

Ratner BD, McElroy BJ. 1986. Electron spectroscopy for chemical analysis: Applications in the biomedical sciences. In Gendreau RM (ed), *Spectroscopy in the Biomedical Sciences,* pp 107–140, CRC Press, Boca Raton, FL.

Ratnoff OD, Menzie C. 1950. A new method for the determination of fibrinogen in small samples of plasma. *J. Lab. Clin. Med.* 37:316.

Ruoslahti E. 1991. Integrins. *J. Clin. Invest.* 87:1.

Ruoslahti E. 1992. The Walter Herbert Lecture: Control of cell motility and tumour invasion by extracellular matrix interactions. *Br. J. Cancer* 66:239.

Ruoslahti E, Pierschbacher MD. 1987. New perspectives in cell adhesion: RGD and integrins. *Science* 238:491.

Sakariassen KS, Bolhuis PA, Sixma JJ. 1979. Human blood platelet adhesion to artery subendothelium is mediated by factor VIII-Von Willebrand factor bound to the subendothelium. *Nature* 279:636.

Sandwick RK, Schray KJ. 1987. The inactivation of enzymes upon interaction with a hydrophobic latex surface. *J. Colloid Interface Sci.* 115:130.

Sandwick RK, Schray KJ. 1988. Conformational states of enzymes bound to surfaces. *J. Colloid Interface Sci.* 121:1.

Shiba E, Lindon JN, Kushner L et al., 1991. Antibody-detectable changes in fibrinogen adsorption affecting platelet activation on polymer surfaces. *Am. J. Physiol.* 260:C965.

Sit PS, Siedlecki CA, Shainoff JR et al. 1998. Substrate-dependent conformations of human fibrinogen visualized by atomic force microscopy under aqueous conditions. *Trans. Soc. Biomater.* 21:101.

Slack SM, Horbett TA. 1989. Changes in the state of fibrinogen adsorbed to solid surfaces: An explanation of the influence of surface chemistry on the Vroman effect. *J. Colloid Interface Sci.* 133:148.

Slack SM, Horbett TA. 1992. Changes in fibrinogen adsorbed to segmented polyurethanes and hydroxymethacrylate-ethylmethacrylate copolymers. *J. Biomed. Mater. Res.* 26:1633.

Slack SM, Horbett TA. 1995. The Vroman effect: A critical review. In TA Horbett, JL Brash (eds), *Proteins at Interfaces II,* pp 112–128, American Chemical Society, Washington, D.C.

Smith JM. 1981. *Chemical Engineering Kinetics,* 3rd ed, McGraw-Hill, New York.

Soria J, Soria C, Mirshahi M et al., 1985. Conformational changes in fibrinogen induced by adsorption to a surface. *J. Colloid Interface Sci.* 107:204.

Stryer L. 1995. *Biochemistry,* 4th ed, W.H. Freeman, New York.

Vroman L, Adams AL. 1969. Identification of rapid changes at plasma-solid interfaces. *J. Biomed. Mater. Res.* 3:43.

Vroman L, Adams AL, Fischer GL et al., 1980. Interaction of high molecular weight kininogen, factor XII and fibrinogen in plasma at interfaces. *Blood* 55:156.

Willems GM, Hermens WT, Hemker HC. 1991. Surface exclusion and molecular mobility may explain Vroman effects in protein adsorption. *J. Biomater. Sci. Polym. Edn.* 1:217.

Wojciechowski P, ten Hove P, Brash JL. 1986. Phenomenology and mechanism of the transient adsorption of fibrinogen from plasma (Vroman effect). *J. Colloid Interface Sci.* 111:455.

Yamada KM. 1991. Adhesive recognition sequences. *J. Biol. Chem.* 266:12809.

Young BR, Lambrecht LK, Cooper SL. 1982. Plasma proteins: Their role in initiating platelet and fibrin deposition on biomaterials. In SL Cooper, NA Peppas (eds), *Biomaterials: Interfacial Phenomena and Applications,* ACS Advances in Chemistry Series, vol 199, pp 317–350, American Chemical Society, Washington, D.C.

Zamarron C, Ginsberg MH, Plow EF. 1990. Monoclonal antibodies specific for a conformationally altered state of fibrinogen. *Thromb. Haemostas.* 64:41.

Zucker MB, Vroman L. 1969. Platelet adhesion induced by fibrinogen adsorbed on glass. *Proc. Soc. Exp. Med.* 131:318.

Further Information

The American Society for Artificial and Internal Organs (ASAIO) (P.O. Box C, Boca Raton, FL 33429-0468, Web address http://www.asaio.com) publishes original articles in ASAIO J through Lippincott-Raven Publishers (227 East Washington Square, Philadelphia, PA 19106-3780) and meeting transactions in *Trans. Am. Soc. Artif. Intern. Organs.*

The Society for Biomaterials (SFB) (6518 Walker St., Ste. 150, Minneapolis, MN 55426-4215, Web address http://www.biomaterials.org) publishes original articles in both *J. Biomed. Mater. Res.* and *J. Biomed. Mater. Res. Appl. Biomater.* through John Wiley and Sons, Inc. (605 Third Ave., New York, NY 10158) and meeting transactions in *Trans. Soc. Biomaterials.* The *J. Colloid Interface Sci.* often contains articles related to protein-surface interactions as well.

The American Association for the Advancement of Science (AAAS) (1200 New York Ave. NW, Washington, D.C. 20002, Web address http://www.aaas.org) publishes original articles in science, and often contains excellent review articles and very current developments in protein research. *Nature*, published through Macmillan Magazines (Porters South, 4 Crinan St., London N1 9XW), is similar in content but provides a decidedly European perspective.

Comprehensive references summarizing applications of protein adsorption and biocompatibility include: 1982. SL Cooper, NA Peppas (eds.), *Biomaterials: Interfacial Phenomena and Applications*, ACS Advances in Chemistry Series, vol 199, Washington, D.C., American Chemical Society; 1987. TA Horbett and JL Brash (eds.), *Proteins at Interfaces: Physicochemical and Biochemical Studies*, ACS Symposium Series, vol 343, Washington, D.C., American Chemical Society; and 1993. SM Factor (ed.), Cardiovascular Biomaterials and Biocompatibility. *Cardiovasc. Pathol.* 2(3) Suppl.

11

Engineering Biomaterials for Tissue Engineering: The 10–100 Micron Size Scale

David J. Mooney
Massachusetts Institute of Technology

Robert S. Langer
Massachusetts Institute of Technology

A significant challenge in tissue engineering is to take a biomaterial and process it into a useful form for a specific application. All devices for tissue engineering transplant cells and/or induce the ingrowth of desirable cell types from the host organism. The device must provide sufficient mechanical support to maintain a space for tissue to form or serve as a barrier to undesirable interactions. Also, the device can be designed to provide these functions for a defined period before biodegradation occurs or on a permanent basis.

Generally speaking, devices can be broken down into two types. Immunoprotective devices contain semipermeable membranes that prevent elements of the host immune system (e.g., IgG antibodies and lymphocytes) from entering the device. In contrast, open devices have large pores (>10 μm) and allow free transport of molecules and cells between the host tissue and transplanted cells. These latter devices are utilized to engineer a tissue that is completely integrated with the host tissue. Both types of devices can range in size from microns to centimeters or beyond, although the larger sizes are usually repetitions on the structure found at the scale of hundreds of microns.

A fundamental question in designing a device is whether to use synthetic or natural materials. Synthetic materials (e.g., organic polymers) can be easily processed into various structures and can be produced cheaply and reproducibly; it also is possible to tightly control various properties such as the mechanical strength, hydrophobicity, and degradation rate of synthetic materials. Whereas natural materials (e.g., collagen) sometimes exhibit a limited range of physical properties and can be difficult to isolate and process, they do have specific biologic activity. In addition, these molecules generally do not elicit unfavorable host tissue responses, a condition which is typically taken to indicate that a material is biocompatible. Some synthetic polymers, in contrast, can elicit a long-term inflammatory response from the host tissue [Bostman, 1991].

A significant challenge in fabricating devices is either to develop processing techniques for natural biomaterials that allow reproducible fabrication on a large-scale basis [Cavallaro et al., 1994] or to develop materials that combine the advantages of synthetic materials with the biologic activity of natural biomaterials [Barrera et al., 1993; Massia and Hubbell, 1991]. Computer-aided-design–computer-aided-manufacturing (CAD-CAM) technology may possibly be employed in the future to custom-fit devices with complex structures to patients.

11.1   Fundamentals

The interaction of the host tissue with the device and transplanted cells can be controlled by both the geometry of the device and the internal structure. The number of inflammatory cells and cellular enzyme activity around implanted polymeric devices has been found to depend on the geometry of the device [Matlaga et al., 1976], with device geometries that contain sharp angles provoking the greatest response. The surface geometry, or microstructure, of implanted polymer devices also has been found to affect the types and activities of acute inflammatory cells recruited to the device as well as the formation of a fibrous capsule [Taylor and Gibbons, 1983].

The pore structure of a device dictates the interaction of the device and transplanted cells with the host tissue. The pore structure is determined by the size, size distribution, and continuity of the individual pores within the device. Porous materials are typically defined as microporous (pore diameter $d < 2$ nm), mesoporous (2 nm $< d <$ 50 nm), or macroporous ($d >$ 50 nm) [Schaeffer, 1994]. Only small molecules (e.g., gases) are capable of penetrating microporous materials. Mesoporous materials allow transport of larger molecules, such as small proteins, but transport of large proteins and cells is prevented. Macroporous materials allow free transport of large molecules, and, if the pores are large enough ($d >$ 10^4 nm), cells are capable of migrating through the pores of the device. The proper design of a device can allow desirable signals (e.g., a rise in serum sugar concentration) to be passed to transplanted cells while excluding molecular or cellular signals which would promote rejections of transplanted cells (e.g., IgG protein).

Fibrovascular tissue will invade a device if the pores are larger than approximately 10 μm, and the rate of invasion will increase with the pore size and total porosity of a device [Mikos et al., 1993c; Weslowski et al., 1961; White et al., 1981]. The degree of fibrosis and calcification of early fabric leaflet valves has been correlated to their porosity [Braunwald et al., 1965], as has the nonthrombogenicity of arterial prosthesis [DeBakey et al., 1964] and the rigidity of tooth implants and orthopedic prosthesis [Hamner et al., 1972; Hulbert et al., 1972].

It is important to realize that many materials do not have a unimodal pore size distribution or a continuous pore structure, and the ability of molecules or cells to be transported through such a device will often be limited by bottlenecks in the pore structure. In addition, the pore structure of a device may change over time in a biologic environment. For example, absorption of water into polymers of the lactic/glycolic acid family results in the formation first of micropores, and eventually of macropores as the polymer itself degrades [Cohen et al., 1991]. The porosity and pore-size distribution of a device can be determined utilizing a variety of techniques [Smith et al., 1994].

Specific properties (e.g., mechanical strength, degradability, hydrophobicity, biocompatibility) of a device are also often desirable. These properties can be controlled both by the biomaterial itself and by the processing technique utilized to fabricate the device. An advantage of fabricating devices from synthetic polymers is the variety of processing techniques available for these materials. Fibers, hollow fibers, and porous sponges can be readily formed from synthetic polymers. Natural biomaterials must be isolated from plant, animal, or human tissue and are typically expensive and suffer from large batch-to-batch variations. Although the wide range of processing techniques available for synthetic polymers is not available for these materials, cells specifically interact with certain types of natural biomaterials, such as extracellular matrix (ECM) molecules [Hynes, 1987]. The known ability of ECM molecules to mediate cell function *in vitro* and *in vivo* may allow precise control over the biologic response to devices fabricated from ECM molecules.

11.2   Applications

The applications of tissue engineering are very diverse, encompassing virtually every type of tissue in the human body. However, the devices utilized in these areas can be divided into two broad types. The first type, immunoprotective devices, utilizes a semipermeable membrane to limit communication between cells in the device and the host. The small pores in these devices ($d < 10$ nm) allow low-molecular-weight proteins and molecules to be transported between the implant and the host tissue, but they prevent large proteins (e.g., immunoglobulins) and host cells (e.g., lymphocytes) of the immune system from entering the device and mediating rejection of the transplanted cells. In contrast, open structures with large pores are typically utilized ($d > 10$ μm) if one desires that the new tissue be structurally integrated with the host tissue. Applications that utilize both types of devices are described below.

Immunoprotective Devices

Devices that protect transplanted cells from the immune system of the host can be broken down into two types, microencapsulation and macroencapsulation systems [Emerich et al., 1992]. Individual cells or small clusters of cells are surrounded by a semipermeable membrane and delivered as a suspension in microencapsulation systems (Fig. 11.1a). Macroencapsulation systems utilize hollow semipermeable membranes to deliver multiple cells or cell clumps (Fig. 11.1b). The small size, thin wall, and spherical shape of microcapsules all optimize diffusional transport to and from the microencapsulated cells. Macroencapsulation devices typically have greater mechanical integrity than microcapsule devices, and they can be easily retrieved after implantation. However, the structure of these devices is not optimal for diffusional transport. Nonbiodegradable materials are the preferred choice for fabricating both types of devices, as the barrier function is typically required over the lifetime of the implant.

A significant effort has been made to cure diabetes by transplanting microencapsulated pancreatic islet cells. Transplantation of nonimmunoprotected islets has led to short-term benefits [Lim and Sun, 1980], but the cells were ultimately rejected. To prevent this, islets have been immobilized in alginate (a naturally occurring polymer derived from seaweed) microbeads coated with a layer of poly(L-lysine) and a layer of polyethyleneimine [Lim and Sun, 1980]. Alginate is ionically cross-linked in the presence of calcium, and the permeability of alginate/poly(L-lysine) microbeads is determined by the formation of ionic or hydrogen bonds between the polyanion alginate and the polycation poly(L-lysine). This processing technique allows cells to be immobilized without exposure to organic solvents or high temperatures. The outer layer of polyethyleneimine was subsequently replaced by a layer of alginate to prevent the formation of fibrous capsules around the implanted microcapsules [O'Shea et al., 1984]. Smaller microbeads (250–400 μm) have been generated with an electrostatic pulse generator [Lum et al., 1992] to improve the *in vivo* survival and the response time of encapsulated cells [Chicheportiche and Reach, 1988]. These devices have been shown to be effective in a variety of animal models [Lim and Sun, 1980; Lum et al., 1992], and clinical trials of microencapsulated islets in diabetic patients are in progress [Soon-Shiong et al., 1994]. Synthetic analogs to alginate have also been developed [Cohen et al., 1990].

The superior mechanical stability of macroencapsulation devices, along with the possibility of retrieving the entire device, makes these types of devices especially attractive when the transplanted cells have limited lifetimes and/or when one needs to ensure that the transplanted cells are not migrating out of the device. Macroencapsulation devices have been utilized to transplant a variety of cell types, including pancreatic cells [Lacy et al., 1991], NGF-secreting cells [Winn et al., 1994], dopamine-secreting cells [Emerich et al., 1992], and Chromaffin cells [Sagen et al., 1993]. The nominal molecular mass cutoff of the devices was 50 kD, allowing immunoprotection without interfering with transport of therapeutic agents from the encapsulated cells. To prevent cell aggregation and subsequent large-scale cell death due to nutrient limitations, macroencapsulated islets have been immobilized in alginate [Lacy et al., 1991].

Devices with Open Structures

Devices with large, interconnected pores ($d > 10$ μm) are utilized in applications where one wishes the transplanted cells to interact directly with host tissue and form a structurally integrated tissue. The open structure of these devices provides little barrier to diffusional transport and often promotes the ingrowth of blood vessels from the host tissue. Degradable materials are often utilized in these applications, since once tissue structures are formed the device is not needed.

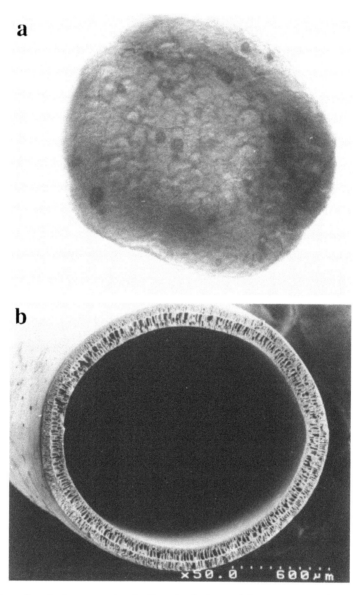

FIGURE 11.1 Examples of microencapsulated cells and a device used for macroencapsulation of cells. (a) Phase contrast photomicrograph of hybridoma cells encapsulated in a calcium cross-linked polyphosphazene gel [Cohen et al., 1993]. Original magnification was 100×. (Used with permission of Editions de Sante.) (b) A SEM photomicrograph of a poly(acrylonitrile-co-vinyl chloride) hollow fiber formed by phase inversion using a dry-jet wet-spinning technique [Schoichet et al., 1994]. (Used with permission of John Wiley and Sons, Inc.)

These types of devices typically fall into two categories. The first types is fabrics, either woven or nonwoven, of small-diameter (approximately 10–40 μm) fibers (Fig. 11.2a). High porosity (>95%) and large average pore size can be easily obtained with this type of material, and these materials can be readily shaped into different geometries. Fibers can be formed from synthetic, crystalline polymers such as polyglycolic acid by melt extrusion [Frazza and Schmitt, 1971]. Fibers and fabrics also can be formed from natural materials such as type I collagen, a type of ECM molecule, by extrusion of soluble collagen into a bath where gelling occurs followed by dehydration of the fiber [Cavallaro et al., 1994]. The tensile strength of fibers is dependent on the extent of collagen cross-linking, which can be controlled by the processing technique [Wang et al., 1994]. Processed collagen fibers can be subsequently spooled and

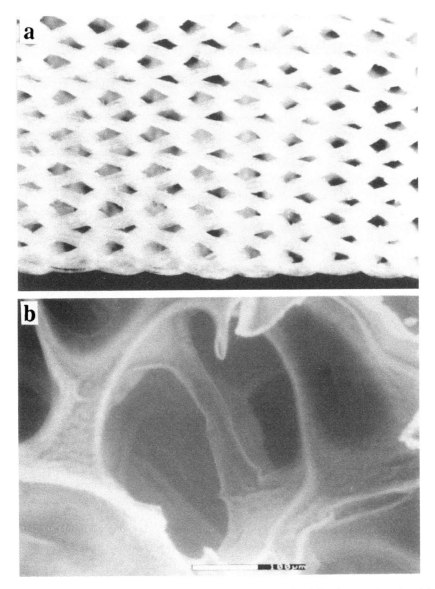

FIGURE 11.2 Examples of a fiber-based fabric and a porous sponge utilized for tissue engineering. (a) A photomicrograph of type I collagen fibers knitted into a fabric. Fiber diameters can be as small as 25 μm, and devices constructed from these fibers can be utilized for a variety of tissue engineering applications [Cavallaro et al., 1994]. (Used with permission of John Wiley and Sons, Inc.) (b) A SEM photomicrograph of a formaldehyde-cross-linked polyvinyl alcohol sponge. These devices have been utilized for a variety of applications, including hepatocyte transplantation [Uyama et al., 1993].

knitted to form fabrics [Cavallaro et al., 1994]. These devices are often ideal when engineering two-dimensional tissues. However, these fabrics typically are incapable of resisting large compressional forces, and three-dimensional devices are often crushed *in vivo*. Three-dimensional fiber-based structures have been stabilized by physically bonding adjacent fibers [Mikos et al., 1993a; Mooney et al., 1994a; Vacanti et al., 1992].

To engineer three-dimensional tissues, porous sponge devices (Fig. 11.2b) are utilized typically in place of fiber-based devices. These devices are better capable of resisting larger compressional forces (approximately 10^4 Pa) [Mikos et al., 1993a] than are unbounded fiber-based devices (approximately 10^2 Pa) [Mooney et al., 1994a] due to the continuous solid phase and can be designed to have complex, three-dimensional forms [Mikos et al., 1993b; White et al., 1972]. Porous sponges can be fabricated from synthetic polymers utilizing a variety of techniques, including performing the polymerization of a hydrophobic polymer in an aqueous solution [Chirila et al., 1993], exploiting phase separation behavior of dissolved polymers in specific solvents [Lo et al., 1994], and combining solvent casting with particulate leaching [Mikos et al., 1993b, 1994]. Porous sponges can be formed from type I collagen and other ECM molecules by chemically cross-linking gels or assembling the collagen in nonnatural polymeric structures [Bell et al., 1981; Chvapil, 1979; Stenzel et al., 1974; Yannas et al., 1982].

Perhaps the most significant clinical effort using open devices has been expended to engineer skin tissue to treat burn victims. Both natural [Bell et al., 1981; Yannas et al., 1982] and synthetic degradable materials [Hansbrough et al., 1992] in the form of porous sponges or fiber-based fabrics have been utilized to transplant various cellular elements of skin. One device fabricated from ECM molecules has also been combined with an outer coat of silicone elastomer to prevent dehydration of the wound site [Yannas et al., 1982]. The various approaches have shown efficacy in animal models, and tissue-engineered skin has progressed to clinical trials [Burke et al., 1981; Compton et al., 1989; Heimbach et al., 1988; Stern et al., 1990].

Another area with great clinical potential is the engineering of bone and cartilage tissue. Various ceramics and biodegradable synthetic polymers have been utilized to fabricate devices for these purposes. Porous calcium phosphate devices loaded with mesenchymal stem cells have been shown to promote bone formation when implanted into soft tissue sites of animals [Goshima et al., 1991; Haynesworth et al., 1992]. Ceramics also have been coated onto prosthetic devices (e.g., hip replacements) to promote bone ingrowth and bonding between the prosthetic device and the host tissue [Furlong and Osborn, 1991]. The degradation rate [de Bruijn et al., 1994] and mechanical properties [Yoshinari et al., 1994] of these ceramics can be controlled by the deposition technique, which determines the crystallinity and chemical structure of the deposited ceramic. The brittleness of ceramic materials limits them in certain applications, and to bypass this problem composite ceramic/polymer devices have been developed [Stupp et al., 1993]. Fiber-based fabrics of biodegradable polymers have also been utilized to transplant cells derived from periosteal tissue and form new bone tissue [Vacanti et al., 1993]. To engineer cartilage tissue with specific structures such as an ear or nasal septum, devices have been fabricated from a nonwoven mesh of biodegradable synthetic polymers molded to the size and shape of the desired tissue. These devices, after seeding with chondrocytes and implantation, have been shown to induce the formation of new cartilage tissue with the same structure as the polymer device utilized as the template [Puelacher et al., 1993; Vacanti et al., 1991, 1992]. After tissue development is complete, the device itself degrades to leave a completely natural tissue.

Liver tissue [Uyama et al., 1993], ligaments [Cavallaro et al., 1994], and neural tissue [Guenard et al., 1992; Madison et al., 1985] also have been engineered with open devices. Tubular tissues, including blood vessels [Weinberg and Bell, 1986], intestine [Mooney et al., 1994b; Organ et al., 1993], and urothelial structures [Atala et al., 1992] have been engineered utilizing open devices fabricated into a tubular structure.

11.3   Conclusions

A variety of issues must be addressed to design and fabricate a device for tissue engineering. Do the transplanted cells need immunoprotection, or should they structurally integrate with the host tissue? If immunoprotection is desired, will a micro- or macroencapsulation device be preferred? If a structurally integrated new tissue is desired, will a fiber-based device or a porous sponge be more suitable? The specific roles that the device will play in a given application and the material itself will dictate the design of the device and the fabrication technique.

Defining Terms

Biocompatible: A material which does not elicit an unfavorable response from the host but instead performs with an appropriate host response in a specific application [Williams, 1987].

Biodegradation: The breakdown of a material mediated by a biologic system [Williams et al., 1992]. Biodegradation can occur by simple hydrolysis or via enzyme- or cell-mediated breakdown.

Extracellular matrix (ECM) molecules: Various substances present in the extracellular space of tissues that serve to mediate cell adhesion and organization.

Immunoprotective: Serving to protect from interacting with the immune system of the host tissue, including cellular elements (e.g., lymphocytes) and proteins (e.g., IgG).

Open devices: Devices with large ($d > 10\ \mu$m) interconnected pores which allow unhindered transport of molecules and cells within the device and between the device and the surrounding tissue.

References

Barrera DA, Zylstra E, Lansbury PT, et al. 1993. Synthesis and RGD peptide modification of a new biodegradable copolymer: poly(lactic acid-co lysine). J Am Chem Soc 115:11010.

Bell E, Ehrlich HP, Buttle DJ, Nakatsuji T. 1981. Living tissue formed in vitro and accepted as skin-equivalent tissue of full thickness. Science 211:1052.

Bostman OM. 1991. Absorbable implants for the fixation of fractures. J Bone Joint Surg 73-A(1):148.

Braunwald NS, Reis RL, Pierce GE. 1965. Relation of pore size to tissue ingrowth in prosthetic heart valves: an experimental study. Surgery 57:741.

Burke JF, Yannas IV, Quinby WC, et al. 1981. Successful use of a physiological acceptable artificial skin in the treatment of extensive burn injury. Ann Surg 194:413.

Cavallaro JF, Kemp PD, Kraus KH. 1994. Collagen fabrics as biomaterials. Biotech Bioeng 43:781.

Chicheportiche D, Reach G. 1988. In vitro kinetics of insulin release by microencapsulated rat islets: effect of the size of the microcapsules. Diabetologia 31:54.

Chirila TV, Constable IJ, Crawford GJ, et al. 1993. Poly(2-hydroxyethyl methacrylate) sponges as implant materials: in vivo and in vitro evaluation of cellular invasion. Biomaterials 14(1):26.

Chvapil M. 1979. Industrial uses of collagen. In DAD Parry, LK Creamer (eds), Fibrous Proteins: Scientific, Industrial, and Medical Aspects, London, Academic Press.

Cohen S, Allcock HR, Langer R. 1993. Cell and enzyme immobilization in ionotropic synthetic hydrogels. In AA Hincal, HS Kas (eds), Recent Advances in Pharmaceutical and Industrial Biotechnology, Paris, Editions de Sante.

Cohen S, Bano MC, Visscher KB, et al. 1990. Ionically cross-linkable phosphazene: a novel polymer for microencapsulation. J Am Chem Soc 112:7832.

Cohen S, Yoshioka T, Lucarelli M, et al. 1991. Controlled delivery systems for proteins based on poly(lactic/glycolic acid) microspheres. Pharm Res 87(6):713.

Compton C, Gill JM, Bradford DA. 1989. Skin regenerated from cultured epithelial autografts on full-thickness wounds from 6 days to 5 years after grafting: A light, electron microscopic, and immunohistochemical study. Lab Invest 60:600.

DeBakey ME, Jordan GL, Abbot JP, et al. 1964. The fate of dacron vascular grafts. Arch Surg 89:757.

De Bruijn JD, Bovell YP, van Blitterswijk CA. 1994. Structural arrangements at the interface between plasma sprayed calcium phosphates and bone. Biomaterials 15(7):543.

Emerich DF, Winn SR, Christenson L, et al. 1992. A novel approach to neural transplantation in Parkinson's disease: Use of polymer-encapsulated cell therapy. Neurosci Biobeh Rev 16:437.

Frazza EJ, Schmitt EE. 1971. A new absorbable suture. J Biomed Mater Res Symp 1:43.

Furlong RJ, Osborn JE. 1991. Fixation of hip prostheses by hydroxylapatite ceramic coatings. J Bone Joint Surg 73-B(5):741.

Goshima J, Goldberg VM, Caplan AI. 1991. The origin of bone formed in composite grafts of porous calcium phosphate ceramic loaded with marrow cells. Clin Orthop Rel Res 191:274.

Guenard V, Kleitman N, Morissey TK, Bunge RP, Aebischer P. 1992. Syngeneic Schwann cells derived from adult nerves seeded in semipermeable guidance channels enhance peripheral nerve regeneration. J Neurosci 12:3310–3320.

Hamner JE, Reed OM, Greulich RC. 1972. Ceramic root implantation in baboons. J Biomed Mater Res Symp 6:1.

Hansbrough JF, Cooper ML, Cohen R, et al. 1992. Evaluation of a biodegradable matrix containing cultured human fibroblasts as a dermal replacement beneath meshed skin grafts on athymic mice. Surgery 111(4):438.

Haynesworth SE, Goshima J, Goldberg VM, et al. 1992. Characterization of cells with osteogenic potential from human marrow. Bone 13:81.

Heimbach D, Luterman A, Burke J, et al. 1988. Artificial dermis for major burns. Ann Surg 208(3):313.

Hulbert SF, Morrison SJ, Klawitter JJ. 1972. Tissue reaction to three ceramics of porous and nonporous structures. J Biomed Mater Res 6:347.

Hynes RO. 1987. Integrins: A family of cell surface receptors. Cell 48:549.

Lacy PE, Hegre OD, Gerasimidi-Vazeou A, et al. 1991. Maintenance of normoglycemia in diabetic mice by subcutaneous xenografts of encapsulated islets. Science 254:1782.

Lim F, Sun AM. 1980. Microencapsulated islets as bioartificial endocrine pancreas. Science 210:908.

Lo H, Kadiyala S, Guggino SE, et al. 1994. Biodegradable foams for cell transplantation. In R Murphy, A Mikos (eds), Biomaterials for Drug and Cell Delivery, Materials Research Society Proceedings, vol 331.

Lum Z, Krestow M, Tai IT, et al. 1992. Xenografts of rat islets into diabetic mice. Transplantation 53(6):1180.

Madison R, Da Silva CR, Dikkes P, et al. 1985. Increased rate of peripheral nerve regeneration using bioresorbable nerve guides and a laminin-containing gel. Exp Neurol 88:767.

Massia SP, Hubbell JA. 1991. An RGD spacing of 440 nm is sufficient for integrin $\alpha_v\beta_3$-mediated fibroblast spreading and 140 nm for focal contact and stress fiber formation. J Cell Biol 115(5):1089.

Matlaga BF, Yasenchak LP, Salthouse TN. 1976. Tissue response to implanted polymers: the significance of sample shape. J Biomed Mater Res 10:391.

Mikos AG, Bao Y, Cima LG, et al. 1993a. Preparation of poly(glycolic acid) bonded fiber structures for cell attachment and transplantation. J Biomed Mater Res 27:183.

Mikos AG, Sarakinos G, Leite SM, et al. 1993b. Laminated three-dimensional biodegradable foams for use in tissue engineering. Biomaterials 14(5):323.

Mikos AG, Sarakinos G, Lyman MD, et al. 1993c. Prevascularization of porous biodegradable polymers. Biotech Bioeng 42:716.

Mikos AG, Thorsen AJ, Czerwonka LA, et al. 1994. Preparation and characterization of poly(L-lactic) foams. Polymer 35(5):1068.

Mooney DJ, Mazzoni CL, Organ GM, et al. 1994a. Stabilizing fiber-based cell delivery devices by physically bonding adjacent fibers. In R Murphy, A Mikos (eds), Biomaterials for Drug and Cell Delivery, Materials Research Society Proceedings, Pittsburgh, PA, vol 331, 47–52.

Mooney DJ, Organ G, Vacanti JP. 1994b. Design and fabrication of biodegradable polymer devices to engineer tubular tissues. Cell Trans 3(2):203.

Organ GM, Mooney DJ, Hansen LK, et al. 1993. Enterocyte transplantation using cell-polymer devices causes intestinal epithelial-lined tube formation. Transplan Proc 25:998.

O'Shea GM, Goosen MFA, Sun AM. 1984. Prolonged survival of transplanted islets of Langerhans encapsulated in a biocompatible membrane. Biochim Biophys Acta 804:133.

Puelacher WC, Vacanti JP, Kim WS, et al. 1993. Fabrication of nasal implants using human shape specific polymer scaffolds seeded with chondrocytes. Surg Forum 44:678–680.

Sagen J, Wang H, Tresco PA, et al. 1993. Transplants of immunologically isolated xenogeneic chromaffin cells provide a long-term source of pain-reducing neuroactive substances. J Neurosci 13(6):2415.

Schaeffer DW. 1994. Engineered porous materials. MRS Bull April 1994:14.

Schoichet MS, Winn SR, Athavale S, et al. 1994. Poly(ethylene oxide)-grafted thermoplastic membranes for use as cellular hydrid bio-artificial organs in the central nervous system. Biotech Bioeng 43:563.

Smith DM, Hua D, Earl WL. 1994. Characterization of porous solids. MRS Bull April 1994:44.

Soon-Shiong P, Sandford PA, Heintz R, et al. 1994. First human clinical trial of immunoprotected islet allografts in alginate capsules. Society for Biomaterials Annual Meeting, Boston, abstract 356.

Stenzel KH, Miyata T, Rubin AL. 1974. Collagen as a biomaterial. Annu Rev Biophys Bioeng 3:231.

Stern R, McPherson M, Longaker MT. 1990. Histologic study of artificial skin used in the treatment of full-thickness thermal injury. J Burn Care Rehab 11:7.

Stupp SI, Hanson JA, Eurell JA, et al. 1993. Organoapatites: Materials for artificial bone: III. Biological testing. J Biomed Mater Res 27(3):301.

Taylor SR, Gibbons DF. 1983. Effect of surface texture on the soft tissue response to polymer implants. J Biomed Mater Res 17:205.

Uyama S, Takeda T, Vacanti JP. 1993. Delivery of whole liver equivalent hepatic mass using polymer devices and hepatotrophic stimulation. Transplantation 55(4):932.

Vacanti CA, Cima LG, Ratkowski D, et al. 1992. Tissue engineered growth of new cartilage in the shape of a human ear using synthetic polymers seeded with chondrocytes. In LG Cima, ES Ron (eds), Tissue Inducing Biomaterials, pp 367–374, Materials Research Society Proceedings, Pittsburgh, vol 252.

Vacanti CA, Kim W, Upton J, et al. 1993. Tissue engineered growth of bone and cartilage. Transplan Proc 25(1):1019.

Vacanti CA, Langer R, Schloo B, et al. 1991. Synthetic polymers seeded with chondrocytes provide a template for new cartilage formation. Plast Reconstr Surg 88(5):753.

Wang MC, Pins GD, Silver FH. 1994. Collagen fibers with improved strength for the repair of soft tissue injuries. Biomaterials 15:507.

Weinberg CB, Bell E. 1986. A blood vessel model constructed from collagen and cultured vascular cells. Science 231:397.

Weslowski SA, Fries CC, Karlson KE, et al. 1961. Porosity: Primary determinant of ultimate fate of synthetic vascular grafts. Surgery 50(1):91.

White RA, Hirose FM, Sproat RW, et al. 1981. Histopathologic observations after short-term implantation of two porous elastomers in dogs. Biomaterials 2:171.

White RA, Weber JN, White EW. 1972. Replamineform: A new process for preparing porous ceramic, metal, and polymer prosthetic materials. Science 176:922.

Williams DF. 1987. Definitions in Biomedicals. Progress in Biomedical Engineering, vol 4, New York, Elsevier.

Williams DF, Black J, Doherty PJ. 1992. Second consensus conference on definitions in biomaterials. In PJ Doherty, RL Williams, DF Williams, et al. (eds), Advances in Biomaterials, vol 10, Biomaterials-Tissue Interactions, pp 525–533, New York, Elsevier.

Winn SR, Hammang JP, Emerich DF, et al. 1994. Polymer-encapsulated cells genetically modified to secrete human nerve growth factor promote the survival of axotomized septal cholinergic neurons. Proc Natl Acad Sci USA 91:2324–2328.

Yannas IV, Burke JF, Orgill DP, et al. 1982. Wound tissue can utilize a polymeric template to synthesize a functional extension of skin. Science 215:174.

Yoshinari M, Ohtsuka Y, Derand T. 1994. Thin hydroxyapatite coating produced by the ion beam dynamic mixing method. Biomaterials 15:529.

Further Information

The Society for Biomaterials, American Society for Artificial Internal Organs, Cell Transplantation Society, and Materials Research Society all sponsor regular meetings and/or sponsor journals relevant to this topic. The following *Materials Research Society Symposium Proceedings* contain a collection of relevant articles: volume 252, *Tissue Inducing Biomaterials* (1992); volume 331, *Biomaterials for Drug and Cell Delivery* (1994). Another good source of relevant material is *Tissue Engineering*, edited by R Skalak and CF Fox, New York, Alan Riss (1988).

12

Regeneration Templates

Ioannis V. Yannas

*Massachusetts Institute
of Technology*

12.1 The Problem of the Missing Organ

Drugs typically replace or correct a missing function at the molecular scale; by contrast, regeneration templates replace the missing function at the scale of tissue or organ. An organ may be lost to injury or may fail in disease: The usual response of the organism is repair, which amounts to contraction and synthesis of scar tissue. Tissues and organs in the adult mammal typically do not regenerate. There are exceptions, such as epithelial tissues of the skin, gastrointestinal tract, genitals, and the cornea, all of which regenerate spontaneously; the liver also shows ability to synthesize substantial organ mass, though without recovery of the original organ shape. There are reports that bone and the elastic ligaments regenerate. These exceptions underscore the fact that the loss of an organ by the adult mammal almost invariably is an irreversible process, since the resulting scar tissue largely or totally lacks the structure and function of the missing organ. The most obvious examples involve losses due to injury such as the loss of a large area of skin following a burn accident or the loss of substantial nerve mass following an automobile accident. However, irreversible loss of function can also occur following disease, although over a lengthy time: Examples are the inability of a heart valve to prevent leakage during diastole as a result of valve tissue response to an inflammatory process (rheumatic fever), and the inability of liver tissue to synthesize enzymes due to its progressive replacement by fibrotic tissue (cirrhosis).

Five approaches have been used to solve the problem of the missing organ. In autografting, a mass of similar or identical tissue from the patient (autograft) is surgically removed and used to treat the area of loss. The approach can be considered to be spectacularly successful until one considers the long-term cost incurred by the patient. An example is the use of sheet autograft to treat extensive areas of full-thickness skin loss; although the patient incorporates the autograft fully with excellent recovery of function, the "donor" site used to harvest the autograft remains scarred. When the autograft is not available, as is common in cases of burns extending over more than 30% of body surface area autograft is meshed in order to make it extensible enough to cover the large wound areas. However, the meshed autograft provides cover only where the graft tissue provides direct cover; where there is no cover, scar forms, and the result is one of low cosmetic value. Similar problems of donor site unavailability and scarring must be dealt with in heart bypass surgery, another widespread example of autografting. In transplantation, the donor tissue is typically harvested from a cadaver, and the recipient has to cope with the problems of rejection and the risk of transmission of viruses from this allograft. Another approach has been based on efforts to synthesize tissues *in vitro* using autologous cells from the patient; this approach has yielded so far a cultured epidermis (a tissue which regenerates spontaneously provided there is a dermal substrate underneath) about 2–3 weeks after the time when the patient was injured. *In vitro* synthesis of the dermis, a tissue which does not regenerate, has not been accomplished so far. Perhaps the most successful approach from the commercial standpoint has been the one in which engineered biomaterials are used; these materials are typically required by their designers to remain intact themselves without interfering with the patient's physiologic functions during the entire lifetime; overwhelmingly, this requirement is observed in its breach. A fifth approach is based on the discovery that an analog of the extracellular matrix (ECM) induces partial regeneration of the dermis, rather than of scar, in full-thickness skin wounds in adult mammals (human, guinea pig, pig) where it is well known that no regeneration occurs spontaneously. This fifth approach of solving the problem of organ loss, *in situ* regeneration, is described in this chapter.

Efforts to induce regeneration have been successful with only a handful of ECM analogs. Evidence of regeneration is sought after the ECM analog has been implanted *in situ*, i.e., at the lesion marking the site of the missing organ. When morphogenesis is clearly evident, based on tests of recovery both of the original tissue structure and function, the matrix which has induced these physiologic or nearly physiologic tissues is named a regeneration template. In the absence of evidence of such morphogenetic activity of the cell-free matrix, the latter is not referred to as a regeneration template.

12.2 Search Principles for Identification of Regeneration Templates

Several parameters have been incorporated in the search for organ regeneration templates. Briefly, these parameters account for the performance of the implant during the early or acute stage following implantation (physicochemical parameters) as well as for the long-term or chronic stage following implantation (biologic parameters).

Immediately upon making contact with the wound bed, the implant must achieve physicochemical nanoadhesion (i.e., adhesion at a scale of 1 nm) between itself and the lesion. Without contact of this type it is not possible to establish and maintain transport of molecules and cells between implant and host tissue. The presence of adequate adhesion can be studied by measurements of the force necessary to peel the implant from the wound bed immediately after grafting.

Empirical evidence has supported a requirement for an implant which is capable of isomorphous tissue replacement, i.e., the synthesis of new tissue at a rate which is of same order as the rate of degradation of the matrix.

$$\frac{t_b}{t_h} = O\left(1\right) \tag{12.1}$$

In Eq. (12.1), t_b denotes a characteristic time constant for biodegradation of the implant *at that tissue site*, and t_h denotes a time constant for healing, the latter occurring by synthesis of new tissue inside the implant.

A third requirement refers to the *critical cell path length* l_c, beyond which migration of a cell into the implant deprives it of an essential nutrient, assumed to be transported from the host tissue by diffusion alone. The emphasis is on the characteristic diffusion path for the nutrient during the early stages of wound healing, before significant angiogenesis occurs several days later. Calculation of the critical cell path can be done by use of the *cell lifeline number,* S, a dimensionless number expressing the relative importance of a chemical reaction, which leads to consumption of an essential nutrient by the cell, and of diffusion of the nutrient which alone makes the latter accessible to the cell. This number is defined as

$$S = \frac{rl^2}{Dc_o} \tag{12.2}$$

where r is the rate of consumption of the nutrient by the cell in mole/cm^3/s, l is the diffusion length, D is the diffusivity of the nutrient in the medium of the implant, and c_o is the nutrient concentration at or near the surface of the wound bed, in mol/cm^3. When $S = O(1)$ the value of l is the critical path length, l_c along which cells can migrate, away from host tissue, without requirement of nutrient in excess of that supplied by diffusion. Equation (12.2) can, therefore, be used to define the maximum implant thickness beyond which cells require the presence of capillaries.

The chemical composition of the implant which has induced regeneration was designed on the basis of studies of wound-healing kinetics. In most mammals, full-thickness skin wounds close partly by contraction of the wounds edges and partly by synthesis of scar tissue. Clearly, skin regeneration over the entire area of skin loss cannot occur unless the wound edges are kept apart and, in addition, the healing processes in the wound bed are modified drastically enough to yield a physiologic dermis rather than scar. Although several synthetic polymers, such as porous (poly)dimethyl siloxane, delay contraction to a small but significant extent, they do not degrade and therefore violate isomorphous tissue replacement, Eq. (12.1). Synthetic biodegradable polymers, such as (poly)lactic acid, can be modified, e.g., by copolymerization with glycolic acid, to yield polymers which satisfy Eq. (12.1); however, evidence is lacking that these synthetic polymers delay contraction and prevent synthesis of scar. By contrast, there is considerable evidence that a certain analog of the extracellular matrix (ECM analogs) not only delays contraction significantly but also leads to synthesis of partly physiologic skin. Systematic use of the delay in contraction as an essay has been made to identify the structural features of the dermis regeneration template (DRT), as shown schematically in Fig. 12.1.

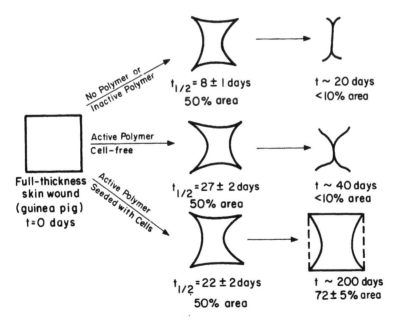

FIGURE 12.1　The kinetics of contraction of full-thickness guinea pig skin wounds can be used to separate collagen-*graft*-glycosaminoglycan copolymers into three classes, as shown. The wound half-life, $t_{1/2}$, is the number of days necessary to reduce the original wound area to 50%. (Courtesy of Massachusetts Institute of Technology.)

Summarized in Fig. 12.1 are three modes of wound-healing behavior, each elicited by an ECM analog of different design. Mode O of healing is described by a very short time for onset of contraction, followed by contraction and definitive closure of the wound with formation of a thin linear scar. Mode I is characterized by a significant delay in onset of contraction, following which contraction proceeds and eventually leads to a linear scar. Mode II is characterized by a significant delay in onset of contraction (somewhat smaller than in mode I), followed by contraction and then by reversal of contraction, with expansion of the original wound perimeter at a rate which exceeds significantly the growth rate of the entire animal. Mode II healing leads to synthesis of a partly physiologic dermis and a physiologic epidermis within the perimeter of the expanded wound bed. Mode O healing occurs when an ECM analog which lacks specificity is used to graft the wound. Mode O is also observed when the wound bed remains ungrafted. Mode I healing occurs when an ECM analog of highly specific structure (the DRT) is grafted on the wound bed. Mode II healing occurs when the DRT, previously identified as the ECM analog which leads to mode I healing, is seeded with autologous epidermal cells before being grafted. Although contraction is a convenient screening method for identification of structural features of ECM analogs which induce skin regeneration, a different procedure has been used to identify the features of an implant that induces regeneration of the peripheral nerve. The structural features of the nerve regeneration template (NRT) were identified using an essay focused on the long-term return of function of the nerve following treatment with candidate ECM analogs.

Recent studies have shown that it is possible to achieve regeneration both of a dermis and an epidermis in sequence, rather than simultaneously, provided that the animal model used is one in which wound closure does not take place almost overwhelmingly by wound contraction. The choice of animal model is, therefore, critical in this respect. Mode I behavior, illustrated in Fig. 12.1, is applicable to wound healing in rodents, such as guinea pigs and rats. In these animals, about 90% of wound closure is accounted for fully by wound contraction; the remainder is accounted for by formation of new tissue. Grafting of a full-thickness skin defect in a rodent with the ECM analog which possesses a highly specific structure (the dermis regeneration template or DRT; see below) leads to lengthy delay of the onset of contraction, eventually followed by contraction and formation of a linear scar-like tissue. Although the gross appearance of the tissue formed is that of a modified linear scar (see Fig. 12.1), there is some histological evidence that the small mass of connective tissue layer formed underneath the epidermis is not scar. In contrast, in animals in which contraction contributes about equally to wound closure as does formation of new tissue, such as the swine, approximately one half of the initial wound area is eventually closed by formation of partly regenerated dermis; soon after that, the new dermis is covered by a new epidermis. In wounds which close in large part by formation of new tissue rather than by contraction, as in the swine, grafting of the cell-free DRT leads, therefore, to sequential formation of a dermis and an epidermis as well, which is the same end result that is arrived at simultaneously by grafting with the keratinocyte-seeded DRT.

Of several ECM analogs that have been prepared, the most commonly studied is a graft copolymer of type I collagen and chondroitin 6-sulfate. The structure of the latter glycosaminoglycan (GAG) is illustrated below in terms of the repeat unit of the disaccharide, an alternating copolymer of D-glucuronic acid and of an O-sulfate derivative of N-acetyl D-galactosamine:

sodium chondroitin 6-sulfate

The principle of isomorphous replacement, Eq. (12.1), cannot be satisfied unless the *biodegradation time constant* of the network, t_b, can be adjusted to an optimal level, about equal to the rate of synthesis of new tissue at that site. Reduction of the biodegradation rate of collagen can be achieved either by grafting GAG chains onto collagen chains or by cross-linking collagen chains to each other. The chemical grafting of GAG chains on polypeptide chains proceeds by previously coprecipitating the two polymers under conditions of acidic pH, followed by covalent cross-linking of the freeze-dried precipitate. A particularly useful procedure for cross-linking collagen chains to GAG, or collagen chains to each other, is a self-cross-linking reaction, requiring no use of cross-linking agent. This condensation reaction principally involves carboxylic groups from glutamyl/aspartyl residues on polypeptide chain P_1 and ϵ-amino groups of lysyl residues on an adjacent chain P_2 to yield covalently bonded collagen chains, as well as condensation of amine groups of collagen with carboxylic groups of glucuronic acid residues on GAG chains to yield *graft*-copolymers of collagen and GAG:

$$P_1-COOH + P_2-NH_2 \rightarrow P_2-NHCO-P_1 + H_2O \qquad (12.3a)$$

$$GAG-COOH + P_2-NH_2 \rightarrow P_2-NHCO-GAG + H_2O \qquad (12.3b)$$

In each case above the reaction proceeds to the right, with formation of a three-dimensional cross-linked network when the moisture content of the protein, or protein-GAG coprecipitate, drops below about 1 wt%. As illustrated by Eq. (12.3), removal of water, the volatile product of the condensation, is favored by conditions which drive the reaction toward the right, with formation of a cross-linked network. Thus, the reaction proceeds to the right when both high temperature and vacuum are used. Another cross-linking reaction, used extensively in preparing implants that have been employed in clinical studies as well as in animal studies, involves use of glutaraldehyde. Dehydration cross-linking, which amounts to self-cross-linking as described above, obviously does not lend toxicity to these implants. Glutaraldehyde, on the other hand, is a toxic substance, and devices treated with it require thorough rinsing before use until free glutaraldehyde cannot be detected in the rinse water. Network properties of cross-linked collagen-GAG copolymers can be analyzed structurally by studying the swelling behavior of small specimens. The method is based on the theory of Flory and Rehner, who showed that the volume fraction of a swollen polymer v_2 depends on the average molecular weight between cross-links, M_c, through the following relationship:

$$\ln\left(1-v_2\right) + v_2 + \chi v_2 - \left(\rho V_1 / M_c\right)\left(v_2^{1/3} - v_2/2\right) = 0 \qquad (12.4)$$

In Eq. (12.4), V_1 is the molar volume of the solvent, ρ is the density of the dry polymer, and χ is a constant characteristic of a specific polymer-solvent pair at a particular temperature.

Although the chemical identify of collagen-GAG copolymers is a necessary element of their biologic activity, it is not a sufficient one. In addition to chemical composition and the cross-link density, biologic activity also depends strongly on the *pore architecture* of these ECM analogs. Pores are incorporated first by freezing a very dilute suspension of the collagen-GAG coprecipitate and then by inducing sublimation of the ice crystals by exposing to vacuum at low temperatures. The resulting pore structure is, therefore, a negative replica of the network of ice crystals (dendrites). It follows that control of the conditions of ice crystal nucleation and growth can lead to a large variety of pore structures. In practice, the average pore diameter decreases with decreasing temperature of freezing while the orientation of pore channel axes also depends on the magnitude of the heat flux vector during freezing. The dependence of pore channel orientation on heat transfer parameters is illustrated by considering the dimensionless Mikic number Mi, a ratio of the characteristic freezing time of the aqueous medium of the collagen-GAG suspension, t_f, to the characteristic time for entry, t_e, of a container filled with the suspension which is lowered at constant velocity into a well-stirred cooling bath:

$$Mi = \frac{t_f}{t_e} = \frac{\rho_w h_{fg} r V}{10 k_j \Delta T} \tag{12.5}$$

In Eq. (12.5), ρ_w is the density of the suspension, h_{fg} is the heat of fusion of the suspension, r is an arbitrary length scale, V is the velocity with which the container is lowered into the bath, k_j is the thermal conductivity of the jacket, and ΔT is the difference between freezing temperature and bath temperature. The shape of the isotherms near the freezing front is highly dependent on the value of Mi. The dominant heat flux vector is normal to these isotherms; i.e., ice dendrites grow along this vector. It has been observed that, for $Mi < 1$ (slow cooling), the isotherms are shallow, flat-shaped parabolae, and the ice dendrites exhibit high axial orientation. For $Mi > 1$ (rapid cooling), the isotherms are steep parabolae, and ice dendrites are oriented along the radial direction.

The structure of the porous matrix is defined by quantities such as the volume fraction, specific surface, mean pore size, and orientation of pores in the matrix. Determination of these properties is based on principles of stereology, the discipline which relates the quantitative statistical properties of three-dimensional structures to those of their two-dimensional sections or projections. In reverse, stereologic procedures allow reconstruction of certain aspects of three-dimensional objects from a quantitative analysis of planar images. A plane which goes through the two-phase structure of pores and collage-GAG fibers may be sampled by random points, by a regular pattern of points, by a near-total sampling using a very dense array of points, or by arranging the sampling points to form a continuous line. The volume fraction of pores, V_V, is equal to the fraction of total test points which fall inside pore regions, P_P, also equal to the total area fraction of pores, A_A, and, finally, equal to the line fraction of pores, L_L, for a linear point array in the limit of infinitely close point spacing

$$V_V = P_P = A_A = L_L \tag{12.6}$$

Whether cells of a particular type should be part of a regeneration template depends on predictions derived from models of developmental biology as well as empirical findings obtained with well-defined wound-healing models. During morphogenesis of a large variety of organs, an interaction between epithelial and mesenchymal cells, mediated by the basal lamina which is interleaved between the two types of cells, is both necessary and sufficient for development of local physiologic structures involving two types of tissue in juxtaposition. In particular, skin morphogenesis in a full-thickness wound model requires the presence of this interaction between the two cell types and the basal lamina over a critical period. In skin wound–healing experiments with adult mammals, wound healing proceeds with formation of scar, rather than physiologic skin, if the wound bed contains epithelial cells and mesenchymal cells (fibroblasts) but no ECM structure which could act temporarily as a basal lamina. If, by contrast, an analog of the basal lamina is present, wound healing proceeds with nearly physiologic morphogenesis of skin. Furthermore, no epidermis is formed unless epithelial cells become involved in wound healing early during wound healing and continue being involved until they have achieved confluence. It is also known that no dermis forms if fibroblasts are not available early during wound healing. These observations suggest the requirements for a DRT which is an analog of the basal lamina and is designed to encourage the migration and interaction of both epithelial cells and fibroblasts within its volume.

Nerve regeneration following injury essentially amounts to elongation of a single nerve cell across a gap resulting from the injury. During nerve development many nerve cells are elongated by processes which eventually become axons. Interaction of elongating processes with basal lamina are credited as being essential in the formation of nerve during development, and it will be assumed here that such interactions are essential in regeneration following adult injury as well. It is also known that Schwann cells, which derive from neural crest cells during development, are essential contributors to regeneration following injury to the adult peripheral nerve. These considerations suggest a nerve regeneration template which is structured as an analog of the basal lamina, interacting with the elongating axons in the presence of Schwann cells.

12.3 Structural Specificity of Dermis Regeneration Template (DRT)

The major events accompanying skin wound healing can be summarized as contraction and scar synthesis. Conventional wisdom prescribes the need for a treatment that accelerates wound healing. A large number of devices that claim to speed various aspects of the healing process have been described in the literature. The need to achieve healing within as short a time as possible is certainly well founded, especially in the clinical setting where the risk to patient's life as well as the morbidity increase with extension of time to heal. However, the discovery of partial skin regeneration by use of the skin regeneration template has introduced the option of a drastically improved healing result for the patient in exchange for a slightly extended hospital stay.

The DRT was optimized in studies with animals in which it was observed that skin regeneration did not occur unless the test ECM analog effectively delayed, rather than accelerated, wound contraction. The length of delay in onset of contraction eventually was used as a quantitative basis for preliminary optimization of the structural features of the DRT. Optimization studies are currently continuing on the basis of a new criterion, namely, the fidelity of regeneration achieved.

Systematic use of the criterion of contraction inhibition has been made to select the biodegradation rate and the average pore diameter of DRT. The kinetics of contraction of full-thickness skin wounds in the guinea pig have been studied for each of the three modes of healing schematically presented in Fig. 12.1. The results, presented in Fig. 12.2, show that mode O healing is characterized by early onset of contraction, whereas mode I and mode II healing show a significant delay in onset of contraction. A measure of the delay is the wound half-life $t_{1/2}$, the time required for the wound area to decrease to 50% of the original value. Use of this index of contraction rate has been made in Figs. 12.3 and 12.4, which present data on the variation of wound half-life with average pore diameter and degradation rate for a

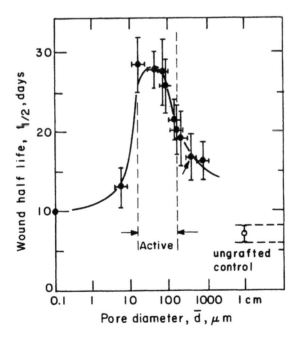

FIGURE 12.2 The kinetics of guinea pig skin wound contraction following grafting with three classes of ECM analogs. Inactive ECM analogs delay the onset of contraction only marginally over the ungrafted wound, whereas active cell-free ECM analogs delay the onset of contraction significantly. When seeded with epithelial cells, not only does an active ECM analog delay the onset of contraction significantly, but it also induces formation of a confluent epidermis and then arrests and reverses the direction of movement of wound edges, leading to expansion of the wound perimeter and to synthesis of partly physiologic skin. (Courtesy of Massachusetts Institute of Technology.)

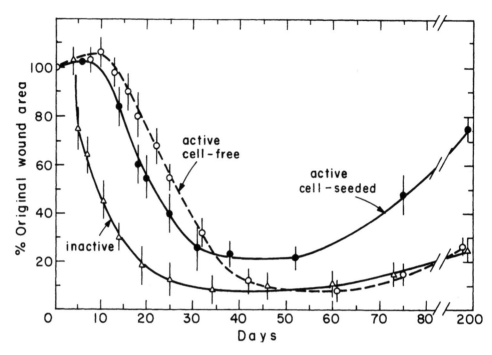

FIGURE 12.3   The half-life of wounds, $t_{1/2}$, grafted with ECM analogs varies with the average pore diameter of the analog. The range of pore diameters where activity is maximal is shown by broken lines. The half-life of the ungrafted wound is shown for comparison. (Courtesy of Massachusetts Institute of Technology.)

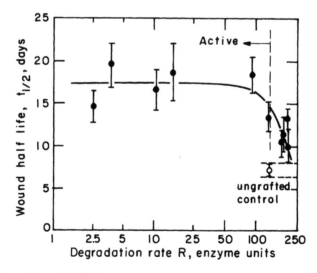

FIGURE 12.4   Variation of wound half-life with degradation rate R of the ECM analog used as graft for a full-thickness guinea pig skin wound. R varies inversely as the biodegradation time constant, t_f. The region of maximal activity is indicated by the broken line. The half-life of the ungrafted wound is shown for comparison. (Courtesy of Massachusetts Institute of Technology.)

type I collagen-chondroitin 6-sulfate copolymer. In Fig. 12.2, mode I kinetics are observed using a cell-free copolymer with average pore diameter and biodegradation rate that correspond to the regions of Figs. 12.3 and 12.4 in which the values of half-life are maximal; these regions characterize the structure of SRT which possesses maximal activity. Maximum delay in wound half-life up to 27 ± 3 days is seen to have occurred when the average pore diameter has ranged from values as low as 20 ± 4 μm to an upper limit of 125 ± 35 μm. In addition, significant delay in wound healing has been observed when the degradation rate has become less than 115 ± 25 enzyme units. The latter index of degradation has been based on the *in vitro* degradation rate of the copolymer in a standardized solution of bacterial collagenase.

The upper limit in degradation rate, defined in Fig. 12.4, is consistent with the requirement of a lower limit in t_b, Eq. (12.1), below which the implant is biodegraded too rapidly to function as a scaffold over the period necessary for synthesis of new tissue; the latter is characterized by t_h. The lower limit in pore diameter, defined in Fig. 12.3, suggests a dimension which is on the order of two cell diameters; adequate space for migration of mesenchymal cells (fibroblasts) from the wound bed into the DRT is thereby guaranteed. At an estimated velocity of 0.2 mm/day for fibroblasts these cells would be expected to migrate across a 0.5-mm thickness of the DRT within very few days, provided that adequate supplies of critical nutrients could be made available to them from host tissue. Use of Eq. (12.2) leads to an estimated critical cell path length l_c of order 100 μm. These estimates suggest that fibroblasts can migrate across at least one-fifth the thickness of the porous implant without requiring the presence of capillaries. However, taking into account the observation that wound exudate (comprising primarily serum, with growth factors and nutrients) fills at least one-half the thickness of the implant within no more than a few hours following grafting, we conclude that the boundary of "host" tissue has moved clearly inside the implant.

Epithelial cells, as well as fibroblasts and a basal lamina analog, also are required for morphogenesis. They can be supplied in a variety of forms. They are always available as epithelial cell sheets, migrating from the wound edges toward the center of the wound bed. However, when the area of skin loss is several centimeters, as with a severely burned patient, these cell sheets, migrating with speeds of about 0.5 mm/day from opposite edges, would not be expected to cover one-half the characteristic wound dimension in less than the time constant t_h for synthesis of new tissue. In the absence of epithelial cells, therefore, at the center of the wound bed, Eq. (12.1) wound be violated. To overcome this limitation, which is imposed by the scale of the wound, it has been necessary to resort to a variety of procedures. In the first, uncultured autologous epidermal cells, extracted from a skin biopsy by controlled enzymatic degradation, have been seeded into ECM analogs by centrifugation into the porous matrix prior to grafting of the latter on the wound bed. Tested with animals, the procedure leads to formation of a confluent epidermis by about 2 weeks, provided that at least 5×10^4 epithelial cells per cm^2 of DRT area have been seeded. In another procedure, a very thin epidermal layer has been surgically removed from an intact area of the patient and has been grafted on the dermal layer which has been synthesized about 2 weeks after grafting with the DRT. The latter procedure has been tested clinically with reproducible success. A third procedure, studied with animals, has made use of cultured epithelia, prepared by a 2- to 3-week period of culture of autologous cells *in vitro* and grafted on the newly synthesized dermal bed. Approximately equivalent fidelity of skin regeneration has been obtained by each of these procedures for supplying epithelial cells to the DRT in the treatment of skin wounds of very large area.

12.4   *In Situ* Synthesis of Skin with DRT

The skin regeneration template DRT induces regeneration of skin to a high degree of fidelity. Fidelity of regeneration has been defined in terms of the degree of recovery of structural and functional features which are present in the intact organ.

The first test of fidelity of skin regeneration following use of the DRT was a study of treatment of full-thickness skin loss in guineas pigs. In this study the lesion was produced by surgery on healthy animals. The characteristic dimension of the wound was about 3 cm, and the desired period for cover by a confluent epidermis was 2 weeks. Covering a wound of such a scale within the prescribed time would have been out of reach of epithelial cells migrating from the wound edges. Accordingly, autologous epithelial cells were extracted from a skin biopsy and seeded into the DRT under conditions of carefully controlled centrifugation.

A clear and unmistakable difference between healing in the presence and absence of DRT was provided by observing the gross anatomy of the wound (Fig. 12.2). In the absence of the DRT, the wound contracted vigorously and closed up with formation of a linear scar by about day 30. In the presence of a cell-seeded DRT, the wound perimeter started contracting with a delay of about 10 days, and contraction was completely arrested and then reversed between days 30 and 40. The wound then continued to expand at a rate that was clearly higher than that expected from the rate of growth of the animal. The long-term appearance of the wound treated with the cell-seeded DRT was that of an organ that appeared grossly identical in color, texture, and touch to intact skin outside the wound perimeter. However, the newly synthesized skin was totally hairless, and the total area of new skin was smaller in area from the original wound area by about 30% (Fig. 12.2).

Morphologic studies of newly synthesized skin in the presence of cell-seeded DRT included comparison with intact skin and scar. Optical microscopy and electron microscopy were supplemented by laser light scattering, the latter used to provide a quantitative measure of collagen fiber orientation in the dermal layer. It was concluded that, in most respects, partly regenerated skin was remarkably similar to intact guinea pig skin. The epidermis in regenerated skin was often hyperplastic; however, the maturation sequence and relative proportion of all cell layers were normal. Keratohyaline granules of the neoepidermis were larger and more irregular in contour than those of the normal granular cell layer. The new skin was characterized by melanocytes and Langerhans cells, as well as a well-formed pattern of rete ridges and interdigitations with dermal papillae, all of which appear in normal skin. Newly synthesized skin was distinctly different morphologically from scar. Scar showed characteristic thinning (atrophy) of the epidermis, with absence of rete ridges and of associated dermal papillae. Elastic fibers in regenerated skin formed a delicate particulate structure, in contrast with scar, where elastic fibers were thin and fragmented. The dermal layer in regenerated skin comprised collagen fibers which were not oriented in the plane of the epidermis, as well as fibroblasts which were not elongated; in scar, collagen fibers were highly oriented in the plane and fibroblasts were elongated. Both normal and regenerated skin comprised unmyelinated nerve fibers within dermal papillae, closely approximated to the epidermis; scar had few, if any, nerves. There were no hair follicles or other skin appendages either in regenerated skin or in scar.

Laser light–scattering measurements of the orientation of collagen fibers in tissue sections of the dermal layer were based on use of the Hermans orientation function

$$f = 2 \left\langle \cos^2 \alpha \right\rangle - 1 \tag{12.7}$$

In Eq. (12.7), α is the angle between an individual fiber and the mean axis of the fibers, and $\langle \cos^2 \alpha \rangle$ is the square cosine of α averaged over all the fibers in the sample. For a random arrangement of fibers, $\langle \cos^2 \alpha \rangle$ equals 1/2, while for a perfectly aligned arrangement it is equal to 1. Accordingly, S varies from 0 (truly random) to 1 (perfect alignment). Measurements obtained by use of this procedure showed that S took the values 0.20 ± 0.11, 0.48 ± 0.05, and 0.75 ± 0.10 for normal dermis, regenerated dermis, and scar dermis, respectively. These results provided objective evidence that regenerated dermis had a morphology of collagen fibers that was clearly not scar ($n = 7$; $p < 0.001$), and was intermediate between that of scar and normal dermis.

Functional studies of regenerated skin showed that the moisture permeability of intact skin and regenerated skin had values of 4.5 ± 0.8 and 4.7 ± 1.9 g/cm/h, insignificantly different from each other ($n = 4$; $p < 0.8$). Mechanical behavior studies showed a positive curvature for the tensile stress-strain curve of regenerated skin as well as of normal skin. However, the tensile strength of regenerated skin was 14 ± 4 MPa, significantly lower than the strength of intact skin, 31 ± 4 MPa ($n = 4$; $p < 0.01$).

The second test of fidelity of skin regeneration was a study of treatment of 106 massively burned humans with the cell-free DRT. The characteristic dimension of the wound in this study was of order 15 cm, and the desired period for cover by a confluent epidermis was 2 weeks. The scale of the wound necessitated the introduction of epithelial cells, and this was accomplished by grafting the newly synthesized dermal layer, 2 weeks after grafting with DRT, with a very thin epidermal layer (epidermal autograft), which was removed from an intact area of the patient. The results of the histologic study of the patient population showed that physiologic dermis, rather than scar, had been synthesized in sites that had been treated with DRT and had later been covered with an epidermal graft.

Progress has been made in clarification of the mechanism by which DRT induces regeneration of the dermis. There is considerable evidence, some of which was presented above, supporting the hypothesis that inhibition of wound contraction is required for regeneration. The evidence also suggests strongly that DRT competitively inhibits formation of specific binding interactions between contractile cells and endogenous ECM.

12.5 Advantages and Disadvantages of Clinical Treatment of Skin Loss with DRT

When skin is the missing organ, the patient faces threats to life posed by severe dehydration and infection. These threats can be eliminated permanently only if the area of missing skin is covered with a device that controls moisture flux within physiologic limits and presents an effective barrier to airborne bacteria. Both of these functions can be returned over a period of about 2 to 4 weeks by use of temporary dressings. The latter include the allograft (skin from a cadaver) and a very large variety of membranes based on synthetic or natural polymers. None of these dressings solves the problem of missing skin over the lifetime of the patient: The allograft does not support synthesis of physiologic skin and must be removed to avoid rejection, and the devices based on the vast majority of engineered membranes do not make effective biologic contact with the patient's tissues, and all lead to synthesis of scar.

Three devices have been tested extensively for their ability to provide long-term physiologic cover to patients with massive skin loss: the patient's own skin (autograft), the dermis regeneration template (DRT), and cultured epithelia (CEA). All three of these treatments have been studied extensively with massively burned patients. Of these, the autograft and DRT are effective even when the loss of skin extends through the full thickness of the dermis (e.g., third-degree burns), whereas CEA is effective when the loss of skin is through part of its thickness only.

The basis for the differences among the three treatments lies in the intrinsic response of skin to injury. Skin comprises three layers: the epidermis, a 100-μm thick cellular layer; the dermis, a 1- to 5-mm layer of connective tissue with very few cells; and the subcutis, a 2- to 4-mm layer of primarily adipose tissue. In the adult mammal, an epidermis lost through injury regenerates spontaneously provided that a dermal substrate is present underneath. When the dermis is lost, whether through part thickness or full thickness, none of the injured mass regenerates; instead, a nonphysiologic tissue, scar, forms. Scar is epithelialized and can, therefore, control moisture flux within physiologic limits as well as provide a barrier to bacterial invasion. However, scar does not have the mechanical strength of physiologic skin. Also, scar synthesis frequently proceeds well beyond what is necessary to cover the wound, and the result of such proliferation is hypertrophic scarring, a cosmetically inferior integument which, when extending over a large area or over hands or face, reduces significantly the mobility of the patient's joints as well as the patient's cosmetic appearance. Autograft can, if used without meshing, provide an excellent permanent cover; if, however, as commonly practiced, autograft is meshed before grafting in order to extend the wound area that becomes covered, the result is new integument which comprises part physiologic skin and part scar and provides the patient with a solution of much lower quality than unmeshed (sheet) autograft. The clinical use of skin regeneration template has led to a new integument comprising a dermal layer, which has been synthesized by the patient, and an epidermal layer, which has been harvested as a very thin epidermal autograft and has been placed on top of the newly synthesized dermis.

The chief advantages DRT over the meshed autograft are the shorter time that it takes to heal the donor site, from which the epidermal graft was harvested, and a superior cosmetic result at the site of the wound. The main disadvantage in the clinical use of DRT is the subjection of the patient to two surgical treatments rather than one (first graft DRT, then graft the epidermal layer after about 2 weeks).

Although it has been shown that a dermis and an epidermis are regenerated sequentially in DRT-treated wounds like that of the swine, in which contraction plays only a modest role in wound closure, the process of sequential skin regeneration is slower than that of simultaneous skin regeneration. Accordingly, the kinetics of wound closure suggest an advantage in the use of keratinocyte-seeded DRT (a two-stage treatment) relative to the unseeded DRT (one-stage treatment). The clinical advantages of CEA are the ability to grow a very large area, about 10,000 times as large as the area of the skin biopsy, thereby providing cover over the entire injured skin area of the patient. The disadvantages of cultured epithelia are the lengthy period required to culture the epidermis from the patient's biopsy and the inability of the CEA to form a mechanically competent bond with the wound bed.

12.6   Modifications of DRT: Use of a Living Dermal Equivalent

The design concept of a skin regeneration template outlined above has been adopted and modified. One modification involves the replacement of the collagen-GAG matrix with a biodegradable mesh consisting of either (poly)glycolic acid (PGA) or polyglactin-910 (PGL) fibers. The latter is used as a matrix for the *in vitro* culture of human fibroblasts isolated from neonatal skin. Fibroblasts synthesize extracellular matrix inside the synthetic polymeric mesh, and this "living dermal equivalent" has been cryopreserved for a specified period prior to use.

The living dermal equivalent has been used to graft full-thickness skin wounds in athymic mice. Following grafting of wounds, these PGA/PGL fibroblast grafts were covered with meshed allograft. The latter is human cadaver skin that was meshed in this study to expand it and achieve coverage of maximum possible wound area. This composite graft became vascularized and that, additionally, epithelial cells from the cadaver graft had migrated to the matrix underneath. After a period of about 100 days following grafting, the reported result was an epithelialized layer covering a densely cellular substratum that resembled dermis. A variant of this design, in which the meshed allograft is not used, has been reported; epidermal cells are cultured with the fibroblast mesh before grafting. Studies of these designs are in progress.

12.7   The Bilayered Skin-Equivalent Graft

In one widely reported development, *in vitro* cell culture procedures have been used to synthesize a bilayered tissue which has been reported to be a useful model of human skin. Briefly, fibroblasts from humans or from rats have been placed inside a collagen gel. Under these conditions, fibroblasts exert contractile forces, trapping the cells inside the contracted collagen lattice. Human epithelial cells, which have been plated onto this contracted dermal equivalent, have been observed to attach to the collagen substrate, multiply, and spread to form a continuous sheet. Differentiation of this sheet has led to formation of specialized epidermal structures, such as a multilayered cell structure with desmosomes, tonofilaments, and keratohyalin granules. Further differentiation events have included the formation of a basement membrane (basal lamina) *in vitro* when a rat epidermis was formed on top of a dermal equivalent produced from rat fibroblasts.

Grafts prepared from the bilayered skin equivalent have been grafted on animals. When grafted on animals, these structures have been reported to become well vascularized with a network of capillaries within 7 to 9 days. It has been reported that the best grafts have blocked wound contraction, but no systematic data have been presented which could be used to compare the *in vivo* performance of these skin equivalents with grafts based on DRT (see above). Gross observations of the area grafted with skin equivalents have shown pink hairless areas which were not hypertrophically scarred. A systematic comparison between scar and the tissue synthesized in sites that have been grafted with skin equivalents has not yet been made.

12.8 Structural Specificity of Nerve Regeneration Template (NRT)

The design principles for regeneration templates presented above have been used to design implants for regeneration of peripheral nerves. The medical problem typically involves the loss of innervation in arms and legs, leading to loss of motor and sensory function (paralysis). The nerves involved are peripheral, and the design problem becomes the regeneration of injured peripheral nerves, with recovery of function.

A widely used animal model for peripheral nerve injury is a surgically generated gap in the sciatic nerve of the rat. Interruption of nerve function in this case is localized primarily in the region of plantar muscles of the foot involved. This relatively well defined area of loss of function can then be studied neurologically in relative isolation from other neurologic events. Furthermore, the rate of recovery of function can be studied by electrophysiologic methods, a procedure which provides continuous data over the entire period of healing. In the peripheral nerve the healing period extends to about 10 weeks, clearly longer than healing in skin, which occurs largely within a period of only 3 weeks.

When the sciatic nerve is cut and a gap forms between the two nerve ends, the distal part of the nerve is isolated from its cell body in the spinal cord. Communication between the central nervous system and the leg is no longer possible. The lack of muscle innervation leads to inactivity, which in turn leads to muscle atrophy. At the site of injury there is degeneration of the myelin sheath of axons, dissociation of Schwann cells, and formation of scar. It has been hypothesized that the formation of scar impedes, more than any other single cause, the elongation of axons across the gap. Axonal elongation through a gap of substantial length becomes, therefore, a parameter of prime importance in the design of a nerve regeneration template (NRT).

Intubation of severed nerve ends is a widely used procedure for isolating axons from the tissue environment of the peripheral nerve. The lumen of the tube serves to isolate the process of nerve regeneration from wound-healing events involving connective tissues outside the nerve; the tube walls, for example, prevent proliferation of scar tissue inside the tube and the subsequent obstruction of the regenerating nerve. Silicone tubes are the most widely used method of intubation. These tubes are both nonbiodegradable and nonpermeable to large molecules. In this isolated environment it is possible to study the substrate preferences of elongating axons by incorporating well-defined ECM analogs and studying the kinetics of functional recovery continuously with electrophysiologic procedures for about 40 weeks following implantation. As in studies of dermal regeneration described above, the ECM analogs which were used in the study of substrate preferences of axons were graft copolymers of type I collagen and chondroitin 6-sulfate. Controls used included the autograft, empty silicone tubes, as well as tubes filled with saline. In these studies, it was necessary to work with a gap dimension large enough to preclude spontaneous regeneration, i.e., regeneration in the absence of an ECM analog. It was observed that a gap length of 10 mm was occasionally innervated spontaneously in the rat, whereas no instances of spontaneous regeneration were observed with a 15-mm gap length. Gap lengths of 10 and 15 mm were used in these studies with rats.

Three structural parameters of ECM analogs were varied systematically. The degradation rate had a significant effect on the fidelity of regeneration, and an abbreviated optimization procedure led to an ECM analog which degraded much faster than the DRT. In combination with Eq. (12.1), this empirical finding suggests that a healing nerve wound contains a much smaller concentration of the degrading enzyme, collagenase; this suggestion is qualitatively consistent with observations of collagenolytic activity in injured nerves. The average diameter also was found to have a significant effect on fidelity of regeneration, and the optimization procedure led to a value of 5 μm, significantly smaller than the average pore diameter in the DRT. Finally, use of Eq. (12.5) led to procedures of preparing ECM analogs, the pore channels of which were either highly aligned along the tube axis, randomly oriented, or radially oriented. ECM analogs with axially aligned pore channels were found to be superior to analogs with other types of alignment.

TABLE 12.1   Design Parameters for Two Regeneration Templates

Design Parameter of ECM Analog	DRT	NRT
Degradation rate, enzyme units	<120	>150
Average pore diameter, μm	20–125	5
Pore channel orientation	Random	Axial

These results have led to a design for an NRT consisting of a specified degradation rate, average pore diameter, and pore channel alignment as shown in Table 12.1 in which the structural parameters of NRT are contrasted to those of DRT.

Studies of Nerve Regeneration Using Degradable Tubes

Porous collagen tubes without matrix content have been extensively studied as guides for peripheral nerve regeneration in rodents and nonhuman primates. The walls of these collagen tubes had an average pore diameter which was considered sufficiently large for transport of molecules as large as bovine serum albumin (MW = 68 kDa). A 4-mm gap in the sciatic nerve of the rat was the standard injury studied. Other injury models that were studied included the 4-mm gap and the 15-mm gap in the adult monkey.

The use of an empty tube did not allow for any degree of optimization of tube parameters to be achieved in this study. Nevertheless, the long-term results showed almost complete recovery of motor and sensory responses, at rates that approximated the recovery obtained following use of the nerve autograft, currently the best conventional treatment in cases of massive loss of nerve mass. The success obtained suggests that collagen tubes can be used instead of autografts, the harvesting of which subject the patient to nerve-losing surgery.

Even more significant improvement in quality of nerve regeneration is obtained when collagen tubes are filled with NRT. Although lower than normal, the histomorphometric and electrophysiologic properties of the regenerate resulting from use of an NRT-filled collagen tube have been statistically indistinguishable from those of the autograft control. Probably, however, the most important effect observed following implantation of the NRT-filled collagen tube has been the observation that, while the total number of myelinated axons in regenerated nerves had reached a plateau by 30 weeks after injury, the number of axons with diameter larger than 6 μm continues to increase at substantial rates through the completion of a recent study (60 weeks). Axons with a diameter larger than 6 μm have been uniquely associated with the A-fiber peak of the action potential, which determines the maximum conduction velocity of the regenerates. Thus, kinetic evidence has been presented which supports the view that the nerve trunk maturation process continues beyond 60 weeks after injury, resulting in a nerve trunk which increasingly approaches the structure of the normal control.

12.9   *In Situ* Synthesis of Meniscus Using a Meniscus Regeneration Template (MRT)

The meniscus of the knee performs a variety of functions which amount to joint stabilization and lubrication, as well as shock absorption. Its structure is that of fibrocartilage, consisting primarily of type I collagen fibers populated with meniscal fibrochondrocytes. The architecture of collagen fibers is complex. In this tissue, which has a shape reminiscent of one-half a doughnut, the collagen fibers are arranged in a circumferential pattern which is additionally reinforced by radially placed fibers. The meniscus can be torn during use, an event which causes pain and disfunction. Currently, the accepted treatments are partial or complete excision of torn tissue. The result of such treatment is often unsatisfactory, since the treated meniscus has an altered shape which is incompatible with normal joint motion and stability. The long-term consequence of such incompatibility is joint degeneration, eventually leading to osteoarthritis.

An effort to induce regeneration of the surgically removed meniscus was based on the use of a type I collagen-chondroitin 6-sulfate copolymer. The precise structural parameters of this matrix have not been reported, so it is not possible to discuss the results of this study in terms of possible similarities and differences with DRT and NRT. The study focused on the canine knee joint, since the latter is particularly sensitive to biomechanical alterations; in this model, joint instabilities rapidly lead to osteoarthritic changes, which can be detected experimentally. Spontaneous regeneration of the canine meniscus following excision is partial and leads to a biomechanically inadequate tissue which does not protect the joint from osteoarthritic changes. The latter condition provides the essential negative control for the study. In this study, knee joints were subjected to 80% removal (resection) of the medial meniscus, and the lesion was treated either by an autograft or by an ECM analog or was not treated at all. Evaluation of joint function was performed by studying joint stability, gait, and treadmill performance and was extended up to 27 months. No evidence was presented to show that the structure of the ECM analog was optimized to deliver maximal regeneration.

The results of this study showed that two-thirds of the joints implanted with the ECM analog, two-thirds of the joints which were autografted, and only 25% of the joints which were resected without further treatment showed regeneration of meniscal tissue. These results were interpreted to suggest that the ECM analog, or meniscus regeneration template (MRT), supported significant meniscal regeneration and provided enough biomechanical stability to minimize degenerative osteoarthritis in the canine knee joint.

Recently, a clinical trial of the feasibility of MRT treatment was conducted on nine patients with either an irreparable tear of the meniscal cartilage or major loss of meniscal cartilage, and who remained in the study for at least 36 months. Following deletion of irreparably damaged meniscal tissue, MRT was implanted at the site of the missing meniscal tissue mass. The results showed that implantation of MRT induced regeneration of meniscal cartilage while the template was undergoing degradation. Compared to patients who were observed during the same period after meniscectomy (removal of damaged meniscal tissue without MRT treatment), patients who were implanted with MRT showed significant reduction in pain as well as greatly improved resumption of strenuous activity.

Defining Terms

Autograft: The patient's own tissue or organ, harvested from an intact area.

Cell lifeline number, *S*: A dimensionless number that expresses the relative magnitudes of chemical reaction and diffusion. This number, defined as S in Eq. (12.2), can be used to compute the maximum path length l_c over which a cell can migrate in a scaffold while depending on diffusion alone for transport of critical nutrients that it consumes. When the critical length is exceeded, the cell requires transport of nutrients by angiogenesis in order to survive.

Cultured epithelia: A mature, keratinizing epidermis synthesized *in vitro* by culturing epithelial cells removed from the patient by biopsy. A relatively small skin biopsy (1 cm²) can be treated to yield an area larger by about 10,000 in 2–3 weeks and can then be grafted on patients.

Dermal equivalent: A term which has been loosely used in the literature to describe a device that replaces, usually temporarily, the functions of the dermis following injury.

Dermis: A 1–5 mm layer of connective tissue populated with quiescent fibroblasts which lies underneath the epidermis. It is separated from the former by a very thin basement membrane. The dermis of adult mammals does not regenerate spontaneously following injury.

Dermis regeneration template (DRT): A graft copolymer of type I collagen and chondroitin 6-sulfate, average pore diameter 20–125 μm, degrading *in vivo* to an extent of about 50% in 2 weeks, which induces partial regeneration of the dermis in wounds from which the dermis has been fully excised. When seeded with keratinocytes prior to grafting, this analog of extracellular matrix has induced simultaneous synthesis both of a dermis and an epidermis.

ECM analog: A model of extracellular matrix, consisting of a highly porous graft copolymer of collagen and a glycosaminoglycan.

Epidermis: The cellular outer layer of skin, about 0.1 mm thick, which protects against moisture loss and against infection. An epidermal graft, e.g., cultured epithelium or a thin graft removed surgically, requires a dermal substrate for adherence onto the wound bed. The epidermis regenerates spontaneously following injury, provided there is a dermal substrate underneath.

Isomorphous tissue replacement: A term used to describe the synthesis of new, physiologic tissue within a regeneration template at a rate of the same order as the degradation rate of the template. This relation, described by Eq. (12.1), is the defining equation for a biodegradable scaffold which couples with, or interacts in this unique manner with, the inflammatory response of the wound bed.

Meniscus regeneration template (MRT):   A graft copolymer of type I collagen and an unspecified glycosaminoglycan, average pore diameter unspecified, which has induced partial regeneration of the knee meniscus in dogs following 80% excision of the meniscal tissue.

Mikic number, *Mi*:   Ratio of the characteristic freezing time of the aqueous medium of the collagen-GAG suspension, t_f, to the characteristic time for entry, t_e, of a container filled with the suspension which is lowered at constant velocity into a well-stirred cooling bath. *Mi*, defined by Eq. (12.5), can be used to design implants which have high alignment of pore channels along a particular axis, or no preferred alignment.

Morphogenesis: The shaping of an organ during embryologic development or during wound healing, according to transcription of genetic information and local environmental conditions.

Nerve regeneration template (NRT):   A graft copolymer of type I collagen and chondroitin 6-sulfate, average pore diameter 5 mm, degrading *in vivo* to an extent of about 50% in 6 weeks, which has induced partial regeneration of the sciatic nerve of the rat across a 15-mm gap.

Regeneration: The synthesis of new, physiologic tissue at the site of a tissue (one cell type) or organ (more than one cell type) which either has been lost due to injury or has failed due to a chronic condition.

Regeneration template: A biodegradable device which, when attached to a missing organ, induces its regeneration.

Scar: The end result of a repair process in skin and other organs. Scar is morphologically different from skin, in addition to being mechanically less extensible and weaker than skin. The skin regeneration template induces synthesis of nearly physiologic skin rather than scar. Scar is also formed at the site of severe nerve injury.

Self-cross-linking: A procedure for reducing the biodegradation rate of collagen, in which collagen chains are covalently bonded to each other by a condensation reaction which is driven by drastic dehydration of the protein. This reaction illustrated by Eqs. (12.3a) and (12.3b), is also used to graft glycosaminoglycan chains to collagen chains without use of an extraneous cross-linking agent.

Stereology: The discipline which relates the quantitative statistical properties of three-dimensional structures to those of their two-dimensional sections or projections. In reverse, stereologic procedures allow reconstruction of certain aspects of three-dimensional objects from a quantitative analysis of planar images. Its rules are used to determine features of the pore structure of ECM analogs.

References

Archibald SJ, Krarup C, Sheffner J, Li S-T, Madison RD. 1991. A collagen-based nerve guide conduit for peripheral nerve repair: An electrophysiological study of nerve regeneration in rodents and non-human primates. J Comp Neurol 306:685–696.

Archibald SJ, Sheffner J, Krarup C, Madison RD. 1995. Monkey median nerve repaired by nerve graft or collagen nerve guide tube. J Neurosci 15:4109–4123.

Butler CE, Orgill DP, Yannas IV, Compton CC. 1998. Effect of keratinocyte seeding of collagen-glycosaminoglycan membranes on the regeneration of skin in a porcine model. Plast Reconstr Surg 101:1572–1579.

Chamberlain LJ, Yannas IV, Hsu H-P, Strichartz G, Spector M. 1998. Collagen-GAG substrate enhances the quality of nerve regeneration through collagen tubes up to level of autograft. Exp Neurol 154(2):315–329.

Chang AS, Yannas IV. 1992. Peripheral nerve regeneration. In B Smith, G Adelman (eds), Neuroscience Year (Supplement 2 to the Encyclopedia of Neuroscience), pp 125–126, Boston, Birkhauser.

Compton CC, Butler CE, Yannas IV, Warland G, Orgill DP. 1998. Organized skin structure is regenerated *in vivo* from collagen-GAG matrices seeded with autologous keratinocytes. J Invest Dermatol 110:908–916.

Hansbrough JF, Boyce ST, Cooper ML, Foreman TJ. 1989. Burn wound closure with autologous keratinocytes and fibroblasts attached to a collagen-glycosaminoglycan substrate. JAMA 262:2125–2141.

Hull BE, Sher SS, Rosen S, Church D, Bell E. 1983. Structural integration of skin equivalents grafted to Lewis and Sprague-Dawley rats. J Invest Dermatol 8:429–436.

Orgill DP, Butler CE, Regan JF. 1996. Behavior of collagen-GAG matrices as dermal replacements in rodent and porcine models, Wounds 8:151–157.

Stone KR, Rodkey WK, Webber RJ, McKinney L, Steadman JR. 1990. Collagen based prostheses for meniscal regeneration, Clin Orth 252:129–135.

Stone KR, Steadman R, Rodkey WG, Li S-T. 1997. Regeneration of meniscal cartilage with use of a collagen scaffold. J Bone Joint Surg 79A:1770–1777.

Yannas IV, Burke JF. 1980. Design of an artificial skin. I. Basic design principles. J Biomed Mater Res 14:65–81.

Yannas IV, Burke JF, Orgill DP, Skrabut EM. 1982. Wound tissue can utilize a polymeric template to synthesize a functional extension of skin. Science 215:174–176.

Yannas IV, Lee E, Orgill DP, Skrabut EM, Murphy GF. 1989. Synthesis and characterization of a model extracellular matrix that induces partial regeneration of adult mammalian skin. Proc Natl Acad Sci USA 86:933–937.

Yannas IV. 1997. Models of organ regeneration processes induced by templates. In A Prokop, D Hunkeler, AD Cherrington (eds), Bioartificial Organs, Ann NY Acad Sci 831:280–293.

Yannas IV. 1998. Studies on the biological activity of the dermal regeneration template. Wound Rep Regen Nov-Dec, 6(6):518–523.

Further Information

Chamberlain LJ, Yannas IV, Arrizabalaga A, Hsu H-P, Norregaard TV, Spector M. 1998. Early peripheral nerve healing in collagen and silicone tube implants. Myofibroblasts and the cellular response. Biomaterials Aug, 19(15):1393–1403.

Chamberlain LJ, Yannas IV, Hsu H-P, Spector M. 1997. Histological response to a fully degradable collagen device implanted in a gap in the rat sciatic nerve. Tissue Eng 3:353–362.

Eldad A, Burt A, Clarke JA, Gusterson B. 1987. Cultured epithelium as a skin substitute. Burns 13:173–180.

FR Noyes (ed), Biology and Biomechanics of the Traumatized Synovial Joint: The Knee as a Model, pp 221–231, AAOS Chicago.

Hansbrough JF, Cooper ML, Cohen R, Spielvogel R, Greemnleaf G, Bartel RL, Naughton G. 1992. Evaluation of a biodegradable matrix containing cultured human fibroblasts as a dermal replacement beneath meshed skin grafts on athymic mice. Surgery 111:438–446.

Heimbach D, Luterman A, Burke J, Cram A, Herndon D, Hunt J, Jordan M, McManus W, Solem L, Warden G, Zawacki B. 1988. Artificial dermis for major burns. Ann Surg 208:313–320.

Madison RD, Archibald SJ, Krarup C. 1992. Peripheral nerve injury. In IK Cohen, RF Diegelmann, WJ Lindblad (eds), Wound Healing, pp 450–487, Philadelphia, Saunders.

Orgill DP, Yannas IV. 1998. Design of an artificial skin. IV. Use of island graft to isolate organ regeneration from scar synthesis and other processes leading to skin wound closure. J Biomed Mater Res 36:531–535.

Rodkey WG, Stone KR, Steadman JR. 1992. Prosthetic meniscal replacement. In GAM Finerman, FR Noyes (eds), Biology and Biomechanics of the Traumatized Synovial Joint: The Knee as a Model, pp 221–231, Amer Acad Orth Surg, Chicago, IL.

Yannas IV, Burke JF, Gordon PL, Huang C. 1977. Multilayer membrane useful as synthetic skin. US patent 4,060,081, Nov. 29.

Yannas IV, Burke JF, Orgill DP, Burke JF. 1982. Regeneration of skin following closure of deep wounds with a biodegradable template. Trans Soc Biomater 5:1–38.

Yannas IV. 1988. Regeneration of skin and nerves by use of collagen templates. In ME Nimni (ed), Collagen, vol 3, pp 87–115, Boca Raton, FL, CRC Press.

Yannas IV. 1989. Skin. Regeneration Templates. Encyclopedia of Polymer Science and Engineering, vol 15, pp 317–334.

Yannas IV. 1990. Biologically active analogues of the extracellular matrix: Artificial skin and nerve. Angew Chem Int Ed Engl 29:20–35.

13

Fluid Shear Stress Effects on Cellular Function

Charles W. Patrick, Jr.
Rice University

Rangarajan Sampath
Rice University

Larry V. McIntire
Rice University

Cells of the vascular system are constantly exposed to mechanical (hemodynamic) forces due to the flow of blood. The forces generated in the vasculature include the frictional force or a fluid shear stress caused by blood flowing tangentially across the endothelium, a tensile stress caused by circumferential vessel wall deformations, and a net normal stress caused by a hydrodynamic pressure differential across the vessel wall. We will restrict our discussion to examining fluid shear stress modulation of vascular cell function. The endothelium is a biologically active monolayer of cells providing an interface between the flowing blood and tissues of the body. It can synthesize and secrete a myriad of vasoconstrictors, vasodilators, growth factors, fibrinolytic factors, cytokines, adhesion molecules, matrix proteins, and mitogens that modulate many physiologic processes, including wound healing, hemostasis, vascular remodeling, vascular tone, and immune and inflammatory responses. In addition to humoral stimuli, it is now well accepted that endothelial cell synthesis and secretion of bioactive molecules can be regulated by the hemodynamic forces generated by the local blood flow. These forces have been hypothesized to regulate neovascularization and the structure of the blood vessel [Hudlicka, 1984]. Clinical findings further show that arterial walls undergo an endothelium-dependent adaptive response to changes in blood flow, with blood vessels in high flow regions tending to enlarge and vessels in the low flow region having reduced lumen diameter, thereby maintaining a nearly constant shear stress at the vessel wall [Zarins et al., 1987]. In addition to playing an active role in the normal vascular biology, hemodynamic

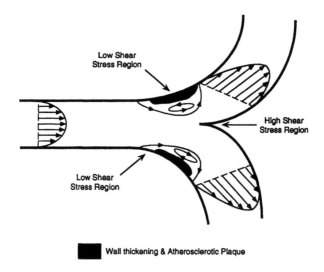

FIGURE 13.1   Atherosclerotic plaques develop in regions of arteries where the flow rate (and resultant wall shear stress) is relatively low, which is often downstream from a vessel bifurcation, where there can be flow separation from the outer walls and regions of recirculation. These regions of low shear stress are pathologically prone to vessel wall thickening and thrombosis.

forces have also been implicated in the pathogenesis of a variety of vascular diseases. Atherosclerotic lesion-prone regions, characterized by the incorporation of Evans blue dye, enhanced accumulation of albumin, fibrinogen, and LDL, increased recruitment of monocytes, and increased endothelial turnover rates exhibit polygonal endothelial cell morphology typically seen in a low-shear environment, as opposed to nonlesion regions that have elongated endothelial cells characteristic of high-shear regions [Nerem, 1993].

In vivo studies of the distribution of atherosclerosis and the degree of intimal thickening have shown preferential plaque localization in low-shear regions. Atherosclerotic lesions were not seen in random locations but were instead found to be localized to regions of arterial branching and sharp curvature, where complex flow patterns develop, as shown in Fig. 13.1 [Asakura and Karino, 1990; Friedman et al., 1981; Gibson et al., 1993; Glagov et al., 1988; Ku et al., 1985; Levesque et al., 1989; Zarins et al., 1983]. Morphologically, intact endothelium over plaque surfaces showed variation in shape and size and loss of normal orientation, characteristic of low-shear conditions [Davies et al., 1988]. Flow in the vascular system is by and large laminar, but extremely complex time dependent flow patterns can develop in localized regions of complex geometry. Zarins and co-workers [1983] have shown that in the human carotid bifurcation, regions of moderate-to-high shear stress where flow remains unidirectional and axially aligned, were relatively free of intimal thickening, whereas extensive plaque localization was seen in the regions where low shear stress, fluid separation from the wall, and complex flow patterns were predominant. Asakura and Karino [1990] presented a technique for flow visualization by using transparent arteries where they directly correlated flow patterns to regions of plaque formation in human coronary arteries. They observed that the flow divider at the bifurcation point, a region of high shear stress, was relatively devoid of plaque deposition, whereas the outer wall, a region of low shear stress, showed extensive plaque formation. Similar patterns were also seen in curved vessels, where the inner wall or the hip region of the curve, a region of low shear and flow separation, exhibited plaque formation. In addition to the direct shear-stress-mediated effects, the regions of complex flow patterns and recirculation also tend to increase the residence time of circulating blood cells in susceptible regions, whereas the blood cells are rapidly cleared away from regions of high wall shear and unidirectional flow [Glagov et al., 1988]. This increased transit time could influence plaque deposition by favoring margination of monocytes and platelets, release of vasoactive agents, or altered permeability at the intercellular junctions to extracellular lipid particles and possible concentration of procoagulant materials [Nollert et al., 1991].

The endothelium forming the interface between blood and the surrounding tissues is believed to act as a sensor of the local hemodynamic environment in mediating both the normal response and the pattern of vascular diseases. *In vivo* studies have shown changes in the actin microfilament localization in a shear-dependent manner. Actin stress fibres have been observed to be aligned with the direction of flow in high-shear regions, whereas they were mostly present in dense peripheral bands in the low-shear regions [Kim et al., 1989]. Langille and Adamson [1981] showed that the cells in large arteries, away from the branches, were aligned parallel to the long axes of the artery in rabbit and mouse. Similar results were shown in coronary arteries of patients undergoing cardiac transplantation [Davies et al., 1988]. Near the branch points of large arteries, however, cells aligned along the flow streamlines. In smaller blood vessels, where secondary flow patterns did not develop, the cell alignment followed the geometry of the blood vessel. In fact, endothelial cell morphology and orientation at the branch may be a natural marker of the detailed features of blood flow [Nerem et al., 1981].

Another cell type that is likely to be affected by hemodynamic forces is the vascular smooth muscle cell (SMC) present in the media. In the early stages of lesion development, SMCs proliferate and migrate into the intima [Ross, 1993; Schwartz et al., 1993]. Since the endothelium is intact in all but the final stages of atherosclerosis, SMCs are unlikely to be directly affected by shear stress. Most of the direct force they experience comes from the cyclical stretch forces experienced by the vessel itself due to pressure pulses [Grande et al., 1989]. Shear forces acting on the endothelium, however, can release compounds such as endothelin, nitric oxide, and platelet-derived growth factors that act as SMC mitogens and can modulate SMC tone. Ono and colleagues [1991] showed that homogenate of shear-stressed endothelial cells contained increased amounts of collagen and stimulated SMC migration *in vitro*, compared to endothelial cells grown under static conditions. The local shear environment could thus act directly or indirectly on the cells of the vascular wall in mediating a physiologic response.

This chapter presents what is currently known regarding how the mechanical agonist of shear stress modulates endothelial cell function in the context of vascular physiology and pathophysiology. In discussing this topic we have adopted an outside-in approach. That is, we first discuss how shear stress affects endothelial cell-blood cell interactions, then progress to how shear stress affects the endothelial cell cytoskeleton, signal transduction, and protein secretion, and finally end with how shear stress modulates endothelial cell gene expression. We close with gene therapy and tissue engineering considerations related to how endothelial cells respond to shear stress. Before proceeding, however, we discuss the devices and methodology used for studying the endothelial cell responses to shear stress *in vitro*.

13.1 Devices and Methodology Used for *in Vitro* Experiments

In vivo studies aimed at understanding cellular responses to shear forces have the inherent problem that they cannot quantitatively define the exact features of the hemodynamic environment. Moreover, it is very difficult to say if the resultant response is due to shear stress or some other feature associated with the hemodynamic environment. Cell culture studies and techniques for exposing cells to a controlled shear environment *in vitro* have been increasingly used to elucidate cellular responses to shear stress and flow. Mechanical-force-induced changes in cell function have been measured *in vitro* using mainly two cell types, cultured monolayers of bovine aortic endothelial cells (BAECs) and human umbilical vein endothelial cells (HUVECs). Shear stress is typically generated *in vitro* by flowing fluid across endothelial cell monolayers under controlled kinematic conditions, usually in the laminar flow regime. Parallel plate and cone-and-plate geometries have been the most common. Physiologic levels of venous and arterial shear stress range between 1–5 dyn/cm² and 6–40 dyn/cm², respectively.

The use of the parallel plate flow chamber allows one to have a controlled and well-defined flow environment based on the chamber geometry (fixed) and the flow rate through the chamber (variable).

In addition, individual cells can be visualized in real time using video microscopy. Assuming parallel plate geometry and Newtonian fluid behavior, the wall shear stress on the cell monolayer in the flow chamber is calculated as

$$\tau_w = \frac{6Q\mu}{\left(bh^2\right)} \tag{13.1}$$

where Q is the volumetric flow rate, μ is the viscosity of the flowing fluid, h is the channel height, b is the channel width, and τ_w is the wall shear stress. The flow chambers are designed such that the entrance length is very small compared to the effective length of the chamber [Frangos et al., 1985]. Therefore, entry effects can be neglected, and the flow is fully developed and parabolic over nearly the entire length of the flow chamber. Flow chambers usually consist of a machined block, a gasket whose thickness determines in part the channel depth, and a glass coverslip to which is attached a monolayer of endothelial cells (Fig. 13.2a). The individual components are held together either by a vacuum, or by evenly torqued screws, thereby ensuring a uniform channel depth. The flow chamber can have a myriad of entry ports, bubble ports, and exit ports. For short-term experiments, media are drawn through the chamber over the monolayer of cells using a syringe pump. For long-term experiments, the chamber is placed in a flow loop. In a flow loop (Fig. 13.2b), cells grown to confluence on glass slides can be exposed to a well-defined shear stress by recirculation of culture medium driven by gravity [Frangos et al., 1985]. Culture medium from the lower reservoir is pumped to the upper reservoir at a constant flow rate such that there is an overflow of excess medium back into the lower reservoir. This overflow serves two purposes: (1) It maintains a constant hydrostatic head between the two reservoirs, and (2) it prevents entry of air bubbles into the primary flow section upstream of the flow chamber that could be detrimental to the cells. The pH of the medium is maintained at physiologic levels by gassing with a humidified mixture of 95% air and 5% CO_2. The rate of flow in the line supplying the chamber is determined solely by gravity and can be altered by changing the vertical separation between the two reservoirs. A sample port in the bottom reservoir allows periodic sampling of the flowing medium for a time-dependent assay.

As mentioned above, cone-and-plate geometries can also be utilized. A schematic of a typical cone-and-plate viscometer is shown in Fig. 13.2c. Shear stress is produced in the fluid contained between the rotating cone and the stationary plate. Cells grown on coverslips can be placed in the shear field (up to 12 at a time). For relatively small cone angles and low rates of rotation, the shear stress throughout the system is independent of position. The cone angle compensates for radial effects seen in plate-and-plate rheometers. The wall shear stress (τ_w) on the cell monolayer in the cone-and-plate viscometer is calculated as

$$\tau_w = \frac{3T}{2\pi R^3} \tag{13.2}$$

where T is the applied torque and R is the cone radius. The flow becomes turbulent, however, at the plate's edge and at high rotational speeds. Modifications from the basic design have allowed use of an optical system with the rheometer, enabling direct microscopic examination and real-time analysis of the cultured cells during exposure to shear stress [Dewey et al., 1981; Schnittler et al., 1993]. For a more complete description of *in vitro* device design and applications, refer to the text edited by Frangos [Transon-Tay, 1993].

13.2   Shear Stress-Mediated Cell-Endothelium Interactions

Cell-cell and cell-substrate interactions in the vascular system are important in a number of physiologic and pathologic situations. Lymphocytes, platelets, or tumor cells in circulation may arrest at a particular site as a result of interaction with the endothelium or the subendothelial matrix. While the margination

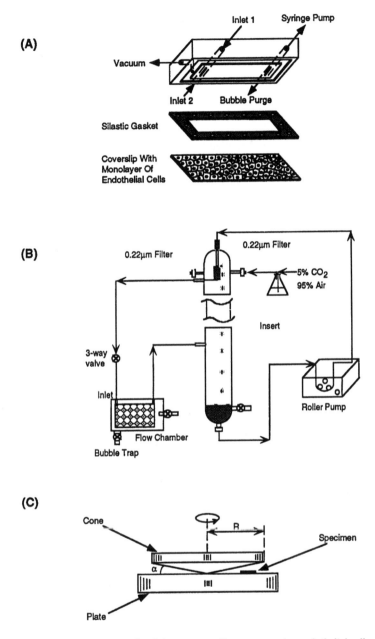

FIGURE 13.2 Devices used for *in vitro* study of shear stress effects on vascular endothelial cells. (a) Parallel plate flow chamber, (b) flow loop, (c) cone-and-plate viscometer.

of leukocyte/lymphocyte to the vessel wall be a normal physiologic response to injury or inflammation, adhesion of blood platelets to the subendothelium and subsequent platelet aggression could result in a partial or complete occlusion of the blood vessel leading to thrombosis or stroke. In addition, the adhesion of tumor cells to the endothelium is often the initial step in the development of secondary metastases. The adhesion of leukocytes, platelets, and tumor cells is not only mediated by adhesion molecules on the endothelium but also mediated by the hemodynamic force environment present in the vasculature. In fact, the specific molecular mechanisms employed for adhesion often vary with the local wall shear stress [Alevriadou et al., 1993; Lawrence et al., 1990].

Targeting of circulating leukocytes to particular regions of the body is an aspect of immune system function that is currently of great research interest. This targeting process consists of adhesion of a specific subpopulation of circulating leukocytes to a specific area of vascular endothelium via cell surface adhesion receptors. The large number of receptors involved and the differential regulation of their expression on particular cell subpopulations make this process very versatile but also quite complicated. An extremely important additional complication arises from the fact that these interactions occur within the flowing bloodstream. Study of these various types of adhesive interactions requires accurate recreation of the flow conditions experienced by leukocytes and endothelial cells. Lawrence and co-workers examined neutrophil adhesion to cytokine-stimulated endothelial cells under well-defined postcapillary venular flow conditions in vitro [Lawrence et al., 1987, 1990; Lawrence and Springer, 1991]. They also demonstrated that under flow conditions neutrophil adhesion to cytokine-stimulated endothelial cells is mediated almost exclusively by CD18-independent mechanisms but that subsequent neutrophil migration is CD18-dependent [Lawrence and Springer, 1991; Smith et al., 1991]. The initial flow studies were followed by many further studies both _in vitro_ [Abbassi et al., 1991, 1993; Anderson et al., 1991; Hakkert et al., 1991; Jones et al., 1993; Kishimoto et al., 1991] and _in vivo_ [Ley et al., 1991; Perry and Granger, 1991; von Andrian et al., 1991; Watson et al., 1991] which clearly distinguish separate mechanisms for initial adhesion/rolling and firm adhesion/leukocyte migration. Research has further shown that in a variety of systems, selectin/carbohydrate interactions are primarily responsible for initial adhesion and rolling, and firm adhesion and leukocyte migration are mediated primarily by integrin/peptide interactions. Methodology discussed for studying receptor specificity of adhesion for leukocytes under flow can also be utilized for studying red cell–endothelial cell interactions [Barabino et al., 1987; Wick et al., 1987, 1993].

The interaction of tumor cells with endothelial cells is an important step in tumor metastasis. To adhere to the vessel wall, tumor cells that come into contact with the microvasculature must resist the tractive force of shear stress that tends to detach them from the vessel wall [Weiss, 1992]. Hence, studies of the mechanisms involved in the process of tumor metastasis must take into account the physical forces acting on the tumor cells. Bastida and co-workers [1989] have demonstrated that tumor cell adhesion depends not only on tumor cell characteristics and endothelial cell adhesion molecule expression but on shear stress in the interaction of circulating tumor cells with the endothelium. The influence of shear stress on tumor cell adhesion suggests that attachment of tumor cells to vascular structures occurs in areas of high shear stress, such as the microvasculature [Bastida et al., 1989]. This is supported by earlier pathologic observations that indicate preferential attachment of tumor cells on the lung and liver capillary system [Warren, 1973]. Some tumor cell types roll and subsequently adhere on endothelial cells using selectin-mediated mechanisms similar to leukocytes, whereas others adhere without rolling using integrin-mediated receptors on endothelial cells [Bastida et al., 1989; Giavazzi et al., 1993; Kojima et al., 1992; Menter et al., 1992; Patton et al., 1993; Pili et al., 1993]. It has been postulated that some tumor cell types undergo a stabilization process prior to firm adhesion that is mediated by transglutaminase cross-linking [Menter et al., 1992; Patton et al., 1993]. Recently, Pili and colleagues [1993] demonstrated that tumor cell contact with endothelial cells increases Ca^{2+} release from endothelial cell intracellular stores, which may have a fundamental role in enhancing cell-cell adhesion. The factors and molecular mechanisms underlying tumor cell and endothelial cell interactions remain largely undefined and are certain to be further explored in the future.

The endothelium provides a natural nonthrombogenic barrier between circulating platelets and the endothelial basement membrane. However, there are pathologic instances in which the endothelium integrity is compromised, exposing a thrombogenic surface. Arterial thrombosis is the leading cause of death in the United States. Among the most likely possibilities for the initiation of arterial platelet thrombi are (1) adhesion of blood platelets onto the subendothelium of injured arteries and arterioles or on ruptured atherosclerotic plaque surfaces, containing collagen and other matrix proteins, with subsequent platelet aggregation, or (2) shear-induced aggregation of platelets in areas of the arterial circulation partially constricted by atherosclerosis or vasospasm. Various experimental models have been developed to investigate the molecular mechanisms of platelet attachment to surfaces (adhesion) and platelet cohesion to each other (aggregation) under shear stress conditions. Whole-blood perfusion studies using annular or parallel-plate perfusion chambers simulate the first proposed mechanism of arterial thrombus formation *in vivo*, that may occur as a result of adhesion on an injured, exposed subendothelial or atherosclerotic plaque surface [Hubbel and McIntire, 1986; Weiss et al., 1978, 1986]. Platelets arriving subsequently could, under the right conditions, adhere to each other, forming aggregates large enough to partially or completely occlude the blood vessel. *In vitro* studies have shown an increase in thrombus growth with local shear rate, an event that is believed to be the result of enhanced arrival and cohesion of platelets near the surface at higher wall shear stresses [Turitto et al., 1987]. Video microscopy provides information on the morphologic characteristics of thrombi and enables the reconstruction of three-dimensional models of thrombi formed on surfaces coated with biomaterials or endothelial cell basement membrane proteins. Macroscopic analysis of thrombi can provide information on platelet mass transport and reaction kinetics with the surface, and microscopic analysis allows dynamic real-time study of cell-surface and intercellular interactions. Such a technology enables the study of key proteins involved in mural thrombus formation, such as vWF [Alevriadou et al., 1993; Folie and McIntire, 1989]. In addition, tests of antithrombotic agents and investigation of the thrombogenicity of various purified components of the vessel wall or polymeric biomaterials can be performed.

13.3 Shear Stress Effects on Cell Morphology and Cytoskeletal Rearrangement

In addition to mediating cell–endothelial cell interactions, shear stress can act directly on the endothelium. It has been demonstrated for almost a decade that hemodynamic forces can modulate endothelial cell morphology and structure [Barbee et al., 1994; Coan et al., 1993; Eskin et al., 1984; Franke et al., 1984; Girard and Nerem, 1991, 1993; Ives et al., 1986; Langille et al., 1991; Levesque et al., 1989; Wechezak et al., 1985]. Conceivably, the cytoskeletal reorganization that occurs in endothelial cells several hours after exposure to flow may, in conjunction with shape change, transduce mechanical signals to cytosolic and nuclear signals (mechanotransduction), thereby playing a role in gene expression and signal transduction [Ingber, 1993; Resnick et al., 1993; Watson, 1991]. In fact, investigators have shown specific gene expression related to cytoskeletal changes [Botteri et al., 1990; Breathnach et al., 1987; Ferrua et al., 1990; Werb et al., 1986]. F-actin has been implicated as the principal transmission element in the cytoskeleton and appears to be required for signal transduction [Watson, 1991]. Actin filaments are anchored in the plasma membrane at several sites, including focal adhesions on the basal membrane, intercellular adhesion proteins, integral membrane proteins at the apical surface, and the nuclear membrane [Davies and Tripathi, 1993]. Substantiating this, Barbee and co-workers [1994] have recently shown, utilizing atomic force microscopy, that F-actin fiber stress bundles are formed in the presence of fluid flow and the fibers are coupled to the apical membrane. Moreover, endothelial cell shape change and realignment with flow can be inhibited by drugs that interfere with microfilament turnover [Davies and Tripathi, 1993]. Although all evidence leads one to believe that the endothelial cell cytoskeleton can respond to flow and that F-actin is involved, the exact mechanism involved remains to be elucidated.

13.4 Shear Stress Effects on Signal Transduction and Mass Transfer

Shear stress and resultant convective mass transfer are known to affect many important cytosolic second messengers in endothelial cells. For instance, shear stress is known to cause ATP-mediated increases in calcium ions (Ca^{2+}) [Ando et al., 1988; Dull and Davies, 1991; Mo et al., 1991; Nollert and McIntire, 1992]. Changes in flow influence the endothelial boundary layer concentration of ATP by altering the convective transport of exogenous ATP, thereby altering ATP's interaction with both the P_{2y}-purinoreceptor and ecto-ATPase. At low levels of shear stress, degradation of ATP by ecto-ATPase exceeds the rate of diffusion, and the steady state concentration of ATP remains low. In contrast, at high levels of shear stress, convection enhances the delivery of ATP from upstream to the P_{2y}-purinoreceptor, and diffusion exceeds the rate of degradation by the ecto-ATPase [Mo et al., 1991]. Whether physiologic levels of shear stress can directly increase intracellular calcium remains unclear. Preceding the calcium increases are increases in inositol-1,4,5 trisphosphate (IP_3) [Bhagyalakshmi et al., 1992; Bhagyalakshmi and Frangos, 1989b; Nollert et al., 1990; Prasad et al., 1993], which binds to specific sites on the endoplasmic reticulum and causes release of Ca^{2+} from intracellular stores, and diacylglycerol (DAG) [Bhagyalakshmi and Frangos, 1989a]. Elevated levels of both DAG and Ca^{2+} can activate several protein kinases, including protein kinase C (PKC). Changes in Ca^{2+}, IP_3, and DAG are evidence that fluid shear stress activated the PKC pathway. In fact, the PKC pathway has been demonstrated to be activated by shear stress [Bhagyalakshmi and Frangos, 1989b; Hsieh et al., 1992, 1993; Kuchan and Frangos, 1993; Milner et al., 1992]. In addition to the PKC pathway, pathways involving cyclic adenosine monophosphate (cAMP) and cyclic guanosine monophosphate (cGMP) may also be modulated by shear stress, as evidenced by increases in cAMP [Bhagyalakshmi and Frangos, 1989b] and cGMP [Kuchan and Frangos, 1993; Ohno et al., 1993] with shear stress. Moreover, it has been shown recently that shear stress causes acidification of cytoslic pH [Ziegelstein et al., 1992]. Intracellular acidification of vascular endothelial cells releases Ca^{2+} into the cytosol [Ziegelstein et al., 1993]. This Ca^{2+} mobilization may be linked to endothelial synthesis and release of vasodilatory substances during the pathological condition of acidosis.

13.5   Shear Stress Effects on Endothelial Cell Metabolite Secretion

The application of shear stress *in vitro* is accompanied by alterations in protein synthesis that are detectable within several hours after initiation of the mechanical agonist. Shear stress may regulate the expression of fibrinolytic proteins by endothelial cells; tPA is an antithrombotic glycoprotein and serine protease that is released from endothelial cells. Once released, it rapidly converts plasminogen to plasmin which, in turn, dissolves fibrin clots. Diamond and co-workers [1989] have shown that venous levels of shear stress do not affect tPA secretion, whereas arterial levels increase the secretion rate of tPA. Arterial flows lead to a profibrinolytic state that would be beneficial in maintaining a clot-free artery. In contrast to tPA, neither venous nor arterial levels of shear stress cause significant changes in plasminogen activator inhibitor-1 (PAI-1) secretion rates [Diamond et al., 1989; Kuchan and Frangos, 1993]. Increased proliferation of smooth muscle cells is one of the early events of arteriosclerosis. The secretion rate of endothelin-1 (ET-1), a potent smooth muscle cell mitogen, has been shown to increase in response to venous levels of shear stress and decrease in response to arterial levels of shear stress [Kuchan and Frangos, 1993; Milner et al., 1992; Nollert et al., 1991; Sharefkin et al., 1991; Yoshizumi et al., 1989]. Both the *in vitro* tPA and ET-1 results are consistent with *in vivo* observations that atherosclerotic plaque development occurs in low shear stress regions as opposed to high shear stress regions. The low shear stress regions usually occur downstream from vessel branches. In these regions we would expect low secretion of tPA and high secretion of ET-1, leading to locally increased smooth muscle cell proliferation (intimal thickening of the vessel) and periodic problems with clot formation (thrombosis). Both of these observations are observed pathologically and are important processes in atherogenesis [McIntire, 1994].

Important metabolites in the arachidonic acid cascade via the cyclooxygenase pathway; prostacylin (PGI_2) and prostaglandin (PGF_{2a}) are also known to increase their secretion rates in response to arterial levels of shear stress [Frangos et al., 1985; Grabowski et al., 1985; Nollert et al., 1989]. In addition, endothelial cells have been shown to increase their production of fibronectin (FN) in response to shear stress [Gupte and Frangos, 1990]. Endothelial cells may respond to shear stress by secreting FN in order to increase their attachment to the extracellular matrix, thereby resisting the applied fluid shear stress. Endothelial cells have been shown to modulate their receptor expression of intercellular adhesion molecule-1 (ICAM-1), vascular cell adhesion molecule-1 (VCAM-1), and monocyte chemotactic peptide-1

(MCP-1) in response to shear stress [Sampath et al., 1995; Shyy et al., 1994]. The adaptive expression of these adhesion molecules in response to hemodynamic shear stress may aid in modulating specific adhesion localities for neutrophils, leukocytes, and monocytes.

13.6 Shear Stress Effects on Gene Regulation

In many cases, the alterations in protein synthesis observed with shear stress are preceded by modulation of protein gene expression. The molecular mechanisms by which mechanical agonists alter the gene expression of proteins are under current investigation. Diamond and colleagues [1990] and Nollert and colleagues [1992] have demonstrated that arterial levels of shear stress upregulate the transcription of tPA mRNA, concomitant with tPA protein secretion. The gene expressions of ET-1 and PDGF, both of which are potent smooth muscle cell mitogens and vasoconstrictors, are also known to be modulated by hemodynamic forces. For instance, arterial levels of shear stress cause ET-1 mRNA to be downregulated [Malek et al., 1993; Malek and Izumo, 1992; Sharefkin et al., 1991]. ET-1 mRNA downregulation is sensitive to the magnitude of the shear stress in a dose-dependent fashion, reaching a saturation at 15 dyn/cm². Conversely, Yoshizumi and co-workers [1989] have shown that venous levels of shear stress cause a transient increase in ET-1 mRNA, peaking at 4 h and returning to basal levels by 12–24 h. However, they had previously reported downregulation of ET-1 mRNA expression [Yanagisawa et al., 1988]. PDGF is expressed as a dimer composed of PDGF-A and PDGF-B subunits. There are conflicting reports as to how arterial shear stresses affect PDGF-B mRNA expression. Malek and colleagues [1993] have shown that arterial levels of shear stress applied to BAECs cause a significant decrease in PDGF-B mRNA expression over a 9-h period. In contrast, Mitsumata and co-workers [1993] and Resnick and co-workers [1993] have shown increases in BAEC mRNA expression of PDGF-B when arterial shear stresses were applied. The discrepancy in the results may be attributed to differences in BAEC cell line origins or differences in the passage number of cells used. In support of the latter two investigators, Hsieh and colleagues [1992] have reported upregulation of PDGF-B mRNA in HUVECs in the presence of arterial shear stress. As with the B chain of PDGF, there are conflicting reports as to the affect of arterial shear stress on PDGF-A. Mitsumata and co-workers [1993] have reported no change in PDGF-A mRNA expression, whereas Hsieh and co-workers [1991, 1992] have reported a shear-dependent increase in the mRNA expression from 0–6 dyn/cm² which then plateaus from 6–51 dyn/cm². Endothelial cell expression of ET-1 and PDGF may be important in blood vessel remodeling. In blood vessels exposed to increased flow, the chronic vasculature response is an increase in vessel diameter [Langille and O'Donnell, 1986]. Hence, it is tempting to postulate that hemodynamic-force-modulated alterations in ET-1 and PDGF mRNA expression may account for much of this adaptive change.

The gene expression of various adhesion molecules involved in leukocyte recruitment during inflammation and disease has also been investigated. ICAM-1 mRNA has been shown to be transiently upregulated in the presence of venous or arterial shear stresses [Nagel et al., 1994; Sampath et al., 1995]. Its time-dependent response peaked at 1–3 h following exposure to shear, before declining below basal levels with prolonged exposure of 6–24 h. In contrast, VCAM-1 mRNA level was downregulated almost immediately upon onset of flow and was found to drop significantly below basal levels within 6 h of initiation of flow at all magnitudes of shear stresses. E-selectin mRNA expression appeared to be generally less responsive to shear stress, especially at the lower magnitudes. After an initial downward trend 1 h following exposure to shear stress (2 dyn/cm²), E-selectin mRNA remained at stable levels for up to 6 h [Sampath et al., 1995]. Recent evidence shows that the expression of MCP-1, a monocyte-specific chemoattractant expressed on endothelial cells, also follows a similar biphasic response with shear stress like ICAM-1 [Shyy et al., 1994]. In addition to adhesion molecules, the gene expression of several growth factors has been investigated. The mRNA expression of heparin-binding epidermal growth factor like growth factor (HB-EGF), a smooth muscle-cell mitogen, transiently increases in the presence of minimal arterial shear stress [Morita et al., 1993]. Transforming growth factor-β1 (TGF-β1) mRNA has been reported to be upregulated in the presence of arterial shear stresses within 2 h and remain elevated for

12 h [Ohno et al., 1992]. In addition, Malek and co-workers [1993] have shown that basic fibroblast growth factor (bFGF) mRNA is upregulated in BAECs in the presence of arterial shear stresses. In HUVECs, however, no significant changes in bFGF message were observed [Diamond et al., 1990]. This difference is probably due to differences in cell source (human versus bovine).

Proto-oncogenes code for binding proteins that either enhance or repress transcription and, therefore, are ideal candidates to act as gene regulators [Cooper, 1990]. Komuro and colleagues [1990, 1991] were the first to demonstrate that mechanical loading causes upregulation of c-*fos* expression. Recently, Hsieh and co-workers [1993] investigated the role of arterial shear stress on the mRNA levels of nuclear proto-oncogenes c-*fos*, c-*jun*, and c-*myc*. Gene expression of c-*fos* was transiently upregulated, peaking at 0.5 h and returning to basal levels within an hour. In contrast, both c-*jun* and c-*myc* mRNA were upregulated to sustainable levels within an hour. The transcribed protein products of c-*fos*, c-*jun*, and c-*myc* may act as nuclear-signaling molecules for mechanically induced gene modulation [Nollert et al., 1992; Ranjan and Diamond, 1993].

13.7 Mechanisms of Shear Stress-Induced Gene Regulation

Although no unified scheme to explain mechanical signal transduction and modulation of gene expression is yet possible, many studies provide insight in an attempt to elucidate which second messengers are involved in gene regulation mediated by hemodynamic forces. There is substantial evidence that the PKC pathway may be involved in the gene regulation. A model of the PKC transduction pathway is shown in Fig. 13.3. Mitsumata and colleagues [1993] have shown that PDGF mRNA modulation by shear stress could be partially attributed to a PKC pathway. Hsieh and co-workers [1992] have shown that shear-induced PDGF gene expression in HUVECs is mainly mediated by PKC activation and requires Ca^{2+} and the involvement of G proteins. In addition, they demonstrated that cAMP and cGMP dependent protein kinases are not involved in PDGF gene expression. Morita and colleagues [1993] have shown that shear-induced HB-EGF mRNA expression is mediated through a PKC pathway and that Ca^{2+} may be involved in the pathway. PKC was also found to be an important mediator in flow-induced c-*fos* expression, with the additional involvement of G proteins, phospholipase C (PLC), and Ca^{2+} [Hsieh et al., 1993]. Moreover, Levin and co-workers [1988] have shown that tPA gene expression is enhanced by PKC activation and Iba and co-workers [1992] have shown that cAMP is not involved in tPA gene expression. As depicted in Fig. 13.3, the PKC pathway may be involved in activating DNA-binding proteins via phosphorylation.

In addition to second messengers, it has been proposed that cytoskeletal reorganization may play a role in regulating gene expression [Ingber, 1993; Resnick et al., 1993]. Morita and colleagues [1993] have shown that shear stress-induced ET-1 gene expression is mediated by the disruption of the actin cytoskeleton and that microtubule integrity is also involved. Gene expression of other bioactive molecules may also be regulated by actin disruption. The actual molecular mechanisms involved in cytoskeletal-mediated gene expression remain unclear. However, the cytoskeleton may activate membrane ion channels and nuclear pores.

In addition to second messengers and the cytoskeletal architecture, it has been postulated by Nollert and others [1992] that transcriptional factors that bind to the DNA may play an active role mediating the signal transduction between the cytosol and nucleus (Fig. 13.4). It is known that nuclear translocation of transcriptional factors and DNA-binding activity of the factors can be mediated by phosphorylation [Bohmann, 1990; Hunter and Karin, 1992]. Many of the transcription factors are protein products of proto-oncogenes. It has previously been stated that shear stress increases expression of c-*fos* and c-*jun*. The gene products of c-*fos* and c-*jun* form protein dimers that bind to transcriptional sites on DNA promoters and act as either transcriptional activators or repressors. Two of the transcriptional sites to which the *fos* and *jun* family dimers bind are the TRE (tumor promoting agent response element) and CRE (cAMP response element). These have consensus sequences of TGACTCA and TGACGTCA, respectively. It is known that the promoter regions of tPA, PAI-1, ET, and TGF-β1 possess sequences of homology to the CRE and TRE [Nollert et al., 1992]. In addition to mediating known transcription factor binding

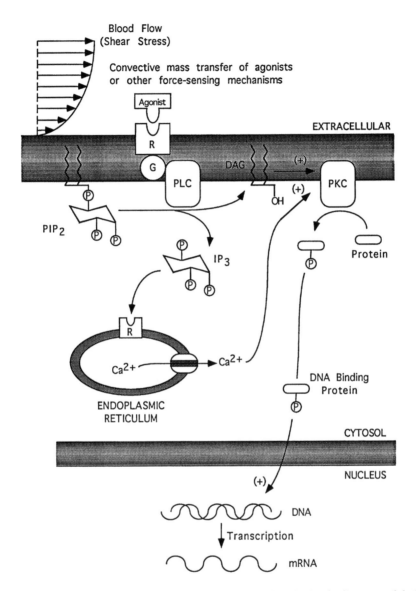

FIGURE 13.3 Model for shear stress induced protein kinase C (PKC) activation leading to modulation of gene expression. Mechanical agonists enhance membrane phosphoinositide turnover via phospholipase C (PLC), producing inositol-1,4,5 trisphosphate (IP_3), and diacylglycerol (DAG). DAG can then activate PKC. IP_3 may also activate PKC via Ca^{2+} release. PKC phosphorylates DNA-binding proteins, thereby making them active. The nuclear binding proteins then alter mRNA transcription. R = receptor, G = G protein, PIP_2 = phosphatidylinositol 4,5-bisphosphate, (+) = activation.

in perhaps novel ways, mechanical perturbations may initiate molecular signaling through specific stress- or strain-sensitive promoters that can activate gene expression. In fact, Resnick and colleagues [1993] have described a *cis*-acting shear stress response element (SSRE) in the PDGF-B promoter, and this sequence is also found in the promoters of tPA, ICAM-1, TGF-β1, *c-fos*, and *c-jun* but not in VCAM-1 or E-selectin promoters. A core-binding sequence of GAGACC was identified that binds to transcriptional factors found in BAEC nuclear extracts. The identify of transcriptional factors that bind this sequence remains unknown. In addition, Malek and co-workers [1993] have shown that shear-stress mediated ET-1 mRNA expression is not dependent on either the PKC or cAMP pathways, but rather shear stress regulates the transcription of the ET-1 gene via an upstream *cis* element in its promoter. It remains to

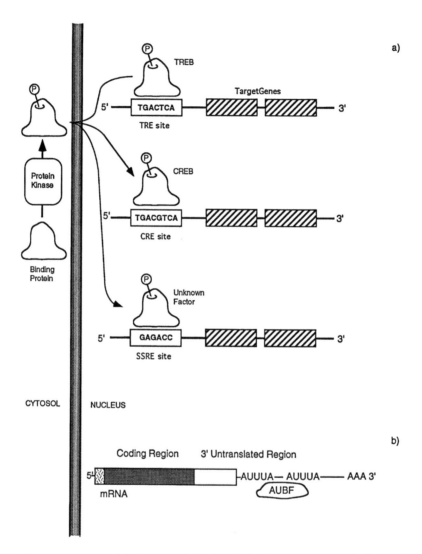

FIGURE 13.4   Gene expression regulated by transcription/translation factors and mechanically sensitive promoters. (a) Phosphorylation of transcription factors allows their translocation to the nucleus and subsequent DNA binding. The transcription factors can activate or inhibit transcription. TRE = tumor promoting agent response element, TREB = tumor promoting agent response element binding protein, CRE = cAMP response element, CREB = cAMP response element binding protein, SSRE = shear sensitive response element. (b) The AU-binding factor binds the AUUUA motif located in the 3' untranslated regions of some mature mRNA and could play an important role in mediating stability and/or transport of these mRNAs; AUBF = AU binding factor.

be seen if ET-1 is shown to have the same response element as that proposed by Resnick and colleagues. As mentioned previously, Mitsumata and co-workers [1993] found that PDGF mRNA modulation was not solely dependent on a PKC pathway. The PKC independent mechanism may very well involve the *cis*-acting shear stress response element that Resnick and colleagues described, though other factors are probably important in controlling the complex temporal pattern of gene expression seen in response to mechanical stimuli. The biphasic response of MCP-1 was shown to be regulated at the transcriptional level, possibly involving activation of AP-1, sites and the subsequent binding to the TRE site. The putative SSRE binding site was also identified in the 5' flanking region of the cloned MCP-1 gene suggesting an interactive mechanism, wherein these *cis*-acting elements collectively regulate the transcriptional activation of MCP-1 gene under shear stress [Shyy et al., 1994].

Another important determinant in the role played by shear stress on gene regulation could be at the level of mRNA stability. It is not known whether the shear-induced downregulation that has been reported, especially in the case of adhesion molecules, is due to a decrease in the transcriptional rate of the gene or due to a decrease in the stability of the transcript. The β-adrenergic receptors, which are part of a large class of G-protein linked cell surface receptors, are also susceptible to desensitization and downregulation [Hadcock and Malbon, 1988]. A study of the molecular basis for agonist-induced instability revealed the existence of an M_r 35,000 protein that specifically binds mRNA transcripts which contain the sequence AUUUA in their 3′ untranslated region (3′-UTR) [Port et al., 1992]. Agonists that decrease the β-adrenergic RNA transcript levels increased the level of this protein. Further, it has been shown that tandem repeats (three or more) of this sequence are needed for efficient binding of the destabilizer protein [Bohjanen et al., 1992]. Recent reports, however, suggest that AUUUA motif alone does not destabilize the mRNA transcripts and that the presence of additional elements in the AU-rich 3′-UTR may be necessary for the observed mRNA instability [Peppel et al., 1991]. Muller and others [1992] also report that binding of certain AU-binding factors (AUBF) to AUUUA motif accelerates the nuclear export of these mRNAs (Fig. 13.4). Further, their study indicates that this AUBF may protect AU-rich mRNAs against degradation by endoribonuclease V, by binding AUUUA motifs, thereby stabilizing the otherwise unstable mRNA.

Analysis of the 3′-UTR of some of the adhesion molecules studied revealed the presence of the AUUUA motif in all three cases. Human VCAM-1 [Cybulsky et al., 1991] has 6 dispersed AUUUA repeats in its 3′-UTR. Human ICAM-1 [Staunton et al., 1988] has 3 AUUUA repeats within 10 bases of each other, and 3-selectin [Hession et al., 1990] has 8 AUUUA repeats, which include 1 tandem repeat and 3 others that are within 10 bases of each other. The constitutively expressed gene human GAPDH [Tokunaga et al., 1987] does not have any AUUUA repeats in the 3′ region analyzed. Of the other shear responsive genes, human PDGF-B (*c-sis*) gene has 1 AUUUA repeat [Ratner et al., 1985]; human endothelin gene [Bloch et al., 1989] has 4, 3 within 10 bases of each other; human tissue plasminogen activator (tPA) [Reddy et al., 1987] has 2; and human thrombomodulin [Jackman et al., 1987] has 9 AUUUA boxes, including 1 tandem repeat. The steady state levels of the tPA and PDGF have been shown to be increased, and those of the adhesion molecules and endothelin have been shown to be decreased by arterial shear stress [Diamond et al., 1990; Hsieh et al., 1992; Sampath et al., 1995], suggesting a possible mechanism of shear-induced destabilization of adhesion molecule mRNA. However, the observed changes can be at the transcriptional level, with the AUUUA motifs playing a role only in the transport of these mRNAs to the cytoplasm. As shown by Muller and colleagues [1992], transport of low-abundance mRNAs like cytokine mRNAs, whose cellular concentrations are one-hundredth or less of that of the high abundance mRNAs, are the ones that are prone to modulation by transport-stimulatory proteins such as AUBF. This can explain the presence of AUUUA boxes in the 3′-UTR of adhesion molecules and other modulators of vascular tone and not in that of the constitutively expressed GADPH, which is an essential enzyme in the metabolic pathway and is expressed in high copy numbers. A more detailed study using transcription run-on assays is needed to address these specific issues.

13.8 Gene Therapy and Tissue Engineering in Vascular Biology

Endothelial cells, located adjacent to the flowing bloodstream, are ideally located for use as vehicles for gene therapy, since natural or recombinant proteins of therapeutic value can be expressed directly into the blood to manage cardiovascular diseases or inhibit vascular pathology. One could drive gene expression only in regions of vasculature where desired by using novel *cis*-acting stress- or strain-sensitive promoter elements or stress-activated transcription factors. For instance, endothelial cells in regions of low shear stress could be modified to express tPA so as to inhibit atherosclerotic plaque formation. An appropriate vector driven by the ET-1 promoter (active at low stress but downregulated at high stress) attached to the tPA gene would be a first logical construct in this application. Likewise, endothelial cells could be modified to increase proliferation rates in order to endothelialize vascular grafts or other vascular prostheses, thereby inhibiting thrombosis. In addition, endothelial cells could be modified to decrease expression of smooth muscle cell mitogens (ET-1, PDGF) to prevent intimal thickening and restenosis. The endothelial cells could even be modified so as to secrete components that would inactivate toxic substances in the bloodstream. Work has already begun to develop techniques to express foreign proteins *in vivo* [Nabel et al., 1989; Wilson et al., 1989; Zwiebel et al., 1989]. Vical and Gen Vec are currently examining ways to express growth factors in coronary arteries to stimulate angiogenesis following balloon angioplasty [Glaser, 1994]. In addition, Tularik Inc. is modifying endothelial cells to overexpress low density lipoprotein (LDL) receptors to remove cholesterol from the bloodstream so as to prevent atherosclerotic plaque formation. The application of gene therapy to cardiovascular diseases is in its infancy and will continue to grow as we learn more about the mechanisms governing endothelial cell gene expression. Since endothelial cells lie in a mechanically active environment, predicting local secretion rates of gene products from transfected endothelial cells will require a knowledge of how these mechanical signals modulate gene expression for each target gene and promoter [McIntire, 1994].

In addition to gene therapy applications, there are tissue engineering applications that can be realized once one gains a fundamental understanding of the function-structure relationship intrinsic to vascular biology. This includes understanding how hemodynamic forces modulate endothelial cell function and morphology. Of primary concern is the development of an artificial blood vessel for use in the bypass and replacement of diseased or occluded arteries [Jones, 1982; Nerem, 1991; Weinberg and Bell, 1986]. This is particularly important in the case of small-diameter vascular grafts (such as coronary bypass grafts), which are highly prone to reocclusion. The synthetic blood vessels must provide the structural support required in its mechanically active environment as well as provide endothelial-like functions, such as generating a nonthrombogenic surface.

13.9 Conclusions

This chapter has demonstrated the intricate interweaving of fluid mechanics and convective mass transfer with cell metabolism and the molecular mechanisms of cell adhesion that occur continuously in the vascular system. Our understanding of these mechanisms and how they are modulated by shear stress is really in the initial stages—but this knowledge is vital to our understanding of thrombosis, atherosclerosis, inflammation, and many other aspects of vascular physiology and pathophysiology. Knowledge of the fundamental cellular and molecular mechanisms involved in adhesion and mechanical force modulation of metabolism under conditions that mimic those seen *in vivo* is essential for real progress to be made in vascular biology and more generally in tissue engineering.

Defining Terms

CRE: *c*AMP *r*esponse *e*lement; its consensus sequence TGACGTCA is found on genes responsive to cAMP agonists such as forskolin.

Gene regulation: Transcriptional and posttranscriptional control of expression of genes in eukaryotes where regulatory proteins bind specific DNA sequences to turn a gene either on (positive control) or off (negative control).

Gene therapy: The modification or replacement of a defective or malfunctioning gene with one that functions adequately and properly, for instance, addition of gene regulatory elements such as specific stress- or strain-sensitive response elements to specifically drive gene expression only in regions of interest in the vasculature so as to control proliferation, fibrinolytic capacity, etc.

Shear: Shear refers to the relative parallel motion between adjacent fluid (blood) planes during flow. The difference in the velocity between adjacent layers of blood at various distances from the vessel wall determines the local shear rate, expressed in cm/s/cm, or s^{-1}.

Shear stress: Fluid shear stress, expressed in dyn/cm^2, is a measure of the force required to produce a certain rate of flow of a viscous liquid and is proportional to the product of shear rate and blood viscosity. Physiologic levels of venous and arterial shear stresses range between 1–5 dyn/cm^2 and 6–40 dyn/cm^2, respectively.

SSRE: Shear stress response element; its consensus GAGACC has been recently identified in genes responsive to shear stress.

Transcription factor: A protein that binds to a *cis*-regulatory element in the promoter region of a DNA and thereby directly or indirectly affects the initiation of its transcription to an RNA.

TRE: Tumor promoting agent response element: its consensus sequence TGACTCA is commonly located in genes sensitive to phorbol ester stimulation.

References

Abbassi O, Kishimoto TK, McIntire LV, et al. 1993. E-selectin supports neutrophil rolling in vitro under conditions of flow. J Clin Invest 92:2719.

Abbassi OA, Lane CL, Krater S, et al. 1991. Canine neutrophil margination mediated by lectin adhesion molecule-1 in vitro. J Immunol 147:2107.

Alevriadou BR, Moake JL, Turner NA, et al. 1993. Real-time analysis of shear-dependent thrombus formation and its blockade by inhibitors of von Willebrand factor binding to platelets. Blood 81:1263.

Anderson DC, Abbassi OA, McIntire LV, et al. 1991. Diminished LECAM-1 on neonatal neutrophils underlies their impaired CD18-independent adhesion to endothelial cells in vitro. J Immunol 146:3372.

Ando J, Komatsuda T, Kamiya A. 1988. Cytoplasmic calcium response to fluid shear stress in cultured vascular endothelial cells. In Vitro Cell Dev 24:871.

Asakura T, Karino T. 1990. Flow patterns and spatial distribution of atherosclerotic lesions in human coronary arteries. Circ Res 66:1045.

Barabino GA, McIntire LV, Eskin SG, et al. 1987. Endothelial cell interactions with sickle cell, sickle trait, mechanically injured, and normal erythrocytes under controlled flow. Blood 70:152.

Barbee KA, Davies PF, Lal R. 1994. Shear stress-induced reorganizations of the surface topography of living endothelial cells imaged by atomic force microscopy. Circ Res 74:163.

Bastida E, Almirall L, Bertomeu MC, et al. 1989. Influence of shear stress on tumor-cell adhesion to endothelial-cell extracellular matrix and its modulation by fibronectin. Int J Cancer 43:1174.

Bhagyalakshmi A, Berthiaume F, Reich KM, et al. 1992. Fluid shear stress stimulates membrane phospholipid metabolism in cultured human endothelial cells. J Vasc Res 29:443.

Bhagyalakshmi A, Frangos JA. 1989a. Mechanism of shear-induced prostacyclin production in endothelial cells. Biochem Biophys Res Commun 158:31.

Bhagyalakshmi A, Frangos JA. 1989b. Membrane phospholipid metabolism in sheared endothelial cells. Proc 2nd Int Symp Biofluid Mechanics and Biorheology, Munich, Germany 240.

Bloch KD, Friedrich SP, Lee ME, et al. 1989. Structural organization and chromosomal assignment of the gene encoding endothelin. J Biol Chem 264:10851.

Bohjanen PR, Petryniak B, June CH, et al. 1992. AU RNA-binding factors differ in their binding specificities and affinities. J Biol Chem 267:6302.

Bohmann D. 1990. Transcription factor phosphorylation: A link between signal transduction and the regulation of gene expression. Cancer Cells 2:337.

Botteri FM, Ballmer-Hofer K, Rajput B, et al. 1990. Disruption of cytoskeletal structures results in the induction of the urokinase-type plasminogen activator gene expression. J Biol Chem 265:13327.

Breathnach R, Matrisian LM, Gesnel MC, et al. 1987. Sequences coding part of oncogene-induced transin are highly conserved in a related rat gene. Nucleic Acid Res 15:1139.

Coan DE, Wechezak AR, Viggers RF, et al. 1993. Effect of shear stress upon localization of the Golgi apparatus and microtubule organizing center in isolated cultured endothelial cells. J Cell Sci 104:1145.

Cooper GM. 1990. Oncogenes, Boston, Jones & Bartlett.

Cybulsky MI, Fries JW, Williams AJ, et al. 1991. Gene structure, chromosomal location, and basis for alternative mRNA splicing of the human VCAM-1 gene. Proc Natl Acad Sci USA 88:7859.

Davies MJ, Woolf N, Rowles PM, et al. 1988. Morphology of the endothelium over atherosclerotic plaques in human coronary arteries. Br Heart J 60:459.

Davies PF, Tripathi SC. 1993. Mechanical stress mechanisms and the cell: An endothelial paradigm. Circ Res 72:239.

Dewey CF Jr, Bussolari SR, Gimbrone MA Jr, et al. 1981. The dynamic response of vascular endothelial cells to fluid shear stress. J Biomech Eng 103:177.

Diamond SL, Eskin SG, McIntire LV. 1989. Fluid flow stimulates tissue plasminogen activator secretion by cultured human endothelial cells. Science 243:1483.

Diamond SL, Sharefkin JB, Dieffenbach C, et al. 1990. Tissue plasminogen activator messenger RNA levels increase in cultured human endothelial cells exposed to laminar shear stress. J Cell Physiol 143:364.

Dull RO, Davies PF. 1991. Flow modulation of agonist (ATP)-response (Ca^{++}) coupling in vascular endothelial cells. Am J Physiol 261:H149.

Eskin SG, Ives CL, McIntire LV, et al. 1984. Response of cultured endothelial cells to steady flow. Microvasc Res 28:87.

Ferrua B, Manie S, Doglio A, et al. 1990. Stimulation of human interleukin-1 production and specific mRNA expression by microtubule-disrupting drugs. Cell Immunol 131:391.

Folie BJ, McIntire LV. 1989. Mathematical analysis of mural thrombogenesis. Biophys J 56:1121.

Frangos JA, Eskin SG, McIntire LV, et al. 1985. Flow effects on prostacyclin production by cultured human endothelial cells. Science 227:1477.

Franke RP, Grafe M, Schnittler H. 1984. Induction of human vascular endothelial stress fibres by shear stress. Nature 307:648.

Giavazzi R, Foppolo M, Dossi R, et al. 1993. Rolling and adhesion of human tumor cells on vascular endothelium under physiological flow conditions. J Clin Invest 92:3038.

Girard PR, Nerem RM. 1991. Fluid shear stress alters endothelial cell structure through the regulation of focal contact-associated proteins. Adv Bioeng 20:425.

Girard PR, Nerem RM. 1993. Endothelial cell signaling and cytoskeletal changes in response to shear stress. Front Med Biol Eng 5:31.

Glagov S, Zarins CK, Giddens DP, et al. 1988. Hemodynamics and atherosclerosis. Arch Pathol Lab Med 112:1018.

Glaser V. 1994. Targeted injectable vectors remain the ultimate goal in gene therapy. Genet Eng News 14:8.

Grabowski EF, Jaffe EA, Weksler BB. 1985. Prostacyclin production by cultured endothelial cell monolayers exposed to step increases in shear stress. J Lab Clin Med 105:36.

Grande JP, Glagov S, Bates SR, et al. 1989. Effect of normolipemic and hyperlipemic serum on biosynthesis response to cyclic stretching of aortic smooth muscle cells. Arteriosclerosis 9:446.

Gupte A, Frangos JA. 1990. Effects of flow on the synthesis and release of fibronectin by endothelial cells. In Vitro Cell Dev Biol 26:57.

Hadcock JR, Malbon CC. 1988. Down-regulation of beta-adrenergic receptors: Agonist-induced reduction in receptor mRNA levels. Biochemistry 95:5021.

Hakkert BC, Kuijipers TW, Leeuwenberg JFM, et al. 1991. Neutrophil and monocyte adherence to and migration across monolayers of cytokine-activated endothelial cells: the contribution of CD18, ELAM-1, and VLA-4. Blood 78:2721.

Hession C, Osborn L, Goff D, et al. 1990. Endothelial leukocyte adhesion molecule-1: Direct expression cloning and functional interactions. Proc Natl Acad Sci USA 87:1673.

Hsieh HJ, Li NQ, Frangos JA. 1991. Shear stress increases endothelial platelet-derived growth factor mRNA levels. Am J Physiol H642.

Hsieh H, Li NQ, Frangos JA. 1992. Shear-induced platelet-derived growth factor gene expression in human endothelial cells is mediated by protein kinase C. J Cell Physiol 150:552.

Hsieh H, Li NQ, Frangos JA. 1993. Pulsatile and steady flow induces c-*fos* expression in human endothelial cells. J Cell Physiol 154:143.

Hubbel JA, McIntire LV. 1986. Technique for visualization and analysis of mural thrombogenesis. Rev Sci Instrum 57:892.

Hudlicka O. 1984. Growth of vessels—historical review. In F Hammerson, O Hudlicka (eds), Progress in Applied Microcirculation Angiogenesis, vol 4, pp 1–8, Basel, Karger.

Hunter T, Karin M. 1992. The regulation of transcription by phosphorylation. Cell 70:375.

Iba T, Mills I, Sumpio BE. 1992. Intracellular cyclic AMP levels in endothelial cells subjected to cyclic strain in vitro. J Surg Res 52:625.

Ingber D. 1993. Integrins as mechanochemical transducers. Curr Opin Cell Biol 3:841.

Ives CL, Eskin SG, McIntire LV. 1986. Mechanical effects on endothelial cell morphology: In vitro assessment. In Vitro Cell Dev Biol 22:500.

Jackman RW, Beeler DL, Fritze L, et al. 1987. Human thrombomodulin gene is intron depleted: Nucleic acid sequences of the cDNA and gene predict protein structure and suggest sites of regulatory control. Proc Natl Acad Sci USA 84:6425.

Jones DA, Abbassi OA, McIntire LV, et al. 1993. P-selectin mediates neutrophil rolling on histamine-stimulated endothelial cells. Biophys J 65:1560.

Jones PA. 1982. Construction of an artificial blood vessel wall from cultured endothelial and smooth muscle cells. J Cell Biol 74:1882.

Kim DW, Gotlieb AI, Langille BL. 1989. In vivo modulation of endothelial F-actin microfilaments by experimental alterations in shear stress. Arteriosclerosis 9:439.

Kishimoto TK, Warnock RA, Jutila MA, et al. 1991. Antibodies against human neutrophil LECAM-1 and endothelial cell ELAM-1 inhibit a common CD18-independent adhesion pathway in vitro. Blood 78:805.

Kojima N, Shiota M, Sadahira Y, Handa K, Hakomori S. 1992. Cell adhesion in a dynamic flow system as compared to static system. J Biol Chem 267:17264–17270.

Komuro I, Kaida T, Shibazaki Y, et al. 1990. Stretching cardiac myocytes stimulates protooncogene expression. J Biol Chem 265:3595.

Komuro I, Katoh Y, Kaida T, et al. 1991. Mechanical loading stimulates cell hypertrophy and specific gene expression in cultured rat cardiac myocytes. J Biol Chem 266:1265.

Kuchan MJ, Frangos JA. 1993. Shear stress regulates endothelin-1 release via protein kinase C and cGMP in cultured endothelial cells. Am J Physiol 264:H150.

Langille BL, Adamson SL. 1981. Relationship between blood flow direction and endothelial cell orientation at arterial branch sites in rabbit and mice. Circ Res 48:481.

Langille BL, Graham JJ, Kim D, et al. 1991. Dynamics of shear-induced redistribution of F-actin in endothelial cells in vivo. Arterioscler Thromb 11:1814.

Langille BL, O'Donnell F. 1986. Reductions in arterial diameter produced by chronic diseases in blood flow are endothelium-dependent. Science 231:405.

Lawrence MB, McIntire LV, Eskin SG. 1987. Effect of flow on polymorphonuclear leukocyte/endothelial cell adhesion. Blood 70:1284.

Lawrence MB, Smith CW, Eskin SG, et al. 1990. Effect of venous shear stress on CD18-mediated neutrophil adhesion to cultured endothelium. Blood 75:227.

Lawrence MB, Springer TA. 1991. Leukocytes roll on a selectin at physiologic flow rates: distinction from and prerequisite for adhesion through integrins. Cell 65:859.

Levesque MJ, Sprague EA, Schwartz CJ, et al. 1989. The influence of shear stress on cultured vascular endothelial cells: The stress response of an anchorage-dependent mammalian cell. Biotech Prog 5:1.

Levin EG, Santell L. 1988. Stimulation and desensitization of tissue plasminogen activator release from human endothelial cells. J Biol Chem 263:9360.

Ley K, Gaehtgens P, Fennie C, et al. 1991. Lectin-like adhesion molecule 1 mediates leukocyte rolling in mesenteric venules in vivo. Blood 77:2553.

Malek AM, Gibbons GH, Dzau VJ, et al. 1993a. Fluid shear stress differentially modulates expression of genes encoding basic fibroblast growth factor and platelet-derived growth factor B chain in vascular endothelium. J Clin Invest 92:2013.

Malek AM, Greene AL, Izumo S. 1993b. Regulation of endothelin 1 gene by fluid shear stress is transcriptionally mediated and independent of protein kinase C and cAMP. Proc Natl Acad Sci USA 90:5999.

Malek A, Izumo S. 1992. Physiological fluid shear stress causes downregulation of endothelin-1 mRNA in bovine aortic endothelium. Am J Physiol 263:C389.

McIntire LV. 1994. Bioengineering and vascular biology. Ann Biomed Eng 22:2.

Menter DG, Patton JT, Updike TV, et al. 1992. Transglutaminase stabilizes melanoma adhesion under laminar flow. Cell Biophys 18:123.

Milner P, Bodin P, Loesch A, et al. 1992. Increased shear stress leads to differential release of endothelin and ATP from isolated endothelial cells from 4- and 12-month-old male rabbit aorta. J Vasc Res 29:420.

Mitsumata M, Fishel RS, Nerem RM, et al. 1993. Fluid shear stress stimulates platelet-derived growth factor expression in endothelial cells. Am J Physiol 263:H3.

Mo M, Eskin SG, Schilling WP. 1991. Flow-induced changes in Ca^{2+} signaling of vascular endothelial cells: Effect of shear stress and ATP. Am J Physiol 260:H1698.

Morita T, Yoshizumi M, Kurihara H, et al. 1993. Shear stress increases heparin-binding epidermal growth factor-like growth factor mRNA levels in human vascular endothelial cells. Biochem Biophys Res Commun 197:256.

Muller WEG, Slor H, Pfeifer K, et al. 1992. Association of AUUUA-binding Protein with A + U-rich mRNA during nucleo-cytoplasmic transport. J Mol Biol 226:721.

Nabel EG, Plautz G, Boyce FM, et al. 1989. Recombinant gene expression in vivo within endothelial cells of the arterial wall. Science 244:1342.

Nagel T, Resnick N, Atkinson W, et al. 1994. Shear stress selectivity upregulates intercellular adhesion molecule-1 expression in cultured vascular endothelial cells. J Clin Invest 94:885.

Nerem RM. 1991. Cellular engineering. Ann Biomed Eng 19:529.

Nerem RM. 1993. Hemodynamics and the vascular endothelium. J Biomech Eng 115:510.

Nerem RM, Levesque MJ, Cornhill JF. 1981. Vascular endothelial morphology as an indicator of the pattern of blood flow. J Biomech Eng 103:172.

Nollert MU, Diamond SL, McIntire LV. 1991. Hydrodynamic shear stress and mass transport modulation of endothelial cell metabolism. Biotech Bioeng 38:588.

Nollert MU, Eskin SG, McIntire LV. 1990. Shear stress increases inositol trisphosphate levels in human endothelial cells. Biochem Biophys Res Commun 170:281.

Nollert MU, Hall ER, Eskin SG, et al. 1989. The effect of shear stress on the uptake and metabolism of arachidonic acid by human endothelial cells. Biochim Biophys Acta 1005:72.

Nollert MU, McIntire LV. 1992. Convective mass transfer effects on the intracellular calcium response of endothelial cells. J Biomech Eng 114:321.

Nollert MU, Panaro NJ, McIntire LV. 1992. Regulation of genetic expression in shear stress stimulated endothelial cells. Ann NY Acad Sci 665:94.

Ohno M, Gibbons GH, Dzau VJ, et al. 1993. Shear stress elevates endothelial cGMP. Role of potassium channel and G protein coupling. Circulation 88:193.

Ohno M, Lopez F, Gibbons GH, et al. 1992. Shear stress induced TGFβ1 gene expression and generation of active TGFβ1 is mediated via a K^+ channel. Circulation 86:I-87.

Ono O, Ando J, Kamiya A, et al. 1991. Flow effects on cultured vascular endothelial and smooth muscle cell functions. Cell Struct Funct 16:365.

Patton JT, Menter DG, Benson DM, et al. 1993. Computerized analysis of tumor cells flowing in a parallel plate chamber to determine their adhesion stabilization lag time. Cell Motility Cytoskel 26:88.

Peppel K, Vinci JM, Baglioni C. 1991. The AU-rich sequences in the 3′ untranslated region mediate the increased turnover of interferon mRNA induced by glucocorticoids. J Exp Med 173:349.

Perry MA, Granger DN. 1991. Role of CD11/CD18 in shear rate-dependent leukocyte-endothelial cell interactions in cat mesenteric venules. J Clin Invest 87:1798.

Pili R, Corda S, Passaniti A, et al. 1993. Endothelial cell Ca^{2+} increases upon tumor cell contact and modulates cell-cell adhesion. J Clin Invest 92:3017.

Port JD, Huang LY, Malbon CC. 1992. β-adrenergic agonists that down-regulate receptor mRNA upregulate a M_r 35,000 protein(s) that selectively binds to β-adrenergic receptor mRNAs. J Biol Chem 267:24103.

Prasad AR, Logan SA, Nerem RM, et al. 1993. Flow-related responses of intracellular inositol phosphate levels in cultured aortic endothelial cells. Circ Res 72:827.

Ranjan V, Diamond SL. 1993. Fluid shear stress induces synthesis and nuclear localization of c-fos in cultured human endothelial cells. Biochem Biophys Res Commun 196:79.

Ratner L, Josephs SF, Jarrett R, et al. 1985. Nucleotide sequence of transforming human c-sis-cDNA clones with homology to platelet derived growth factor. Nucleic Acids Res 13:5007.

Reddy VB, Garramone AJ, Sasak H, et al. 1987. Expression of human uterine tissue-type plasminogen activator using BPV vectors. DNA 6:461.

Resnick N, Collins T, Atkinson W, et al. 1993. Platelet-derived growth factor B chain promoter contains a cis-acting fluid shear-stress-responsive-element. Proc Natl Acad Sci USA 90:4591.

Ross R. 1993. The pathogenesis of atherosclerosis: a perspective for the 1990s. Nature 362:801.

Sampath R, Kukielka GL, Smith CW, et al. 1995. Shear stress mediated changes in the expression of leukocyte adhesion receptors on human umbilical vein endothelial cells in vitro. Ann Biomed Eng May-June, 23(3):247–256.

Schnittler HJ, Franke RP, Akbay U, et al. 1993. Improved in vitro rheological system for studying the effect of fluid shear stress on cultured cells. Am J Physiol 265:C289.

Schwartz CJ, Valente AJ, Sprague EA. 1993. A modern view of atherogenesis. Am J Cardiol 71:9B.

Sharefkin JB, Diamond SL, Eskin SG, et al. 1991. Fluid flow decreases preproendothelin mRNA levels and suppresses endothelin-1 peptide release in cultured human endothelial cells. J Vasc Surg 14:1.

Shyy YJ, Hsieh HJ, Usami S, et al. 1994. Fluid shear stress induces a biphasic response of human monocyte chemotactic protein 1 gene expression in vascular endothelium. Proc Natl Acad Sci USA 91:4678.

Smith CW, Kishimoto TK, Abbassi OA, et al. 1991. Chemotactic factors regulate LECAM-1 dependent neutrophil adhesion to cytokine-stimulated endothelial cells in vitro. J Clin Invest 87:609.

Staunton DE, Marlin SD, Stratowa C, et al. 1988. Primary structure of ICAM-1 demonstrates interaction between members of the immunoglobulin and integrin supergene families. Cell 52:925.

Tokunaga K, Nakamura Y, Sakata K, et al. 1987. Enhanced expression of a glycearldehyde-3-phosphate dehydrogenase. Cancer Res 47:5616.

Tran-son-Tay R. 1993. Techniques for studying the effects of physical forces on mammalian cells and measuring cell mechanical properties. In JA Frangos (ed), Physical Forces and the Mammalian Cell, p 1, New York, Academic Press.

Turitto VT, Weiss HJ, Baumgartner HR, et al. 1987. Cells and aggregates at surfaces. In EF Leonord, VT Turitto, L Vroman (eds), Blood in Contact with Natural and Artificial Surfaces, vol 516, pp 453–467, New York, Annals of the New York Academy of Sciences.

Von Andrian UH, Chambers JD, McEvoy LM, et al. 1991. Two-step model of leukocyte-endothelial cell interaction in inflammation. Proc Natl Acad Sci USA 88:7538.

Warren BA. 1973. Evidence of the blood-borne tumor embolus adherent to vessel wall. J Med 6:150.

Watson PA. 1991. Function follows form: Generation of intracellular signals by cell deformation. FASEB J 5:2013.

Watson SR, Fennie C, Lasky LA. 1991. Neutrophil influx into an inflammatory site inhibited by a soluble homing receptor-IgG chimaera. Nature 349:164.

Wechezak AR, Viggers RF, Sauvage LR. 1985. Fibronectin and F-actin redistribution in cultured endothelial cells exposed to shear stress. Lab Invest 53:639.

Weinberg CB, Bell E. 1986. A blood vessel model constructed from collagen and cultured vascular cells. Science 231:397.

Weiss HJ, Turitto VT, Baumgartner HR. 1978. Effect of shear rate on platelet interaction with subendothelium in citrated and native blood. J Lab Clin Med 92:750.

Weiss HJ, Turitto VT, Baumgartner HR. 1986. Platelet adhesion and thrombus formation on subendo-thelium in platelets deficient in GP IIb-IIIa, Ib, and storage granules. Blood 67:905.

Weiss L. 1992. Biomechanical interactions of cancer cells with the microvasculature during hematogenous metastasis. Cancer Metastasis Rev 11:227.

Werb Z, Hembry RM, Murphy G, et al. 1986. Commitment to expression of metalloendopeptidases, collagenase, and stromelysin: Relationship of inducing events to changes in cytoskeletal architecture. J Cell Biol 102:697.

Wick TM, Moake JL, Udden MM, et al. 1987. ULvWF multimers increase adhesion of sickle erythrocytes to human endothelial cells under controlled flow. J Clin Invest 80:905.

Wick TM, Moake JL, Udden MM, et al. 1993. ULvWF multimers preferentially promote young sickle and non-sickle erythrocyte adhesion to endothelial cells. Am J Hematol 42:284.

Wilson JM, Birinyi LK, Salomon RN, et al. 1989. Implantation of vascular grafts lined with genetically modified endothelial cells. Science 244:1344.

Yanagisawa M, Kurihara H, Kimura S, et al. 1988. A novel potent vasoconstrictor peptide produced by vascular endothelial cells. Nature 332:411.

Yoshizumi M, Kurihara H, Sugiyama T, et al. 1989. Hemodynamic shear stress stimulates endothelin production by cultured endothelial cells. Biochem Biophys Res Commun 161:859.

Zarins C, Zatina MA, Giddens DP. 1987. Shear stress regulation of artery lumen diameter in experimental atherogenesis. J Vasc Surg 5:413.

Zarins CK, Giddens DP, Bharadvaj BK, et al. 1983. Carotid bifurcation atherosclerosis. Circ Res 53:502.

Ziegelstein RC, Cheng L, Blank PS, et al. 1993. Modulation of calcium homeostasis in cultured rat aortic endothelial cells by intracellular acidification. Am J Physiol 265:H1424.

Ziegelstein RC, Cheng L, Capogrossi MC. 1992. Flow-dependent cytosolic acidification of vascular endothelial cells. Science 258:656.

Zwiebel JA, Freeman SM, Kantoff PW, et al. 1989. High-level recombinant gene expression in rabbit endothelial cells transduced by retroviral vectors. Science 243:220.

The Roles of Mass Transfer in Tissue Function

Edwin N. Lightfoot
University of Wisconsin

Karen A. Duca
University of Wisconsin

Mass transfer lies at the heart of physiology and provides major constraints on the metabolic rates and anatomy [Pries et al., 1996; Bunk, 1998] of living organisms, from the organization of organ networks to intracellular structures. Limitations on mass transport rates are major constraints for nutrient supply, waste elimination and information transmission at all of these levels. The primary functional units of metabolically active tissue, e.g., the Krogh tissue cylinders of muscle and brain, liver lobules and kidney nephrons, have evolved to just eliminate significant mass transfer limitations in the physiological state [Lightfoot, 1974]. Turnover rates of highly regulated enzymes are just on the slow side of diffusional limitations [Weisz, 1973]. Signal transport rates are frequently mass transport limited [Lauffenburger and Linderman, 1993], and very ingenious mechanisms have evolved to speed these processes [Berg and von Hippel, 1985; Bray, 1998; Francis and Palsson, 1997; Valee and Sheets, 1996]. In contrast elaborate membrane barriers organize and control intracellular reactions in even the simplest organisms.

Understanding tissue mass transport is important both for the engineer and scientist. Examples of engineering interest include the design of extracorporeal devices and biosensors [Fishman et al., 1998]. For the scientist it is important to understand the sometimes complex interactions of transport and reaction to interpret transport based experiments [Bassingthwaighte et al., 1998]. Here we shall concentrate on qualitative behavior and orders of magnitude, with particular emphasis on time constants. These are the normal starting points of any serious study. A general background in biology [Campbell, 1996] and physiology [Johnson, 1998] will be helpful.

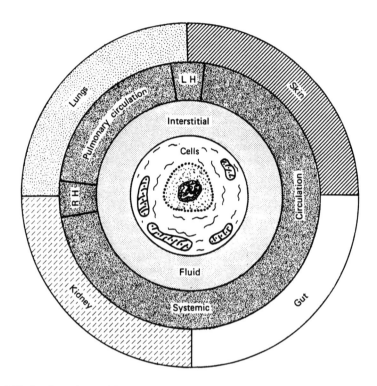

FIGURE 14.1 Diffusional topology of the mammalian body. Convective transport (bulk flow) dominates in the major blood vessels and airways but becomes comparable to diffusion and reaction in the functional units surrounding capillaries and sinusoids. At the cellular and subcellular levels concentration diffusion complicated by electrical effects and a wide variety of carrier transport processes, interacts in complex ways with enzymatic and genetic reactions. (Inspired by Dr. Peter Abbrecht, University of Michigan. Reprinted with permission from Lightfoot (1974). Copyright 1974 by John Wiley & Sons, Inc.)

14.1   Topology and Transport Characteristics of Living Organisms [Schmidt-Nielsen, 1983, 1984; Calder, 1984; Berg, 1993; Bassingthwaighte et al., 1994]

If one includes viruses, the size scales of living systems range from nanometers to meters: spanning a linear ratio of 10^9 and a mass ratio of 10^{27}, which is greater than Avogadro's number! As indicated in Fig. 14.1, the higher animals are organized into spatial hierarchies of discrete structures, which span this whole size range (Table 14.1). At the largest scales animals may be considered as organ networks connected by major blood vessels, with each organ carrying out its own set of specialized tasks.

Organs are in turn composed essentially of large numbers of microcirculatory *functional units* organized in parallel and perfused by capillaries or other microscopic ducts which supply oxygen and other nutrients, carry away waste products, and interchange via a variety of chemical messengers [Lauffenburger and Linderman, 1993]. The Krogh tissue cylinder of Fig. 14.2 is representative and corresponds approximately to the functional units of the brain (see, however, Federspiel and Popel, 1986; Popel, 1989; Hellums et al., 1996; Vicini et al., 1998; Bassingthwaighte et al., 1998).

Nutrients and metabolic end products are transported at the size scale of the tissue cylinder axially by convection.

TABLE 14.1   The Spatial Hierarchy in Mammals, Characteristic Lengths

Entity	Length Scale, m
Whole body	10^{-1}–10^{0}
Organs	10^{-2}–10^{-1}
Microcirculatory units	10^{-4}
Cells	10^{-5} (eukaryots)
	10^{-6} (prokaryots)
Intracellular organelles	10^{-6}
Molecular complexes	10^{-8}

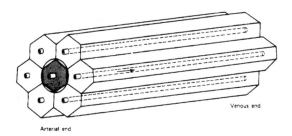

FIGURE 14.2 Krogh tissue cylinder. A circular cylinder is used as an approximation to close-packed hexagonal elements.

Radial transport is primarily by concentration diffusion or *Brownian motion* [Lightfoot and Lightfoot, 1997] and, to a lesser extent by *Starling flow*, slow seepage across the *proximal* region of the capillary driven by the relatively high pressure of entering capillary blood. Flow takes place through clefts between the *endothelial cells* forming the capillary wall and between the *parenchymal* cells forming the tissue cylinder. The clefts are narrow and *permselective*, rejecting large solutes. Starling flow was once thought to reverse direction in the *distal* (downstream) regions of the tissue cylinder as a result of lower hydro-dynamic pressure and increased colloid osmotic pressure caused by the permselectivity of the clefts. However, it is now accepted that such reverse flow does not occur to a significant extent and that the seepage ends up primarily in the lymph ducts and on to the venous blood.

The microcirculatory units are in turn comprised of cells which are themselves complex structures. Sketched in Fig. 14.3 is a pancreatic beta cell, which produces, stores, and secretes insulin. Its organization is similar to that of a chemical plant, with raw materials and energy input at the bottom where mito-chondria produce the chemical energy for cell metabolism, a synthesis and transport area, plus the control

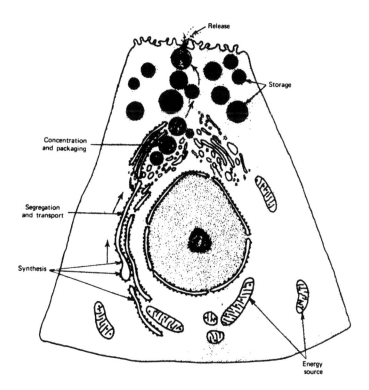

FIGURE 14.3 Structure and organization of a representative eukaryotic cell. Schematic cross-section of a pancreatic beta cell. (Reprinted with permission from Lightfoot (1974). Copyright 1974 by John Wiley & Sons.)

region of the cell nucleus, at the center, and packaging, storage, and export at the top. All of this is accomplished in about 10 μm.

The cell contains smaller structures known collectively as *organelles* that segregate and coordinate the many processes required for its operation and maintenance. Prominent in the diagram are mitochondria, which use various carbon sources and oxygen to form high-energy phosphate bonds as in ATP—the energy sources needed for cell metabolism. Also shown are the cell nucleus where DNA is stored, ribosomes in which RNA is used to produce individual proteins, and the endoplasmic reticulum which holds the ribosomes and channels the proteins produced by them to Golgi apparatus (not shown) for packaging. Also not shown are *microtubules* and other filaments comprising the *cytoskeleton* [Alberts et al., 1945; Campenot et al., 1996; Maniotis et al., 1997]. The latter provide for chromosome segregation, help to maintain cellular shape, and in some cases provide mobility [Vallee and Sheetz]. They also act as transport networks along with motor proteins, discussed below. Organization and structure of the cells is described in standard works [Alberts et al., 1945].

At the smallest level are enzyme clusters and substructures of cell membranes used for selective transport across the cell boundary [Lauffenberger and Linderman, 1993]. Underlying these structures are biochemical reaction networks that are largely shared by all species, and all are composed of the same basic elements, primarily proteins, carbohydrates, and lipids. As a result there are a great many interspecies similarities [Schmidt-Nielsen, 1983].

This elaborate organization just described is constrained to a very large extent by mass transfer considerations and in particular by the effect of characteristic time and distance scales of the effectiveness of different mass transport mechanisms. At the larger size scales, only flow or convection is fast enough to transport oxygen and major metabolites, and convective transport is a major function of the larger blood vessels. Diffusive transport begins to take precedence at the level of microcirculatory units. At the cellular level and below, diffusion may even be too fast and undirected, and selectively permeable membranes, have evolved to maintain spatial segregation against the randomizing forces of diffusion.

14.2   Fundamentals: The Basis of a Quantitative Description

Underneath the bewildering complexity of living organisms are some very simple underlying principles which make a unified description of mass transport feasible. Of greatest utility are observed similarities across the enormous range of system sizes and common magnitudes of key thermodynamic, reaction, and transport parameters. Some simplifying features must still be accepted as justified by repeated observation, and others can be understood from the first principles of molecular kinetic theory. Here we summarize some of the most useful facts and approximations in preparation for the examples of the next section.

Self-Similarity and Cross-Species Correlations

It is a striking characteristic of life-forms that each increase in our mathematical sophistication has shown new regularity in their anatomic and physiologic characteristics. The ability of simple geometric forms to describe morphology has been recognized at least since Leonardo da Vinci, and the definitive work of D'Arcy Thompson summarizes much of this early work. The next step was the concept of *allometry*, first introduced by J. S. Huxley in 1927 [Schmidt-Nielsen, 1984; Calder, 1984; Lightfoot, 1974]. This is a rudimentary form of self similarity usually expressed as

$$P = aM^b \qquad (14.1)$$

where P is any property, M is average species mass, and a and b are constants specific to the property. A large number of allometric relations are available, and those of most interest to us deal with metabolic rate. For example, total basal rates of oxygen consumption for whole animals is given to a good approximation by:

$$R_{O,tot} \times 3.5 M^{3/4} \tag{14.2}$$

Here $R_{O,tot}$ is the oxygen consumption rate in ml O_2 (STP)/h, and M is body mass in grams. Under basal conditions, fat is the primary fuel and heat generation is about 4.7 kcal per milliliter of oxygen (STP) consumed. Small animals have higher specific metabolic rates than large ones, but this is in part because a higher proportion of their body mass is made up of highly active body mass, and for the important case of brain tissue it is invariant at about:

$$R_{O_2}(\text{brain}) \approx 3.72 \cdot 10^{-5} \text{ mmols } O_2/\text{cm}^3, \text{s} \tag{14.3}$$

for all species. For the liver and kidneys, specific metabolic activity is somewhat lower and falls off slowly with an increase in animal size, but this may be due to an increasing proportion of supporting tissue such as blood vessels and connective tissue. Accurate data valid under physiologic conditions are difficult to find, and to a first approximation specific metabolic activity of parenchymal cells, those actually engaged in the primary activity of the organ, may be close to that of brain for both liver and kidneys.

The sizes of both microcirculatory units and cells in vertebrates are also very insensitive to animal size. Capillaries are typically about 3 to 4 μm in radius and about 50 to 60 μm apart. Typical mammalian cells are about 10 to 50 μm in diameter, and organelles such as mitochondria are about the size of prokaryotic cells, about 1 μm in diameter. Approximate characteristics of a cerebral tissue cylinder are given in Table 14.2. The oxygen-carrying capacity of blood, ionic makeup of body fluids, solubility of gases, and oxygen diffusivities in body fluids are also largely invariant across species, and some representative data are provided in Tables 14.3, 14.4, and 14.5.

TABLE 14.2 Characteristic Cerebral Tissue Cylinder

Item	Magnitude
Outer radius	30 μm
Capillary radius	3 μm
Length	180 μm
Blood velocity	400 μm/s
Arterial oxygen tension	0.125 atm
Arterial oxygen concentration (total)	8.6 mM
Arterial oxygen concentration (dissolved O_2)	0.12
Venous oxygen tension	0.053 atm
Venous oxygen concentration (total)	5.87 mM
Venous oxygen concentration (dissolved O_2)	0.05
Tissue oxygen diffusivity	1.5 E-5 cm²/s (estd.)
Oxygen respiration rate (zero order)	0.0372 mmols O_2/liter-s

TABLE 14.3 Oxygen Solubilities

Solvent	Temperature, °C	O_2 Pressure, atm	Concentration, mM/atm
Water	25		1.26
	30		1.16
	35		1.09
	40		1.03
Plasma	37		1.19
Red cell interior (dissolved O_2 only)	37		1.18
Extracellular tissue (estd.)	37		1.1
Oxygen gas	37		39.3
Alveolar air	37	0.136	
Air (0.21 atm of oxygen)	37	0.21	

TABLE 14.4 Effective Oxygen Diffusivities

Solvent	Temperature, °C	Pressure	Diffusivity, cm²/s
Water	25		2.1 E-5
Water	37		3.0 E-5
Blood plasma	37		2.0 E-5
Normal blood	37		1.4 E-5
Red cell interior	37		0.95 E-5
Air	25	1 atm	0.20

TABLE 14.5 Intracellular Diffusion Coefficients

Compound	MW	Radius, Å	Diffusivity in Water cm²/s × 10⁷	Intracell Diffusivity; cm²/s × 10⁷	Diffusivity Ratio
Sorbitol	170	2.5	94	50	1.9
Methylene blue	320	3.7	40	15	2.6
Sucrose	324	4.4	52	20	2.6
Eosin	648	6.0	40	8	5.0
Dextran	3600	12.0	18	3.5	5.0
Inulin	5500	13.0	15	3.0	5.0
Dextran	10,000	23.3	9.2	2.5	3.7
Dextran	24,000	35.5	6.3	1.5	4.2
Actin	43,000	23.2	5.3	0.03	167
Bovine serum albumin	68,000	36.0	6.9	0.10	71

Allometric correlations are essentially empirical and cannot be predicted from any fundamental physical principles. Moreover, most measurements, except solubility and diffusivity data, are of doubtful accuracy.

Recently a more sophisticated form of self-similarity, fractal geometry, has been found useful for the description of a wide variety of biological applications of mass transfer interest [Bassingthwaighte et al., 1994]; applications of nonlinear dynamics are fast increasing [Griffith, 1996].

Time Constants: The Key to Quantitative Modeling

The first step in system modeling is to establish orders of magnitudes of key parameters, and most particularly time constants: estimates of the time required for a given transient process to be "effectively complete." Time constant or order of magnitude analysis is useful because dynamic response times are insensitive to geometric detail and boundary conditions at the order of magnitude level of approximation, i.e., within a factor of ten. Time constants are, however, essentially heuristic quantities and can only be understood on the basis of experience [Lightfoot and Lightfoot, 1997].

Once characteristic system time scales are established, one can restrict attention to processes with response times of the same order: Those an order of magnitude faster can be treated as instantaneous and those ten times slower as not happening at all. Both fast and slow terms in system description, e.g., the diffusion equation of transport phenomena [Bird et al., 1960], can then be eliminated. Such simplification often provides valuable insights as well as simplifying integration. Quantitative descriptions are particularly valuable at the microcirculatory level, for example, in diagnostic procedures, and they have been well studied [Bassingthwaighte and Goresky]. Here we shall stay with relatively simple examples to illustrate selected characteristics of tissue mass transfer, and we begin with diffusion. We then briefly introduce time constants characterizing flow, chemical reaction, and boundary conditions.

Brownian Motion and Concentration Diffusion

The basis of most species selective transport is the relatively slow observable motion of molecules or particles resulting from intermolecular collisions [Lightfoot and Lightfoot, 1997]. Such *Brownian motion* does not take any predictable direction, but the particles under observation do tend to move farther from their starting point with increasing time. The extent of diffusional motion can be described as the probability of finding any reference particle a distance r from its initial position. For an unbounded quiescent fluid this is [Einstein, 1905]:

$$P(r) = e^{-r^2/4D_{PF}t} \Big/ \Big[8\big(\pi D_{PF}t\big)^{3/2}\Big]; \quad 4\pi \int_0^\infty P(r)r^2\,dr = 1 \qquad (14.4a, 4b)$$

This equation defines the *Brownian* diffusivity, D_{PF}, of a particle or molecule relative to a surrounding fluid. Here P is a spherically symmetrical normalized probability density. Here r is distance (in spherical coordinates) from the initial position, and t is time. The mean net distance traveled from the initial point in unbounded quiescent three-dimensional space is easily determined from the above distribution as:

$$r_m^2 = 4\pi \int_0^\infty r^2 \cdot r^2 P(r)\,dr = 6D_{PF}t, \quad r_m^2 = 4D_{PF}t, \quad x_m^2 = 2D_{PF}t \ (14.5a, 5b, 5c)$$

for distances from a point, line, and plane, respectively. These results provide useful insight in suggesting characteristic diffusion times t as the time required for "most" of a transient diffusion process to be complete. Some commonly accepted values are shown in Table 14.6. The numbers in the last column are the fractional changes in solute inventory for a sudden change in surface concentration on a particle initially at a different uniform concentration. For the hollow cylinder, the outer surface of radius R_T is assumed impermeable to diffusion, and the inner surface of radius R_C is permeable. The length L is assumed large compared to either radius. Fractional completion depends in a complex way on the radius ratio, but the diffusion time given is a good approximation.

For large numbers of particles or molecules nonuniformly distributed in a moving fluid, following the Brownian motion of individual molecules becomes too cumbersome to use. We must then average behavior over large numbers of molecules to obtain a *continuum approximation* known as Fick's law [Bird et al., 1960], which describes the relative motion of solute and solvent and may be written in the form

$$\big(v_P - v_F\big)\left(\frac{x_P x_F}{D_{PF}}\right) = -\nabla x_P \qquad (14.6)$$

Here v_p is observable velocity of species P in a mixture of P and F, x_p is mole fraction of species P in the mixture, and D_{PF} is binary mutual mass diffusivity of solute P relative to solvent fluid F. For situations of interest here, the Fick's law diffusivity may be considered equal to the Brownian diffusivity.

TABLE 14.6 Characteristic Diffusional Response Times

Shape	T_{dif}	L	Fractional Completion
Sphere	$L^2/6D_{PF}$	Radius	>0.99
Cylinder	$L^2/4D_{PF}$	Radius	>0.99
Slab	$L^2/2D_{PF}$	Half-thickness	>0.93
Hollow cylinder	$(L^2/2D_{PF})\ln(R_T/R_c)$	Outer radius, R_T	

Equation 14.6 is valid for binary or dilute solutions of liquids, gases, and homogeneous, and some typical magnitudes for biologic situations are shown in Tables 14.4 and 14.5. For dilute solutions, hydrodynamic diffusion theory [Bird et al., 1960] provides useful insight:

$$\pi R_P D_{PF} \mu_F / \kappa T = C \tag{14.7}$$

where C is equal to $(1/6)$ if the molecular radius of the solute P is much less than that of the solvent F and $(1/4)$ if they are about equal. Here μ is solvent viscosity, R_P and R_F are effective spherical solute and solvent radii, κ is the Boltzmann constant, and T is absolute temperature. Hydrodynamic diffusion theory has been extended to solutes in small fluid-filled pores [Deen, 1987] for characterizing transport in microporous membranes.

More Complex Situations

Most biologic transport processes occur in multicomponent solutions. A generalized diffusion equation [Hirschfelder et al., 1954; Lightfoot and Lightfoot, 1997; Taylor and Krishna, 1993] is available, but lack of data usually forces neglect of multicomponent effects. For our purposes transport of both molecules and particles is adequately described by the simplified equations in Table 14.7, which simply state that relative velocity of a particle or molecule P through a fluid F is proportional to the sum of "driving forces" acting on it.

Flow, Chemical Reaction, and Boundary Conditions

We now introduce additional time constants in order to characterize the interactions of diffusion with flow and chemical reaction and to show that boundary conditions can have an important bearing on

TABLE 14.7 Particle-Molecular Analogs Dilute Binary Diffusion in a Quiescent Continuum

Particles

$$\left(v_p - v_F\right) = D_{PF}\left\{\nabla \ln n_p + \frac{1}{\kappa T}\left[V_P\left(1 - \rho_P^0/\rho\right)(\nabla p)_\infty - F_{em} + \left(\rho_P^o + \tfrac{1}{2}\rho_f\right)V_P\frac{dv_P}{dt}\right.\right.$$

$$\left.\left. - 6\left(\pi\mu\rho_F^o\right)^{1/2}R_P^2 I + \text{thermal diffusion}\right]\right\}$$

where:

$$I = \int_0^t \left[v_p'(\tau)\big/(t-\tau)^{1/2}\right]d\tau$$

Molecules (interdiffusion of species P and F)

$$\left(v_P - v_F\right) = -D_{PF}\left\{\nabla \ln x_p + \left(1/RT\right)\left[V_P\left(1 - \rho_P^o/\rho\right)\nabla_p - F_{em}\right]\right\}$$

Both:

$$D_{PF} = \frac{\kappa T}{6\pi\mu R_p}$$

Here:

κ = the Boltzmann constant, or molecular gas constant
n_p = number concentration of particles
R_p = particle or molecular radius
V_p = particle volume or partial molal volume of species P
F_{em} = total electromagnetic force per particle
F_{em} = molar electromagnetic force on species P
ρ = density of fluid phase
ρ_P^o = density of particle or reciprocal of partial specific volume of species P in solution
v' = instantaneous acceleration of particle P
The subscript ∞ refers to conditions near the particle but outside its hydrodynamic boundary layer.

system behavior. We begin with flow where mean solute residence time, T_m, forms a convenient time scale. For flow through a cylindrical duct of length L with constant volumetric average velocity $<v>$, we may write:

$$T_m \equiv L/<v> \tag{14.8}$$

More generally, for constant volumetric flow at a rate Q through a system of volume V with a single inlet and outlet and no significant diffusion across either, T_m is equal to V/Q. For chemical reactions we choose as our system, a reactive solid open to diffusion over at least part of its surface where concentration of solute i under consideration is maintained at a uniform value c_{i0} and where the average volumetric rate of consumption of that solute is $<R_i>$. We then define a reaction time constant as:

$$T_{rxn} \equiv c_{i0}/<R_i> \tag{14.9}$$

Note that both c_{i0} and $<R_i>$ are measurable, at least in principle [Damköhler, 1937; Weisz, 1973]. Finally we consider as an illustrative situation decay of solute concentration c_i in the inlet stream to a flow system according to the expression

$$c_i(t, \text{ inlet}) = c_i(0, \text{ inlet}) \exp\left(-t/T_{BC}\right) \tag{14.10}$$

where t is time and T_{BC} is a constant. We now have enough response times for the examples we have selected below, and we turn to illustrating their utility.

14.3 Characteristic Behavior: Selected Examples

We now consider some representative examples to illustrate the mass transfer behavior of living tissues.

Alveolar Transients and Pulmonary Mass Transport: At the distal ends of the pulmonary network are the alveoli, irregular sacs of air surrounded by blood-filled capillaries, with effective diameters of about 75 to 300 μm. The blood residence time is of the order of a second, and it is desired to determine whether gas-phase mass transfer resistance is appreciable. To answer, we take the worst possible scenario: flat-plate geometry with a half-thickness of 150 μm or 0.0105 cm. From Table 14.4 we find the oxygen diffusivity to be about 0.2 cm²/s. It follows that alveolar response time is

$$T_{dif} \approx (0.015)/0.4 = 0.56 \, \text{ms}$$

This is extremely fast, with respect to both the 1-s residence time assumed for alveolar blood and the $^1/_{12}$ of a minute between breaths: gas-phase mass transfer resistance is indeed negligible. This is typical for absorption of sparingly soluble gases, and a similar situation occurs in cell culture vessels.

Mass Transfer between Blood and Tissue: We next identify blood vessels capable of transferring dissolved solute between blood and surrounding tissue. To be effective we assume that mean blood residence time should at least equal the radial diffusion time:

$$\frac{L}{<v>} \geq \frac{R^2}{4D_{PB}} = \frac{D^2}{16D_{PB}} \, ; \, \frac{LD_{PB}}{D^2 <v>} \geq 1/16 = 0.0625$$

where D is vessel diameter. From the data for a 13-kg dog in Table 14.8, we find the great majority of vessels much too short and that only the three smallest classes—arterioles, capillaries, and venules—are at all capable of transferring appreciable mass. These, especially the capillaries, are quite effective. They

TABLE 14.8 Mass Transfer Effectiveness of Blood Vessels (13-kg Dog, #39)

Vessel	Radius, cm	Lenght, cm	$<v>$, cm/s	$LD^2/d_{PF}<v>$
Aorta	0.5	10	50	0.00003
Larger arteries	0.15	20	13.4	0.00003
Secondary arteries	0.05	10	8	0.005
Terminal arteries	0.03	1.0	6.0	0.002
Arterioles	0.001	0.2	0.032	6.25
Capillaries	0.0004	0.1	0.07	89.4
Venules	0.0015	0.2	0.07	12.7
Terminal veins	0.075	1.0	1.3	0.0014
Secondary veins	0.12	10	1.48	0.0047
Larger veins	0.3	20	3.6	0.0006
Venae cavae	0.625	40	33.4	0.00003

have long been classified as the microcirculation on the basis of being invisible to the unaided eye. This simple order of magnitude analysis provides a functional definition and a guide to the design of hollow fiber cell culture vessels. More refined analyses [Lightfoot, 1974] based on the parameter magnitudes of Table 14.2 shows that lateral diffusional resistance of capillaries is in fact rather small, but recent analyses [Popel, 1989] suggest a more complex picture.

Convection and diffusion in parallel [Lightfoot and Lightfoot, 1997] is also of interest, but it is more complicated because of convective dispersion [Lightfoot and Lightfoot, 1997]. However, the lung shows a sharp transition between convective ducts and those which can be assumed well-mixed by axial diffusion [Hobbs and Lightfoot, 1979; Hubal, 1996; Farhi]. This has long been known to pulmonary physiologists who often model the adult human lung as a plug-flow channel ("dead space") of about 500 ml leading to a well-mixed volume of about 6000 ml.

Intercapillary Spacing in the Microcirculation: It has been shown [Damköhler, 1937; Weisz, 1973] that optimized commercial catalysts normally exhibit ratios of diffusion to reaction times, as defined in Table 14.6 in the relatively narrow range:

$$1/3 < T_{dif}/T_{rxn} < 1$$

Moreover, Weisz has shown that this ratio holds for many biologic systems as well, so that enzyme activities can often be inferred from their location and function. Here we compare this expectation for cerebral tissue cylinders using the data of Tables 14.2 and 14.6. Throughout the tissue cylinder:

$$T_{dif} = \frac{9 \cdot 10^{-6}\ cm^2}{3 \cdot 10^{-5}\ cm^2/s} \cdot \ln(10) = 0.69\ s$$

For venous conditions, which are the most severe,

$$T_{rxn} = \frac{0.0372}{0.0584} = 0.64\ s \quad \text{and} \quad T_{dif}/T_{rxn} \approx 1$$

These numbers are reasonable considering the uncertainty in the data and the approximation used for diffusion time. The brain, for example, is far from homogeneous. More elaborate calculations suggest somewhat more conservative design. However, these figures are correct in suggesting that the brain is "designed" for oxygen transport and that the safety factor is small [Neubauer and James, 1998]. Sections of the brain become anoxic at about 2/3 of normal blood flow. The body's control mechanisms will shut down other vital organs such as the gut, liver, and kidneys when blood cardiac output oxygen supply drops to keep the brain as well supplied as possible. All of these comments are for the physiologic (normal) state. Lowering brain temperature can greatly decrease oxygen demand and permit survival under otherwise fatal conditions. This effect is important in cryosurgery and drowning: whereas about 6 min of anoxia damages the adult brain at normal temperature, about 1 h is required at 62°F.

Intracellular Dispersion: We now ask how long it will take a protein initially concentrated in a very small region to disperse through the interior of a cell, and we shall assume the cell to be a sphere with a 1 μm radius. We begin by noting that the cell interior or cytoplasm is a concentrated solution of polymeric species and that the diffusivity of large molecules is considerably slowed relative to water. We therefore assume a diffusivity of 10^{-8} cm²/s as suggested by the last entry in Table 14.5. If the protein is originally at the center of the sphere, the dispersion time is

$$T_{dis} \equiv T_{dif} = \frac{R_{cell}^2}{6D_{pc}^-}\left(1 \cdot 10^{-4}\right)^2 \Big/ \left(6 \cdot 10^{-8}\right) \approx \left(1/6\right) s$$

If the protein is initially near the cell periphery, diffusion will take about four times as long, or about 2/3 s. Reliable *intracellular* diffusion coefficients are important: the corresponding numbers for aqueous solution would have been about 2.4 ms and 10 ms, respectively! Cell interiors—the *cytoplasm*—are crowded.

Diffusion Controlled Reaction: We now calculate the rate at which a very dilute protein of 2.5 nm radius solution in a cell of 1 μm radius is adsorbed on a spherical adsorbent particle of radius 2.5 nm if the adsorption is *diffusion controlled*. That is, we assume that the free protein concentration immediately adjacent to the adsorbent surface is always effectively zero because of the speed and strength of the adsorption reaction. In diffusion only the region within a few diameters of a sphere's surface offers effective resistance to transport [Carslaw and Jaeger, 1959; see also Özisik, 1993]. We can thus assume rapid equilibration over the entire cell volume, except for a thin diffusional boundary layer adjacent to the target surface: the ratio of protein plus adsorbent to cell diameter is only about 0.05. The rate at which protein is adsorbed on the sphere surface per unit area is then [Lightfoot, 1974]:

$$N_P = \frac{D_{PF} c_{P\infty}}{\left(R_P + R_{ads}\right)} \cdot \left(1 + \frac{1}{\sqrt{\pi \tau}}\right)$$

where $C_{P\infty}$ is the protein concentration far from the sphere, assumed uniform over the bulk of cell volume since we are about to see that it adjusts rapidly on the time scale of the adsorption process. The radius of the protein is R_P, that of the adsorbent R_{ads}, and the dimensionless time τ defined by

$$\tau \equiv \frac{t D_{PF}}{\left(R_P + R_{ads}\right)^2} = \frac{t}{2.5 \cdot 10^{-5} s}$$

Adsorption rate is within 10% of its asymptotic value when $\pi\tau = 100$, and

$$t_{1/10} = \left(2.5 \cdot 10^{-5} s\right)\left(100/\pi\right) \approx 0.8\,ms$$

This is much smaller than distribution time, and transients can be neglected: the time scales of the transient and distribution are *well separated*. We now write a mass balance for the rate of change of bulk protein concentration:

$$-V_{cell}\frac{dc_{P\infty}}{dt} \approx -V_{cell}\frac{dc_P}{dt} = A_{ads}N_P; \quad d\ln c_P/dt = 3\Big[\left(R_P + R_{ads}\right)/R_{cell}^3\Big]Ð_{PF} = 1/T_{rxn}$$

Here V_{cell} is the volume of the cell, and A_{ads} is the effective area of the adsorbent; T is the characteristic reaction time, that required to reduce cellular concentration by a factor e or about 2.7. For our conditions, reasonably representative of a prokaryotic cell,

$$T_{rxn} = \left[\frac{3 \cdot 5 \cdot 10^{-7}}{\left(10^{-4}\right)^3} \cdot 10^{-8} \right]^{-1} s = 67s$$

This is clearly a long time compared to the dispersion time of the last example, and the assumed time scale separations of all three adsorption and dispersion processes are amply justified. Using time scale separations has greatly simplified what was originally a major numerical task [Berg and von Hipple, 1985].

If the protein concentration is now interpreted as the probability of finding a protein in any position, and the target is a DNA site, T_{rxn} is the time required for gene expression, and it can be seen that it is very slow! Comparison of these predictions with experiment showed that both prokaryotic cells respond much faster and this led to a major discovery [Berg and von Hipple, 1985]: DNA exhibits a general binding affinity for promoter molecules which permits the adsorbed protein to undergo one-dimensional diffusion along the DNA chain—thus increasing effective binding site size. Eukaryotes, which are roughly ten times larger in diameter, have elaborate internal barriers [Holsstege et al., 1998] and are much more complex diffusionally.

Many other diffusion controlled reactions occur in living systems, for example, protein folding, and here brute force molecular dynamic calculations are difficult even with supercomputers. One can greatly speed calculation by taking judicious time scale separation [Rojnuckarin et al., 1998].

The Energy Cost of Immobility

Many cell constituents, from small metabolites to organelles, are free to move in the cytoplasm and yet must be limited in their spatial distribution. Many such entities are transported by mechanochemical enzymes known as *protein motors* which depend upon consumption of metabolic energy. Here we estimate the energy cost of such processes to maintain spatial segregation, without detailed knowledge of the mechanisms used. The basis of our analysis [Okamoto and Lightfoot, 1992] is the Maxwell-Stefan equation of Table 14.7 and more particularly the fact that migration velocities are related to the motive force of Brownian motion and any mechanically transmitted force through the diffusivity. The heart of our argument is that the mechanical force applied by the protein motors must produce a migration equal and opposite to that resulting from the dispersive force of Brownian motion:

$$\left(v_P - v_F\right)_{tot} = \left(v_P - v_F\right)_{dif} + \left(v_P - v_F\right)_{mech} = 0,$$

$$\left(v_P - v_F\right)_{dif} = D_{PF} \nabla \ln n_P \qquad \left(v_P - v_F\right)_{mech} = F D_{PF}/\kappa T$$

where n_P is the number concentration of proteins, and F is the mechanical force required to produce the motion. Now the power P_P required for transporting a particle back against diffusional motion is the product of the mechanical force and mechanical migration velocity:

$$P_P = F \cdot \left(v_P - v_F\right)_{mech} = \kappa T \left(\nabla \ln n_P\right)^2$$

For a particle of mass $\mathbf{m}_P = (4/3)\pi R_P^3 \rho_P$ where ρ_P is particle density, the power requirement per unit mass is:

TABLE 14.9 Energetics of Forced Diffusion

| Particle | Radius, Å | Dilute Solution | | Cytoplasm | |
		Rel. Diff.	$\hat{P}/\Delta G$	Rel. Diff.	Estimated $\hat{P}/\Delta G$
Small metabolite	3	1	7×10^6	1	7×10^6
Globular protein	30	1	7×10^2	0.01	7
Typical organelle	10^4	1	6×10^{-8}	$10^{-1/2}$	6×10^{-12}

$$P_p / m_p \equiv \hat{P} = \frac{\left(\kappa T \nabla \ln n_p\right)^2}{8 \pi \mu_{\text{eff}} \rho_p R_P^4}$$

Here μ_{eff} is the effective viscosity of the cytoplasm, ρ_p is particle density, and R_p is effective particle radius. This very strong effect of particle radius suggests that protein motors will be most effective for larger particles, and calculations of Okamoto and Lightfoot [1992] bear out this suggestion.

If the particle is to be held for the most part within 1 μm of the desired position and the free energy transduction of the cell as a whole corresponds to that of brain tissue, Table 14.9 shows the cost of mechanical motion is negligible for organelles, prohibitive for small metabolites and problematic for proteins. However, for small amounts of critically important metabolites and problematic for proteins. However, for small amounts of critically important metabolites, mechanical transport may still take place. The quantity, $\hat{P}/\Delta G$, is the ratio of power consumption to mean cellular energy transduction, both per unit mass.

It remains to be noted that estimating the cost of organelle transport accurately requires additional information, and some is available in [Okamoto and Lightfoot, 1992]. It is impossible for the cell to transport the large number of small metabolites, and a number of alternate means of segregation have developed. Among them are permselective membranes and compact enzyme clusters, making it difficult for intermediate metabolites to escape into the general cytoplasmic pool. These topics must be discussed elsewhere.

Defining Terms[1]

Allometry: A special form of similarity in which the property of interest scales across species with some constant power of species mass.

Alveolus: A pulmonary air sac at the distal end of an airway.

Arterioles: The smallest subdivision of the arterial tree proximal to the capillaries.

ATP: Abbreviation of adenosine triphosphate, the source of chemical energy for a wide variety of metabolic reactions.

Capillaries: The smallest class of blood vessel, between an arteriole and venule, whose walls consist of a single layer of cells.

Cell: The smallest unit of living matter capable of independent functioning, composed of protoplasm and surrounded by a semipermeable plasma membrane.

Convection: Mass transport resulting directly from fluid flow.

Cytoplasm: The protoplasm or substance of a cell surrounding the nucleus, carrying structures within which most of the life processes of the cell take place.

Cytoskeleton: An intracellular network of microtubules.

---

[1]For more complete definitions see the *Oxford Dictionary of Biochemistry and Molecular Biology,* 1997.

Distal: At the downstream end of a flow system.
Endothelium: A single layer of thin flattened cells lining blood vessels and some body cavities.
Microcirculation: The three smallest types of blood vessels—arterioles, capillaries, and venules.
Microtubule: Long, generally straight elements of the cytoskeleton, formed of the protein tubulin.
Mitochondrion: Compartmentalized double-membrane self-reproducing organelle responsible for generating usable energy by formation of ATP. In the average cell there are several hundred mitochondria each about 1.5 μm in length.
Organelle: A specialized cytoplasmic structure of a cell performing a specific function.
Parenchyma: The characteristic tissue of an organ or a gland, as distinguished from connective tissue.
Proximal: At the upstream end of a flow system.
Venules: The smallest vessels of the venous tree, distal to the capillaries.

References

Adolph EF. 1949. Quantitative relations in the physiological constitutions of mammals, *Science* 109: 579.

Alberts, B et al., 1945. *The Molecular Biology of the Cell*, 3rd ed., Garland, New York.

Bassingthwaighte JB, Goresky CA. Modeling in the analysis of solute and water exchange in the microvasculature, Chap. 13, *Handbook of Physiology—The Cardiovascular System IV.*

Bassingthwaighte, JB, Liebovitch, LS, and West, BJ, 1994. *Fractal Physiology*, Oxford University Press, Oxford.

Bassingthwaighte, JB, Goresky, CA, and Linehan, JH. 1998. *Whole Organ Approaches to Cellular Metabolism*, Springer, New York.

Berg, OG. 1993. *Random Walks in Biology*, expanded edition, Princeton University Press, Princeton, NJ.

Berg OG, von Hippel PH. 1985. Diffusion controlled macromolecular interactions. *Annu. Rev. Biophys. Chem.* 14:13 1.

Bird RB, Stewart WE, Lightfoot EN. 1960. *Transport Phenomena*, Wiley, New York.

Bray, D. 1998. Signaling complexes: biophysical constraints on intracellular communication, *Annu. Rev. Biophys. Biomol. Struct.* 27:59-75.

Bunk, S. 1998. Do energy transport systems shape organisms? *The Scientist*, Dec. 14-15.

Calder WA. 1984. *Size, Function and Life History*, Harvard University Press, Cambridge, MA.

Campenot RB, Lund K, Senger DL. 1996. Delivery of newly synthesized tubulin to rapidly growing distal axons of rat sympathetic neurons in compartmented cultures, *J. Cell Biol.* 135:701-709.

Campbell, NA, 1996. *Biology*, 4th ed, Benjamin/Cummins.

Carslaw HS, Jaeger JC. 1959. *Conduction of Heat in Solids*, 2nd ed, Oxford University Press, Oxford.

Damköhler G. 1937. Einfluss von Diffusion, Strömung und Wärmetransport auf die Ausbeute bei chemische-technische Reaktionen, *Chemieingenieur* 3:359.

Deen WM. 1987. Hindered transport of large molecules in liquid-filled pores, *AIChEI* 33 (9): 1409.

Einstein A. 1905. *Ann. Phys.* 17:549.

Farhi LE. Ventilation-perfusion relationships, Chap. 11. In *Handbook of Physiology—the Respiratory System IV.*

Federspiel WJ, Popel AS. 1986. A theoretical analysis of the effect of the particulate nature of blood on oxygen release in capillaries, *Microvasc. Res.* 32:164-189.

Fishman, HA, Greenwald DR, Zare RN. 1998. Biosensors in chemical separations, *Annu. Rev. Biophys. Biol. Mol. Struct.* 27:165-198.

Francis K, Palsson BO. 1997. Effective intercellular communication distances, etc., *Proc. Natl. Acad. Sci. U.S.A.* 94:12258-12262.

Griffith, TM. 1996. Temporal chaos in the microcirculation, *Cardiovasc. Res.* 31(3):342-358.

Gruenberg J, Maxfield FR. 1995. Membrane transport in the endocytic pathway, *Curr. Opin. Cell Biol.* 7:552-563.

Hellums, JD et al., 1996. Simulation of intraluminal gas transport processes in the microcirculation, *Ann. Biomed. Eng.* 24:1-24.

Hirschfelder JO, Curtiss CF, Bird RB. 1954. *Molecular Theories of Gases and Liquids,* Wiley, New York.

Hobbs SH, Lightfoot EN. 1979. A Monte-Carlo simulation of convective dispersion in the large airways. *Resp. Physiol.* 37:273.

Holsstege FCP et al., 1998. Dissecting the regulatory circuitry of a eukaryotic genome, *Cell* 95:717-728.

Hubal EA et al., 1996. Mass transport models to predict toxicity of inhaled gases in the upper respiratory tract, *J. Appl. Physiol.* 80(4):1415-1427.

Johnson LR. 1998. *Essential Medical Physiology,* 2nd ed., Lippincott-Raven, Philadelphia.

Lauffenberger DA, Linderman JJ. 1993. *Receptors,* Oxford University Press, Oxford.

Lightfoot EN. 1974. *Transport Phenomena and Living Systems,* Wiley-Interscience, New York.

Lightfoot EN, Lightfoot EJ. 1997. *Mass Transfer in Kirk-Othmer Encyclopedia of Separation.*

Maniotis AJ, Chen CS, Ingber DE. 1997. Demonstration of mechanical connections between integrins, cytoskeletal filaments, and nucleoplasm that stabilize nuclear structure, *Proc. Natl. Acad. Sci. U.S.A.* 94:849-854.

Neubauer RA, James P. 1998. Cerebral oxygenation and the recovereable brain, *Neurol. Res.* 20, Supplement 1, S33-36.

Okamoto GH, Lightfoot EN. 1992. Energy cost of intracellular organization. *Ind. Eng. Chem. Res.* 31 (3):732.

Ozisik MN. 1993. *Heat Conduction,* 2nd ed., Wiley, New York.

Popel AS. 1989. Theory of oxygen transport to tissue. *Clin. Rev. Biomed. Eng.* 17 (3):257.

Pries AR, TW Secomb, P Gaeghtgens, 1996. Biophysical aspects of blood flow in the microvasculature, *Cardiovasc. Res.* 32:654-667.

Rojnuckarin A, Kim S, Subramanian S. 1998. Brownian dynamic simulation of protein folding: Access to milliseconds time scale and beyond, *Proc. Natl. Acad. Sci. U.S.A.* 95:4288-4292.

Schmidt-Nielsen K. 1983. *Animal Physiology: Adaptation and Environment,* 3rd ed., Cambridge University Press, Cambridge, U.K.

Schmidt-Nielsen K. 1984. *Scaling: Why Is Animal Size So Important?* Cambridge University Press, Cambridge, U.K.

Suominen, PK et al., 1997. Does water temperature affect outcome of nearly drowned children? *Resuscitation* 35(2):111-115.

Taylor R, Krishna R. 1993. *Multicomponent Mass Transfer,* New York, Wiley.

Thompson DW. 1961. *On Growth and Form* (an abridged edition, JT Bonner, ed.), Cambridge University Press, Cambridge, U.K.

Vallee RB, Sheetz MP. 1996.Targeting of motor proteins, *Science* 271:1539-1544.

Vicini, P et al. 1998. Estimation of blood flow heterogeneity in skeletal muscle. *Ann. Biomed. Eng.* 26:764-774.

Weisz PB. 1973. Diffusion and chemical transformation—an interdisciplinary excursion. *Science* 179:433.

Welling PG. 1997. *Pharmacokinetics,* American Chemical Society, Washington, D.C.

15

The Biology of Stem Cells

Craig T. Jordan
Somatix Therapy Corp.

Gary Van Zant
University of Kentucky Medical Center

Life for most eukaryotes, and certainly all mammals, begins as a single totipotent stem cell, the zygote. This cell contains the same complement of genes—no more and no less—as does every adult cell that will make up the organism once development is complete. Nonetheless, this cell has the unique characteristic of being able to implement every possible program of gene expression and is thus totipotent. How is this possible? It is now known that the selective activation and repression of genes distinguishes cells with different developmental potentials. Unraveling this complex series of genetic changes accompanying the progressive restriction of developmental potential during ontogeny is the realm of modern developmental biology. In contrast to the zygote, which has unlimited developmental potential, an intestinal epithelial cell or a granulocyte, for example, is a highly developed cell type that is said to be differentiated. These cells are fixed with respect to their developmental potential and thus no longer possess the ability to contribute to other tissue types. Indeed, intestinal epithelial cells and granulocytes are incapable of undergoing further division and are said to be terminally differentiated. These mature cells have therefore undergone a process whereby they each have acquired a unique and complex repertoire of functions. These functions are usually associated with the cellular morphologic features and/or enzymatic profiles required to implement a specific developmental or functional program. We will come back to the tissue dynamics of these two cell types in a later section of this chapter.

Between the extremes of developmental potency represented by the zygote and terminally differentiated cells, there is obviously a tremendous number of cell divisions (roughly 2^{44}) and an accompanying restriction of this potential in zygotic progeny. The human body, for example, is composed of greater than 10^{13} cells—all ultimately derived from one, the zygote. Where during the developmental sequence does restriction occur? Is it gradual or quantal? These questions are fundamental to an understanding of developmental biology in general and stem cell biology in particular.

15.1 Embryonic Stem Cells

Let us consider first the ultimate human stem cell, the zygote, in more detail. As cellular growth begins, the early embryonic cells start to make a series of irreversible decisions to differentiate along various developmental pathways. This process is referred to as developmental commitment. Importantly, such decisions do not occur immediately; rather, the zygote divides several times and proceeds to the early blastocyst stage of development while maintaining totipotency in all its daughter cells. This is evident most commonly in the phenomenon of identical twins, where two distinct yet genetically matched embryos arise from the same zygote. The ability of early embryonic cells to maintain totipotency has been utilized by developmental biologists as a means to experimentally manipulate these embryonic stem cells, or ES cells, as they are commonly known. In 1981, two scientists at Cambridge, Evans and Kaufman, were able to isolate ES cells from a blastocyst-stage mouse embryo and demonstrate that such cells could be cloned and grown for many generations *in vitro* [Kaufman et al., 1983]. Remarkably, under the appropriate culture conditions, such cells remained completely totipotent. That is to say, upon reimplantation into another embryo, the stem cells could grow and contribute to the formation of an adult mouse. Importantly, the ES cells retained the developmental potential to differentiate into all the possible adult phenotypes, thereby proving their totipotency.

Thus, in culture, the ES cells were said to self-renew without any subsequent loss of developmental potential. Upon reintroduction into the appropriate environment, the ES cells were able to differentiate into any of the various mature cell types. The basic decision of whether to self-renew or differentiate is a common theme found in stem cells of many developmental systems. Generally self-renewal and differentiation go hand in hand; i.e., the two events are usually inseparable. The important findings of Evans and Kaufman demonstrated that self-renewal and differentiation could be uncoupled and that an extended self-renewal phase of growth was attainable for mammalian embryonic cells.

The advent of ES cell technology has had an enormous impact on the field of mammalian molecular genetics. The ability to culture ES cells was quickly combined with molecular techniques which allow for the alteration of cellular DNA. For example, if an investigator were interested in the function of a gene, he or she might elect to mutate the gene in ES cells so that it was no longer functional. The genetically altered ES cells would then be used to generate a line of mice which carry the so-called gene knockout [Koller and Smithies, 1992; Robertson, 1991]. By examining the consequences of such a mutation, clues to the normal function of a gene may be deduced. Techniques such as these have been widely used over the past 10 years and continue to develop as even more powerful means of studying basic cellular function become available.

15.2 Control of Stem Cell Development

The concepts of self-renewal and differentiation are central to the description of a stem cell; indeed, the potential to manifest these two developmental options is the only rigorous criterion used in defining what constitutes a true stem cell. Consequently, in studying stem cells, one of the most important questions to consider is how the critical choice whether to self-renew or differentiate is made. As seen in the case of ES cells, the environment of the stem cell or extrinsic signals determine the outcome of the self-renewal decision. In other words, such cells are not intrinsically committed to a particular developmental fate; rather, their environment mediates the differentiation decision. Surprisingly, for ES cells this decision is dictated by a single essential protein, or growth factor, known as Leukemia inhibitory factor (LIF) [Hilton and Gough, 1991; Smith et al., 1992]. In the presence of sufficient concentrations of LIF, ES cells will self-renew indefinitely in culture. Although ES cells eventually lose their totipotency *in vitro*, this is thought to be due to technical limitations of *ex vivo* culture rather than developmental decisions by the cells themselves.

Interestingly, the default decision for ES cells appears to be differentiation; i.e., unless the cells are prevented from maturing by the presence of LIF, they will quickly lose their totipotent phenotype. Upon beginning the differentiation process, ES cells can be steered along a variety of developmental pathways simply by providing the appropriate extrinsic signal, usually in the form of a growth factor.

Unfortunately, the control of other types of stem cells has proved more difficult to elucidate. In particular, the control of blood-forming, or hematopoietic stem cells, has been extensively studied, but as yet the developmental control of these cells is poorly understood.

15.3   Adult Stem Cells

As the mammalian embryo develops, various organ systems are formed, and tissue-specific functions are elaborated. For the majority of mature tissues, the cells are terminally differentiated and will continue to function for extended periods of time. However, some tissues operate in a much more dynamic fashion, wherein cells are continuously dying and being replenished. These tissues require a population of stem cells in order to maintain a steady flow of fresh cells as older cells turn over. Although there are several examples of such tissue types, perhaps the best characterized are the hematopoietic system and the intestinal epithelia. These two cell types have population parameters that call for their continuous and rapid production: Both cell types occur in very large numbers (approximately 10^{11} to 10^{12} for the human hematopoietic system) and have relatively short life spans that can often be measured in days or sometimes even hours [Kroller and Pallson, 1993]. These two tissues in adults are therefore distinct (along with skin epithelium) in that they require tissue-specific stem cells in order to satisfy the inherent population dynamics of the system.

Stem cells of this nature represent a population arrested at an intermediate level of developmental potency that permits them to perform the two classic stem cell functions: They are able to replenish and maintain their own numbers through cell divisions that produce daughter cells of equivalent potency, that is, self-renew. And they have the capacity, depending on need, to differentiate and give rise to some, if not all, of the various mature cell types of that tissue. Stem cells of the small intestine, to the best of our knowledge, give rise to at least four highly specialized lineages found in the epithelium: Paneth, goblet, enteroendocrine, and enterocytes; these stem cells are therefore pluripotent (i.e., they have the potential to give rise to many different, but not all, lineages) [Potten and Loeffler, 1990]. Similarly, pluripotent stem cells of the hematopoietic system give rise to an even wider variety of mature cells, including at least eight types of blood cells: the various lymphocytes, natural killer cells, megakaryocytes, erthroid cells, monocytes, and three types of granulocytes [Metcalf and Moore, 1971].

Proof of the existence of gut and hematopoietic stem cells came from studies of the effects of ionizing radiation on animals. This research, in the 1940s and 1950s, was spurred by concern over military and peaceful uses of atomic energy. It became recognized that the organ/tissue systems most susceptible to radiation damage were those that normally had a high turnover rate and were replenished by stem cell populations, i.e., the gut lining and the hematopoietic system. In particular, the latter was found to be the radiation dose-limiting system in the body. It was subsequently discovered that mice could be rescued from imminent death from radiation "poisoning" by the transfusion of bone marrow cells following exposure [Barnes et al., 1959]. Initially it was not clear whether the survival factor was humoral or cellular, but mounting evidence pointed to a cell-mediated effect, and, as the dose of bone marrow cells was titrated to determine the number required for survival, it was found that low numbers of cells resulted in the development of macroscopic nodules on the spleens of irradiated mice.[1] These nodules were composed of cells of some but not all lineages of blood formation—lymphopoiesis was notably missing [Till and McCulloch, 1961]. Low-level radiation was then used to induce unique chromosomal aberrations in bone marrow cells prior to transplantation into lethally irradiated recipients. In this way, unique microscopically identifiable translocations would be passed on to all progeny of an altered cell. It was found that the spleen nodules were, in fact, colonies of hematopoietic cells, all possessing an identical chromosomal marker [Becker et al., 1963]. This observation strongly suggested that the nodule was a clonal population, derived from a single stem cell. Since several lineages were represented in the spleen colony, the stem cell responsible was pluripotent. Moreover, single spleen colonies could be isolated and injected into secondary irradiated recipients and give rise to additional spleen colonies. This suggested that the cell giving rise to a spleen colony was capable of some degree of self-renewal as well as multilineage

---

[1]Injected bone-marrow-derived stem cells lodge and develop in several types of hematopoietic tissue, including spleen. Apparently, the splenic microenvironment can at least transiently support stem cell growth and development.

differentiation [Till et al., 1964]. The cells which give rise to spleen colonies were termed CFU-S for colony-forming unit-spleen and have been studied extensively in the characterization of pluripotent hematopoietic stem cells.

More recent studies employing a similar strategy have used retroviruses to mark stem cells. The site of viral integration in an infected host cell genome is random and is passed with high fidelity to all progeny, thus by molecular means stem cell clones may be identified. Such an approach allows for the analysis not only of spleen colonies but of all anatomically dispersed lymphohematopoietic sites, including bone marrow, spleen, thymus, lymph nodes, and mature blood cells in the circulation [Dick et al., 1985; Keller et al., 1985; Lemischka et al., 1986]. These analyses unequivocally showed that the same stem cell may give rise to all lineages, including lymphocytes. Repetitive blood cell sampling and analysis gave a temporal picture of the usage and fate of the stem cell population. In the first few weeks and months after transplant of nonlimiting numbers of stem cells, polyclonal hematopoiesis was the rule; however, after approximately 4 to 6 months, the number of stem cell clones was reduced. In fact, in some cases, a single stem cell clone was responsible for all hematopoiesis for over a year—about half the mouse's lifetime [Jorday and Lemischka, 1990]. These data were interpreted to mean that many stem cell clones were initially active in the irradiated recipient mice, but over time a subset of stem cells grew to dominate the hematopoietic profile. This implies either that not all the stem cells were equivalent in their devel-opmental potential or that the stem cells were not all seeded in equivalent microenvironments and therefore manifest differing developmental potentials. Both these possibilities have been supported by a variety of subsequent experiments; however, the details of this observation remain cloudy.

One piece of evidence suggesting intrinsic differences at the stem cell level comes from studies of allophenic mice [Mintz, 1971]. These artificially generated strains of laboratory mice are created by aggregating the early embryos of two distinguishable mouse strains. As mentioned previously, early embryonic cells are totipotent; thus, upon combining such cells from two strains, a chimeric mouse will arise in which both cell sources contribute to all tissues, including the stem cell population. Patterns of stem cell contribution in allophenic mice show that one strain can cycle more rapidly and thus contribute to mature blood cells early in life, whereas the other slow-growing strain will arise to dominate at later times. Importantly, upon reimplantation of allophenic bone marrow into a secondary irradiated recipient, the two phases of stem cell activity are recapitulated. Thus, the stem cells which had become completely quiescent in the primary animal were reactivated initially, only to be followed by a later phase of activity from the second strain [Van Zant, 1992]. These data suggest that intrinsic differences at the stem cell level rather than the local microenvironment can mediate differences in stem cell activity.

Unlike most organ systems, mature cells of the lymphohematopoietic system are dispersed either in the circulation or in scattered anatomic sites such as the thymus, lymph, nodes, spleen, and, in the case of macrophages, in virtually all tissues of the body. The site of production of most of the mature cells, the bone marrow, is a complex tissue consisting of stromal elements, stem and progenitor cells, maturing cells of multiple lineages, and capillaries and sinusoids of the circulatory system into which mature cells are released. Spatial relationships between these different components are not well understood because of their apparently diffuse organization and because of the paucity of some of the critical elements, most notably the stem cells and early progenitors.

In contrast, the small intestinal epithelium has a much more straightforward organization that has expedited the understanding of some of the critical issues having to do with stem cell differentiation. Numerous fingerlike projections of the epithelium, called *villi*, extend into the intestinal lumen to effectively increase the surface area available for absorption. Each villus is covered with approximately 3500 epithelial cells, of which about 1400 are replaced on a daily basis [Potten and Loeffler, 1990]. Surrounding each villus are 6–10 crypts from which new epithelial cells are produced. They subsequently migrate to villi, and as senescent cells are shed from the villus tip, a steady progression of epithelial cells proceed unidirectionally to replace them. Crypts consist of only about 250 cells, including what is now estimated to be 16 stem cells. Since there are about 16 cells in the circumference of the crypt, stem cells occupy one circumferential ring of the crypt interior. This ring has been identified as the fourth from the bottom, directly above the Paneth cells. In addition, the fifth circumferential ring is occupied by direct progeny of stem cells which retain pluripotency and, in emergencies, may function as stem cells. Given the detailed quantitative information available regarding stem cell numbers and epithelial cell turnover rates, the number of stem cell doublings occurring during a human life span of 70 years has been estimated to be about 5000. Whether this demonstrates that tissue-specific stem cells are immortal is the topic of the following section.

15.4   Aging of Stem Cells

Given the zygote's enormous developmental potential and that ES cells represent cells of apparently equivalent potency that can be propagated as cell lines, it is reasonable to ask whether aging occurs at the cellular level. Put another way, can normal cells, other than ES cells, truly self-replicate without differentiation or senescence? Or do ES cells represent unique examples of cells capable of apparently indefinite self-renewal without differentiation? One of the definitions of hematopoietic stem cells alluded to above is that they self-replicate. Without self-renewal, it might be argued, a stem cell population may be exhausted in a time-frame less than a lifetime of normal hematopoiesis or in far less time in the event of unusually high hematopoietic demands associated with disease or trauma. If, for example, hematopoietic stem cells can be propagated *in vitro* without differentiation, it could have tremendous impact on a number of clinically important procedures including bone marrow transplantation and gene therapy.

In classic experiments studying fibroblast growth *in vitro*, Hayflick [1965] observed that there were a finite number of divisions (about 50) that a cell was capable of before reaching senescence. It has been thought that totipotent and pluripotent stem cells may be exempt from this constraint. An analysis above of intestinal epithelial stem cells suggested that in a lifetime they undergo several thousand replications, apparently without any loss in developmental potential. However, several lines of evidence call into question the immortality of hematopoietic stem cells and point to at least a limited self-renewal capacity. For example, studies in which marrow was serially transplanted from primary recipients to secondary hosts, and so on, the number of effective passages is only about four to five [Siminovitch et al., 1964]. After the first transplant, normal numbers of relatively late progenitors are produced, but the number of repopulating stem cells is either diminished or the cells' developmental potential attenuated, or both, resulting in a requirement for successively larger numbers of transplanted cells to achieve engraftment. Another interpretation of these results is that the transplantation procedure itself is responsible for the declining repopulating ability of marrow, rather than an intrinsic change in the self-renewal capacity of the stem cells. According to this argument, the repetitive dissociation of stem cells from their normal microenvironmental niches in the marrow, and the required reestablishment of those contacts during seeding and serial engraftment, irreversibly alter their self-renewal capacity [Harrison et al., 1978]. A mechanistic possibility for this scenario is that differentiation is favored when stem cells are not in contact with their stromal microenvironment. In this context, exposure to growth factors has an overwhelming differentiating influence on stem cells in suspension that is normally tempered by stromal associations.

Recently, an intriguing series of findings has emerged which may at least partially explain cellular aging. At the end of chromosomes there is a specialized region of DNA known as a telomere. This segment of DNA is comprised of hundreds of short six-nucleotide repeats of the sequence TTAGGG. It has been found that the length of telomeres varies over the life of a cell. Younger cells have longer telomeres, and as replication occurs the telomeres can be seen to shorten. It is thought that via the normal DNA replication process, the last 50 to 200 nucleotides of the chromosome fail to be synthesized, and thus telomeres are subject to loss with every cell division (reviewed in Blackburn [1992] and Greider [1991]). Consequently, telomeric shortening may act as a type of molecular clock. Once a cell has undergone a certain number of divisions, i.e., aged to a particular extent, it becomes susceptible to chromosome destabilization and subsequent cell death. Importantly, the rate at which telomeric sequence is lost may not be constant. Rather, some cells have the ability to regenerate their telomeres via an enzymatic activity known as telomerase. By controlling the loss of telomeric sequence, certain cell types may be able to extend their ability to replicate. Perhaps primitive tissue such as ES cells, when cultured with LIF, are able to express high levels of telomerase and thereby maintain their chromosomes indefinitely. Similarly, perhaps early hematopoietic stem cells express telomerase, and as differentiation occurs, the telomerase activity is downregulated. Although intriguing, these hypotheses are very preliminary, and much more basic research will be required to elucidate the mechanisms of the stem cell replication and aging.

In contrast to normal mechanisms of preserving replicative ability, a type of aberrant self-renewal is observed in the phenomenon of malignant transformation, or cancer. Some hematopoietic cancers are thought to originate with a defect at an early stem or progenitor cell level (e.g., chronic myelogenous leukemia). In this type of disease, normal differentiation is blocked, and a consequent buildup of immature, nonfunctional hematopoietic cells is observed. Malignant or neoplastic growth comes as a consequence of genetic damage or alteration. Such events range from single nucleotide changes to gross chromosomal deletions and translocations. Mechanistically, there appear to be two general types of mutation which cause cancer. One, activation of so-called oncogenes, is a dominant event and only needs to occur in one of a cell's two copies of the gene. Second, inactivation of tumor-suppressor genes removes the normal cellular control of growth and results in unchecked replication. These two categories of genetic alteration are analogous to stepping on a car's accelerator versus releasing the brake; both allow movement forward. Importantly, malignancy often comes as the result of a multistep process, whereby a series of genetic alterations occur. This process has been shown to involve different combinations of genes for different diseases [Vogelstein and Kinzler, 1993].

15.5   Other Types of Stem Cells

Other tissues may also have stem cell populations contributing to the replacement of effete mature cells. For example, in the liver only a very small faction (2.5–5×10^{-5}) of hepatocytes is dividing at any given time, resulting in a complete turnover time of about 1 year [Sell, 1994]. This compares with the complete turnover of intestinal epithelia or granulocytes in a period of a few days. Nonetheless, growing evidence, some of which remains controversial, suggests that hepatic stem cells play a role in this tissue turnover. A moderate loss of liver tissue due to mild or moderate insult is probably replaced by the division of mature hepatocytes. However, a severe loss of hepatic tissue is thought to require the enlistment of the putative stem cell population, morphologically identified as oval cells.

Similarly, Noble's group in London has identified cells in the rat optic nerve that have the requisite functions of stem cells [Wren et al., 1992]. These cells, called *oligodendrocyte-type 2 astrocyte (O-2A) progenitors*, are capable of long-term self-renewal *in vitro* and give rise to oligodendrocytes through asymmetric divisions resulting in one new progenitor and one cell committed to differentiation. Conversion *in vitro* of O-2A progenitors into rapidly dividing and differentiating cells has been shown to be regulated extrinsically by platelet-derived growth factor (PDGF) and the basic form of fibroblast growth factor (bFGF) [Wolswijk and Noble, 1992]. Since these two growth factors are known to be produced *in vivo* after brain injury, a mechanism is suggested for generation of the large numbers of new oligodendrocytes required subsequent to trauma and demyelination.

15.6   Summary

- The zygote is the paradigm of a totipotent stem cell.
- ES cells derived from early embryos can be propagated indefinitely and maintain totipotency when cultured in the presence of LIF. Experimental control of differentiation and self-renewal in adult stem cells is being extensively investigated.
- Stem cells are defined by two characteristic traits: (1) Stem cells can self-renew, and (2) they can produce large numbers of differentiated progeny. Stem cells possess the intrinsic ability to manifest either trait; however, extrinsic factors mediate their developmental fate.
- Tissue-specific stem cells are pluripotent but not totipotent.

- Intestinal, epithelial, and hematopoietic tissues are classical self-renewing systems of the adult. In addition, recent studies have indicated the presence of stem cells in several other tissues (e.g., liver, nervous system).
- Although stem cells clearly have an extensive replication potential, it is not clear whether they are truly immortal. Stem cells may possess the ability to circumvent normal cellular processes that determine aging at the cellular level.
- Mutations at the DNA level can alter normal cellular control of stem cell replication and differentiation. This type can lead to aberrant development and subsequent malignancy.

Defining Terms

Commitment: The biologic process whereby a cell decides which of several possible developmental pathways to follow.

Differentiation: Expression of cell- or tissue-specific genes which results in the functional repertoire of a distinct cell type.

ES cells: Mouse stem cells originating from early embryonic tissue, capable of developing into any of the adult cell types.

Gene knockout: Deletion or alteration of a cellular gene using genetic engineering technology (generally performed on ES cells).

Hematopoietic: Blood forming.

Ontogeny: The process of development, generally referring to development from the zygote to adult stages.

Pluripotent: Capable of differentiation into multiple cell types.

Self-renew: Term describing cellular replication wherein no developmental commitment or differentiation takes place.

Terminally differentiated: The final stage of development in which all cell-specific features have been attained and cell division is no longer possible.

Totipotent: Capable of differentiation into all possible cell types.

References

Barnes DWH, Ford CE, Gray SM, et al. 1959. Progress in Nuclear Energy, series VI: Spontaneous and Induced Changes in Cell Populations in Heavily Irradiated Mice, London, Pergamon Press.

Becker AJ, McCulloch EA, Till JE. 1963. Cytological demonstration of the clonal nature of spleen colonies derived from transplanted mouse marrow cells. Nature 197:452.

Blackburn EH. 1992. Telomerases. Annu Rev Biochem 61:113.

Dick JE, Magil MC, Huszar D, et al. 1985. Introduction of a selectable gene into primitive stem cells capable of long-term reconstruction of the hemopoietic system of W/W^v mice. Cell 42:71.

Evans MJ, Kaufman MH. 1981. Establishment in culture of pluripotent cells from mouse embryos. Nature 292:154.

Greider CW. 1991. Telomeres. Curr Opin Cell Biol 3(3):444.

Harrison DE, Astle CM, Delaittre JA. 1978. Loss of proliferative capacity in immohemopoietic stem cells caused by serial transplantation rather than aging. J Exp Med 147:1526.

Hayflick L. 1965. The limited in vitro lifetime of human diploid cell strains. Exp Cell Res 37:614.

Hilton DJ, Gough NM. 1991 Leukemia inhibitory factor: A biological perspective. J Cell Biochem 46(1):21.

Jordan CT, Lemischka IR. 1990. Clonal and systemic analysis of long-term hematopoiesis in the mouse. Genes Dev 4:220.

Kaufman MH, Robertson EJ, Handyside AH, et al. 1983. Establishment of pluripotential cell lines from haploid mouse embryos. J Embryol Exp Morphol 73:249.

Keller G, Paige C, Gilboa E, et al. 1985. Expression of a foreign gene in myeloid and lymphoid cells derived from multipotent hematapoietic precursors. Nature 318:149.

Koller BH, Smithies O. 1992. Altering genes in animals by gene targeting. Annu Rev Immunol 10:705.

Koller MR, Palsson BØ. 1993. Tissue engineering: Reconstitution of human hematopoiesis ex vivo. Biotechnol Bioeng 42:909.

Lemischka IR, Raulet DH, Mulligan RC. 1986. Developmental potential and dynamic behavior of hematopoietic stem cells. Cell 45:917.

Metcalf D, Moore MAS. 1971. Haemopoietic Cells, Amsterdam, Elsevier/North-Holland.

Mintz B. 1971. Methods in Mammalian Embryology, San Francisco, WH Freeman.

Potten CS, Loeffler M. 1990. Stem cells: Attributes, cycles, spirals, pitfalls and uncertainties. Lessons for and from the crypt. Development 110:1001.

Robertson EJ. 1991. Using embryonic stem cells to introduce mutations into the mouse germ line. Biol Reprod 44(2):238.

Sell S. 1994. Liver stem cells. Mod Pathol 7(1):105.

Siminovitch L, Till JE, McCulloch EA. 1964. Decline in colony-forming ability of marrow cells subjected to serial transplantation into irradiated mice. J Cell Comp Physiol 64:23.

Smith AG, Nichols J. Robertson M, et al. 1992. Differentiation inhibiting activity (DIA/LIF) and mouse development. Dev Biol 151(2):339.

Till JE, McCulloch EA. 1961. A direct measurement of the radiation sensitivity of normal mouse bone marrow cells. Radiat Res 14:213.

Till JE, McCulloch EA, Siminovitch L. 1964. A stochastic model of stem cell proliferation based on the growth of spleen colony-forming cells. Proc Natl Acad Sci USA 51:29.

Van Zant G, Scott-Micus K, Thompson BP, et al. 1992. Stem cell quiescence/activation is reversible by serial transplantation and is independent of stromal cell genotype in mouse aggregation chimeras. Exp Hematol 20:470.

Vogelstein B, Kinzler KW. 1993. The multistep nature of cancer. Trends Genet 9(4):138.

Wolswijk G, Noble M. 1992. Cooperation between PDGF and FGF converts slowly dividing O-2A adult progenitors cells to rapidly dividing cells with characteristics of O-2A perinatal progenitor cells. J Cell Biol 118(4):889.

Wren D, Wolswijk G, Noble M. 1992. In vitro analysis of the origin and maintenance of O-2A adult progenitor cells. J Cell Biol 116(10):167.

16

Cell Motility
and Tissue Architecture

Graham A. Dunn
King's College London

The characteristic architecture of a tissue results from an interplay of many cellular processes. In addition to the secretion of extracellular matrix, we may distinguish between processes related to the cell cycle—cell growth, division, differentiation, and death—and processes related to cell motility—cell translocation, directed motile responses, associated movements, and remodeling of the extracellular matrix. These processes are controlled and directed by cell-cell interactions, by cell-matrix interactions, and by cellular interactions with the fluid phase of the tissue. It is known that all three types of interactions can control both the speed and direction of cell translocation. This control results in the directed motile responses, which are the main subject of this chapter. Learning how to manipulate these motile responses experimentally will eventually become an essential aspect of tissue engineering.

Probably the greatest challenge to tissue engineering lies in understanding the complex dynamic systems that arise as a result of feedback loops in these motile interactions. Not only is cell translocation controlled by the fluid phase, by the matrix, and by other cells of the tissue, but cell motility can profoundly influence the fluid phase, remodel the matrix, and influence the position of other cells by active cell-cell responses or by associated movements. It is often forgotten that, especially in "undifferentiated" types of tissue cells such as fibroblasts, the function of the cell's motile apparatus is not only to haul the cell through the extracellular matrix of the tissue spaces but also to remodel this matrix and to change the positions of other cells mechanically by exerting tension on cell-matrix and cell-cell adhesions. These complex dynamic systems lie at the heart of pattern formation in the tissue, and indeed in the developing embryo, and understanding them will require not only a knowledge of the motile responses but also an understanding of the mechanism of cell motility itself.

In the study of cell motility, a great deal is now known about the relative dispositions of specific molecules that are thought to contribute to the motile process, and the dynamics of their interactions are beginning to be unraveled; yet there appears to have been comparatively little progress toward a satisfactory explanation of how a cell moves. There are some molecular biologists who still believe that it is just a question of time before the current molecular genetic thrust will alone come up with the answers. But there is a rapidly growing climate of opinion, already prevalent among physicists and engineers, that nonlinear dynamic processes such as cell motility have emergent properties that can never be completely understood solely from a knowledge of their molecular basis. Cell locomotion, like muscle contraction, is essentially a mechanical process, and a satisfactory explanation of how it works will inevitably require a study of its mechanical properties. Unlike muscle, the cellular motile apparatus is a continuously self-organizing system, and we also need to know the overall dynamics of its capacity for reorganization. These outstanding areas of ignorance are essentially problems in engineering. There is a nice analogy for this conceptual gap between the molecular and engineering aspects of biologic pattern formation in Harrison's new book on the kinetic theory of living pattern [Harrison, 1993]: "one cannot supplant one end of a bridge by building the other. They are planted in different ground, and neither will ever occupy the place of the other. But ultimately, one has a bridge when they meet in the middle." This chapter is intended to encourage the building of that bridge.

16.1 Directed Motile Responses *in Vivo*

Cellular Interactions with the Fluid Phase

Cellular responses to the fluid phase of tissue spaces are thought to be mediated largely by specific diffusible molecules in the fluid phase. By far the most important directed response is chemotaxis: the unidirectional migration of cells in a concentration gradient of some chemoattractant or chemorepellent substance. Its study dates back to long before the advent of tissue culture, since it is a widespread response among the free-living unicellular organisms. The most widely studied system in vertebrates is the chemotaxis of neutrophil leukocytes in gradients of small peptides. In the case of tissue cells, it has long been conjectured, usually on the basis of surprisingly little evidence, that the direction of certain cell migrations also might be determined by chemotaxis, and it is recently becoming clear that chemotaxis can in fact occur in several vertebrate tissue cells in culture, particularly in gradients of growth factors and related substances. Yet whether it does occur naturally, and under what circumstances, is still an area of dispute. The concentration gradients themselves are usually speculated to arise by molecular diffusion from localized sources, although a nonuniform distribution of sinks could equally explain them, and they are only likely to arise naturally in conditions of very low convective flow. Besides controlling the migration of isolated cells, there is some evidence that gradients of chemoattractants also may control the direction of extension of organized groups of cells such as blood capillary sprouts, and of cellular processes, such as nerve axons. Although the mechanisms of these responses may be closely allied to those chemotaxis, they should more properly be classed as chemotropism, since the effect is to direct the extension of a process rather than the translocation of an isolated cell. The *influence on tissue architecture* of chemotaxis and chemotropism is possibly to determine the relative positions of different cell types and to determine the patterns of angiogenesis and innervation—though this is still largely conjectural. Chemotaxis is potentially a powerful pattern generator if the responding cells can modify and/or produce the gradient field.

Apart from chemotaxis, there also exists the possibility of mechanically mediated cellular responses to flow conditions in the fluid phase. The principal situation *in vivo* where this is likely to be important is in the blood vessels, and the mechanical effects of flow on the endothelial cells that line the vessel walls has been investigated.

Cellular Interactions with the Acellular Solid Phase

In a tissue, the cellular solid phase is the extracellular matrix, which is usually a fibrillar meshwork, though it may take the laminar form of a basement membrane. One directed response to the fibrillar extracellular matrix is the guidance of cell migrations, during embryonic development, for example, along oriented matrix fibrils. The discovery of this response followed soon after the dawn of tissue culture and is generally attributed to Paul Weiss, who named it contact guidance in the 1930s, though Loeb and Fleisher had already observed in 1917 that cells tend to follow the "path of least resistance" along oriented matrix fibrils (see Dunn [1982]). In culture, contact guidance constrains cell locomotion to be predominantly bidirectional, along the alignment axis of the matrix, whereas many embryonic migrations are predominantly unidirectional. This raises the question of whether contact guidance alone can account for these directed migrations *in vivo* or whether other responses are involved. The *influence on tissue architecture* of contact guidance is less conjectural than that of chemotaxis, since matrix alignment is more easily observed than chemical gradients, and the cells themselves are often coaligned with the matrix. Directed motion can be inferred since, in culture, this orientation of the cell shape on aligned surfaces is strongly correlated with an orientation of locomotion. In conjunction with cellular remodeling of the matrix, contact guidance becomes a potentially powerful generator of pattern. Since the cells, by exerting tension, can align the matrix, and the matrix alignment can guide the cells, a mutual interaction can arise whereby cells are guided into regions of higher cell density. Harris and colleagues [1984] have shown that such a feedback loop can result in the spontaneous generation of a regular array of cell clusters from a randomly distributed field of cells and matrix. The pattern of feather formation in birds' skin, for example, might arise by just such a mechanism.

Several other types of directed response may be mediated by the properties of the solid phase of the cell's environment. One is chemoaffinity, which Sperry [1963] proposed could account for the specific connections of the nervous system by guiding nerve fibers along tracks marked out by specific molecules adsorbed to the surface of substratum. A similar response has been proposed to account for the directional migration of primordial germ cells.

Cellular Interactions with Other Cells

Neighboring cells in the tissue environment may be considered as part of the solid phase. Thus it has been reported that when cells are used as a substratum for locomotion by other cells, directed responses such as contact guidance or chemoaffinity may occur, and these responses may persist even if the cells used as a substratum are killed by light fixation. However, the reason that cell-cell interactions are dealt with separately here is that cells show a directed response on colliding with other living cells that they do not show on colliding with cells that have been lightly fixed. Contact inhibition of locomotion, discovered by Abercrombie and Heaysman [1954], is a response whereby a normal tissue cell, on collision with another, is halted and eventually redirected in its locomotion. The effect of the response is to prevent cells from using other cells as a substratum, and a distinguishing feature of the response to living cells is a temporary local paralysis of the cell's active leading edge at the site of contact, which does not generally occur with a chemoaffinity type of response. The *influence on tissue architecture* of contact inhibition is probably profound but not easily determined. It is possibly the main response by which cells are kept more or less in place within a tissue, rather than milling around, and a failure of contact inhibition is thought to be responsible for the infiltration of a normal tissue by invasive malignant cells. Contact inhibition can cause cell locomotion to be directed away from centers of population and thus gives rise to the radial pattern of cell orientation that is commonly observed in the outgrowths from explant cultures. A major question is whether this motile response is related, mechanistically, to the so-called contact inhibition of growth, which is also known to fail in malignant cells but which is probably mediated by diffusion of some signal rather than by cell-cell contact.

16.2 Engineering Directed Motile Responses *in Vitro*

The investigation of the directed motile responses, using tissue culture, can reveal many aspects of the mechanisms that control and direct cell motility *in vivo* and also give a valuable insight into the mechanism of cell motility. In fact, most of what we know about these responses *in vivo* is deduced from experiments in culture. On the other hand, many of the responses discovered in culture may never occur naturally, and yet their study is equally important because it may yield further clues to the mechanism of cell motility and result in valuable techniques for tissue engineering. However, responses to properties of the culture environment, such as electric or magnetic fields, that are not yet known to have any counterparts *in vivo* will not be dealt with here.

A general experimental approach to engineering motile responses is first to try to reproduce in culture some response that appears to occur *in vivo*. The main reason is that the cell behavior can be observed *in vitro*, whereas this is possible *in vivo* only in very few instances. Another important reason is that once achieved *in vitro*, the response may be "dissected," by progressively simplifying the culture environment, until we isolate one or more well-defined properties that can each elicit a response. To be successful, this approach not only requires the design of culture environments that each isolate some specific environmental property and simultaneously allow the resulting cell behavior to be observed but also requires methods for adequately quantifying this resulting behavior.

When designing an artificial environment, it is important to consider its information content. Obviously, a uniform field of some scalar quantity is isotropic and cannot, therefore, elicit a directed motile response. A nondirected motile response, such as a change in speed caused by a change in some scalar property, is generally called a kinesis. Anisotropic uniform fields may be vector fields or may be able to distinguish opposite directions in the field and exhibit a unidirectional response, generally known as a taxis. Or cell movement perpendicular to the vector may predominate, which is sometimes known as a diataxis. In the case of a uniform field of some symmetric second-order tensor, such as strain or surface curvature, there is simply no information to distinguish opposite directions in the field, and yet orthogonal axes may be distinguished. This can give rise to a bidirectional response or, in three-dimensional fields, also to a response where translocation along one axis is suppressed. There is no generally agreed on name to cover all such possible responses, but the term *guidance* will be used here. Some examples of culture environments with specific physiocochemical properties are given below.

Environments with Specific Properties of the Fluid Phase

A Linear Concentration Gradient

The most common method of reproducing the chemotaxis response *in vitro* is to use a Boyden chamber in which a gradient of some specific chemical is formed by diffusion across a membrane filter. The resulting directed cell translocation is inferred from the relative number of cells that migrate through the pores of the filter from its upper to its lower surface. While this system is very useful for screening for potential chemoattractants, its usefulness for investigating the mechanism of the motile response is strictly limited, since it does not fulfill our two main criteria for an *in vitro* system. In the Boyden chamber, the properties of the environment are not well defined (since the gradient within the narrow, often tortuous pores of the filter is unpredictable), and the cell response cannot be observed directly. The Zigmond chamber was introduced to overcome these difficulties, by allowing the cell behavior to be observed directly, but the gradient is very unstable and cannot be maintained reliably for longer than an hour or two. Zicha and colleagues [1991] have recently developed a direct viewing chemotactic chamber with much greater stability and better optical properties. The chamber is constructed from glass and has an annular bridge separating concentric wells (Fig. 16.1). When covered by a coverslip carrying the cells,

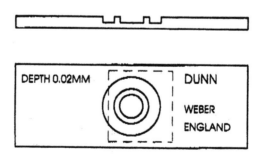

FIGURE 16.1   The Dunn chemotaxis chamber.

a gap of precisely 20 μm is formed between coverslip and bridge in which the gradient develops. The blind central well confers the greater stability, which allows chemotactic gradients to be maintained for many hours and thus permits the chemotactic responses of slowly moving tissue cells and malignant cells to be studied for the first time. Weber Scientific International, Ltd., manufactures this as the Dunn chamber.

In use, both wells of the chamber are initially filled with control medium. The coverslip carrying the cells is then inverted over the wells, firmly seated, and sealed with wax in a slightly offset position (shown by the dashed lines) to allow access to the outer well. The outer well is then emptied using a syringe, refilled with medium containing the substance under test at known concentration, and the narrow opening is sealed with wax.

Assuming that diffusion is the only mechanism of mass transport in the 20-μm gap between coverslip and bridge, whereas convection currents keep the bulk contents of the two wells stirred, then the concentration in the 20-μm gap as a function of distance r from the center of the inner well is given by

$$C(r) = \frac{C_i \ln(b/r) + C_o \ln(r/a)}{\ln(b/a)} \tag{16.1}$$

where C_i and C_o are the concentrations in the inner and outer wells, respectively, and a and b are the inner and outer radii of the bridge. Because the bridge is annular, the gradient is slightly convex, but the deviation from linearity is very small.

Figure 16.2 shows the formation of the gradient during the first hour for a molecule with diffusion coefficient $D = 13.3 \times 10^{-5}$ mm²/s, such as a small globular protein of molecular weight 17 kDa and chamber dimensions $a = 2.8$ mm, $b = 3.9$ mm. The equations describing gradient formation are given in Zicha et al. [1991], but it suffices here to show that the gradient is almost linear after 30 min. The flux from outer to inner well though the gap of height h (= 20 μm) is given by

$$\frac{dQ}{dt} = \frac{2\pi h D (C_o - C_i)}{\ln(b/a)} \tag{16.2}$$

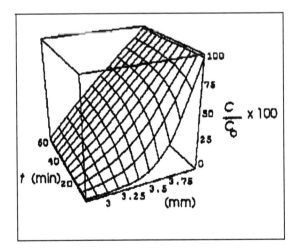

FIGURE 16.2 Formation of the gradient in the Dunn chemotaxis chamber (see text).

This flux tends to destroy the gradient, and the half-life of the gradient is equal to $(\ln 2)/kD$, where k is a constant describing the geometric properties of the chamber. For a chamber with volumes v_o and v_i of the outer and inner wells, respectively, k is given by

$$k = \frac{2\pi h(v_i + v_o)}{\ln(b/a)v_i v_o}$$

(16.3)

Thus, for our small protein, a chamber with $v_o = 30$ μl, $v_i = 14$ μl, and other dimensions as before gives a gradient with a half-life of 33.6 h. This is ample time to study the chemotaxis of slowly moving tissue cells, with typical speeds of around 1 μm per minute, as well as permitting the study of long-term chemotaxis in the more rapidly moving leukocytes with typical speeds around 10 μm per minute.

From the point of view of information content, a linear concentration gradient may be viewed as a nonuniform scalar field of concentration or as a uniform vector field of concentration gradient. Thus, if the cell can distinguish between absolute values of concentration, as well as being able to detect the gradient, then the chemotaxis response may be complicated by a superimposed *chemokinesis* response. A stable linear concentration gradient is a great advantage when trying to unravel such complex responses. Other sources of complexity are the possibilities that cells can modify the gradient by acting as significant sinks, can relay chemotactic signals by releasing pulses of chemoattractant, or can even generate chemotactic signals in response to nonchemotactic chemical stimulation. These possibilities offer endless opportunities for chaotic behavior and pattern generation.

A Gradient of Shear Flow

The flow conditions in the fluid phase of the environment can have at least two possible effects on cell motility. First, by affecting mass transport, they can change the distribution of molecules, and second, they can cause a mechanical shear stress to be exerted on the cells. Figure 16.3 shows a culture chamber designed by Dunn and Ireland [1985] that allows the behavior of cells to be observed under conditions of laminar shear flow. If necessary, the cells may be grown on the special membrane in Petriperm culture dishes (Heraeus), which allows gaseous exchange into the medium beneath the glass disk. Laminar shear

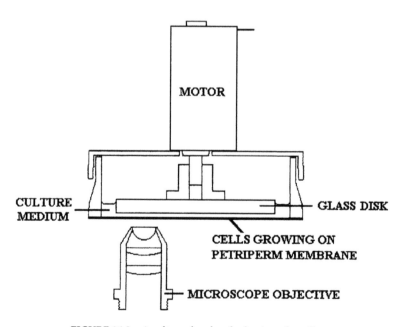

FIGURE 16.3 A culture chamber for laminar shear flow.

flow is probably the simplest and best defined flow regime, and the shear flow produced by an enclosed rotating disk has been described in detail [Daily and Nece, 1960]. Very low flow rates, caused by rotating the disk at around 1 rpm with a separation of about 1 mm between disk and cells, are useful for causing a defined distortion to diffusion gradients arising as a result of cell secretion or adsorption of specific molecules. Much information about, for example, chemoattractants produced by cells may be obtained in this way. Higher shear stresses, around 100 times greater, are known to affect the shape and locomotion of cells mechanically, and higher rotational speeds and/or smaller separations will be needed to achieve these.

Environments with Specific Properties of the Solid Phase

Aligned Fibrillar Matrices

The bidirectional guidance of cells by oriented fibrillar matrices is easily replicated in culture models. Plasma clots and hydrated collagen lattices are the most commonly used substrates, and alignment may be achieved by shear flow, mechanical stress, or strong magnetic fields during the gelling process. The magnitude and direction of orientation may be monitored, after suitable calibration, by measuring the birefringence in a polarizing microscope equipped with a Brace-Köhler compensator. These methods of alignment result in environments that are approximately described as uniform tensor fields, since mechanical strain is a familiar second-order tensor, and they generally give rise to bidirectional motile responses. In three dimensions, the strain tensor that results from applying tension along one axis can be described as a prolate ellipsoid, whereas applying compression along one axis results in an oblate ellipsoid. Thus we might distinguish between prolate guidance, in which bidirectional locomotion predominates along a single axis, and oblate guidance, in which locomotion is relatively suppressed along one of the three axes. But unidirectional information can be imposed on an oriented fibrillar matrix. Boocock [1989] achieved a unidirectional cellular response, called desmotaxis, by allowing the matrix fibrils to form attachments to the underlying solid substratum before aligning them using shear flow. This results in an asymmetrical linkage of the fibrils, and similar matrix configurations may well occur *in vivo*.

Fibrillar environments in culture are probably good models for the type of cell guidance that occurs *in vivo*, but they are so complex that it is difficult to determine which anisotropic physicochemical properties elicit the cellular response. Among the possibilities are morphologic properties (the anisotropic shape or texture of the matrix), chemical properties (an oriented pattern of adhesiveness or specific chemical affinity), and mechanical properties (an anisotropic viscoelasticity of the matrix). One approach to discovering which properties are dominant in determining the response is to try to modify each in turn while leaving the others unaffected. This is difficult, though some progress has been made. Another approach is to design simpler environments with better defined properties, as described in the sections that follow.

Specific Shapes and Textures

Ross Harrison, the inventor of tissue culture, placed spiders' webs in some cultures and reported in 1912 that "The behavior of cells ... shows not only that the surface of a solid is a necessary condition but also that when the latter has a specific linear arrangement, as in the spider web, it has an action in influencing the direction of movement." It is hardly surprising to us today that a cell attached to a very fine fiber, in a fluid medium, is constrained to move bidirectionally. Nevertheless, such stereotropism or guidance by substratum availability is a guidance response and may have relevance to the problem of guidance by aligned fibrillar matrices. Moreover, in the hands of Paul Weiss, the guidance of cells on single cylindrical glass fibers was shown to have a more subtle aspect and it is now known that fibers up to 200 μm in diameter, which have a circumference approximately 10 times greater than the typical length of a fibroblast, will still constrain the locomotion to be parallel with the fiber axis. And so we may distinguish guidance by substratum shape, sometimes known as topographic or morphographic guidance, from guidance by substratum availability. The surface curvature of a cylinder is a uniform tensor field, and since opposite directions within the surface are always equivalent, the cellular response must be bidirectional.

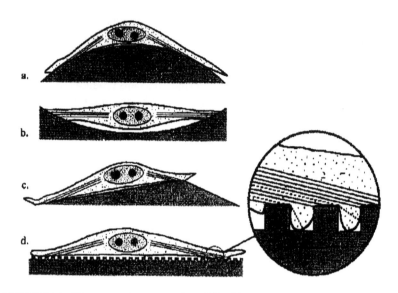

FIGURE 16.4   Diagrammatic cross section of fibroblasts on substrata of various shapes.

Figure 16.4a is a diagrammatic cross section of a fibroblast attached to a convex cylindrical surface. These surfaces are easily made to any required radius of curvature by pulling glass rod in a flame. Dunn and Heath [1976] speculated that a cell must have some form of straightedge in order to detect slight curvatures of around 100 μm in radius. Obvious candidates were the actin cables that extend obliquely into the cytoplasm from sites of adhesion. These cables or stress fibers are continually formed as the fibroblast makes new adhesions to the substratum during locomotion and are known to contact and thereby to exert a tractive force on the substratum. The bundles of actin filaments are shown in the diagram as sets of parallel straight lines meeting the substratum at a tangent, and it is clear that the cables could not be much longer than this without being bent around the cylinder. Dunn and Heath proposed as an explanation of cell guidance along cylinders that the cables do not form in a bent condition and hence the traction exerted by the cell is reduced in directions of high convex curvature.

Further evidence for this hypothesis was found by observing cell behavior on substrata with other shapes. On concave cylindrical surfaces made by drawing glass tubing in a flame, the cells are not guided along the cylindrical axis but tend to become bipolar in shape and oriented perpendicular to the axis [Dunn, 1982]. This is to be expected, since, as shown in Fig. 16.4b, concave surfaces do not restrict formation of unbent cables but allow the cells to spread up the walls, which lifts the body of the cell clear of the substratum and thus prevents spreading along the cylinder axis. On substrata made with a sharp change in inclination like the pitched roof of a house, the hypothesis predicts that locomotion across the ridge is inhibited when the angle of inclination is greater than the angle at which the actin cables normally meet a plane substratum, as in Fig. 16.4c. These substrata are more difficult to make than cylinders and require precision optical techniques for grinding and polishing a sharp and accurate ridge angle. Fibroblasts behaved as predicted on these substrata, the limiting angle being about 4°, and high-voltage electron microscopy revealed the actin cables terminate precisely at the ridge on substrata with inclinations greater than this.

Substrata with fine parallel grooves have long been known to be very effective for eliciting morphographic guidance and are interesting because they can be a well-defined mimicry of some of the shape properties of an aligned fibrillar matrix while being mechanically rigid. Effective substrata can easily be made by simply scratching a glass surface with a very fine abrasive, but such substrata are not well defined and their lack of uniformity may give rise to variations in macroperties such as wettability, that cannot be ruled out as causing the guidance. Early attempts to make better-defined substrata used ruling engines such as those used to make diffraction gratings, but Dunn and Brown [1986] introduced electron beam lithography followed by ion milling to make grooves of rectangular cross section down to about 1 μm in width. Clark and colleagues [Clark et al., 1991] have now achieved rectangular grooves with spacings as low as 260 nm using the interference of two wavefronts, obtained by splitting an argon laser beam, to produce a pattern of parallel fringes on a quartz slide coated with photoresist. Groove depths a small as 100 nm can elicit a guidance response from certain cell types, and the main reason for pursuing this line of inquiry is now to discover the molecular mechanism responsible for this exquisite sensitivity.

Figure 16.4c shows a diagrammatic cross section of a fibroblast on a substratum consisting of a parallel array of rectangular grooves. One question that has been debated is whether the cells generally sink into the grooves, as shown here, or bridge across them. In the latter case, the wall and floor of the grooves are not an available substratum, and the cellular response might be a form of guidance by substratum availability. Ohara and Buck [1979] have suggested that this might occur, since the focal adhesions of fibroblasts are generally elongated in the direction of cell movement, and if they are forced to become oriented by being confined to the narrow spaces between grooves, this may force the locomotion into the same orientation. On the other hand, if the cells do generally sink into the grooves, then the Dunn and Heath hypothesis also could account for guidance even by very fine grooves, since individual actin filaments in the bundles, shown as dashed lines in the inset to the figure, would become bent and possibly disrupted if the cell made any attempt to pull on them other than in a direction parallel with the grooves. It is still therefore an unresolved issue whether different mechanisms operate in the cases of cylinders and grooves or whether a common mechanism is responsible for all cases of guidance by the shape of the substratum. Other groove profiles, particularly asymmetrical ones such as sawtooth profiles, will be needed for testing these and other rival hypotheses, and an intriguing possibility is that a unidirectional cell response might be achieved on microfabricated substrata with two orthogonal arrays of parallel sawtooth grooves, as shown in Fig. 16.5.

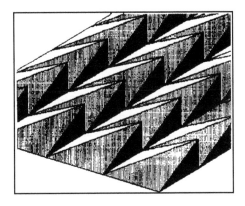

FIGURE 16.5 A proposed microfabricated substratum with two orthogonal arrays of parallel sawtooth grooves.

Specific Patterns of Adhesiveness

The equivalent in culture of the chemoaffinity response is *guidance by differential adhesiveness*, in which cell locomotion is confined to regions of higher adhesiveness patterned on the substrate. As with grooved surfaces, adhesive tracks that guide cells effectively are easily made by a variety of methods, including physically streaking nonadhesive viscous materials on an adhesive substratum or scratching through a nonadhesive film overlying an adhesive substratum. Again, however, these easily made surfaces are not well defined, and in particular, their anisotropic adhesiveness tends to be contaminated by anisotropic surface texture and sometimes by anisotropic mechanical properties. Carter [1965] was probably the first to describe a method of printing a well-defined pattern of adhesiveness onto a substratum; he used the vacuum evaporation of palladium, through a mask, onto a glass substratum made nonadhesive by first coating it with cellulose acetate. Clark and colleagues [1992] have now described a method for fabricating any required pattern of differential adhesiveness by using photolithography to obtain a hydrophobic pattern of methyl groups covalently coupled to a hydrophilic quartz substratum. The most recent developments in their laboratories are to use these patterns of hydrophobicity as templates for patterning specific proteins onto the substratum, and it seems that soon it will be possible to make almost any required pattern in any combination of proteins.

The explanation of the guidance of cells along tracks of higher adhesiveness appears to be obvious. In extreme cases, when the cells cannot adhere at all to the substrate outside the track, then the response is equivalent to guidance by substratum availability, and if the track happens to be sufficiently narrow, cell locomotion is restricted to the two directions along the track. But guidance along tracks of higher adhesiveness may still be very pronounced even when the cells can also adhere to and move on the regions of lower adhesiveness. The explanation in this case is that on encountering boundaries between regions of different adhesiveness, cells will cross them far more frequently in the direction from lower to higher adhesiveness. It is generally assumed that this results from a tug-of-war competition, since traction can be applied more effectively by the parts of the cell overlapping the region of higher adhesiveness. It is not known, however, how the traction fails in those parts of the cell which lose the competition, whether by breakage or slipping of the adhesions or by a relative failure of the contractile apparatus. Another possibility is simply that the cell spreads more easily over the more highly adhesive regions.

One reason for studying guidance by differential adhesiveness is to discover whether it can account for guidance by oriented extracellular matrices. An array of very narrow, parallel stripes of alternately high and low adhesiveness mimics the linear arrangement of substratum availability in an aligned matrix. Dunn [1982] found that if the repeat spacing is so small that a cell can span several stripes, there is no detectable cell orientation or directed locomotion even though an isolated adhesive stripe can strongly guide cells. Clark and colleagues [1992] confirmed this observation with one cell type (BHK) but found that cells of another type (MDCK) could become aligned even when spanning several stripes but would become progressively less elongated as the repeat spacing decreased. It is not yet clear, therefore, whether the linear arrangement of substratum availability in an aligned matrix might contribute to the guidance response in some cell types. It is clear from work of Clark and colleagues, however, that the adhesive stripes become less effective in eliciting guidance as their repeat spacing decreases, whereas the opposite is true for grooved surfaces. Thus it seems unlikely that substratum availability is the mechanism of guidance by grooved surfaces and, conversely, unlikely that adhesive stripes guide cells by influencing the orientation of the focal adhesions as suggested for grooved surfaces by Ohara and Buck [1979].

Binary patterns of adhesiveness were not the only ones studied by Carter [1965]. His technique of shadowing metallic palladium by vacuum evaporation onto cellulose acetate also could produce a graded adhesiveness. By placing a rod of 0.5 mm diameter on the substratum before shadowing, he found that the penumbral regions of the rod's shadow acted as steep gradients of adhesiveness that would cause cultured cells to move unidirectionally in the direction of increasing adhesiveness. This is therefore a taxis as distinct from a guidance response, and he named it haptotaxis. It is still not clear whether haptotaxis plays any role *in vivo*.

Specific Mechanical Properties

As yet, there has been no demonstration that anisotropic mechanical properties of the substratum can elicit directed motile responses. However, it is known that isotropic mechanical properties, such as the viscosity of the substratum, can influence cell locomotion [Harris, 1982], and it appears that changing the mechanical properties of aligned matrices can reduce cell guidance [Dunn, 1982; Haston et al., 1983], although it is probable that other properties are altered at the same time. Moreover, the phenomenon of desmotaxis suggest that it is the asymmetrical mechanical linkage of the fibrils that biases the locomotion. Guidance by anisotropic mechanical properties therefore remains a distinct possibility, but further progress is hampered by the difficulty of fabricating well-defined substrata. An ideal substratum would be a flat, featureless, and chemically uniform surface with anisotropic viscoelastic properties, and it is possible that liquid crystal surfaces will provide the answer.

Environments with Specific Arrangements of Neighboring Cells

Although contact inhibition of locomotion is of primary importance in determining patterns that develop in populations of cells, it is not easy to control the effects of contact inhibition in culture. If the cells are seeded on the substratum at nonuniform density, the response will generally cause cell locomotion to be biased in the direction of decreasing cell density. This can give a unidirectional bias if superimposed on a guidance response, and it has been conjectured that certain cell migrations *in vivo* are biased in this way. Cellular contact responses also can lead to the mutual orientation of confluent neighboring cells, and this can lead to wide regions of cooriented cells arising spontaneously in uniformly seeded cultures.

A typical culture arrangement from studying contact inhibition is to seed two dense populations of cells, often primary explants of tissue, about 1 mm apart on the substratum [Abercrombie and Heaysman, 1976]. Homologous contact inhibition causes the cells to migrate radially from these foci, usually as confluent sheets, until the two populations collide. With noninvasive cells, their locomotion is much reduced after the populations have met, and there is little intermixing of the population boundary. If one of the two populations is of an invasive type, however, failure of heterologous contact inhibition will cause it to infiltrate the other population, and their invasiveness can be measured by the depth of interpenetration.

Defining Terms

Associated movements: Occur when cells passively change position as a result of external forces, generated by cell motility elsewhere, that are transmitted either through the extracellular matrix or through cell-cell contacts.

Cell motility: A blanket term that covers all aspects of movement actively generated by a cell. It includes changes in cell shape, cell contraction, protrusion and retraction of processes, intracellular motility, and cell translocation.

Cell translocation, cell locomotion, or cell migration: All describe active changes in position of a cell in relation to its substratum. The translocation of tissue cells always requires a solid or semisolid substratum. In seeking a more rigorous definition, *positions* must first be defined for both the cell and its substratum. This is not always easy, since both may change continually in shape.

Chemoaffinity: The directional translocation of cells or extension of cellular protrusions along narrow tracks of specific molecules adsorbed to the substratum.

Chemokinesis: A *kinesis* (q.v.) in which the stimulating scalar property is the concentration of some chemical.

Chemotaxis: The directional translocation of cells in a concentration gradient of some chemoattractant or chemorepellent substance.

Chemotropism: The directional extension of a cellular protrusion or multicellular process in a concentration gradient of some chemoattractant or chemorepellent substance.

Contact guidance: The directional translocation of cells in response to some anisotropic property of the substratum.

Contact inhibition of locomotion: Occurs when a cell collides with another and is halted and/or redirected so that it does not use the other cell as a substratum.

Desmotaxis: Describes a unidirectional bias of cell translocation in a fibrillar matrix that is allowed to attach to a solid support and then oriented by shear flow.

Diataxis: A *taxis* (q.v.) in which translocation perpendicular to the field vector predominates. This leads to a bidirectional bias in two dimensions.

Directed motile responses: The responses of cells to specific properties of their environment that can control the direction of cell translocation or, in the case of nerve growth, for example, can control the direction of extension of a cellular protrusion.

Guidance: Used here to indicate a directed response to some high-order-tensor-like property of the environment in which opposite directions are equivalent. Translocation is biased bidirectionally in two dimensions.

Guidance by differential adhesiveness: A form of *guidance by substratum availability* (q.v.) in which cell locomotion is wholly or largely confined to narrow tracks of higher adhesiveness on the substratum. The response may be absent or much reduced if the cell spans several parallel tracks.

Guidance by substratum availability: Occurs when the translocation of a cell is confined to an isolated narrow track either because no alternative substratum exists or because the cell is unable to adhere to it.

Guidance by substratum shape, topographic guidance, or morphographic guidance: All refer to the guidance of cells by the shape or texture of the substratum. It is not known whether all types of morphographic guidance are due to a common mechanism.

Haptotaxis: The tendency of cells to translocate unidirectionally up a steep gradient of increasing adhesiveness of the substratum.

Heterologous contact inhibition: The *contact inhibition of locomotion* (q.v.) that may occur when a cell collides with another of different type. Contact inhibition is called nonreciprocal when the responses of the two participating cells are different. A cell type that is invasive with respect to another will generally fail to show contact inhibition in heterologous collisions.

Homologous contact inhibition: The *contact inhibition of locomotion* (q.v.) that may occur when a cell collides with another of the same type. It is not always appreciated that invasive cell types can show a high level of homologous contact inhibition.

Kinesis: The dependence of some parameter of locomotion, usually speed or rate of turning, on some scalar property of the environment. In an adaptive kinesis, the response is influenced by the rate of change of the scalar property, and if the environment is stable but spatially nonuniform, this can lead to behavior indistinguishable from a *taxis* (q.v.). Current nomenclature is inadequate to deal with such situations [Dunn, 1990].

Oblate guidance: A form of guidance in three dimensions in which translocation is suppressed along a single axis.

Prolate guidance: A form of guidance in three dimensions in which translocation along a single axis predominates.

Stereotropism: A form of *guidance by substratum availability* (q.v.) in which the only solid support available for locomotion consists of isolated narrow fibers.

Taxis: A directed response to some vectorlike property of the environment. Translocation is usually biased unidirectionally, either along the field vector or opposite to it, except in the case of *diataxis* (q.v.).

References

Abercrombie M, Heaysman JEM. 1954. Observations on the social behaviour of cells in tissue culture. Exp Cell Res 6:293.

Boocock CA. 1989. Unidirectional displacement of cells in fibrillar matrices. Development 107:881.

Carter SB. 1965. Principles of cell motility: The direction of cell movement and cancer invasion. Nature 208:1183.

Clark P, Connolly P, Curtis ASG, et al. 1991. Cell guidance by ultrafine topography in vitro. J Cell Sci 99:73.

Clark P, Connolly P, Moores GR. 1992. Cell guidance by micropatterned adhesiveness in vitro. J Cell Sci 103:287.

Daily JW, Nece RE. 1960. Chamber dimension effects on induced flow and frictional resistance of enclosed rotating disks. Trans AM Soc Mech Eng D82:217.

Dunn GA. 1982. Contact guidance of cultured tissue cells: A survey of potentially relevant properties of the substratum. In R Bellairs, A Curtis, G Dun (eds), Cell Behaviour: A Tribute to Michael Abercrombie, pp 247–280. Cambridge, Cambridge University Press.

Dunn GA. 1990. Conceptual problems with kinesis and taxis. In JP Armitage, JM Lackie (eds), Biology of the Chemotactic Response, pp 1–13. Society for General Microbiology Symposium, 46. Cambridge, Cambridge University Press.

Dunn GA, Brown AF. 1986. Alignment of fibroblasts on grooved surfaces described by a simple geometric transformation. J Cell Sci 83:313.

Dunn GA, Heath JP. 1976. A new hypothesis of contact guidance in tissue cells. Exp Cell Res 101:1.

Dunn GA, Ireland GW. 1984. New evidence that growth in 3T3 cell cultures is a diffusion-limited process. Nature 312:63.

Harris AK. 1982. Traction and its relation to contraction in tissue cell locomotion. In R Bellairs, A Curtis, G Dunn (eds), Cell Behaviour: A Tribute to Michael Abercrombie, pp 109–134. Cambridge, Cambridge University Press.

Harris AK, Stopak D, Warner P. 1984. Generation of spatially periodic patterns by a mechanical instability: A mechanical alternative to the Turning model. J Embryol Exp Morphol 80:1.

Harrison LG. 1993. Kinetic Theory of Living Pattern, Cambridge, Cambridge University Press.

Haston WS, Shields JM, Wilkinson PC. 1983. The orientation of fibroblasts and neutrophils on elastic substrata. Exp Cell Res 146:117.

Ohara PT, Buck RC. 1979. Contact guidance in vitro: A light, transmission and scanning electron microscopic study. Exp Cell Res 121:235.

Sperry RW. 1963. Chemoaffinity in the orderly growth of nerve fiber patterns and connections. Proc Natl Acad Sci USA 50:703.

Zicha D, Dunn GA, Brown AF. 1991. A new direct-viewing chemotaxis chamber. J Cell Sci 99:769.

17

Tissue Microenvironments

Michael W. Long
University of Michigan

Tissue development is regulated by a complex set of events in which cells of the developing organ interact with each other, with general and specific growth factors, and with the surrounding extracellular matrix (ECM) [Long, 1992]. These interactions are important for a variety of reasons such as localizing cells within the microenvironment, directing cellular migration, and initiating growth-factor-mediated developmental programs. It should be realized, however, that simple interactions such as those between cells and growth factor are not the sole means by which developing cells are regulated. Further complexity occurs via interactions of cells and growth factors with extracellular matrix or via other interactions which generate specific developmental responses.

Developing tissue cells interact with a wide variety of regulators during their ontogeny. Each of these interactions is mediated by defined, specific receptor-ligand interactions necessary to stimulate both the cell proliferation and/or motility. For example, both chemical and/or extracellular matrix gradients exist which signal the cell to move along "tracks" of molecules into a defined tissue area. As well, high concentrations of the attractant, or other signals, next serve to "localize" the cell, thus stopping its nonrandom walk. These signals which stop and/or regionalize cells in appropriate microenvironments are seemingly complex. For example, in the hematopoietic system, complexes of cytokines and extracellular matrix molecules serve to localize progenitor cells [Long et al., 1992], and similar mechanisms of cell/matrix/cytokine interactions undoubtedly exist in other developing systems. Thus, the regulation of cell development, which ultimately leads to tissue formation is a complex process in which a number of elements work in cohort to bring about coordinated organogenesis: stromal and parenchymal cells, growth factors and extracellular matrix. Each of these is a key component of a localized and highly organized microenvironmental regulatory system.

Cellular interactions can be divided into three classes: cell-cell, cell-extracellular matrix, and cell-growth factor, each of which is functionally significant for both mature and developing cells. For example, in a number of instances blood cells interact with each other and/or with cells in other tissues. Immunologic cell-cell interactions occur when lymphocytes interact with antigen-presenting cells, whereas neutrophil or lymphocyte egress from the vasculature exemplifies blood cell-endothelial cell recognition. Interactions between cells and the extracellular matrix (the complex prontinaceous substance surrounding

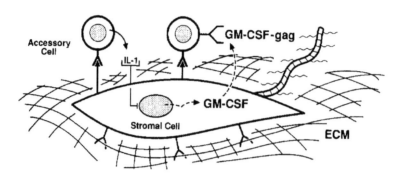

FIGURE 17.1 Hematopoietic cellular interactions. This figure illustrates the varying complexities of putative hematopoietic cell interactions. A conjectural complex is shown in which accessory cell–stromal cell, and stromal cell–PG-growth factor complexes localize developmental signals. ECM = extracellular matrix, gag = glycosaminoglycan side chain bound to proteoglycan (PG) core protein (indicated by cross-hatched curved molecule); IL-1 = interleukin-1; GM-CSF = granulocyte-macrophage colony-stimulating factor. Modified from Long [1992] and reprinted with permission.

cells) also play an important role. During embryogenesis matrix molecules are involved both in cell migration and in stimulating cell function. Matrix components are also important in the growth and development of precursor cells; they also serve either as cytoadhesion molecules for these cells or to compartmentalize growth factors within specific microenvironmental locales. For certain tissues such as bone marrow, a large amount of information exists concerning the various components of the nature of the microenvironment. For others such as bone, much remains to be learned of the functional microenvironment components. Many experimental designs have examined simple interactions (e.g., cell-cell, cell-matrix). However, the situation *in vivo* is undoubtedly much more complex. For example, growth factors are often bound to matrix molecules which, in turn, are expressed on the surface of underlying stromal cells. Thus, very complex interactions occur (e.g., accessory cell–stromal cell–growth factor–progenitor cell–matrix, see Fig. 17.1), and these can be further complicated by a developmental requirement for multiple growth factors.

The multiplicity of tissue-cell interactions requires highly specialized cell surface structures (i.e., receptors) to both mediate cell adhesion and transmit intracellular signals from other cells, growth factors, and/or the ECM. Basically, two types of receptor structures exist. Most cell surface receptors are proteins which consist of an extracellular ligand-binding domain, a hydrophobic membrane-spanning region, and a cytoplasmic region which usually functions in signal transduction. The amino acid sequence of these receptors often defines various families of receptors (e.g., immuno-globulin and integrin gene superfamilies). However, some receptors are not linked to the cell surface by protein, as certain receptors contain phosphotidylinositol-based membrane linkages. This type of receptor is usually associated with signal transduction events mediated by phospholipase C activation [Springer, 1990]. Other cell surface molecules important in receptor-ligand interactions are surface proteins which function as a coreceptors. Coreceptors function with a well-defined receptor, usually to amplify stimulus-response coupling.

The goal of this chapter is to examine the common features of each component of the microenvironment (cellular elements, soluble growth factors, and extracellular matrix). As each tissue or organ undergoes its own unique and complex developmental program, this review cannot cover these elements for all organs and tissue types. Rather, two types of microenvironments (blood and bone) will be compared in order to illustrate commonalties and distinctions.

17.1   Cellular Elements

Cells develop in a distinct hierarchical fashion. During the ontogeny of any organ, cells migrate to the appropriate region for the nascent tissue to form and there undergo a phase of rapid proliferation and differentiation. In tissues which retain their proliferative capacity (bone marrow, liver, skin, the gastrointestinal lining, and bone), the complex hierarchy of proliferation cells is retained throughout life. This is best illustrated in the blood-forming (hematopoiesis) system. Blood cells are constantly produced, such that approximately 70 times an adult human's body weight of blood cells is produced through the human life span. This implies the existence of a very primitive cell type that retains the capacity for self-renewal. This cell is called a *stem cell*, and it is the cell responsible for the engraphment of hematopoiesis in recipients of bone marrow transplantation. Besides a high proliferative potential, the stem cell also is characterized by its multipotentiality in that it can generate progeny (referred to as *progenitor cells*) which are committed to each of the eight blood cell lineages. As hematopoietic cells proliferate, they progressively lose their proliferative capacity and become increasingly restricted in lineage potential. As a result, the more primitive progenitor cells in each lineage produce higher colony numbers, and the earliest cells detectable *in vitro* produce progeny of two to three lineages (there is no *in vitro* assay for transplantable stem cells*)*. Similar stem cell hierarchies exist for skin and other regenerating tissues, but fewer data exist concerning their hierarchical nature.

The regulation of bone cell development is induced during bone morphogenesis by an accumulation of extracellular and intracellular signals [Urist et al., 1983a]. Like other systems, extracellular signals are known to be transferred from both cytokines and extracellular matrix molecules [Urist et al., 1983a] to responding cell surface receptors, resulting in eventual bone formation. The formation of bone occurs by two mechanisms. Direct development of bone from mesenchymal cells (referred to as *intramembranous ossification*, as observed in skull formation) occurs when mesenchymal cells directly differentiate into bone tissue. The second type of bone formation (the endochondrial bone formation of skeletal bone) occurs via an intervening cartilage model. Thus, the familiar cell hierarchy exists in the development and growth of long bones, beginning with the proliferation of mesenchymal stem cells, their differentiation into ostogenic progenitor cells, and then into osteoblasts. The osteoblasts eventually calcify their surrounding cartilage and/or bone matrix to form bone. Interestingly, the number of osteoporgenitor cells in adult bone seems too small to replace all the large mass of bone normally remodeled in the process of aging of the skeleton [Urist et al., 1983a]. Observations from this laboratory confirm this concept by showing that one (unexpected) source of bone osteoprogenitor cells is the bone marrow [Long et al., 1990; Long and Mann, 1993]. This reduced progenitor cell number also implies that there is a disassociation of bone progenitor cell recruitment from subsequent osteogenic activation and bone deposition and further suggests multiple levels of regulation in this process (*vide infra*).

As mentioned, cell-cell interactions mediate both cellular development and stimulus-response coupling. When coupled with other interactions (e.g., cell-ECM), such systems represent a powerful mechanism for directing and/or localizing developmental regulation. Further, combinations of these interactions potentially can yield lineage-specific or organ-specific information. Much of our understanding of cell-cell interactions comes from the immune system and from the study of developing blood cells and their interactions with adjacent stromal cells [Dexter, 1982; Gallatin et al., 1986; Springer, 1990]. For example, the isolation and cloning of immune cell ligands and receptors resulted in the classification of gene families which mediate cell-cell interactions within the immune and hematopoietic systems, and similar systems undoubtedly play a role in the development of many tissues.

There are three families of molecules which mediate cell-cell interactions (Table 17.1). The immunoglobulin superfamily is expressed predominantly on cells mediating immune and inflammatory responses (and is discussed only briefly here). The integrin family is a large group of highly versatile proteins which is involved in cell-cell and cell-matrix attachment. Finally, the selectin family is comprised of molecules which are involved in lymphocyte, platelet, and leukocyte interactions with endothelial cells. Interestingly, this class of cell surface molecules utilizes specific glycoconjungates (encoded by glycoslytransferase genes) as their ligands on endothelial cell surfaces.

Immunoglobulin Gene Superfamily

These molecules function in both antigen recognition and cell-cell communication. The immunglobulin superfamily (Table 17.2) is defined by a 90–100 base pair immunoglobulinlike domain found within a

TABLE 17.1 Cell Adhesion Molecule Superfamilies

Immunoglobulin superfamily of adhesion receptors

LFA 2 (CD2)	T-Cell receptor (CD3)
LFA 3 (CD58)	CD4 (TCR coreceptor)
ICAM 1 (CD54)	CD8 (TCR coreceptor)
ICAM 2	MHC class I
VCAM-1	MHC class II

Integrins

β_1 Integrins (VLA proteins)

P150,95 (CD11$_c$/CD18)

VLA 1–3,6

VLA 4(LPAM 1, CO49d/CO29)

Fibronectin receptor (VLA 5, CD-/CD29)

LPAM 2

β_2 Integrins

LFA 1 (CD11$_a$/ CD18)

Mac 1 or Mo l (CD11$_b$/CD18)

β_3 Integrins

Vitronectin receptor

Platelet gp-IIb/IIa

Selectin/LEC-CAMS

Mel14 (LE-CAM-1, LHR, LAM-1, Leu 8, Ly 22, gp90 MEL)

ELAM-1 (LE-CAM-2)

GMP 140 (LE-CAM 3, PADGEM, CD 62)

Source: Originally adapted from Springer [1990] and Brandley and co-workers [1990] and reprinted from Long [1992] with permission.

dimer of two antiparallel β strands [Sheetz et al., 1989; Williams and Barclay, 1988]; for a review, see Springer [1990]. Two members of this family, the T-cell receptor and immunoglobulin, function in antigen recognition. The T-cell receptor recognizes antigenic peptides in the context of two other molecules on the surface of antigen-presenting cells: major histocompatibility (MHC) class I and class II molecules [Bierer et al., 1989; Sheetz et al., 1989; Springer, 1990]. Whereas the binding of T-cell receptor to MHC/antigenic peptide complexes seems sufficient for cell-cell adhesion, cellular activation also requires the binding of either of two coreceptors, CD8 or CD4. Neither coreceptor can directly bind the MHC complex, but, rather, each seems to interact with the T-cell receptors to synergistically amplify intercellular signaling [Shaw et al., 1986; Spits et al., 1986; Springer, 1990].

Integrin Gene Superfamily

Integrin family members are involved in interactions between cells and extracellular matrix proteins [Giancotti and Ruoslahti, 1990]. Cell attachment to these molecules occurs rapidly (within minutes) and is a result of increased avidity rather than increased expression (see Lawrence and Springer [1991] and references therein). The binding sequence within the ligand for most, but not all, integrins is the tripeptide sequence arganine-glycine-asparagine (RGD) [Ruoslahti and Pierschbacher, 1987]. Structurally, integrins consist of two membrane-spanning alpha and beta chains. The alpha subunits contain three to four tandem repeats of a divalent-ion-binding motif and require magnesium or calcium to function. The alpha chains are (usually) distinct and bind with common or related β subunits to yield functional receptors [Giancotti and Ruoslahti, 1990]. The β subunits of integrins have functional significance, and integrins can be subclassified based on the presence of a given beta chain. Thus, integrins containing β1 and β3 chains are involved predominantly in cell-extracellular matrix interactions, whereas molecules containing the β2 subunits function in leukocyte-leukocyte adhesion (Tables 17.1 and 17.2). The cytoplasmic domain of many integrin receptors interacts with the cytoskeleton. For example, several integrins

TABLE 17.2   Cell Surface Molecules Mediating Cell-Cell Interactions

Cell Receptor	Receptor: Cell Expression	Ligand, Co-, or Counter-Receptor	Ligand Co- or Counter-Receptor Cell Expression	References
Ig superfamily				
MHC I	Macroph, T cell	CD8,TCR	T cells	Springer 1990
MHC II	Macroph, T cell	CD4, TCR	T cells	Springer 1990
ICAM-1	Endo, neut. HPC, B cells, T cells, macroph*	LFA-1	Mono, T and B cells	Springer 1990
ICAM-2	Endo	LFA-1	Mono, T and B cells	Springer 1990
LFA-2	T cells	LFA-3	T cells, eryth	Springer 1990
Integrins				
Mac1	Macroph, neut	Fibrinogen, C3bi	Endo, plts	Springer 1990
LFA-1	Macroph, neut	(See above)	(See above)	
VCAM	Endo	VLA4	Lymphocytes, monocytes B cells	Brandley et al. 1990 Miyamake 1990
gp150,95	Macro, neut	(See above)	(See above)	
FN-R	Eryth lineage	Fibronectin	N.A.	see Table 17.3
IIb/IIIa	Plts, mk	Fibrinogen, TSP, VN vWF	Endo	Springer 1990
Selectins				
LEC-CAM-1 (Mel 14)	Endo	Addressins, neg. charged oligosaccrides	Lymphocytes	Brandley et al. 1990
ELAM-1 (LE-CAM-2)	Endo	sialyl-Lewis X[†]	Endo[‡] Neut, tumor cells	Lowe et al. 1990
LEC-CAM-3 (GMP-140)	Plt gran Weible-Palade bodies, endo	Lewis X (CD15)	Endo Neut	Brandley et al. 1990

Source: Modified from Long [1992] and reprinted with permission. Macroph = macrophage; Mono = monocyte; Endo = endothelial cell; Eryth = erythroid cells; Plts = platelets; Neut = neutrophil; Mk = megakarocyte.
[†]Constituatively expressed by few cells, upregulated by TNF-β and IL-1.
[‡]Sialylated, fucosylated lactosaminoglycans. Modified from Long [1992] and reprinted with permission.

are known to localize near focal cell contacts were actin bundles terminate [Giancotti and Ruoslahti, 1990; Springer, 1990]. As a result, changes in receptor binding offer an important mechanism for linking cell adhesion to cytoskeletal organization.

Selectins

The selectin family of cell-adhesion receptors contains a single N-terminus, calcium-dependent, lectin-binding domain, an EGF receptor (EFGR) domain, and a region of cysteine-rich tandem repeats (from two to seven) which are homologous to complement-binding proteins [Bevilacqua et al., 1989; Springer, 1990; Stoolman, 1989]. Selectins (e.g., MEL14, gp90MEL, ELAM-1, and GMP140/PADGEM, Table 17.2) are expressed on neutrophils and lymphocytes. They recognize specific glycoconjugate ligands on endothelial and other cell surfaces. Early studies demonstrated that fucose or mannose could block lymphocyte attachment to lymph node endothelial cells [Brandley et al., 1990]. Therefore, the observation that the selectin contain a lectin-binding domain [Bevilacqua et al., 1989] led to the identification of the ligands for two members of this family; for review see Brandley and co-workers [1990]. Lowe and co-workers first demonstrated that alpha (1,3/1,4) fucosyltransferase cDNA converted nonmyeloid COS or CHO cells to selectin (sialyl-Lewis X) positive cells which bound to both HL60 cells and neutrophils in an ELAM-1-dependent manner [Lowe et al., 1990]. Conversely, Goelz and co-workers screened an expression library using a monoclonal antibody which inhibited ELAM-mediated attachment which yielded a novel alpha (1,3) fucosyltransferase whose expression conferred ELAM binding activity on target cells [Goelz et al., 1990].

Unlike mature neutrophils and lymphocytes, information on cell-cell interactions among hematopoietic progenitor cells is less well developed (see Table 17.3). Data concerning the cytoadhesive capacities

TABLE 17.3   Hematopoietic Cell–Stromal Cell Interactions (Unknown Receptor-Ligand)

Cell Phenotype	Stromal Cell	References
B cells	Fibroblasts	Ryan et al., 1990; Witte et al., 1987
Pre-B cell	Heter stroma	Palacios et al., 1989
BFC-E	Fibroblasts	Tsai et al., 1986, Tsai et al., 1987
CFC-S	Fibroblasts (NIH 3T3)	Roberts et al., 1987
CFC-S, Bl-CFC	Heter stroma*	Gordon et al., 1985, 1990a, 1990b
CFC-GM	Heter stroma	Tsai et al., 1987; Campbell et al., 1985
CFC-Mk	Heter stroma	Tsai et al., 1987; Campbell et al., 1985

*Methylprednisolone stimulated stromal cells, unstimulated fail to bind—see Gordon and co-workers [1985]. Heter = heterologous; BFC-E = burst forming cell-erythroid; CFC = colony-forming cell; S = spleen; Bl = blast; GM = granulocyte/macrophage; Mk = megakaryocyte.
Source: From Long [1992]. Reprinted with permission.

of hematopoietic progenitor cells deal with the interaction of these cells with underlying, preestablished stromal cell layers [Dexter, 1982]. Gordon and colleagues documented that primitive hematopoietic human blast-colony forming cells (Bl-CFC) adhere to performed stromal cell layers [Gordon et al., 1985, 1990b] and showed that the stromal cell ligand is not one of the known cell adhesion molecules [Gordon et al., 1987a]. Other investigators have shown that hematopoietic (CD34-selected) marrow cell populations attach to stromal cell layers and that the attached cells are enriched for granulocyte-macrophage progenitor cells [Liesveld et al., 1989]. Highly enriched murine spleen colony-forming cells (CFC-S) attach to stromal cell layers, proliferate, and differentiate into hematopoietic cells [Spooncer et al., 1985]. Interestingly, underlying bone marrow stromal cells can be substituted for by NIH 3T3 cells [Roberts et al., 1987], suggesting that these adherent cells supply the necessary attachment ligand for CFU-S attachment [Roberts et al., 1987; Yamazaki et al., 1989].

17.2   Soluble Growth Factors

Soluble specific growth factors are an obligate requirement for the proliferation and differentiation of developing cells. These growth factors differ in effects from the endocrine hormones such as anabolic steroids or growth hormone. Whereas the endocrine hormones affect general cell function and are required and/or important to tissue formation, their predominant role is one of homeostasis. Growth *factors*, however, specifically drive the developmental programs of differentiating cells. Whether these function in a permissive or an inductive capacity has been the subject of considerable past controversy, particularly with respect to blood cell development. However, the large amount of data demonstrating linkages between receptor-ligand interaction and gene activation argues persuasively for an inductive/direct action on gene expression and, hence, cell proliferation and differentiation.

Again, a large body of knowledge concerning growth factors comes from the field of hematopoiesis (blood cell development). Hematopoietic cell proliferation and differentiation are regulated by numerous growth factors; for reviews see Metcalf [1989] and Arai and colleagues [1990]. Within the last decade approximately 29 stimulatory cytokines (13 interleukins, M-CSF, erythroprotein, G-CFS, GM-CSF, c-kit ligand, gamma-interferon, and thrombopoietin) have been molecularly cloned and examined for their function in hematopoiesis. Clearly, this literature is beyond the scope of this review. However, the recent genetic cloning of eight receptors for these cytokines has led to the observation that a number of these receptors have amino acid homologies [Arai et al., 1990], showing that they are members of one or more gene families (Table 17.4). Hematopoietic growth factor receptors structurally contain a large extracellular domain, a transmembrane region, and a sequence-specific cytoplasmic domain [Arai et al., 1990]. The extracellular domains of interleukin-1, interleukin-6, and gamma-interferon are homologous with the immunoglobulin gene superfamily, and weak but significant amino-acid homologies exist among the interleukin-2 (beta chain), IL-6, IL-3, IL-4, erythropoietin, and GM-CSF receptors [Arai et al., 1990].

TABLE 17.4 Hematopoietic Growth Factor Receptor Families

Receptors with homology to the immunoglobulin gene family
Interleukin-1 receptor
Interleukin-6 receptor
Gamma-interferon receptor
Hematopoietic growth factor receptor family
Interleukin-2 receptor (β-chain)
Interleukin-3 receptor
Interleukin-4 receptor
Interleukin-6 receptor
Erythropoietin receptor
G/M-CSF receptor

Source: Modified from Long [1992]. Reprinted with permission.

Like other developing tissues, bone responds to bone-specific and other soluble growth factors. TGF-β is a member of a family of polypeptide growth regulators which affects cell growth and differentiation during developmental processes such as embryogenesis and tissue repair [Sporn and Roberts, 1985]. TGF-β strongly inhibits proliferation of normal and tumor-derived epithelial cells and blocks adipogenesis, myogenesis, and hematopoiesis [Sporn and Roberts, 1985]. However, in bone, TGF-β is a positive regulator. TGF-β is localized in active centers of bone differentiation (cartilage canals and osteocytes) [Massague, 1987], and TGF-β is found in high quantity in bone, suggesting that bone contains the greatest total amount of TGF-β [Gehron Robey et al., 1987; Massague, 1987]. During bone formation, TGF-β promotes chrondrogenesis [Massague, 1987]—an effect presumably related to its ability to stimulate the deposition of extracellular matrix (ECM) components [Ignotz and Massague, 1986]. Besides stimulating cartilage formation, TGF-β is synthesized and secreted in bone cell cultures and stimulates the growth of subconfluent layers of fetal bovine bone cells, thus showing it to be an autocrine regulator of bone cell development [Sporn and Roberts, 1985].

In addition to TGF-β, other growth factors or cytokines are implicated in bone development. Urist and co-workers have been able to isolate various regulatory proteins which function in both *in vivo* and *in vitro* models [Urist et al., 1983b]. Bone morphogenic protein (BMP), originally an extract of demineralized human bone matrix, has now been cloned [Wozney et al., 1988] and, when implanted *in vivo*, results in a sequence of events leading to functional bone formation [Muthukumaran and Reddi, 1985; Wozney et al., 1988]. The implanting of BMP is followed by mesenchymal cell migration to the area of the implant, differentiation into bone progenitor cells, deposition of new bone, and subsequent bone remodeling to allow the establishment of bone marrow [Muthukumaran and Reddi, 1985]. A number of additional growth factors which regulate bone development exist. In particular, bone-derived growth factors (BDGF) stimulate bone cells to proliferate in serum-free media. [Hanamura et al., 1980; Linkhart et al., 1986]. However, these factors seem to function at a different level from BMP [Urist et al., 1983a].

17.3 Extracellular Matrix

The extracellular matrix (ECM) varies in its tissue composition throughout the body and consists of various molecules such as laminin, collagens, proteoglycans, and other glycoproteins [Wicha et al., 1982]. Gospodarowicz and co-workers demonstrated that ECM components greatly affect corneal endothelial cell proliferation *in vitro* [Gospodarowicz et al., 1980; Gospodarowicz and Ill, 1980]. Studies by Reh and co-workers indicate that the ECM protein laminin is involved in inductive interactions which give rise to retinal-pigmented epithelium [Reh and Gretton, 1987]. Likewise, differentiation of mammary epithelial cells is profoundly influenced by ECM components; mammary cell growth *in vivo* and *in vitro* requires type IV collagen [Wicha et al., 1982]. A number of investigations elucidated a role for ECM and its components in hematopoietic cell function. These studies have identified the function of both previously known and newly identified ECM components in hematopoietic cell cytoadhesion (Table 17.5).

TABLE 17.5 Protiens and Glycoprotiens Mediating Hematopoietic Cell–Extracellular Matrix Interactions

Matrix Component	Cell Surface Receptor	Cellular Expression	References
Fibronectin	FnR	Erythroid; BFC-E; B cells; Lymphoid cells; HL60 cells	Patel, 1984, 1986, 1987; Patel et al., 1985; Ryan et al., 1990; Tsai et al., 1987; Van de Water et al., 1988
	IIb/IIIa	Platelets and megakaryocytes	Giancotti et al., 1987
Thrombospondin	TSP-R	Monocytes and platelets	Silverstein and Nachman, 1987; Leung, 1984
		Human CFC	Long and Dixit, 1990
		CFC-GEMM	Long and Dixit, 1990
Hyaluronic acid	CD44	T and B cells	Aruffo et al., 1990, Dorshkind, 1989; Horst et al., 1990; Miyake et al., 1990
		Neutrophils Tumor Cells	
Hemonectin	Unk	CFC-GM, BFC-E Immat. neutr. BFU-E	Campbell et al., 1985, 1987, 1990
Proteoglycans:			
Heparan sulfate	Unk	Bl-CFC	Gordon, 1988; Gordon et al., 1988
Unfract ECM	Unk	Bl-CFC, bm Stroma	Gordon et al., 1988; Campbell et al., 1985

R = receptor; BFC-E = the burst-forming cell-erythrocyte; HL60 = a promyelocytic leukemia cell line; CFC = colony-forming cell; GEMM = granulocyte erythrocyte macrophage megakarocyte; GM = granulocyte/macrophage; unk = unknown; Bl = blast cell; bm = bone marrow. Modified and reprinted from Long [1992] with permission.

As mentioned, soluble factors, stromal cells, and extracellular matrix (the natural substrate surrounding cells *in vivo*) are critical elements of the hematopoietic microenvironment. Work by Wolf and Trenton on the hematopoietic microenvironment *in vivo* provided the first evidence that (still unknown) components of the microenvironment are responsible for the granulocytic predominance of bone marrow hematopoiesis and the erythrocytic predominance of spleen [Wolf and Trentin, 1968]. Dexter and co-workers observed that the *in vitro* development of adherent cell populations is essential for the continued proliferation and differentiation of blood cells in long-term bone marrow cell cultures [Dexter and Lajtha, 1974; Dexter et al., 1976]. These stromal cells elaborate specific ECM components such as laminin, fibronectin, and various collagens and proteoglycans, and the presence of these ECM proteins coincided with the onset of hematopoietic cell proliferation [Zuckerman and Wicha, 1983]. The actual roles for extracellular matrix versus stromal cells in supporting cell development remains somewhat obscure, as it often is difficult to disassociate stromal cell effects from those of the ECM, since stromal cells are universally observed to be enmeshed in the surrounding extracellular matrix.

Bone extracellular matrix contains both collagenous and noncollagenous proteins. A number of non-collagenous matrix proteins, isolated from demineralized bone, are involved in bone formation. Osteonectin is a 32 kDa protein which, binding to calcium, hydroxypatite, and collagen, is felt to initiate nucleation during the mineral phase of bone deposition [Termine et al., 1981]. *In vivo* analysis of osteonectin message reveals its presence in a variety of developing tissues [Holland et al., 1987; Nomura et al., 1988]. However, osteonectin is present in its highest levels in bones of the axial skeleton, skull, and the blood platelet (megakaryocyte) [Nomura et al., 1988]. Bone gla protein (BGP, osteocalcin) is a vitamin K-dependent, 5700 Da calcium-binding bone protein which is specific for bone and may regulate $Ca^2 +$ deposition [Price et al., 1976, 1981; Termine et al., 1981]. Other bone proteins seem to function as cytoadhesion molecules [Oldberg et al., 1986; Somerman et al., 1987] or have unresolved functions [Reddi, 1981]. Moreover, bone ECM also contains a number of the more common mesenchymal growth factors such as PDGF, basic, and acidic fibroblast growth factor [Canalis, 1985; Hauschka et al., 1986; Linkhart et al., 1986; Urist et al., 1983a]. These activities are capable of stimulating the proliferation of mesenchymal target cells (BALB/c 3T3 fibroblasts, capillary endothelial cells, and rat fetal osteoblasts). As well, bone-specific proliferating activities such as the BMP exist in bone ECM. Although these general and specific growth factors undoubtedly play a role in bone formation, little is understood concerning the direct inductive/permissive capacity of bone-ECM or bone proteins themselves on human bone cells or their progenitors. Nor is the role of bone matrix in presenting growth factors understood—such "matricrine" (factor-ECM) interactions may be of fundamental importance in bone cell development.

When bone precursor cells are cultured on certain noncollagenous proteins, they show an increase in proliferation and bone protein expression (MWL, unpublished observation). Moreover, we have shown, using the hematopoietic system as a model, that subpopulations of primitive progenitor cells require both a mitogenic cytokine and a specific extracellular matrix (ECM) molecule in order to proliferate [Long et al., 1992]. Indeed, without this obligate matrix-cytokine ("matricrine") signal, the most primitive of blood precursor cells fail to develop *in vitro* [Long et al., 1992]. Although poorly understood, a similar requirement exists for human bone precursor cells, and complete evaluation of osteogenic development (or that of other tissues) thus requires additional studies of ECM molecules. For example, we have demonstrated the importance of three bone ECM proteins in human bone cell growth: osteonectin, osteocalcin, and type I collagen [Long et al., 1990, 1994]. Additional bone proteins such as bone sialo-protien and osteopontin are no doubt important to bone structure and function, but their role is unknown [Nomura et al., 1988; Oldberg et al., 1986].

The above observations on the general and specific effects of ECM on cell development have identified certain matrix components which seem to appear as a recurrent theme in tissue development. These are proteoglycans, thrombospondin, fibronectin, and the collagens.

Proteoglycans and Glycosaminoglycans

Studies on the role of proteoglycans in blood cell development indicate that both hematopoietic cells [Minguell and Tavassoli, 1989] (albeit as demonstrated by cell lines) and marrow stromal cells [Gallagher et al., 1983; Kirby and Bentley, 1987; Spooncer et al., 1983; Wight et al., 1986] produce various proteoglycans. Proteoglycans (PG) are polyanionic macromolecules located both on the stromal cell surface and within the extracellular matrix. They consist of a core protein containing a number of covalently linked glycosaminoglycan (GAG) side chains, as well as one or more O- or N-linked oligosaccharides. The GAGs consist of nonbranching chains of repeating *N*-acetylglucosamine or *N*-acetylglactosamine disaccharide units. With the exception of hyaluronic acid, all glycosaminoglycans are sulfated. Interesting, many extracellular matrix molecules (fibronectin, laminin, and collagen) contain glycosaminoglycan-binding sites, suggesting that complex interactions occur within the matrix itself.

Proteoglycans play a role in both cell proliferation and differentiation. Murine stromal cells produce hyaluronic acid, heparan sulfate, and chondroitin sulfate [Gallagher et al., 1983], and *in vitro* studies show PG to be differentially between stromal cell surfaces and the media, with heparan sulfate being the primary cell-surface molecule and chondroitin sulfate the major molecular species in the aqueous phase [Spooncer et al., 1983]. In contrast to murine cultures, the human hematopoietic stromal cells *in vitro* contain small amounts of heparan sulfate and large amounts of dermatin and chondroitin sulfate, which seem to be equally distributed between the aqueous phase and extracellular matrix [Wight et al., 1986]. The stimulation of proteoglycan/GAG synthesis is associated with an increased hematopoietic cell proliferation, as demonstrated by an increase in the percentage of cells in S-phase [Spooncer et al., 1983]. Given the general diversity of proteoglycans, it is reasonable to expect that they may encode both lineage-specific and organ-specific information. For example, organ-specific PGs stimulate differentiation, as marrow-derived ECM directly stimulates differentiation of human progranulocytic cells (HL60), whereas matrix derived from skin fibroblasts lacks this inductive capacity [Luikart et al., 1987]. Moreover, organ-specific effects are seen in studies of human blood precursor cell adhesion to marrow-derived heparan sulfate but not to heparan sulfates isolated from bovine kidney [Gordon et al., 1988].

Interestingly, cell-surface-associated PGs are involved in the compartmentalization or localization of growth factors within the microenvironment. Thus, the proliferation of hematopoietic cells in the presence of hematopoietic stroma is associated with a glycosaminoglycan-bound growth factor (GM-CSF) [Gordon et al., 1987b], and determination of the precise GAG molecules involved in this process (i.e., heparan sulfate) has showed that heparan sulfate side chains bind two blood cell growth factors: GM-CSF and interleukin-3 [Roberts et al., 1988]. These data imply that ECM components and growth factors combine to yield lineage-specific information and indicate that, when PG- or GAG-bound, growth factor is presented to the progenitor cells in a biologically active form.

Thrombospondin (TSP)

Thrombospondin is a large, trimeric disulfide-linked glycoprotein (molecular weight 450,000, subunit molecular weight 180,000) having a domainlike structure [Frazier, 1987]. Its protease-resistant domains are involved in mediating various TSP functions such as cell binding and binding of other extracellular matrix proteins [Frazier, 1987]. Thrombospondin is synthesized and secreted into extracellular matrix by most cells; for review, see Lawler [1986] and Frazier [1987]. Matrix-bound TSP is necessary for cell adhesion [Varian et al., 1986], cell growth [Majack et al., 1986], and carcinoma invasiveness [Riser et al., 1988] and is differentially expressed during murine embryogenesis [O'Shea and Dixit, 1988].

Work from our laboratories shows that thrombospondin functions within the hematopoietic microenvironment as a cytoadhesion protein for a subpopulation of human hematopoietic progenitor cells [Long et al., 1992; Long and Dixit, 1990]. Interestingly, immunocytochemical metabolic labeling studies show that hematopoietic cells (both normal marrow cells and leukemic cell lines) synthesize TSP, deposit it within the ECM, and are attached to it. The attachment of human progenitor cells to thrombospondin is not mediated by its integrin-binding RGD sequence because this region of the TSP molecule is cryptic, residing within the globular carboxy-terminus of the molecule. Thus, excess concentrations of a tetrapeptide containing the RGD sequence did not inhibit attachment of human progenitor cells [Long and Dixit, 1990], and similar observations exist in other cell systems [Asch et al., 1987; Roberts et al., 1987; Varian et al., 1988]. Other studies from this author's laboratories show that bone marrow ECM also plays a major role in hematopoiesis in that complex ECM extracts greatly augment LTBMC cell proliferation [Campbell et al., 1985] and that marrow-derived ECM contains specific cytoadhesion molecules [Campbell et al., 1987, 1990; Long et al., 1990, 1992; Long and Dixit, 1990].

Fibronectin

Fibronectin is a ubiquitous extracellular matrix molecule that is known to be involved in the attachment of paryenchymal cells to stromal cells [Bentley and Tralka, 1983; Zuckerman and Wicha, 1983]. As with TSP, hematopoietic cells synthesize, deposit, and bind to fibronectin [Zuckerman and Wicha, 1983]. Extensive work by Patel and co-workers shows that erythroid progenitor cells attach to fibronectin in a developmentally regulated manner [Patel et al., 1985; Patel and Lodish, 1984, 1986, 1987]. In addition to cells of the erythroid lineage, fibronectin is capable of binding lymphoid precursor cells and other cell phenotypes [Bernardi et al., 1987; Giancotti et al., 1986]. Structurally, cells adhere to two distinct regions of the fibronectin molecule, one of which contains the RGD sequence; the other is within the carboxy terminal region and contains a high-affinity binding site for heparan [Bernardi et al., 1987].

Collagen

The role of various collagens in blood cell development remains uncertain. *In vitro* marrow cells produce types I, III, IV, and V collagen [Bentley, 1982; Bentley and Foidart, 1981; Castro-Malaspina et al., 1980; Zuckerman and Wicha, 1983], suggesting a role for these extracellular matrix components in the maintenance of hematopoiesis. Consistent with this, inhibition of collagen synthesis with 6-hydroxyprolene blocks or reduces hematopoiesis *in vitro* [Zuckerman et al., 1985]. Type I collagen is the major protein of bone, comprising approximately 90% of its protein.

17.4 Considerations for *ex Vivo* Tissue Generation

The microenvironmental complexities discussed above suggest that the *ex vivo* generation of human (replacement) tissue (e.g., marrow, liver) will be a difficult process. However, many of the needed tissues (liver, marrow, bone, and kidney) have a degree of regenerative or hyperplastic capacity which allows their *in vitro* cultivation. Thus, *in vivo* growth of many of these tissues types is routinely performed, albeit at varying degrees of success. The best example of this is bone marrow. If unfractionated human bone marrow is established in culture, the stromal and hematopoietic cells attempt to recapitulate *in vivo* hematopoiesis. Both soluble factors and ECM proteins are produced [Dexter and Spooncer, 1987; Long and Dixit, 1990; Zuckerman and Wicha, 1983], and relatively long-term hematopoiesis occurs. However, if long-term bone marrow cultures are examined closely, they turn out to not faithfully reproduce the *in vivo* microenvironment [Dexter and Spooncer, 1987; Spooncer et al., 1985; Schofield and Dexter, 1985]. Over a period of 8–12 weeks (for human cultures) or 3–6 months (for murine cultures), cell proliferation ceases, and the stromal/hematopoietic cells die. Moreover, the pluripotentiality of these cultures is rapidly lost. In vivo, bone marrow produces a wide variety of cells (erythroid, megakaryocyte/platelet, four types of myeloid cells, and B-lymphocytes). Human long-term marrow cultures produce granulocytes and megakaryocytes for 1–3 weeks, and erythropoiesis is seen only if exogenous growth factors are added. Thereafter, the cultures produce granulocytes and macrophages. These data show that current culture conditions are inadequate and further suggest that other factors such as rate of fluid exchange (perfusion) or that the three-dimensional structure of these cultures is limiting.

Recent work by Emerson, Palsson, and colleagues demonstrated the effectiveness of altered medium exchange rates in the expansion of blood cells *in vitro* [Caldwell et al., 1991; Schwartz et al., 1991a, 1991b]. These studies showed that a daily 50% medium exchange affected stromal cell metabolism and stimulated a transient increase in growth factor production [Caldwell et al., 1991]. As well, these cultures underwent a 10-fold expansion of cell numbers [Schwartz et al., 1991b]. While impressive, these cultures nonetheless decayed after 10–12 weeks. Recently, this group utilized continuous-perfusion bioreactors to achieve a longer *ex vivo* expansion and showed a 10 to 20-fold expansion of specific progenitor cell types [Koller et al., 1993]. These studies demonstrate that bioreactor technology allows significant expansion of cells, presumably via better mimicry of *in vivo* conditions.

Another aspect of tissue formation is the physical structure of the developing organ. Tissues exist as three-dimensional structures. Thus, the usual growth in tissue culture flasks is far removed from the *in vivo* setting. Essentially, cells grown *in vitro* proliferate at a liquid/substratum interface. As a result, primary tissue cells grow until they reach confluence and then cease proliferating, a process known as *contact inhibition*. This, in turn, severely limits the degree of total cellularity of the system. For example, long-term marrow cultures (which do not undergo as precise a contact inhibition as do cells from solid tissues) reach a density of $1–2 \times 10^6$ per milliliter. This is three orders of magnitude less than the average bone marrow density *in vivo*. A number of technologies have been applied to this three-dimensional growth problem (e.g., hollow fibers). However, the growth of cells on or in a nonphysiologic matrix is less than optimal in terms of replacement tissue, since such implants trigger a type of immune reaction (foreign body reaction) or are thrombogenic.

Recently, another type of bioreactor has been used to increase the *ex vivo* expansion of cells. Rotating wall vessels are designed to result in constant, low-shear suspension of tissue cells during their development. These bioreactors thus simulate a microgravity environment. The studies of Goodwin and associates document a remarkable augmentation of mesenchymal cell proliferation in low-shear bioreactors. Their data show that mesenchymal cell types show an average three- to sixfold increase in cell density in these bioreactors, reaching a cellularity of approximately 10^7 cells/ml [Goodwin et al., 1993a, 1993b]. Importantly, this increase in cell density was associated with a 75% reduction in glucose utilization as well as an approximate 85% reduction in the enzymatic markers of anabolic cellular metabolism (SGOT and LDH) [Goodwin et al., 1993a]. Importantly, further work by Goodwin and colleagues shows that the growth of mesenchymal cells (kidney and chondrocyte) under low-shear conditions leads to the formation of tissuelike cell aggregates which is enhanced by growing these cells on collagen-coated microcarriers [Duke et al., 1993; Goodwin et al., 1993a].

The physical requirements for optimal bone precursor cell (i.e., osteoprogenitor cells and preosteoblasts) proliferation both *in vivo* and *ex vivo* are poorly understood. *In vivo*, bone formation most often occurs within an intervening cartilage model (i.e., a three-dimensional framework referred to as endochondral ossification). This well-understood bone histogenesis is one of embryonic and postnatal chondrogenesis, which accounts for the shape of bone and the subsequent modification and calcification of bone cell ECM by osteoblasts. Recent work in this laboratory has examined the physical requirements for bone cell growth. When grown in suspension cultures (liquid/substratum interface), bone precursor cells develop distinct, clonal foci. These cells, however, express low amounts of bone-related proteins, and they rapidly expand as "sheets" of proliferating cells. As these are nontransformed (i.e., primary) cells, they grow until they reach confluence and then undergo contact inhibition and cease proliferating. We reasoned that growing these cells in a three-dimensional gel might augment their development. It is known from other systems that progenitor cell growth and development in many tissues requires the presence of at least one mitogenic growth factor, and that progenitor cell growth in a three-dimensional matrix results in the clonal formation of cell colonies by restricting the outgrowth of differentiated progeny [Metcalf, 1989]. Thus, bone precursor cells were overlayered with chemically defined, serum-free media containing a biopolymer, thus providing the cells with a three-dimensional scaffold in which to proliferate. In sharp contrast to bone precursor cell growth at a planar liquid/substratum interface, cells grown in a three-dimensional polymer gel show a marked increase in proliferative capacity and an increased per-cell production of the bone-specific proteins (MWL, unpublished observations).

17.5 Conclusions and Perspectives

As elegantly demonstrated by the composite data above, the molecular basis and function of the various components of tissue microenvironments are becoming well understood. However, much remains to be learned regarding the role of these and other, as yet unidentified molecules in tissue development. One of the intriguing questions to be asked is how each interacting molecule contributes to defining the molecular basis of a given microenvironment—for example, the distinct differences in hematopoiesis as it exists in the marrow versus the spleen (i.e., a predominance granulopoiesis and erythropoiesis, respectively) [Wolf and Trentin, 1968]. Another rapidly advancing area is the dissection of the molecular basis of cell trafficking into tissues. Again, the immune system offers for the assessment of this process. Thus, interaction of the lymphocyte receptors with specific glycoconjugates of vascular addressins [Goldstein et al., 1989; Idzerda et al., 1989; Lasky et al., 1989] suggests that similar recognition systems are involved in other tissues, particularly the bone marrow. Another interesting observation is that hematopoietic progenitor cells synthesize and bind to their own cytoadhesion molecules, independent of the matrix molecules contributed by the stromal cells. For example, developing cells *in vitro* synthesize and attach to fibronectin, thrombospondin, and hemonectin, suggesting that these molecules function solely in an autochthonous manner to localize or perhaps stimulate development. Such a phenomenon may be a generalized process, as we have noted similar patterns of ECM expression/attachment in osteopoietic cell cultures. Coupled with data from the bioreactor studies, this suggests that under appropriate biology/physical conditions tissue cells may spontaneously reestablish their structure. Finally, the elucidation of the various requirements for optimal progenitor cell growth (cell interactions, specific growth factors and matrix components, and/or accessory cells which supply them) should allow the improvement of *ex vivo* culture systems to yield an environment in which tissue reconstitution is possible. Such a system would have obvious significance in organ-replacement therapy.

References

Arai K, Lee F, Miyajima A, et al. 1990. Cytokines: Coordinators of immune and inflammatory responses. Annu Rev Biochem 59:783.

Aruffo A, Staminkovic I, Melnik M, et al. 1990. CD44 is the principal cell surface receptor for hyaluronate. Cell 61:1303.

Asch AS, Barnwell J, Silverstein RL, et al. 1987. Isolation of the thrombospondin membrane receptor. J Clin Invest 79:1054.

Bentley SA. 1982. Collagen synthesis by bone marrow stromal cells: A quantitative study. Br J Haematol 50:491.

Bentley SA, Froidart JM. 1981. Some properties of marrow derived adherent cells in tissue culture. Blood 56:1006.

Bentley SA, Tralka TS. 1983. Fibronectin-mediated attachment of hematopoietic cells to stromal elements in continuous bone marrow cultures. Exp Hematol 11:129.

Bernardi P, Patel VP, Lodish HF. 1987. Lymphoid precursor cells adhere to two different sites on fibronectin. J Cell Biol 105:489.

Bevilacqua MP, Stengelin S, Gimbrone MA, et al. 1989. Endothelial leukocyte adhesion molecule 1: An inducible receptor for neutrophils related to complement regulatory proteins and lectins. Science 243:1160.

Bierer BE, Sleckman BP, Ratnofsky SE, et al. 1989. The biologic roles of CD2, CD4, and CD8 in T-cell activation. Annu Rev Immunol 7:579.

Brandley BK, Sweidler SJ, Robbins PW. 1990. Charbohydrate ligands of the LEC cell adhesion molecules. Cell 63:861.

Caldwell J, Palsson PB, Locey B, et al. 1991. Culture perfusion schedules influence the metabolic activity and granulocyte-macrophage colony-stimulating factor production rates of human bone marrow stromal cells. J Cell Physiol 147:344.

Campbell A, Sullenberger B, Bahou W, et al. 1990. Hemonectin: A novel hematopoietic adhesion molecule. Prog Clin Biol Res 352:97.

Campbell A, Wicha MS, Long MW. 1985. Extracellular matrix promotes the growth and differentiation of murine hematopoietic cells in vitro. J Clin Invest 75:2085.

Campbell AD, Long MW, Wicha MS. 1987. Haemonectin, a bone marrow adhesion protein specific for cells of granuolocyte lineage. Nature 329:744.

Campbell AD, Long MW, Wicha MS. 1990. Developmental regulation of granulocytic cell binding to hemonectin. Blood 76:1758.

Canalis E. 1985. Effect of growth factors on bone cell replication and differentiation. Clin Orthop Rel Res 193:246.

Castro-Malaspina H, Gay RE, Resnick G, et al. 1980. Characterization of human bone marrow fibroblast colony-forming cells and their progeny. Blood 56:289.

Coulombel L, Vuillet MH, Tchernia G. 1988. Lineage- and stage-specific adhesion of human hematopoietic progenitor cells to extracellular matrices from marrow fibroblasts. Blood 71:329.

Dexter TM. 1982. Stromal cell associated haemopoiesis. J Cell Physiol 1:87.

Dexter TM, Allen TD, Lajtha LG. 1976. Conditions controlling the proliferation of haemopoietic stem cells in vitro. J Cell Physiol 91:335.

Dexter TM, Lajtha LG. 1974. Proliferation of haemopoietic stem cells in vitro. Br J Haematol 28:525.

Dexter TM, Spooncer E. 1987. Growth and differentiation in the hemopoietic system. Annu Rev Cell Biol 3:423.

Dorshkind K. 1989. Hemopoietic stem cells and B-lymphocyte differentiation. Immunol Today 10:399.

Duke PJ, Danne EL, Montufar-Solis D. 1993. Studies of chondrogenesis in rotating systems. J Cell Biochem 51:274.

Frazier WA. 1987. Thrombospondin: A modular adhesive glycoprotein of platelets and nucleated cells. J Cell Biol 105:625.

Gallagher JT, Spooncer E, Dexter TM. 1983. Role of the cellular matrix in haemopoiesis: I. Synthesis of glycosaminoglycans by mouse bone marrow cell cultures. J Cell Sci 63:155.

Gallatin M, St John TP, Siegleman M, et al. 1986. Lymphocyte homing receptors. Cell 44:673.

Gehron Robey P, Young MF, Flanders KC, et al. 1987. Osteoblasts synthesize and respond to transforming growth factor-type beta (TGF-beta) in vitro. J Cell Biol 105:457.

Giancotti FG, Comoglio PM, Tarone G. 1986. Fibronectin-plasma membrane interaction in the adhesion of hemopoietic cells. J Cell Biol 103:429.

Giancotti FG, Languino LR, Zanetti A, et al. 1987. Platelets express a membrane protein complex immunologically related to the fibroblast fibronectin receptor and distinct from GPIIb/IIIa. Blood 69:1535.

Giancotti FG, Ruoslahti E. 1990. Elevated levels of the alpha 5 beta 1 fibronectin receptor suppress the transformed phenotype of Chinese hamster ovary cells. Cell 60:849.

Goelz SE, Hession C. Goff D, et al. 1990. ELFT: A gene that directs the expression of an ELAM-1 ligand. Cell 63:1349.

Goldstein LA, Zhou DF, Picker LJ, et al. 1989. A human lymphocyte homing receptor, the hermes antigen, is related to cartilage proteoglycan core and link proteins. Cell 56:1063.

Goodwin TJ, Prewett TI, Wolf DA, et al. 1993a. Reduced shear stress: A major component in the ability of mammalian tissues to form three-dimensional assemblies in simulated microgravity. J Cell Biochem 51:301.

Goodwin TJ, Schroeder WF, Wolf DA, et al. 1993b. Rotating vessel coculture of small intestine as a prelude to tissue modeling: Aspects of simulated microgravity. Proc Soc Exp Biol Med 202:181.

Gordon MY. 1988. The origin of stromal cells in patients treated by bone marrow transplantation. Bone Marrow Transplant 3:247.

Gordon MY, Bearpark AD, Clarke D, et al. 1990a. Haemopoietic stem cell subpopulations in mouse and man: Discrimination by differential adherence and marrow repopulation ability. Bone Marrow Transplant 5:6.

Gordon MY, Clarke D, Atkinson J, et al. 1990b. Hemopoietic progenitor cell binding to the stromal microenvironment in vitro. Exp Hematol 18:837.

Gordon MY, Dowding CR, Riley GP, et al. 1987a. Characterization of stroma-dependent blast colony-forming cells in human marrow. J Cell Physiol 130:150.

Gordon MY, Hibbin JA, Dowding C, et al. 1985. Separation of human blast progenitors from granulocytic, erythroid, megakaryocytic, and mixed colony-forming cells by "panning" on cultured marrow-derived stromal layers. Exp Hematol 13:937.

Gordon MY, Riley GP, Clarke D. 1988. Heparan sulfate is necessary for adhesive interactions between human early hemopoietic progenitor cells and the extracellular matrix of the marrow microenvironment. Leukemia 2:804.

Gordon MY, Riley GP, Watt SM, et al. 1987b. Compartmentalization of a haematopoietic growth factor (GM-CSF) by glycosaminoglycans in the bone marrow microenvironment. Nature 326:403.

Gospodarowicz D, Delgado D, Vlodasvsky I. 1980. Permissive effect of the extracellular matrix on cell proliferation in vitro. Proc Natl Acad Sci USA 77:4094.

Gospodarowicz D, Ill C. 1980. Extracellular matrix and control of proliferation of vascular endothelial cells. J Clin Invest 65:1351.

Hanamura H, Higuchi Y, Nakagawa M, et al. 1980. Solubilization and purification of bone morphogenetic protein (BMP) from Dunn osteosarcoma. Clin Orthop Rel Res 153:232.

Hauschka PV, Marvrakos AE, Iafarati MD, et al. 1986. Growth factors in bone matrix: Isolation of multiple types by affinity chromatography on heparinsepharose. J Biol Chem 261:12665.

Holland PWH, Harmper SJ, McVey JH, et al. 1987. In vivo expression of mRNA for the Ca++-binding protein SPARC (osteonectin) revealed by in situ hybridization. J Cell Biol 105:473.

Horst E, Meijer CJML, Radaskiewicz T, Ossekoppele GP, VanKrieken JHJM, Pals ST. 1990. Adhesion molecules in the prognosis of diffuse large-cell lymphoma: expression of a lymphocyte homing receptor (CD44), LFA-1 (CD11a/18), and ICAM-1 (CD54). Leukemia 4:595-599.

Idzerda RL, Carter WG, Nottenburg C, et al. 1989. Isolation and DNA sequence of a cDNA clone encoding a lymphocyte adhesion receptor for high endothelium. Proc Natl Acad Sci USA 86:4659.

Ignotz RA, Massague J. 1986. Transforming growth factor-beta stimulates the expression of fibronectin and collagen and their incorporation into the extracellular matrix. J Biol Chem 261:4337.

Kirby SL, Bentley SA. 1987. Proteoglycan synthesis in two murine bone marrow stromal cell lines. Blood 70:1777.

Koller MR, Emerson SG, Palsson BO. 1993. Large-scale expansion of human stem and progenitor cells from bone marrow mononuclear cells in continuous perfusion cultures. Blood 82:378.

Lasky LA, Singer MS, Yednock TA, et al. 1989. Cloning of a lymphocyte homing receptor reveals a lectin domain. Cell 56:1045.

Lawler J. 1986. The structural and functional properties of thrombospondin. Blood 67:1197-1209.

Lawrence MB, Springer TA. 1991. Leukocytes roll on a selectin at physiologic shear flow rates: Distinction from and prerequisite for adhesion through integrins. Cell 65:859.

Leung LLK. 1984. Role of thrombospondin in platelet aggregation. J Clin Invest 74:1764.

Liesveld JL, Abbound CN, Duerst RE, et al. 1989. Characterization of human marrow stromal cells: Role in progenitor cell binding and granulopoiesis. Blood 73:1794.

Linkhart TA, Jennings JC, Mohan S, et al. 1986. Characterization of mitogenic activities extracted from bovine bone matrix. Bone 7:479.

Long, MW. 1992. Blood cell cytoadhesion molecules. Exp Hematol 20:288.

Long MW, Ashcraft A, Mann KG. 1994. Regulation of human bone marrow-derived osteoprogenitor cells by osteogenic growth factors. Submitted.

Long MW, Briddell R, Walter AW, et al. 1992. Human hematopoietic stem cell adherence to cytokines and matrix molecules. J Clin Invest 90:251.

Long MW, Dixit VM. 1990. Thrombospondin functions as a cytoadhesion molecule for human hematopoietic progenitor cells. Blood 75:2311.

Long MW, Mann KG. 1993. Bone marrow as a source of osteoprogenitor cells. In MW Long, MS Wicha (eds), The Hematopoietic Microenvironment, pp 110–123, Baltimore, Johns Hopkins University Press.

Long MW, Williams JL, Mann KG. 1990. Expression of bone-related proteins in the human hematopoietic microenvironment. J Clin Invest 86:1387.

Lowe JB, Stoolman LM, Nair RP, et al. 1990. ELAM-1-dependent cell adhesion to vascular endothelium determined by a transfected human fucosyl transferase cDNA. Cell 63:475.

Luikart SD, Sackrison JL, Maniglia CA. 1987. Bone marrow matrix modulation of HL-60 phenotype. Blood 70:1119.

Majack RA, Cook SC, Bornstein P. 1986. Control of smooth muscle cell growth by components of the extracellular matrix: Autocrine role for the thrombospondin. Proc Natl Acad Sci USA 83:9050.

Massague J. 1987. The TGF-beta family of growth and differentiation factors. Cell 49:437.

Metcalf D. 1989. The molecular control of cell division, differentiation commitment and maturation in haematopoietic cells. Nature 339:27.

Minguell JJ, Tavassoli M. 1989. Proteoglycan synthesis by hematopoietic progenitor cells. Blood 73:1821.

Miyake K, Medina KL, Hayashi S, et al. 1990. Monoclonal antibodies to Pgp-1/CD44 block lymph-hemopoiesis in long-term bone marrow cultures. J Exp Med 171:477.

Miyake K, Weissman IL, Greenberger JS, et al. 1991. Evidence for a role of the integrin VLA-4 in lympho-hematopoiesis. J Exp Med 173:599.

Miyamake K, Medina K, Ishihara K, et al. 1991. A VCAM-like adhesion molecule on murine bone marrow stromal cells mediates binding of lymphocyte precursors in culture. J Cell Biol 114:557.

Muthukumaran N, Reddi AH. 1985. Bone matrix-induced local bone induction. Clin Orthop Rel Res 200:159.

Nomura S, Wills AJ, Edwards DR, et al. 1988. Developmental expression of 2ar (osteopontin) and SPARC (osteonectin) RNA as revealed by in situ hybridization. J Cell Biol 106:441.

O'Shea KS, Dixit VM. 1988. Unique distribution of the extracellular matrix component thrombospondin in the developing mouse embryo. J Cell Biol 107:2737.

Oldberg A, Franzen A, Heinegard D. 1986. Cloning and sequence analysis of rat bone sialoprotein (osteopontin) cDNA reveals an Arg-Gly-Asp cell-binding sequence. Proc Natl Acad Sci USA 83:8819.

Palacios R, Stuber S, Rolink A. 1989. The epigenetic influences of bone marrow and fetal liver stroma cells on the developmental potential of pre-B lymphocyte clones. Eur J Immunol 19:347.

Patel VP, Ciechanover A, Platt O, et al. 1985. Mammalian reticulocytes lose adhesion to fibronectin during maturation to erythrocytes. Proc Natl Acad Sci USA 82:440.

Patel VP, Lodish HF. 1984. Loss of adhesion of murine erythroleukemia cells to fibronectin during erythroid differentiation. Science 224:996.

Patel VP, Lodish HF. 1986. The fibronectin receptor on mammalian erythroid precursor cells: Characterization and developmental regulation. J Cell Biol 102:449.

Patel VP, Lodish HF, 1987. A fibronectin matrix is required for differentiation of murine erythroleukemia cells into reticulocytes. J Cell Biol 105:3105.

Ploemacher RE, Brons NHC. 1988. Isolation of hemopoietic stem cell subsets from murine bone marrow: II. Evidence for an early precursor of day-12 CFU-S and cells associated with radioprotective ability. Exp Hematol 16:27.

Price PA, Ostuka AS, Poser JW, et al. 1976. Characterization of a gamma-carboxyglutamic acid-containing protein from bone, Proc Natl Acad Sci USA 73:1447.

Price PA, Lothringer JW, Baukol SA, et al. 1981. Developmental appearance of the vitamin K-dependent protein of one during calcification. Analysis of mineralizing tissues in human, calf, and rat. J Biol Chem 256:3781.

Reddi AH. 1981. Cell biology and biochemistry of endochondral bone development. Coll Res 1:209.

Reh TA, Gretton H. 1987. Retinal pigmented epithelial cells induced to transdifferentiate to neurons by laminin. Nature 330:68.

Riser BL, Varani J, Carey TE, et al. 1988. Thrombospondin binding and thrombospondin synthesis by human squamous carcinoma and melanoma cells: Relationship to biological activity. Exp Cell Res 174:319.

Roberts DD, Sherwood JA, Ginsburg V. 1987a. Platelet thrombospondin mediates attachment and spreading of human melanoma cells. J Cell Biol 104:131.

Roberts RA, Spooncer E, Parkinson EK, et al. 1987b. Metabolically inactive 3T3 cells can substitute for marrow stromal cells to promote the proliferation and development of multipotent haemopoietic stem cells. J Cell Physiol 132:203.

Roberts R, Gallagher J, Spooncer E, et al. 1988. Heparan sulphate bound growth factors: A mechanism for stromal cell mediated haemopoiesis. Nature 332:376.

Ruoslahti E, Pierschbacher MD. 1987. New perspectives in cell adhesion: RGD and integrins. Science 238:491.

Ryan DH, Nuccie Bl, Abbound CN, et al. 1990. Maturation-dependent adhesion of human B cell precursors to the bone marrow microenvironment. J Immunol 145:477.

Schofield R, Dexter TM. 1985. Studies on the self-renewal ability of CFU-S which have been serially transferred in long-term culture or in vivo. Leuk Res 9:305.

Schwartz RM, Emerson SG, Clarke MF, et al. 1991a. In vitro myelopoiesis stimulated by rapid medium exchange and supplementation with hematopoietic growth factors. Blood 78:3155.

Schwartz RM, Palsson BO, Emerson SG. 1991b. Rapid medium perfusion rate significantly increases the productivity and longevity of human bone marrow cultures. Proc Natl Acad Sci USA 88:6760.

Shaw S, Luce GE, Quinones R, et al. 1986. Two antigen-independent adhesion pathways used by human cytotoxic T-cell clones. Nature 323:262.

Sheetz MP, Turney S, Qian H, et al. 1989. Nanometre-level analysis demonstrates that lipid flow does not drive membrane glycoprotein movements. Nature 340:248.

Silverstein RL, Nachman RL. 1987. Thrombospondin binds to monocytes-macrophages and mediates platelet-monocyte adhesion. J Clin Invest 79:867.

Somerman MJ, Prince CW, Sauk JJ, et al. 1987. Mechanism of fibroblast attachment to bone extracellular matrix: Role of a 44kilodalton bone phosphoprotein. J Bone Miner Res 2:259.

Sits H, van Schooten W, Keizer H, et al. 1986. Alloantigen recognition is preceded by nonspecific adhesion of cytotoxic T cells and target cells. Science 232:403.

Spooncer E, Gallagher JT, Krizsa F, et al. 1983. Regulation of haemopoiesis in long-term bone marrow cultures: IV. Glycosaminoglycan synthesis and the stimulation of haemopoiesis by beta-D-xylosides. J Cell Biol 96:510.

Spooncer E, Lord BI, Dexter TM. 1985. Defective ability to self-renew in vitro of highly purified primitive haematopoietic cells. Nature 316:62.

Sporn MB, Roberts AB. 1985. Autocrine growth factors and cancer. Nature 313:745.

Springer TA. 1990. Adhesion receptors of the immune system. Nature 346:425.

Stoolman LM. 1989. Adhesion molecules controlling lymphocyte migration. Cell 56:907.

Termine JD, Kleinman HK, Whison SW, et al. 1981. Osteonectin, a bone-specific protein linking mineral to collagen. Cell 26:99.

Tsai S, Sieff CA, Nathan DG. 1986. Stromal cell-associated erythropoiesis. Blood 67:1418.

Tsai S, Patel V, Beaumont E, et al. 1987. Differential binding of erythroid and myeloid progenitors to fibroblasts and fibronectin. Blood 69:1587.

Urist MR, DeLange RJ, Finerman GAM. 1983a. Bone cell differentiation and growth factors. Science 220:680.

Urist MR, Sato K, Brownell AG, et al. 1983b. Human bone morphogenic protein (hBMP). Proc Soc Exp Biol Med 173:194.

Van de Water L, Aronson D, Braman V. 1988. Alteration of fibronectin receptors (integrins) in phorbol ester-treated human promonocytic leukemia cells. Cancer Res 48:5730.

Varani J, Dixit VM, Fligiel SEG, et al. 1986. Thrombospondin-induced attachment and spreading of human squamous carcinoma cells. Exp Cell Res 156:1.

Varani J, Nickloff BJ, Risner BL, et al. 1988. Thrombospondin-induced adhesion of human kertinocytes. J Clin Invest 81:1537.

Wicha MS, Lowrie G, Kohn E, et al. 1982. Extracellular matrix promotes mammary epithelial growth and differentiation in vitro. Proc Natl Acad Sci USA 79:3213.

Wight TN, Kinsella MG, Keating A, et al. 1986. Proteoglycans in human long-term bone marrow cultures: Biochemical and ultrastructural analyses. Blood 67:1333.

Williams AF, Barclay AN. 1988. The immunoglobulin superfamily—domains for cell surface recognition. Annu Rev Immunol 6:381.

Witte PL, Robbinson M, Henley A, et al. 1987. Relationships between B-lineage lymphocytes and stromal cells in long-term bone marrow cultures. Eur J Immunol 17:1473.

Wolf NS, Trentin JJ. 1968. Hemopoietic colony studies: V. Effect of hemopoietic organ stroma on differentiation of pluripotent stem cells. J Exp Med 127:205.

Wozney JM, Rosen V, Celeste AJ, et al. 1988. Novel regulators of bone formation: Molecular clones and activities. Science 242:1528.

Yamazaki K, Roberts RA, Spooncer E, et al. 1989. Cellular interactions between 3T3 cells and interleukin-3-dependent multipotent haemopoietic cells: A model system for stromal-cell-mediated haemopoiesis. J Cell Physiol 139:301.

Zuckerman KS, Rhodes RK, Goodrum DD, et al. 1985. Inhibition of collagen deposition in the extra cellular matrix prevents the establishment of a stroma supportive of hematopoiesis in long-term murine bone marrow cultures. J Clin Invest 75:970.

Zuckerman KS, Wicha MS. 1983. Extracellular matrix production by the adherent cells of long-term murine bone marrow cultures. Blood 61:540.

18

The Importance of Stromal Cells

Brian A. Naughton
Advanced Tissue Sciences, Inc.

All tissue is composed of *parenchymal* (from Greek, *that poured in beside*) and *stromal* (Greek, *framework or foundation*) cells. Parenchyma are the functional cells of a tissue (e.g., for liver, hepatic parenchymal cells or hepatocytes; for bone marrow, hematopoietic cells), where stroma comprises primarily connective tissue elements which, together with their products, form the structural framework of tissue. Parenchymal cells can be derivatives of any of the three germ layers, and during development they usually grow into areas populated by stromal cells or their progenitors. Under the strictest definition, stromal cells are derivatives of mesenchyme and include fibroblasts, osteogenic cells, myofibroblasts, and fat cells which appear to arise from a common stem/progenitor cell [Friedenstein et al., 1970; Owen, 1988] (Fig. 18.1). Some investigators apply the term *stromal cell* to all the nonparenchymal cells that contribute to the microenvironment of a tissue and include endothelial cells and macrophages (histiocytes) in this classification as well [Strobel et al., 1986]. However, the ontogeny of both endothelial cells and macrophages is distinct from that of mesenchymal tissue-derived cells [Wilson, 1983]. In this chapter, the more expansive definition of stroma will be used. A partial listing of tissue cells that may influence the function of organ parenchyma is in Table 18.1. For the sake of brevity, migrating cells of bone marrow origin will not be discussed in the text (e.g., mast cells, B lymphocytes, natural killer cells), although these cells can influence parenchyma either directly or via cytokine-mediated modulation of stromal cell function.

Stromal and parenchymal cell components are integrated to form a multifunctional tissue *in vivo*. This chapter will focus on the contribution of stromal cells to the microenvironment and their use in culture to support parenchymal function.

18.1   Tissue Composition and Stromal Cells

Some similarities in the spatial organization of cells of different tissues are apparent. Epithelial cells are a protective and regulatory barrier not just for skin but for all surfaces exposed to blood or to the external environment (e.g., respiratory tract, tubular digestive tract). These cells rest atop a selectively permeable

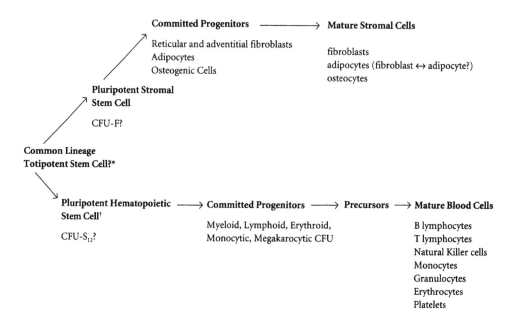

FIGURE 18.1 Hypothetical relationship between the ontogeny of stromal and parenchymal (hematopoietic) cells of the bone marrow. Note that stromal cell is defined in this chart as only those cells that are derivatives of mesenchyme. Hematopoietic stem and progenitor cells express CD 34. This epitope also is expressed by stromal cell precursors (CFU-F) [Simmons and Torok-Storb, 1991] and adherent stromal cells develop from cell populations selected for the CD 34 antigen. In addition, fetal marrow elements with CD 34 +, CD 38–, HLA-DR-phenotypes were reported to develop not only the hematopoietic microenvironment but also the hematopoietic cells themselves [Huang and Terstappen, 1992]. *Indicates the possibility that, at least in the fetus, there may be a common stem cell for bone marrow stromal and hematopoietic elements. †There are several schools of thought relating to single or multiple stem cell pools for the lymphoid versus the other lineages.

TABLE 18.1 Cells That Contribute to the Tissue Microenvironment

Stromal cells: derivatives of a common precursor cell
  Mesenchyme
  Fibroblasts
  Myofibroblasts
  Osteogenic/chondrogenic cells
  Adipocytes
Stromal-associated cells: histogenically distinct from stromal cells, permanent residents of a tissue
  Endothelial cells
  Macrophages
Transient cells: cells that migrate into a tissue for host defense either prior to or following an inflammatory stimulus
  B lymphocytes/plasma cells
  Cytotoxic T cells and natural killer (NK) cells
  Granulocytes
Parenchymal cells: cells that occupy most of the tissue volume, express functions that are definitive for the tissue, and interact with all other cell types to facilitate the expression of differentiated function

basement membrane. The composition of the underlying tissue varies, but it contains a connective tissue framework for parenchymal cells. If the tissue is an artery or a vein, the underlying connective tissue is composed of circularly arranged smooth-muscle cells which in turn are surrounded by an adventitia of loose connective tissue. Tissues within organs are generally organized into functional units around capillaries which facilitate metabolite and blood gas transport by virtue of their lack of a smooth muscle layer (*tunica media*) and the thinness of their adventitial covering. Connective tissue cells of the tissue underlying capillaries deposit extracellular matrix (ECM) which is a mixture of fibrous proteins (collagens) embedded in a hydrated gel of glycosaminoglycans (GAGs). The GAGs, as distinguished by their sugar residues, are divided into five groups: hyaluronic acid, the chondiotin sulfates, dermatan sulfate, heparan and heparin sulfate, and keratan sulfate. All the GAGs except hyaluronic acid link with proteins to form proteoglycans. These proteoglycans bind to long-chained hyaluronic acid cores that interweave the cross-linked collagen fibers that form the framework of the tissue. The basic composition and density of deposition of stromal cell-derived ECM varies from tissue to tissue [Lin and Bissel, 1993]. Figure 18.2 is a scanning electron micrograph (SEM) depicting the intricacies of the ECM deposited by human bone marrow-derived stromal cells growing on a three-dimensional culture template. The ECM forms a sieve-like arrangement for diffusion in an aqueous environment and a number of bone marrow-derived migratory cells are present as well. Such an arrangement dramatically enhances the surface area for cell growth. Although these voids are primarily filled by parenchymal cells, normal tissue interstitium also contains migratory immunocompetent cells such as B lymphocyte/plasma cells, T cells, and natural killer cells as well as the ubiquitous macrophage (histiocyte). The numbers of these cells are enhanced during inflammatory episodes when neutrophils or other granulocytes and/or mononuclear leukocytes infiltrate the tissue. Cytokines and other proteins released by these leukocytes recruit stromal cells in the tissue repair process. This phenomenon can be exploited by tumor cells to enhance their invasiveness (see Section 18.2 Tumor Cells). Although tissue function *in toto* is measured by parenchymal cell output (e.g., for liver, protein synthesis, metabolism; for bone marrow, blood cell production), this is profoundly influenced by and in some instances orchestrated by the stromal cell microenvironment.

Stromal cells contribute to parenchymal cell function by synthesizing the unique mix of ECM proteins necessary for cell seeding/attachment of specific types of tissue cells, the modulation of gene expression in parenchymal cells by events triggered by cytoskeleton-mediated transduction [Ben-Ze'ev et al., 1988], the deposition of ECM proteins to sequester growth and regulatory factors for use by developing parenchyma [Roberts et al., 1988], deposition of ECM of the right density to permit diffusion of nutrients, metabolites, and oxygen (and egress of CO_2 and waste) to the extent necessary to maintain the functional state of the tissue, by forming the appropriate barriers to minimize cell migration or intrusion, and by synthesizing and/or presenting cytokins that regulate parenchymal cell function, either constituitively or following induction by other humoral agents (see Table 18.2).

Creating cultures that contain the multiplicity of cell types found *in vivo* presents a daunting task for several reasons: (1) Culture media that are rich in nutrients select for the most actively mitotic cells at the expense of more mitotically quiescent cells. (2) Cell phenotypic expression and function is related to its location in tissue to some extent. It is difficult, especially using a flat (i.e., two-dimensional) culture template, to create a microenvironment that is permissive or inductive for the formation of tissue-like structures. (3) Localized microenvironmental niches regulate different parenchymal cell functions or, in the case of bone marrow, hematopoietic cell differentiation. These milieus are difficult to reproduce in culture, since all cells are exposed to essentially the same media components. However, a major goal of tissue culture is to permit normal cell-cell associations and the reestablishment of tissue polarity so that parenchymal cell function is optimized. The question of three dimensionality will be addressed later in this chapter. A brief survey of the various types of stromal elements follows.

Fibroblasts

Fibroblasts are responsible for the synthesis of many GAGs and for the deposition and organization of collagens. Although present in most tissues, fibroblasts exhibit specialization with respect to the type of ECM that they secrete. For example, liver tissue contains type I and type IV collagen, whereas type II collagen is found in cartilaginous tissues. Bone marrow contains types I, III, IV, and V collagen [Zuckerman, 1984]. Heterogeneity of collagen deposition as well as GAG composition exists not only between different tissues but in developmentally different stages of the same tissue [Thonar and Kuettner, 1987].

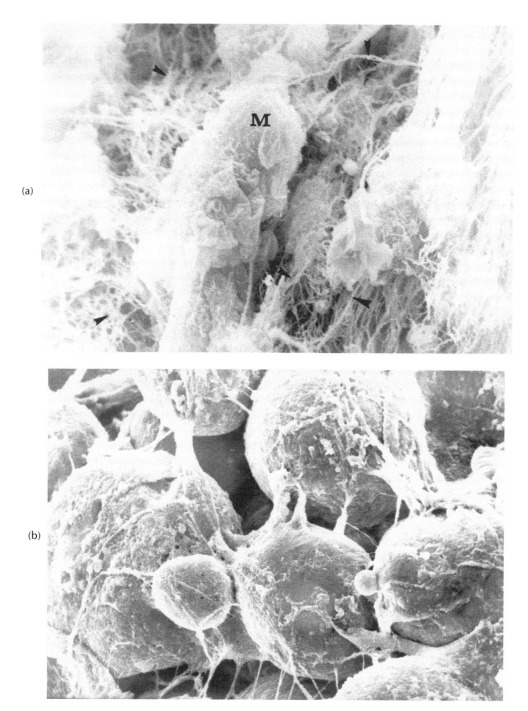

FIGURE 18.2 Scanning electron micrographs of bone marrow cultures on nylon screen templates (a) Photograph depicting a portion of a macrophage (M) associated with the numerous, delicate, interweaving strands of ECM (arrows) that are deposited between the openings of the nylon screen of a bone marrow stromal cell culture. (b) Myeloid cells of a hematopoietic colony growing in a coculture of human stromal cells and hematopoietic cells. Note the pattern of attachment of individual cells to matrix and the large open area between the cells for nutrient access. (c) The photograph depicts the intimate association of cells of a myeloid or mixed myeloid/monocytic colony (arrow) with enveloping fibroblastic cells (F) in a bone marrow coculture. A filament of the nylon (n) screen is also present in the field. (d) An erythroid colony (E) in a human bone marrow coculture on nylon screen. Note that the more mature erythroid cells are on the periphery of the colony and that it is in close apposition to a macrophage (M). A nylon filament is also present (n).

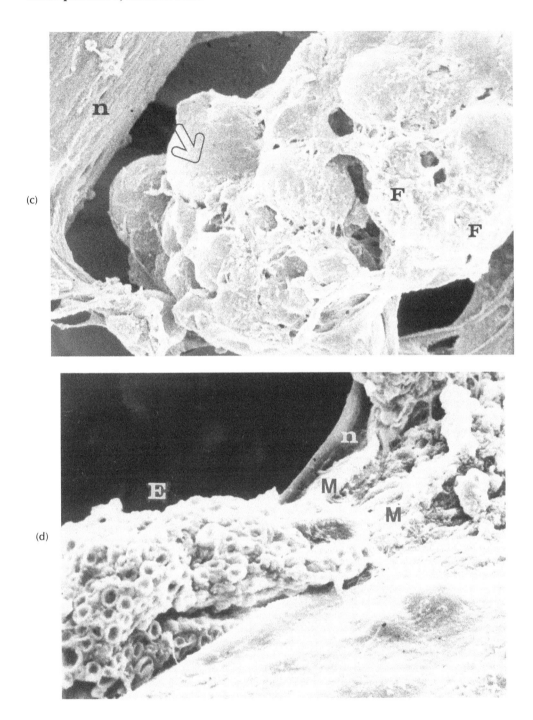

(c)

(d)

FIGURE 18.2 (continued)

In addition to matrix deposition, fibroblasts synthesize the cytokines of the fibroblast growth factor (FGF) family, a variety of interleukins, and GM-CSF as well as other regulatory cytokines (Table 18.2). Fibroblast activity can be modulated by circulating or locally diffusable factors including IL-1, TGFβ, TNFα, and a host of other factors [Yang et al., 1988]. For example, IL-1 activated splenic stroma supported the growth of rat natural killer cells in long-term culture [Tjota et al., 1992]. In addition, treatment of bone

TABLE 18.2 Stromal Cell Phenotypes and Secretory Profiles

Phenotypes[a]	Cytokine/Protein Secretion
MHC I (all)	Il-1β (mφ, E, F, A)
MHC II (E, mφ)	M-CSF (mφ, E, F)
CD 10 (Neural endopeptidase)[b]	G-CSF (mφ, F)
CD 29 (β₂ integrin) (all)	GM-CSF (mφ, E)
CD 34 (CFU-F)	LIF (mφ, F)
CD 36 (IA 7 (mφ)	GM-colony enhancing factor (mφ)
CD 44 (H-CAM)[b]	TGFβ (mφ, F)
CD 49b (α₂ chain of VLA-2)[b]	TNFα (mφ, F)
CD 49d (α₄ chain of VLA-4)[b]	PAF (E)
CD 49e (α₅ chain of VLA-5)[b]	BPA (mφ, E)
CD 51 (vitronectin receptor)[b]	IFNα (mφ, F, E)
CD 54 (ICAM-1) (all)	IFNγ (F)
CD 58 (LFA-3) (all)	Il-6 (mφ)
CD 61 (GP 111a)	c-kit ligand (mφ, F)
VCAM-1 (E)	Acidic and basic FGF (F)
α SM actin (F)	Angiotensinogen (A)
Vimentin (F)	Lipoprotein lipase (A)
Decorin (Mes)	Adipocyte P2 (A)
Fibronectin (F, mφ)	MIP-1α (mφ)
Laminin (E)	Complement proteins C1-C5 (mφ)
Collagen I (F)	Factor B, properdin (mφ)
Collagen III (F)	Transcobalamin II (mφ)
Collagen IV (F)	Transferrin (mφ)
von Willebrand factor (E)	Arachidonic acid metabolites (mφ, E)
Adipsin (A)	HGF/SF (F)
	flt3-ligand (S)
	Prolactin (F)
	LIF (S)[c]
	STR-3 (F)
	(IL-3, IL-7, IL-9, IL-11, IL-15, neuroleukin)[b]

[a] Phenotypic expression of stroma in bone marrow cultures. Parentheses indicate localization according to cell type (mφ = Macrophage, F = Fibroblast, E = endothelial, A = adipocyte, Mes = mesenchyme). Many of these phenotypes were identified in the original work of Cicuttini et al. [1992] and Moreau et al. [1993].

[b] Indicates the presence of mRNA and /or protein expression in bone marrow cultures but not localized to a particular cell type.

[c] Found in fallopian tube stroma [Keltz et al., 1997].

Abbreviations: BPA—erythroid burst promoting activity, CD—cluster determinant, MHC—major histocompatibility complex, M—monocyte, G—granulocyte, CSF—colony stimulating factor, CFU-F—colony forming unit-fibroblast, MIP—macrophage inflammatory protein, IL—interleukin, IFN—interferon, TGF—transforming growth factor, TNF—tumor necrosis factor, PAF—platelet activating factor, FGF—fibroblast growth factor/scatter factor, LIF—leukemia inhibitory factor, STR-3—stromelysin 3.

marrow stromal cell cultures with the steroid methylprednisolone reduced the concentration of hyaluronic acid and heparan sulfate relative to other proteins [Siczkowski et al., 1993], perhaps making them more conducive to hematopoietic support. Horse serum, presumably because of its high content of hydrocortisone and other steroids, was an essential component of medium used to maintain hematopoiesis in early long-term bone marrow cultures [Greenberger et al., 1979]. In our experience, medium supplementation with hydrocortisone or other corticosteroids enhances the ability of liver-derived stromal cells to support parenchymal hepatocyte function for longer-terms *in vitro* [Naughton et al., 1994], although the precise mechanism(s) has not been defined.

Fibroblastic cells in tissue appear to be heterogeneous with respect to support function. Early morphometric studies of bone marrow indicated that stroma supporting different types of hematopoiesis exhibited different staining patterns. The development of highly specific monoclonal antibodies in the intervening years made possible a much more detailed analysis of stromal cells of bone marrow and other tissues and provided a number of avenues to isolate these cells for study. Whereas bone marrow stromal cells can be separated from hematologic cells by virtue of their adherence to plastic, this technique was not optimal for all tissues. Monoclonal antibodies can now be used to "dissect" cells from the stromal microenvironment using a variety of techniques including flow cytometry, immune panning, immuno-magnetic microspheres, and affinity column methodologies. Monoclonal antibodies also make it possible to select for stromal cell progenitors like the fibroblast-colony forming unit (CFU-F) which is CD 34 positive.

Endothelial Cells

For nonglandular tissues such as bone marrow, the endothelial cells are vascular lining cells and can be distinguished by the expression of or the message for von Willebrand factor and surface major histo-compatibility complex-II (MHC-II) antigens. As cells of the vascular *tunica intima*, they, along with the basement membrane, form a selective barrier to regulate the transport of substances to and from the blood supply. In addition, their expression of integrins following stimulation with IL-1 or other mediators regulates the attachment of immunocompetent cells during acute (neutrophils) or chronic (T lympho-cytes, monocytes) inflammation. Endothelial cells also regulate other vascular functions. They synthesize the vasodilatory effector nitric oxide after induction with acetylcholine [Furchgott and Zawadzki, 1980] and secrete regulatory peptides, the endothelins, which counteract this effect [Yanagisawa et al., 1988]. Specialized vascular endothelia are present in bone marrow, where they permit the egress of mature leukocytes from the marrow into the sinusoids, and in the liver, where the surfaces of the cells lining sinusoids are fenestrated to facilitate transport. In a more general context, endothelial cells also produce collagen IV for basement membranes and secrete several cytokines including IL-1, fibronectin, M-CSF, and GM-CSF and release platelet-activating factor (Table 18.2). Vascular endothelia are nonthrombogenic and contribute to angiogenesis by mitotically responding to locally secreted factors such as bFGF and aFGF. These endothelia possess LDL receptors and degrade this lipoprotein at substantially higher rates than other types of cells. These cells also have receptors for Fc, transferrin, mannose, galactose, and Apo-E, as well as for scavenger receptors [Van Eyken and Desmet, 1993]. Endothelia tend to assemble into tubular structures in culture, but their contribution to parenchymal cell growth *in vitro* is contingent on the generation of the proper tissue polarity.

In addition to vascular endothelial cells, some organs possess nonvascular endothelial cells such as the bile duct lining cells of the liver. These cells possess antigenic profiles and secretory potentials that are similar to vascular endothelia.

Adipocytes, Fat-Storing Cells

These cells are represented in varying concentrations in different tissues. They are related to fibroblasts (Fig. 18.2), and transformation of fibroblasts to adipocytes *in vitro* can be induced by supplementation of the medium with hydrocortisone or other steroids [Brockband and van Peer, 1983; Greenberger, 1979] which induce the expression of lipoproteinlipase and glycerolphosphate dehydrogenase as well as an increase in insulin receptors [Gimble et al., 1989]. Like fibroblasts, marrow adipocytes are heterogeneous and display different characteristics related to their distribution in red or yellow marrow [Lichtman, 1984]. These characteristics include insulin independence but glucocorticoid dependence *in vitro*, positive staining with perfomic acid-Schiff, and higher concentrations of neutral fats and unsaturated fatty acids in triglycerides. In bone marrow *in vivo*, there appears to be an inverse relationship between adipogenesis and erythropoiesis: phenylhydrazine-induced anemia causes a rapid conversion of yellow marrow (con-taining adipocytes) to red marrow due to compensatory erythroid heperplasia [Maniatis et al., 1971]. However, the role of the adipocyte in supporting hematopoiesis in culture is controversial. Although Dexter and co-workers [1977] associated declining myelopoiesis in long-term murine bone marrow cultures with the gradual disappearance of adipocytes from the stromal layer, these cells may not be necessary to support hematopoiesis in human bone marrow cultures [Touw and Lowenberg, 1983]. In this regard, IL-11 suppressed adipogenesis but simulated human CD34+ HL-DR + progenitor cells cocultured with human bone marrow stroma and enhanced the numbers of myeloid progenitor cells [Keller et al., 1993]. Hematopoiesis *in vivo* requires the proper ECM for cell attachment and differentiation as well as regulation by cytokines elaborated by stromal cells [Metcalf, 1993]. Although there is considerable redundancy in the synthesis of regulatory factors by different stromal cell populations, no single cell population has been identified that can provide an entire hematopoietic microenvironment. Further complicating the issue is a recent report indicating that CD 34+ hematopoietic progenitors produce soluble factors that control the production of some cytokines by stromal cells [Gupta et al., 1998]. If "cross-talk" between parenchyma and stroma is established as an important regulatory mechanism, the ratio between the relative numbers of stroma and parenchyma in a tissue culture will assume paramount importance. The use of cell lines to provide hematopoietic support will be discussed later in this chapter.

In the liver, purified fat-storing cells are capable of broad-scale synthetic activity that includes collagens I, III, IV, fibronectin, heparan sulfate, chondroitin sulfate, and dermatan sulfate [DeLeeuw et al., 1984]. Adipocytes also synthesize colony-stimulating factors and other regulatory cytokines (Table 18.2). In addition to the above characteristics, adipocytes are desmin positive and therefore are phenotypically related to myogenic cells or myofibroblasts. The function of adipocytes may vary depending on their location. Adipocytes in the bone marrow are in close apposition to the sinusoidal endothelial cells and in the liver are found in the space of Disse under the endothelial cells. Hepatic fat-storing cells are finely integrated into several contiguous parenchymal cells and contain fat droplets that are qualitatively different from those found in hepatic parenchymal cells in that they contain high levels of retinols. Liver adipocytes are responsible for the metabolism and storage of vitamin A [DeLeeuw et al., 1984], provide some of the raw materials for the synthesis of biologic membranes, and also contribute to local energy metabolism needs. Adeipocytes of other tissues also act as a type of "progenitor" cell that can be converted to different phenotypes (e.g., osteoblasts or chondroblasts) under the appropriate conditions and are capable of stimulating osteogenesis via their secretion of cytokines [Benayahu et al., 1993].

Macrophages

Macrophages are derivatives of peripheral blood monocytes and are, therefore, bone-marrow-derived. They seed and remain on the surfaces of sinusoidal vessels in organs such as the liver and the spleen or migrate into the interstitial spaces of virtually all tissues. Macrophages are quintessential immunocompetent cells and are central components of many defense strategies, including randomized microbial phagocytosis and killing; antibody-dependent cellular cytotoxicity (ADCC), where they are directed against microbial or other cells that are opsonized with antibody; nonrandomized (specific) phagocytosis mediated by the association of immunoglobulins with a multiplicity of F_c receptors on their surfaces; the presentation of processed antigen to lymphocytes; secretion of and reaction to chemotaxins; and an enzymatic profile enabling them to move freely through tissue. The secretory capacity of macrophages is prodigious. In addition to plasma components such as complement proteins C1 through C5, they synthesize the ferric iron- and vitamin B_{12}–building proteins, transferrin and transcobalamin II, as well as a host of locally acting bioreactive metabolites of arachidonic acid. Macrophage secretory activity appears to influence two simultaneous events *in vivo*, inflammation and tissue repair. One monokine, IL-1, enhances the adhesion of neutrophils to vascular endothelial cells and activates B and T lymphocytes and other macrophages while stimulating the formation of acute phase proteins inducing collagen, ECM, and cytokine synthesis by fibroblasts and other stromal cells. IL-1, as well as a host of other humoral regulatory factors, originates in macrophages, including TNFα, IFNα, GM-CSF, and MIP-1α (Table 18.2). The ability of macrophages to secrete regulatory cytokines makes them an important contributor to the tissue microenvironment.

Macrophages have been intrinsically associated with erythropoiesis in the bone marrow [Bessis and Breton-Gorius, 1959] and [Naughton et al., 1979]. As such, these "nurse cells" destroy defective erythroblasts and the fetal and regenerating liver, and provide recycled iron stores for hemoglobin synthesis by developing red cells. They also synthesize and/or store erythropoietin.

18.2 Stromal Cells as "Feeder Layers" for Parenchymal Cell Culture

Irradiated stromal feeder layers were first used by Puck and Marcus [1955] to support the attachment and proliferation of HeLa cells in culture. Direct contact with feeder layers of cells also permits the growth of glioma cells and epithelial cells derived from breast tissue and colon [Freshney et al., 1982]. Enhanced attachment of parenchymal cells and production of factors to regulate growth and differentiation are two important benefits of coculturing parenchymal and stromal cells.

Bone Marrow

Bone marrow was the first tissue to be systematically investigated in regard to the influence of ECM and stromal cells on the production of blood cells. By the mid-1970s, the influence of microenvironmental conditions [Trentin, 1970; Wolf and Trentin, 1968] and ECM deposition [McCuskey et al., 1972; Schrock et al., 1973] upon hematopoiesis was well established in the hematology literature. Dexter and co-workers [1977] were the first to apply the feeder-layer-based coculture technology to hematopoietic cells by inoculating mouse bone marrow cells into preestablished, irradiated feeder layers of marrow-derived stromal (adherent) cells. These cultures remained hematopoietically active for several months. By comparison, bone marrow cells cultured in the absence of feeder layers or supplementary cytokines terminally differentiated within the first 2 weeks in culture; stromal cells were the only survivors [Brandt et al., 1990; Chang and Anderson, 1971]. If the cultures are not supplemented with exogenous growth factors, then myeloid cells, monocytic cells, and nucleated erythroblasts are present for the first 7–10 days of culture. This trilineage pattern is narrowed over successive weeks in culture so that from about 2–4 weeks myeloid and monocytic cells are produced, and, if cultured for longer terms, the products of the culture are almost entirely monocytic. However, the nature of hematopoietic support can be modulated by changing the environmental conditions. In this regard, cocultures established under identical conditions as the above produce B lymphocytes if the steroid supplementation of the medium is removed and the ambient temperature is increased [Whitlock and Witte, 1982]. Static bone marrow coculture systems are generally categorized as declining because of this and the finding that the hematopoietic progenitor cell concentrations decrease as a function of time in culture. However, this trend can be offset by coculturing bone marrow in bioreactors that provide constant media exchange and optimize oxygen delivery [Palsson et al., 1993] or by supplementing the cocultures with cocktails of the various growth factors elaborated by stromal cells [Keller et al., 1993]. Connective tissue feeder layers had originally been hypothesized to act by conditioning medium with soluble factors that stimulated growth and by providing a substratum for the selective attachment of certain types of cells [Puck and Marcus, 1955]. These are functions that have since been proven for bone marrow and other tissue culture systems.

It is very difficult to recreate the marrow microenvironment *in vitro*. One reason is that the marrow stromal cell populations proliferate at different rates; if expanded vigorously using nutrient-rich medium, the culture selects for fibroblastic cells at the expense of the more slowly dividing types of stroma. We established rat bone marrow cocultures using stromal cells that were passaged for 6 months, and these cultures produced lower numbers of progenitor cells (CFU-C) in the adherent zone as compared to cocultures established with stroma that was only passed three to four times (Fig. 18.3). Cells released from cultures using the older stroma were almost entirely monocytic, even at earlier terms of culture. In a related experiment, we suspended nylon screen cocultures of passage 3–4 stroma and bone marrow hematopoietic cells in flasks containing confluent, 6-month-old stromal cell monolayers and found that these monolayer cells inhibited hematopoiesis in the coculture [Naughton et al., 1989].

We use early passage stroma for our cocultures in order to retain a representation of all the stromal cell types. If hematopoietic cells from cocultures are removed after about a month *in vitro* and reinoculated onto a new template containing passage 3–4 stromal cells and cultured for an additional month, the progenitor cell concentrations of the adherent zones are considerably higher than in cocultures where no transfer took place [Naughton et al., 1994]. This experiment indicated that continued access to "fresh"

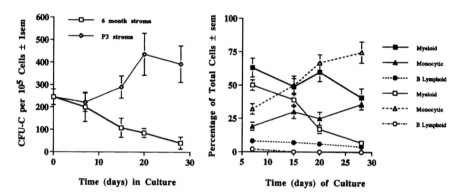

FIGURE 18.3   *Left*. Mean CFU-C progenitor concentration of the adherent zone of a three-dimensional coculture of rat bone hematopoietic cells and rat bone marrow stroma. Stock cultures to generate the stromal cells for the cocultures were seeded onto the three-dimensional template either after passage (P3) or following expansion in monolayer culture for 6 months. Stroma at early passage is substantially more supportive of CFU-C progenitor cells than "old" stroma that is primarily fibroblastic in nature. Vertical lines through the means = ±1 standard error of the mean (sem). *Right*. Analysis of the cellular content of the nonadherent zone of rat bone marrow hematopoietic cell: stromal cell cocultures on three-dimensional templates by flow cytometry. Cocultures were established either with P3 stroma (closed figures) or stroma that was grown in monolayer culture for 6 months (open figures). The mean percentages of cells recognized by the phenotyping antibodies MOM/3F12/F2 (myeloid), ED-1 (monocytic), and OX-33 (B lymphoid) (Serotec, UK) are depicted. Vertical lines through the means = ±1 sem. Whereas low passage stroma generates myeloid, B lymphoid, and monocytic cells in cocultures and releases them into the nonadherent zone, 6-month-old stroma supports mainly the production of macrophages.

stroma enhances hematopoiesis. The maintenance of mixed populations of stromal cells are desirable for a number of reasons. The same cytokine may be synthesized by different stromal cells, but its mode of action is usually synergistic with other cytokines for the differentiation of a specific blood cell lineage(s). Differentiation may not occur in the absence one of these cytokines, although some degree of redundancy in cytokine expression is intrinsic to the stromal system [Metcalf, 1993]. The fibroblastic cells that "grow out" of later passage human and rodent bone marrow stroma share some phenotypic properties with muscle cells (αSM actin+, CD34–, STRO-1–). These cells (endothelial cells and macrophages are absent or present in negligible quantities) supported hematopoietic progenitors for up to 7 weeks of culture but no longer [Moreau et al., 1993], indicating that other types of cells are necessary for long-term hematopoiesis *in vitro*.

Stromal cells derived from spleen or bone marrow were also shown to support the growth and maturation of rat natural killer cells in long-term three-dimensional culture [Tjota et al., 1992]. Natural killer cells produced by the cultures for more than 2 months *in vitro* continued to kill YAC-1 (NK sensitive) target cells when activated by IL-2. In more recent experiments, fetal thymus-derived stroma supported the production of CD45+/CD56+ human natural killer cells when cocultured with CD34+lin- progenitors [Vaz et al., 1998]. In related work, stromal cell-derived IL-15 was found to enhance the production of CD56+/CD3– natural killer cells from human CD34+ hematopoietic progenitors [Mrózek et al., 1996]. In addition, the process of natural killer cell maturation (but not early progenitor cell proliferation) appears to require direct contact with stromal cells [Tsuji and Pollack, 1995].

Cytoadhesive molecule expression and its modulation is also an important consideration for the engineering of bone marrow and other tissues. In the case of bone marrow, this regulates "homing" or seeding, restricting cells in specific areas within tissues both to expose them to regulatory factors and to the release of cells from the supportive stroma upon maturation. For example, the sequential expression of hemonectin, a cytoadhesion molecule of myeloid cells, in yolk sac blood islands, liver, and bone marrow during embryonic and fetal life parallels the granulopoiesis occurring in these respective organs [Peters et al., 1990]. Hematopoietic stem cells [Simmons et al., 1992] and B-cell progenitors [Ryan et al., 1991]

TABLE 18.3 Cells Contributing to the Hepatic Microenvironment

Cell Type	Size, μm	Relative Percent of Total Cells	Characteristics
Stroma			
Kupffer cells	12–16	8	MHC-1+, MHC-II+, Fcr, C3r, mannose and D-acetrylglucosamine receptors, acid phosphatase+, density = 1.076 gm/ml,* 1.036 gm/ml[†]
Vascular endothelia	11-12	9	MHC-1+, MHC II+, vWF+, F$_c$r, TF$_r$, mannose, apo-E, and scavenger receptors, density = 1.06–1.08 gm/ml,* 1.036 gm/ml[†]
Biliary endothelia	10–12	5	MHC-1+, Positive for cytokeratins 7, 8, 18, 19, β2 microglobulin+, positive for VLA-2,3,6 integrins, agglutinate with UEA, WGA, SBA, PNA, density = 1.075–1.1 gm/ml,* 1.0363gm/ml[†]
Fat-storing cells	14–18	3	MHC-1+, desmin+, retinol+, ECM expression, collagen I, IV expression, density =1.075–1.1 gm/ml*
Fibroblasts	11–14	7	MHC-1+, ECM expression, collagen I, IV expression, density = 1.025 gm/ml,* 1.063 gm/ml[†]
Pit cells	11-15	1-2(variable)	MHC-1+, asialo-GM+, CD8+, CD-5-
Parenchymal cells			
Mononuclear (type 1)	17-22	35	MHC-I-, MHC-II-, blood group antigen-, density = 1.10–1.14 gm/ml,* 1.067 gm/ml[†]
Binuclear (type II)	20-27	27	MHC-I±, MHC-II-, blood group antigen-, density = 1.10-1.14 gm/ml,* 1.071 gm/ml[†]
Acidophilic (type III)	25-32	5	MHC-1±, MHC-II-, blood group antigen-, density = 1.038 gm/ml[†]

Abbreviations: ECM = extracellular matrix, MHC = major histocompatibility complex, PNA = peanut agglutinin, SBA = soybean agglutinin, WGA = wheat germ agglutinin, UEA = *Ulex europaeus* agglutinin.

bind to VCAM-1 on cultures stromal cells by expression of VLA-4. In addition, erythroid progenitor cells bind preferentially to the fibronectin component of the ECM and remain bound throughout their differentiation [Tsai et al., 1987]. A basic requirement of stromal feeder layers is the expression of the proper cytoadhesion molecule profile to permit attachment of parenchyma; in this instance these are hematopoietic stem and progenitor cells.

Liver

Liver is an hematopoietic organ during fetal life, and it contains many of the same stromal cell populations found in bone marrow (Table 18.3). Research trends in liver cell and bone marrow culture have followed a somewhat parallel course. Both tissues are difficult to maintain *in vitro*; the parenchymal cell numbers either declined (hematopoietic progenitors) or lost function and dedifferentiated (hepatocytes) over time in culture. When mixed suspensions of hepatic cells are inoculated into liquid medium, approximately 20% of the total cells attach. The nonadherent population remains viable for about 72 h. The adherent cells, although they proliferate for only 24–48 h after inoculation, can survive for substantially longer periods. However, many of these adherent parenchymal cells undergo drastic phenotypic alterations, especially if the medium is conditioned with serum. These changes include a flattening and spreading on plastic surfaces as well as a propensity to undergo nuclear division in the absence of concomitant cytoplasmic division. The appearance of these bizarre, multinucleated, giant cells herald the loss of liver-specific functions such as albumin synthesis and the metabolism of organic chemicals by cytochrome P450 enzymes. The percentage of hepaocytes attaching to the flask, the maintenance of rounded parenchymal cell phenotype, and the expression of specialized hepatic function *in vitro* can be enhanced by precoating the flasks with ECM components such as type I collagen [Michalopoulos and Pitot, 1975], fibronectin [Deschenes et al., 1980], homogenized liver tissue matrix [Reid et al., 1980], laminin, and type IV collagen [Bissell et al., 1987]. Hepatocyte survival and functional expression also improved when hepatocytes were cocultured with liver-derived [Fry and Bridges, 1980] and murine 3T3 [Kuri-Harcuch and Mendoza-Figueroa, 1989] fibroblasts as well as a preestablished layer of adherent liver epithelial cells [Guguen-Guillouzo et al., 1983]. As with bone marrow culture on feeder layers, cells derived from the liver itself usually provide the best support in culture. However, we have found that hepatic parenchyma will express a differentiated function *in vitro* if supported by bone marrow stroma. Conversely, liver-derived stromal cells support hematopoiesis in culture but his microenvironment favors erythropoisis (unpublished observations).

In contrast to the role of bone marrow stroma on hematopoiesis, the influence of hepatic stromal cells on the function and/or growth of parenchymal hepatocytes has not been exhaustively investigated. However, several studies indicate the Kupffer cells, fat-strong cells, and perhaps other stroma influence parenchymal cell cytochrome P450 enzyme expression [Peterson and Renton, 1984] and act in tandem with parenchymal cells to metabolize lipopolysaccharide [Treon et al., 1979]. In addition, adipocytes and hepatic fibroblasts synthesize collagen type I and the proteoglycans heparan sulfate, dermatan sulfate, and chondroitin sulfate as well as hyaluronic acid, which is unsulfated in the liver and occurs as a simple GAG. Stromal cells as well as parenchyma deposit fibronectin. Liver adipocytes, like their relatives in bone marrow, express phenotypes (vimentin+, actin+, tubulin+) linking them histogenically to fibro-blasts and mogenic cells [DeLeeuw et al, 1984]. Fat-storing cells as well as vascular endothelia apparently synthesize the type IV collagen found in the space of Disse, and fibrin originating from parenchymal cell fibrinogen synthesis is a significant part of liver matrix, at least in culture. As with the hematopoietic cells in bone marrow cultures, hepatic parenchymal cell gene expression is modulated by attachment to ECM and influenced by factors released by stromal cells. For example, parenchymal cells attaching to laminin-coated surfaces express the differentiation-associated substance α-fetoprotein, whereas the synthesis of albumin synthesis is favored when parenchymal cells bind to type IV collagen [Michalopoulous and Pitot, 1975]. Hepatocytes bind to fibronectin using the $\alpha_5\beta$ integrin heterodimer and AGp110, a nonintegrin glycoprotein. Cytoadhesion molecule expression by heapatic cells and cells of other tissues changes with and perhaps controls development [Stamatoglou and Hughes, 1994]. Just as differential hemonectin expression occurred during the development of the hematopoietic system [Peters et al., 1990], a differential expression of liver proteins occurs during ontogeny. Although fibronec-tin and its receptor are strongly expressed in liver throughout life, AGp110 appears later in development and may guide the development of parenchyma into a polarized tissue. It will probably be necessary to incorporate the various stromal support cells found in liver into hepatocyte cultures.

Tumor Cells

Stromal cells contribute to the process of neoplastic invasion of tissue by responding in a paracrine fashion to signals released by tumor cells. This includes the tumor-stimulated release of angiogenic factors from fibroblasts such as acid and basic FGF and the release of vascular endothelia growth factor/vascular proliferation factor (VEGF/VPF) by tumor cells to recruit endothelial cells and stimulate their prolifer-ation and development into blood vessels to feed the growing neoplasm (reviewed by Wernert [1997]). In addition to cooperating in the establishment of tumors, stromal cells also contribute to their invasive-ness. Activation and/or release of stromal cell-derived tissue factor (TF) (whose release by damaged tissue initiates the extrinsic limb of the protease coagulation cascade) has been associated with the progression from early to invasive breast cancer [Vrana et al., 1996]. In this regard, upon direct contact with tumor cells, stromal cells produce stromelysin 3 (STR-3), a matrix metalloproteinase that accelerates the migra-tion of metastatic cells through tissue by degrading tissue matrix [Mari et al., 1998]. STR-3 is overex-pressed in a wide variety of tumor stroma in breast, lung, colon, and other cancers. It would be appropriate to include coculture studies (i.e., tumor and stroma) in the investigation of the biology of cancer in vitro as well as its reponsivity to potential treatments. We have previously demonstrated that the presence of stroma alters the hematologic responsiveness to chemotherapy agents such as cyclophosphamide [Naugh-ton et al., 1992]. In related work, primary cultures of murine plasmacytomas require a feeder layer.

Alteration of ECM composition and other support functions of the stroma by anti-inflammatory drugs prevented plasmacytoma growth *in vivo* and *in vitro* [De Grassi et al., 1993].

18.3 Support of Cultured Cells Using Cell Lines

The precise roles of the various cellular constituents of the tissue microenvironment have not been fully defined. One approach to understanding these mechanisms is to develop stroma cell lines with homogeneous and well-defined characteristics and then ascertain the ability of these cells to support parenchyma in coculture. A brief survey of some of these lines is found in Table 18.4. Stromal cell lines derived from bone marrow are usually either fibroblastic (F) or a mixture of fibroblastic and adipocytic cells which contain a subpopulation of fibroblastic cells that can be induced to undergo lipogenesis with dexamethasone or hydrocortisone (A) (reviewed by Gimble [1990]). In general, fibroblastic lines support myelopoiesis and monocytopoiesis and stroma with both fibroblastic and adipocytic cells supports myelopoiesis as well as B lymphopoiesis. The MBA-14 cell line, which consists of stroma bearing fibroblastic as well as monocytic phenotypes, stimulated the formation of CFU-C (bipotential myeloid/monocytic) progenitors in coculture. Different cell lines that were transformed using the large T oncogene of simian virus 40 (U2) were used as feeder layers for bone marrow hematopoietic cells. Cocultures established using bone-marrow-derived stroma exhibited considerably better maintenance of the primitive stem cell CFU-S$_{12}$ in culture than similarly transfected skin, lung, or kidney tissue cells [Rios and Williams, 1990]. Although feeder layers share a number of characteristics (cytokine production, ECM deposition), it is probably best to derive your feeder cells from the tissue that you wish to coculture rather than use xenogeneic feeder cells or cells derived from a completely dissimilar tissue. In this respect, we found that total cell output and progenitor cell concentrations were substantially higher in rat bone marrow cocultures supported with rat bone marrow stroma as compared to those established using immortalized human skin fibroblasts or fetal lung cell lines [Naughton and Naughton, 1989].

TABLE 18.4 Some Representative Stromal Cell Lines Used to Support Hematopoietic Cells or Hepatocytes

Cell Line	Species	Phenotype[*]	Support Capability
Bone marrow			
AC-4	Mouse	A	Myeloid, monocytic, B lymphoid
ALC	Mouse	A	Myeloid, monocytic, B lymphoid
GM 1380	Human	F	Short-term myelo- + monopoiesis
GY-30	Mouse	A	Myeloid, monocytic, B lymphoid myelopoiesis
K-1	Mouse	A	
MBA-14	Mouse	F/M	Enhances CFU-C numbers myelopoiesis
MS-1	Mouse	F	
U2	Mouse	F[†]	Maintenance of CFU-S$_{12}$, myelopoiesis
3T3	Mouse	F	
10 T1/2	Mouse	F	Stimulates CFU-GEMM, -GM
10T1/2 clone D	Mouse	A	Stimulates CFU-GM only
266 AD	Mouse	A	Myeloid, monocytic, B lymphoid
Liver			
3T3	Mouse	F	Enhanced lipid metabolism, extends period of cytochrome P450 activity†
Detroit 550	Human	F	Prolonged cytochrome P450 and NADPH-cytochrome C reductase activity‡

Source: Adapted from Anklesaria et al. [1987] and Gimble [1990].

[*]Major phenotype of the cell line (F = fibroblastic, M = monocytic, A = capable of supporting adipocyte phenotypes).

[†]A bone marrow-derived cell line that was transformed with the large T oncogene of simian virus 40.

[‡]Support functions are compared to liquid cultures of rat hepatocytes without stroma.

Abbreviations: CFU = colony-forming unit; G = granulocyte; M = macrophage; S = spleen; GEMM = granulocyte, erythrocyte, megakaryoctye, monocyte; NADPH = nicotinamide adenine dinucleotide phosphate.

18.4 Stereotypic (Three-Dimensional) Culture versus Monolayer Culture

Tissue is a three-dimensional arrangement of various types of cells that are organized into a functional unit. These cells also are polarized with respect to their position within tissue and the microenvironment, and therefore the metabolic activity and requirements of the tissue are not uniform throughout. Three-dimensional culture was first performed successfully by Leighton [1951] using cellulose sponge as a template. Collagen gel frameworks [Douglas, 1980] also have been and are currently being employed to culture tissues such as skin, breast epithelium, and liver. In addition, tumor tissue cocultured with stroma in collagen gels respond to drugs in a manner similar to that observed *in vivo* [Rheinwald and Beckett, 1981].

We developed three-dimensional coculture templates using nylon filtration screens and felts made of polyester or bioresorbably polyglycolic acid polymers [Naughton et al., 1987, 1994]. Rodent or human bone marrow cocultures retained multilineage hematopoietic expression in these stereotypic cultures, a phenomenon that is possible in plastic flask or suspension cultures only if the medium is supplemented with cocktails of cytokines [Peters et al., 1993]. Cocultures of rat hepatic parenchymal and stromal cells on three-dimensional templates also displayed a number of liver-specific functions for at least 48 days in culture, including the active synthesis of albumin, fibrinogen, and other proteins and the expression of dioxin-inducible cytochrome P450 enzyme activity for up to 2 months in culture [Naughton et al., 1994]. Furthermore, hepatic parenchyma in these stereotypic cocultures proliferated in association with stromal elements and the ECM they deposited until all "open" areas within the template were utilized. Our method is different from others because we use stromal cells derived from the tissue we wish to culture to populate the three-dimensional template. These cells secrete tissue-specific ECM and other matrix components that are indigenous to the normal microenvironment of the tissue. Parenchymal cells associate freely within the template after their inoculation and bind to other cells and/or matrix based upon their natural cytoadhesion molecule profiles. We do not add exogenous proteins.

Three-dimensional scaffolds such as nylon screen or polyester felt provide large surface areas for cell attachment and growth. Although mass transfer limitations of diffusion dictate the maximum thickness (density) of a tissue culture, suspended three-dimensional cultures have the advantage of being completely surrounded by medium. This arrangement effectively doubles the maximum tissue thickness that is possible with a plastic flask-based culture. These stereotypic cultures also appear to form tissuelike structure *in vitro* and, when implanted after coculture on bioresorbable polymer templates, *in vivo*.

Defining Terms

When hematopoietic cells are inoculated into semisolid or liquid medium containing the appropriate growth factors, some of the cells are clonal and will form colonies after approximately 2 weeks in culture. These colonies arise from hematopoietic progenitor cells and are called **colony-forming units** or **CFU**. These colonies can consist of granulocytic cells (**G**), monocytic cells (**M**), a mixture of these two cell types (**GM**), or erythroid cells (**E**). Less mature progenitor cells have a greater potential for lineage expression. For example, a **CFU-GEMM** contains granulocytic, erythroid, megakaryocytic, and mono-cytic cells and is therefore the least mature progenitor of this group.

The text also mentions **CFU-S**. Whereas the other assays quantify colony formation *in vitro*, this is an *in vivo* assay. Briefly, irradiated mice are infused with meatopoietic cells. Some of these cells will colonize the spleen and will produce blood cells that "rescue" the animal. As with the *in vitro* assays, colonies that arise later in culture originate from less mature cells. The **CFU-S**$_{12}$ therefore is a more primitive hemato-poietic cell than the **CFU-S**$_9$.

References

Anklesaria P, Kase K, Glowacki J, et al. 1987. Engraftment of a clonal bone marrow stromal cell line *in vivo* stimulates hematopoietic recovery from total body irradiation. Proc Natl Acad Sci USA 84:7681.

Beneyahu D, Zipori D, Wientroub S. 1993. Marrow adipocytes regulate growth and differentiation of osteoblasts. Biochem Biophys Res Commun 197:1245.

Ben-Ze'ev A, Robinson GS, Bucher NLR, et al. 1988. Cell-cell and cell-matrix interactions differentially regulate the expression of hepatic and cytoskeletal genes in primary cultures of rat hepatocytes. Proc Natl Acad Sci USA 85:2161.

Bessis M, Breton-Gorius J. 1959. Nouvelles observations sur l'ilot erythroblastique et la rhopheocytose de la ferritin. Rev Hematol 14:165.

Bissell DM, Arenson DM, Maher JJ, et al. 1987. Support of cultured hepatocytes by a laminin-rich gel: Evidence for a functionally significant subendothelial matrix in normal rat liver. J Clin Invest 790:801.

Brandt J, Srour EF, Van Besien K, et al. 1990. Cytokine-dependent long term culture of highly enriched precursors of hematopoietic progenitor cells from human bone marrow. J Clin Invest 86:932.

Brockbank KGM, van Peer CMJ. 1983. Colony stimulating activity production by hemopoietic organ fibroblastoid cells in vitro. Acta Haematol 69:369.

Chang VT, Anderson RN. 1971. Cultivation of mouse bone marrow cells: I. Growth of granulocytes. J Reticuloendoth Soc 9:568.

Cicuttini FM, Martin M, Ashman L., et al. 1992. Support of human cord blood progenitor cells on human stromal cell lines transformed by SV_{40} large T antigen under the influence of an inducible (metallothionein) promoter. Blood 80:102.

Degrassi A, Hilbert DM, Rudikoff S, et al. 1993. In vitro culture of primary plasmacytomas requires stromal cell feeder layers. Proc Natl Acad Sci USA 90:2060.

DeLeeuw AM, McCarthy SP, Geerts A, et al. 1984. Purified rat liver fat-storing cells in culture divide and contain collagen. Hepatology 4:392.

Dexter TM, Allen TD, Lajtha LG. 1977. Conditions controlling the proliferation of haematopoietic stem cells in vitro. J Cell Physiol 91:335.

Douglas WHJ, Moorman GW, Teel RW. 1980. Visualization of cellular aggregates cultured on a three-dimensional collagen sponge matrix. In Vitro 16:306.

Freshney RI, Hart E, Russell JM. 1982. Isolation and purification of cell cultures from human tumours. In E Reid, GMW Cook, DJ Moore (eds), Cancer Cell Organelles. Methodological Surveys: Biochemistry, pp 97–110, Chichester, England, Horwood Press.

Friedenstein AJ, Chailakhyan RK, Gerasimov UV. 1970. Bone marrow osteogenic stem cells: In vitro cultivation and transplantation in diffusion chambers. Cell Tiss Kinet 20:263.

Furchgott RF, Zawadzki JV. 1980. The obligatory role of endothelial cells in the relaxation of arterial smooth muscle by actylcholine. Nature 286:373.

Gallagher JT, Spooncer E, Dexter TM. 1982. Role of extracellular matrix in haemopoiesis: I. Synthesis of glycosaminoglycans by mouse bone marrow cultures. J Cell Sci 63:155.

Gimble JM. 1990. The function of adipocytes in the bone marrow stroma. New Biol 2:304.

Gimble JM, Dorheim MA, Cheng Q, et al. 1989. Response of bone marrow stromal cells to adipogenetic antagonists. Mol Cell Biol 9:4587.

Greenberger JS. 1979. Corticosteroid-dependent differentiation of human marrow preadipocytes in vitro. In Vitro 15:823.

Guguen-Guilluozo C, Clement B, Baffet G, et al. 1983. Maintenance and reversibility of active albumin secretion by adult rat hepatocytes co-cultured with another cell type. Exp Cell Res 143:47.

Gupta P, Blazar BR, Gupta K, et al. 1998. Human CD34+ bone marrow cells regulate stromal production of interleukin-6 and granulocyte colony-stimulating factor and increase the colony-stimulating activity of stroma. Blood 91:3724.

Huang S, Terstappen LWMM. 1992. Formation of haematopoietic microenvironment and haematopoietic stem cells from single human bone marrow cells. Nature 360:745.

Keller D, Ou XX, Rour EF, et al. 1993. Interleukin-II inhibits adipogenesis and stimulates myelopoiesis in human long-term marrow cultures. Blood 82:1428.

Keltz MD, Atton E, Buradagunta S, et al. 1996. Modulation of leukemia inhibitory factor gene expression and protein biosynthesis in human fallopian tube. Am J Gynecol Obstet 175:1611.

Kuri-Harcuch W, Mendoza-Figueroa T. 1989. Cultivation of adult rat hepatocytes on 3T3 cells: Expression of various liver differentiated functions. Differentiation 41:148.

Leighton J. 1951. A sponge matrix method for tissue culture: Formation of organized aggregates of cells in vitro. J Natl Cancer Inst 12:545.

Lictman MA. 1984. The relationship of stromal cells to hemopoietic cells in marrow. In DG Wright, JS Greenberger (eds), Long-Term Bone Marrow Culture, pp 3–30, New York, A.R. Liss.

Lin CQ, Bissell MJ. 1993. Multi-faceted regulation of cell differentiation by extracellular matrix. FASEB J 7:737.

Maniatis A, Tavassoli M, Crosby WH. 1971. Factors affecting the conversion of yellow to red marrow. Blood 37:581.

Mari BP, Anderson IC, Mari SE, et al. 1998. Stromelysin-3 is induced in tumor/stroma cocultures and inactivated via a tumor-specific and basic fibroblast growth factor-dependent mechanism. J Biol Chem 273:618.

McCuskey RS, Meineke HA, Townsend SF. 1972. Studies of the hemopoietic microenvironment: I. Changes in the microvascular system and stroma during erythropoietic regeneration and suppression in the spleens of CF_1 mice. Blood 5:697.

Metcalf D. 1993. Hematopoietic growth factors. Redundancy or subtlety? Blood 82:3515.

Michalopoulos G, Pitot HC. 1975. Primary culture of parenchymal liver cells on collagen membranes. Exp Cell Res 94:70.

Moreau I, Duvert V, Caux C, et al. 1993. Myofibroblastic stromal cells isolated from human bone marrow induce the proliferation of both early myeloid and B-lymphoid cells. Blood 82:2396.

Mrózek E, Anderson P, and Aligiuri MA. 1996. Role of interleukin-15 in the development of human CD56+ natural killer cells from CD34+ human progenitor cells. Blood 87:2632.

Naughton BA, Kolks GA, Arce JM, et al. 1979. The regenerating liver: A site of erythropoiesis in the adult long-evans rat. Am J Anat 156:159.

Naughton BA, Naughton GK. 1989. Hematopoiesis on nylon mesh templates. Ann NY Acad Sci 554:125.

Naughton BA, San Roman J, Sibanda B, et al. 1994. Stereotypic culture systems for liver and bone marrow: Evidence for the development of functional tissue in vitro and following implantation in vivo. Biotech Bioeng 43:810.

Naughton BA, Sibanda B, San Román J, et al. 1992. Differential effects of drugs upon hematopoiesis can be assessed in long-term bone marrow cultures established on nylon screens. Proc Soc Exp Biol Med 199:481.

Owen ME. 1988. Marrow stromal stem cells. J Cell Sci 10:63.

Palsson BO, Paek S-H, Schwartz RM, et al. 1993. Expansion of human bone marrow progenitor cells in a high cell density continuous perfusion system. Biotechnology 11:368.

Peters C, O'Shea KS, Campbell AD, et al. 1990. Fetal expression of hemonectin: An extracellular matrix hematopoietic cytoadhesion molecule. Blood 75:357.

Peterson TC, Renton KW. 1984. Depression of cytochrome P-450-dependent drug biotransformation in hepatocytes after the activation of the reticuloendothelial system by dextran sulfate. J Pharmacol Exp Ther 229:229.

Puck TT, Marcus PI. 1955. A rapid method for viable cell titration and clone production with HeLa cells in tissue culture: The use of X-irradiated cells to supply conditioning factors. Proc Natl Acad Sci USA 41:432.

Reid LM, Gaitmaitan Z, Arias I, et al. 1980. Long-term cultures of normal rat hepatocytes on liver biomatrix. Ann NY Acad Sci 349:70.

Rios M, Williams DA. 1990. Systematic analysis of the ability of stromal cell lines derived from different murine adult tissues to support maintenance of hematopoietic stem cells in vitro. J Cell Physiol 145:434.

Roberts R, Gallagher J, Spooncer E, et al. 1988. Heparan sulfate bound growth factors: A mechanism for stromal cell-mediated haemopoiesis. Nature 332:376.

Ryan DH, Nuccie BL, Abboud CN, et al. 1991. Vascular cell adhesion molecule-1 and the integrin VLA-4 mediate adhesion of human B cell precursors to cultured bone marrow adherent cells. J Clin Invest 88:995.

Schrock LM, Judd JT, Meineke HA, et al. 1973. Differences in concentration of acid mucopolysaccharides between spleens of normal and polycythemic CF1 mice. Proc Soc Exp Biol Med 144:593.

Siczkowski M, Amos A, Gordon MY. 1993. Hyaluronic acid regulates the function and distribution of sulfated glycosaminoglycans in bone marrow stromal cultures. Exp Hematol 21:126.

Simmons PJ, Masinovsky B, Longenecker BM, et al. 1992. Vascular cell adhesion molecule-1 expressed by bone marrow stromal cells mediates the binding of hematopoietic progenitor cells. Blood 80:388.

Simmons PJ, Torok-Storb B. 1991. CD 34 expression by stromal precursors in normal human adult bone marrow. Blood 78:2848.

Strobel E-S, Gay RE, Greenberg PL. 1986. Characterization of the in vitro stromal microenvironment of human bone marrow. Int J Cell Cloning 4:341.

Stamatoglou SC, Hughes RC. 1994. Cell adhesion molecules in liver function and pattern formation. FASEB J 8:420.

Thonar EJ-MA, Kuttner KE. 1987. Biochemical basis of age-related changes in porteoglycans. In TN Wight, RP Mecham (eds), Biology of Proteoglycans, pp 211–246, New York, Academic Press.

Tjota A, Rossi Tm, Naughton BA. 1992. Stromal cells derived from spleen or bone marrow support the proliferation of rat natural killer cells in long-term culture. Proc Soc Exp Biol Med 200:431.

Touw I, Lowenberg B. 1983. No simulative effect of adipocytes on hematopoiesis in long-term human bone marrow cultures. Blood 61:770.

Trentin JJ. 1970. Influence of hematopoietic organ stroma (Hematopoietic inductive microenvironment) on stem cell differentiation. In AS Gordon (ed), Regulation of Hematopoiesis, New York, Appleton-Century-Crofts.

Treon SP, Thomas P, Baron J. 1979. Lippopolysaccharide (LPS) processing by Kupffer cells releases a modified LPS with increased hepatocyte binding and decreased tumor necrosis-α stimulatory capacity. Proc Soc Exp Biol Med 202:153.

Tsai S, Patel V. Beaumont E, et al. 1987. Differential binding to erythroid and myeloid progenitors to fibroblasts and fibronectin. Blood 69:1587.

Tsuji JM, Pollack SB. 1995. Maturation of murine natural killer cells in the absence of exogenous cytokines requires contact with bone marrow stroma. Nat Immun 14:44.

Van Eyken P, Desmet VJ. 1993. Bile duct cells. In AV Le Bouton (ed), Molecular and Cell Biology of the Liver, pp 475-524, Boca Raton, FL, CRC Press.

Vaz F, Srour EF, Almeida-Porada G, et al. 1998. Human thymic stroma supports natural killer (NK) cell development from immature progenitors. Cell Immunol 186:133.

Vrana JA, Stang MT, Grande JP, et al. 1996. Expression of tissue factor in tumor stroma correlates with progression to invasive human breast cancer: Paracrine regulation by carcinoma cell-derived members of the transforming growth factor beta family. Cancer Res 56:5063.

Wernert N. 1997. The multiple roles of tumor stroma. Virchows Arch 430:433.

Whitlock CA, Witte ON. 1982. Long term culture of B lymphocytes and their precursors from murine bone marrow. Proc Natl Acad Sci USA 77:4756.

Wight TN, Kinsella MG, Keating A, et al. 1986. Proteoglycans in human long-term bone marrow cultures: Biochemical and ultrastructural analysis. Blood 67:1333.

Wilson D. 1983. The origin of the endothelium in the developing marginal vein of the chick wing-bud. Cell Differ 13:63.

Wolf NS, Trentin JJ. 1968. Hematopoietic colony studies: V. Effects of hemopoietic organ stroma on differentiation of pluripotent stem cells. J Exp Med 127:205.

Yanagisawa M, Jurihara HJ, Kimura S, et al. 1988. A novel potent vasoconstrictor peptide produced by vascular endothelial cells. Nature 332:411.

Yang Y-C, Tsai S, Wong GG, et al. 1988. Interleukin-1 regulation of hematopoietic growth factor production by human stromal fibroblasts. J Cell Physiol 134:292.

Zuckerman KS. 1984. Composition and function of the extracellular matrix in the stroma of long-term bone marrow cell cultures. In DG Wright, JS Greenberger (eds), Long-Term Bone Marrow Culture, pp 157–170, New York, A.R. Liss.

Zuckerman KS, Rhodes RK, Goodrum DD, et al. 1985. Inhibition of collagen deposition in the extracellular matrix prevents the establishment of stroma supportive of hematopoiesis in long term murine bone marrow cultures. J Clin Invest 75:970.

Further Information

There are a number of different methodologies for isolating cells including gradient density centrifugation, sedimentation at unit gravity, lectin agglutination, and reaction with specific antibodies followed by immunoselection via panning or immunomagnetic microspheres. These methods are described and illustrated well in volumes 1–5 of *Cell Separation: Methods and Selected Applications*, New York, Academic Press, 1987. For additional details concerning the relevance of ECM deposition to the development and functional expression of various types of tissue cells, the reader is referred to the serial reviews of this subject that appeared in *The FASEB Journal* from volume 7, number 9 (1993) to volume 8, number 4 (1994). Information about the various cell types of the liver, their interaction with matrix components, and their mechanisms of gene expression can be found in *Molecular and Cell Biology of the Liver*, Boca Raton, Florida, CRC Press (1993). Similarly, for more details concerning bone marrow cells and the mechanisms of hematopoiesis, consult *The Human Bone Marrow*, volume 1, Boca Raton, Florida, CRC Press (1992).

19

Tissue Engineering of Bone Marrow

Manfred R. Koller
Oncosis

Bernhard Ø. Palsson
University of California–San Diego

The human body consumes a staggering 400 billion mature blood cells every day, and this number increases dramatically under conditions of stress such as infection or bleeding. A complex scheme of multilineage proliferation and differentiation, termed *hematopoiesis* (Greek for blood forming), has evolved to meet this demand. This regulated production of mature blood cells from immature stem cells, which occurs mainly in the bone marrow (BM) of adult mammals, has been the focus of considerable research effort. *Ex vivo* models of human hematopoiesis now exist that have significant scientific value and promise to have an impact on clinical practice in the near future. This endeavor is spread across many fields, including cell biology, molecular biology, bioengineering, and medicine.

This chapter introduces the reader to the fundamental concepts of hematopoiesis, the clinical applications which drive much of the effort to reconstitute hematopoiesis *ex vivo*, and the progress made to date toward achieving this goal.

19.1 Biology of Hematopoiesis

The Hematopoietic System: Function and Organization

There are eight major types of mature blood cells which are found in the circulation (Fig. 19.1). The blood cell population is divided into two major groups; the myeloid and lymphoid. The myeloid lineage

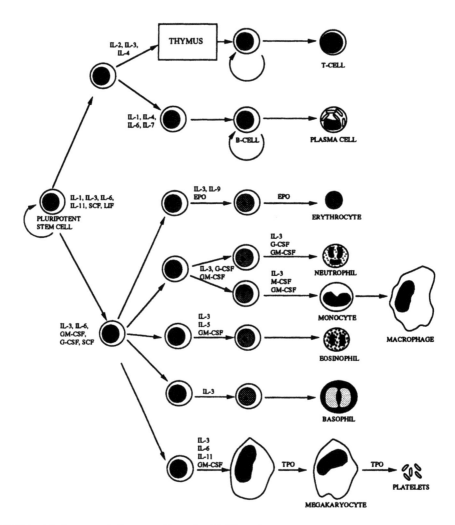

FIGURE 19.1 The hematopoietic system hierarchy. Dividing pluripotent stem cells may undergo self-renewal to form daughter stem cells without loss of potential or may experience a concomitant differentiation to form daughter cells with more restricted potential. Continuous proliferation and differentiation along each lineage results in the production of many mature cells. This process is under the control of many growth factors (GFs). The site of action of some of the better-studied GFs are shown. The mechanisms that determine which lineage a cell will develop into are not understood, although many models have been proposed.

includes erythrocytes (red blood cells), monocytes, the granulocytes (neutrophils, eosinophils, and basophils), and platelets (derived from noncirculating megakaryocytes). Thymus-derived (T) lymphocytes and BM-derived (B) lymphocytes constitute the lymphoid lineage. Most mature blood cells exhibit a limited lifespan *in vivo*. Although some lymphocytes are thought to survive for many years, it has been shown that erythrocytes and neutrophils have lifespans of 120 days and 8 h, respectively [Cronkite, 1988]. As a result, hematopoiesis is a highly prolific process which occurs throughout our lives to fulfill this demand.

Mature cells are continuously produced from *progenitor cells*, which in turn are produced from earlier cells which originate from *stem cells*. There are many levels in this hierarchical system, which is usually diagrammed as shown in Fig. 19.1. At the left are the very primitive stem cells, the majority of which are in a nonproliferative state (G_0) [Lajtha, 1979]. These cells are very rare (1 in 100,000 BM cells) but collectively have enough proliferative capacity to last several lifetimes [Boggs et al., 1982; Spangrude et al., 1988]. Through some unknown mechanism, at any given time a small number of these cells are actively proliferating, differentiating, and self-renewing, thereby producing more mature progenitor cells while maintaining the size of the stem cell pool. Whereas stem cells (by definition) are not restricted to any lineage, their progenitor cell progeny do have a restricted potential and are far greater in number. The restricted nature of these progenitors has led to a nomenclature which describes their potential outcome. Those that develop into erythrocytes are called colony-forming unit-erythrocyte (CFU-E, the term colony-forming unit relates to the biological assay which is used to measure progenitor cells). Similarly, progenitors which form granulocytes and macrophages are called CFU-GM. Therefore, as the cells differentiate and travel from left to right in Fig. 19.1, they become more numerous, lose self-renewal ability, lose proliferative potential, become restricted to a single lineage, and finally become a mature cell of a particular type. The biology of stem cells is discussed in Chapter 15. The need for identification of the many cell types present in the hematopoietic system has led to many types of assays. Many of these are biologic assays (such as *colony-forming assays*), which are performed by culturing the cells and examining their progeny, both in number and type [Sutherland et al., 1991a]. Another example is the *long-term culture-initiating cell* (LTC-IC) assay which measures a very early cell type through 5–16 weeks of *in vitro* maintenance [Koller et al., 1998a]. In contrast to these biologic assays, which are destructive to the cells being measured, is the real-time technique of *flow cytometry*. Flow cytometry has been used extensively in the study of the hematopoietic system hierarchy. Antibodies to antigens on many of the cell types shown in Fig. 19.1 have been developed (see Brott et al. [1995]). Because of the close relation of many of the cell types, often combinations of antigens are required to definitively identify a particular cell. Recently, much effort has been focused on the identification of primitive stem cells, and this has been accomplished by analyzing increasingly smaller subsets of cells using increasingly complex antibody combinations. The first such antigen that was found in CD34, which identifies all cells from the stem through progenitor stage (typically about 2% of BM mononuclear cells (MNC), see Fig. 19.2) [Civin et al., 1984]. The CD34 antigen is stage-specific but not lineage-specific and therefore identifies cells that lead to repopulation of all cell lineages in transplant patients [Berenson et al., 1991]. However, the CD34 antigen is not restricted to hematopoietic cells because it is also found on certain stromal cells in the hematopoietic microenvironment (see Chapters 17 and 18). Although CD34 captures a small population which contains stem cells, this cell population is itself quite heterogeneous and can be fractionated by many other antigens. Over the past several years, many different combinations of antibodies have been used to fractionate the CD34$^+$ population. CD34$^+$ fractions which lack CD33, HLA-DR, CD38, or CD71 appear to be enriched in stem cells [Civin and Gore, 1993]. Conversely, CD34$^+$ populations which coexpress Thy-1 or *c-kit* appear to contain the primitive cells [Civin and Gore, 1993]. These studies have revealed the extreme rarity of stem cells within the heterogeneous BM population (see Fig. 19.2). Of the *mononuclear cell* (MNC) subset (~40% of whole BM), only ~2% are CD34$^+$, and of those, only ~5% may be CD38$^+$. Furthermore, this extremely rare population is still heterogeneous with respect to stem cell content. Consequently, stem cells as single cells have not yet been identified.

Molecular Control of Hematopoiesis: The Hematopoietic Growth Factors

A large number of hematopoietic growth factors (GFs) regulate both the production and functional activity of hematopoietic cells. The earliest to be discovered were the colony-stimulating factors (CSFs, because of their activity in the colony-forming assay), which include interleukin-3 (IL-3), granulocyte-macrophage (GM)-CSF, granulocyte (G)-CSF, and monocyte (M)-CSF. These GFs, along with erythropoietin, have been relatively well characterized because of their obvious effects on mature cell production and/or activation. The target cells of some of the better-studied GFs are shown in Fig. 19.1. Subsequent intensive research continues to add to the growing list of GFs that affect hematopoietic cell proliferation, differentiation, and function (Table 19.1). However, new GFs have been more difficult to find and characterize because their effects are more subtle, often providing a synergistic effect which potentiates other known GFs. In addition, there appears to be a significant amount of redundancy and pleotropy in this GF network, which makes the discovery of new GFs difficult [Metcalf, 1993]. In fact, more recent

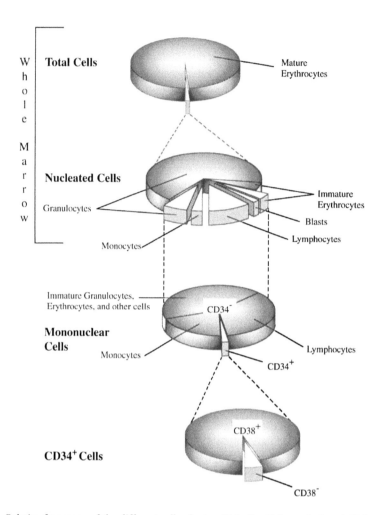

FIGURE 19.2 Relative frequency of the different cell subsets within the BM population. A BM aspirate typically contains 99% mature erythroid cells (mostly from blood contamination), and therefore usually only the nucleated cell fraction is studied. Simple density gradient centrifugation techniques, which remove most of the mature erythrocytes and granulocytes, yield what is known as the mononuclear cell (MNC) fraction (about 40% of the nucleated cells). CD34+ cells, about 2% of MNC, can be isolated by a variety of methods to capture the primitive cells, although the population is quite heterogeneous. The most primitive cells are found in subsets of CD34+ cells (e.g., CD38−), which identify about 5% of the CD34+ population. These rare subsets can be obtained by flow cytometry but are still somewhat heterogeneous with respect to stem cell content. Consequently, although methods are available to fractionate BM to a great extent, individual stem cells have not yet been identified. This diagram conveys the heterogeneous nature of different BM populations as well as the incredible rarity of the primitive cell subset, which is known to contain the stem cells.

discoveries have focused on potential receptor molecules on the target cell surface, which then have been used to isolate the appropriate ligand GF. Examples of such recently discovered GFs which exhibit synergistic interactions with other GFs to act on primitive cells include *c-kit* ligand and *flt-3* ligand. Another example is *thrombopoietin*, a stimulator of platelet production, a factor whose activity was described over 30 years ago but was cloned only recently [De Sauvage et al., 1994]. These and other GFs that act on primitive cells are the subject of intense study because of their potential scientific and commercial value. Already, several of the GFs have been developed into enormously successful pharmaceuticals, used in patients who have blood cell production deficiencies due to many different causes (see below).

TABLE 19.1 Hematopoietic Growth Factors

Growth Factor Name	Other Names	Abbreviations	Reference
Interleukin-1	Hemopoietin-1	IL-1	Dinarello et al., 1981
Interleukin-2		IL-2	Smith, 1988
Interleukin-3	Multicolony-stimulating factor	IL-3, Multi-CSF	Ihle et al., 1981
Interleukin-4	B-cell-stimulatory factor-1	IL-4, BSF-1	Yokota et al., 1988
Interleukin-5		IL-5	Yokota et al., 1988
Interleukin-6	B-cell-stimulatory factor-2	IL-6, BSF-2	Kishimoto, 1989
Interleukin-7		IL-7	Tushinski et al., 1991
Interleukin-8	Neutrophil activating peptide-1	IL-8, NAP-1	Herbert and Baker, 1993
Interleukin-9		IL-9	Donahue et al., 1990
Interleukin-10	Cytokine synthesis inhibitory factor	IL-10, CSIF	Zlotnik and Moore,1991
Interleukin-11		IL-11	Du and Williams, 1994
Interleukin-12	NK cell stimulatory factor	IL-12, NKSF	Wolf et al., 1991
Interleukin-13		IL-13	Minty et al., 1993
Interleukin-14	High molecular weight B cell growth factor	IL-14, HMW-BCGF	Ambrus et al., 1993
Interleukin-15		IL-15	Grabstein et al., 1994
Interleukin-16	Lymphocyte chemoattractant factor	IL-16; LCF	Center et al., 1997
Interleukin-17		IL-17	Yao et al., 1995
Interleukin-18	IFN-gamma-inducing factor	IL-18; IGIF	Ushio et al., 1996
Erythropoietin		Epo	Krantz, 1991
Monocyte-CSF	Colony-stimulating factor-1	M-CSF, CSF-1	Metcalf, 1985
Granulocyte-CSF		G-CSF	Metcalf, 1985
Granulocyte-macrophage-CF		GM-CSF	Metcalf, 1985
Stem cell factor	*c-kit* ligand, Mast cell growth factor	SCF, KL, MGF	Zsebo et al., 1990
Interferon-gamma	Macrophage activating factor	IFN-γ; MAF	Virelizier et al., 1985
Macrophage inflammatory protein-1	Stem cell inhibitor	MIP-1, SCI	Graham et al., 1990
Leukemia inhibitory factor		LIF	Metcalf, 1991
Transforming growth factor-beta		TGF-β	Sporn and Roberts, 1989
Tumor necrosis factor-alpha	Cachetin	TNF-α	Pennica et al., 1984
flk-2 ligand	*flk*-3 ligand	Fl	Lyman et al., 1994
Thrombopoietin	c-mpl ligand; Megakaryocyte growth and development factor	Tpo, ML; MGDF	de Sauvage et al., 1994

The Bone Marrow Microenvironment

Hematopoiesis occurs in the BM cavity in the presence of many accessory and support cells (or *stromal cells*). In addition, like all other cells *in vivo*, hematopoietic cells have considerable interaction with the extracellular matrix (ECM). These are the chief elements of what is known as the BM microenvironment. Further details on the function of stroma and the microenvironment, and their importance in tissue engineering, are found in Chapters 17 and 18.

Bone Marrow Stromal Cells

Due to the physiology of marrow, hematopoietic cells have a close structural and functional relationship with stromal cells. Marrow stroma includes fibroblasts, macrophages, endothelial cells, and adipocytes. The ratio of these different cell types varies at different places in the marrow and as the cells are cultured *in vitro*. The term stromal layer therefore refers to an undefined mixture of different adherent cell types which grow out from a culture of BM cells. *In vitro*, stem cells placed on a stromal cell layer will attach to and often migrate underneath the stromal layer [Yamakazi et al., 1989]. Under the stromal layer, some of the stem cells will proliferate, and the resulting progeny will be packed together, trapped under the stroma, forming a characteristic morphologic feature known as a cobblestone area (see below). It is widely believed that primitive cells must be in contact with stromal cells to maintain their primitive state. However, much of the effect of stromal cells has been attributed to the secretion of GFs. Consequently, there have been reports of successful hematopoietic cell growth with the addition of numerous soluble

GFs in the absence of stroma [Bodine et al., 1989; Brandt et al., 1990, 1992; Haylock et al., 1992; Koller et al., 1992a; Verfaillie, 1992]. However, this issue is quite controversial, and stromal cells are still likely to be valuable because they synthesize membrane-bound GFs [Toksoz et al., 1992], ECM components [Long, 1992], and probably some as yet undiscovered cytokines. In addition, stromal cells can modulate the GF environment in a way that would be very difficult to duplicate by simply adding soluble GFs [Koller et al., 1995]. This modulation may be responsible for the observations that stroma can be both stimulatory and inhibitory [Zipori, 1989].

The Extracellular Matrix

The ECM of BM consists of collagens, laminin, fibronectin [Zuckerman and Wicha, 1983], victronectin [Coulombel et al., 1988], hemonectin [Campbell et al., 1987], and thrombospondin [Long and Dixit, 1990]. The heterogeneity of this system is further complicated by the presence of various proteoglycans, which are themselves complex molecules with numerous glycosaminoglycan chains linked to a protein core [Minguell and Tavassoli, 1989; Spooncer et al., 1983; Wight et al., 1986]. These glycosaminoglycans include chondroitin, heparan, dermatan, and keratan sulfates and hyaluronic acid. The ECM is secreted by stromal cells of the BM (particularly endothelial cells and fibroblasts) and provides support and cohesion for the marrow structure.

There is a growing body of evidence indicating that ECM is important for the regulation of hematopoiesis. Studies have shown that different glycosaminoglycans bind and present different GFs to hematopoietic cells in an active form [Gordon et al., 1987; Roberts et al., 1988]. This demonstrates that ECM can sequester and compartmentalize certain GFs in local areas and present them to hematopoietic cells, creating a number of different hematopoietically inductive microenvironments. Another important ECM function is to provide anchorage for immature hematopoietic cells. Erythroid precursors have receptors which allow them to attach to fibronectin. As cells mature through the BFU-E to the reticulocyte stage, adherence to fibronectin is gradually lost, and the cells are free to enter the circulation [Patel et al., 1985]. It has also been shown that binding to fibronectin renders these erythroid precursors more responsive to the effects of Epo [Weinstein et al., 1989]. Another adhesion protein termed hemonectin has been shown to selectively bind immature cells of the granulocyte lineage in an analogous fashion [Campbell et al., 1987]. This progenitor binding by ECM has led to the general concept for stem cell homing. When BM cells are injected into the circulation of an animal, a sufficient number are able to home to the marrow and reconstitute hematopoiesis [Tavassoli and Hardy, 1990]. It is therefore likely that homing molecules are present on the surface of the primitive cells. Studies suggest that lectins and CD44 on progenitor cells may interact with ECM and stromal elements of the marrow to mediate cellular homing [Aizawa and Tavassoli, 1987; Kansas et al., 1990; Lewinsohn et al., 1990; Tavassoli and Hardy, 1990]. These concepts have been reviewed in detail [Long, 1992].

19.2   Applications of Reconstituted *ex Vivo* Hematopoiesis

The hematopoietic system, as described above, has many complex and interacting features. The reconstitution of functional hematopoiesis, which has long been desired, must address these features to achieve a truly representative *ex vivo* system. A functioning *ex vivo* human hematopoietic system would be a valuable analytic model to study the basic biology of hematopoiesis. The clinical applications of functional *ex vivo* models of human hematopoiesis are numerous and are just beginning to be realized. Most of these applications revolve around cancer therapies and, more recently, gene therapy. The large-scale production of mature cells for transplantation represents an important goal that may be realized in the more distant future.

Bone Marrow Transplantation

In 1980, when *bone marrow transplantation* (BMT) was still an experimental procedure, fewer than 200 BMTs were performed worldwide. Over the past decade, BMT has become an established therapy for many diseases. In 1996, over 40,000 BMTs were performed, primarily in the United States and Western

Europe, for more than a dozen different clinical indications [Horowitz and Rowling, 1997]. The number of BMTs performed annually is increasing at a rate of 20–30% per year and is expected to continue to rise in the foreseeable future.

BMT is required as a treatment in a number of clinical settings because the highly prolific cells of the hematopoietic system are sensitive to many of the agents used to treat cancer patients. Chemotherapy and radiation therapy usually target rapidly cycling cells, so hematopoietic cells are ablated along with the cancer cells. Consequently, patients undergoing these therapies experience neutropenia (low neutrophil numbers), thrombocytopenia (low platelet numbers), and anemia (low red blood cell numbers), rendering them susceptible to infections and bleeding. A BMT dramatically shortens the period of neutropenia and thromobocytopenia, but the patient may require repeated transfusions. The period during which the patient is neutropenic represents the greatest risk associated with BMT. In addition, some patients do not achieve *engraftment* (when cell numbers rise to safe levels). As a result, much effort is focused on reducing the severity and duration of the blood cell nadir period following chemotherapy and radiation therapy.

There are several sources of hematopoietic cells for transplantation. BMT may be performed with patient marrow (autologous) that has been removed and cryopreserved prior to administration of chemotherapy or with donor marrow (allogeneic). The numbers of autologous transplants outnumber allogenic transplants by a 2:1 ratio, but there are advantages and disadvantages with both techniques.

Autologous Bone Marrow Transplantation

Autologous BMTs have been used in the treatment of a variety of diseases including acute lymphoblastic leukemia (ALL), acute myelogenous leukemia (AML), chronic myelogenous leukemia (CML), various lymphomas, breast cancer, neuroblastoma, and multiple myeloma. Currently, autologous BM transplantation is hampered by the long hospital stay that is required until engraftment is achieved and the possibility of reintroducing tumor cells along with the cryopreserved marrow. In fact, retroviral marking studies have proved that tumor cells reinfused in the transplant can contribute to disease relapse in the patient [Rill et al., 1994; Deisseroth et al., 1994]. Long periods of neutropenia, anemia, and thrombocytopenia require parenteral antibiotic administration and repeated blood component transfusions.

Autologous transplantation could also be used in gene therapy procedures. The basic concept underlying gene therapy of the hematopoietic system is the insertion of a therapeutic gene into the hematopoietic stem cell, so that a stable transfection is obtained. Engineered retroviruses are the gene carriers currently used. However, mitosis of primitive cells is required for integration of foreign DNA [Bodine et al., 1989]. A culture system which contains dividing stem cells is therefore critical for the enablement of retroviral-based gene therapy of the hematopoietic system. This requirement holds true whether or not the target stem cell population has been purified prior to the transfection step. To date, only very limited success has been achieved with retroviral transfection of human BM cells, whereas murine cells are routinely transfected. A comprehensive and accessible accounting of the status of gene therapy has been presented elsewhere [Mulligan, 1993].

Allogeneic Bone Marrow Transplantation

In patients with certain hematologic malignancies, or with genetic defects in the hematopoietic population, allogeneic transplants are currently favored when suitable matched donors are available. With these leukemias, such as CML, it is likely that the patient's marrow is diseased and would not be suitable for autotransplant. A major obstacle in allogeneic transplantation, however, is the high incidence of *graft-versus-host disease* (GVHD), in which the transplanted immune cells attack the host's tissues as foreign.

Alternative Sources of Hematopoietic Cells for Transplantation

Although hematopoiesis occurs mainly in the BM of adult mammals, during embryonic development, pluripotent stem cells first arise in the yolk sac, are later found in the fetal liver, and at the time of delivery are found in high concentrations in umbilical cord blood. In adults, stem cells are found in peripheral blood only at very low concentrations, but the concentration increases dramatically after stem cell mobilization. Mobilization of stem cells into peripheral blood is a phenomenon that occurs in response to chemotherapy or GF administration. Therefore, hematopoietic stem cells can be collected from cord blood [Gluckman et al., 1989; Wagner et al., 1992] or from mobilized peripheral blood [Schneider et al., 1992] as well as from BM. Disadvantages of cord blood are the limited number of cells that can be obtained from the one individual and the question of whether this amount is sufficient to repopulate an adult patient. Mobilized peripheral blood results in more rapid patient engraftment than BM, and as a consequence, its use is becoming more prevalent, particularly in the autologous setting.

Tissue Engineering and Improved Transplantation Procedures

BMT would be greatly facilitated by reliable systems and procedures for *ex vivo* stem cell maintenance, expansion, and manipulation. For example, the harvest procedure, which collects 1–2 liters of marrow, is currently a painful and involved operating room procedure. The complications and discomfort of marrow donation are not trivial and can affect donors for a month or more [Stroncek et al., 1993]. Through cell expansion techniques, a small marrow specimen taken under local anesthesia in an outpatient setting could be expanded into the large number of cells required for transplant, thereby eliminating the large harvest procedure. Engraftment may be accelerated by increasing the numbers of progenitors and immature cells available for infusion. In addition, it may be possible to cryopreserve expanded cells to be infused at multiple time points, thereby allowing multiple cycles of chemotherapy (schedule intensification). Finally, the use of expanded cells may allow increasing doses of chemotherapy (dose intensification), facilitating tumor reduction while ameliorating myeloablative side effects.

The expansion of alternative hematopoietic cell sources would also facilitate transplant procedures. For example, multiple rounds of apheresis, each requiring ~4 h, are required to collect enough mobilized peripheral blood cells for transplant. Expansion of a small amount of mobilized peripheral blood may reduce the number of aphereses required or eliminate them altogether by allowing the collection of enough cells from a volume of blood that has not been apheresed. With cord blood, there is a limit on the number of cells that can be collected from a single donor, and it is currently thought that this number is inadequate for an adult transplant. Consequently, cord blood transplants to date have been performed on children. Expansion of cord blood cells may therefore enable adult transplants from the limited number of cord blood cells available for collection.

Large-Scale Production of Mature Blood Cells

Beyond the ability to produce stem and progenitor cells for transplantation purposes lies the promise to produce large quantities of mature blood cells. Large-scale hematopoietic cultures could potentially provide several types of clinically important mature blood cells. These include red blood cells, platelets, and granulocytes. About 12 million units of red blood cells are transfused in the United States every year, the majority of them during elective surgery and the rest in acute situations. About 4 million units of platelets are transfused every year into patients who have difficulty exhibiting normal blood clotting. Mature granulocytes, which constitute a relatively low-usage market of only a few thousand units administered each year, are involved in combating infections. This need arises in situations when a patient's immune system has been compromised and requires assistance in combating opportunistic infections, such as during chemotherapy and the healing of burn wounds.

All in all, the market for these blood cells totals about $1–1.5 billion in the United States annually, with a worldwide market that is about three to four times larger. The ability to produce blood cells on demand *ex vivo* would alleviate several problems with the current blood cell supply. The first of these problems is the availability and stability of the blood cell supply. The availability of donors has traditionally been a problem, and, coupled with the short shelf-life of blood cells, the current supply is unstable and cannot meet major changes in demand. The second problem is the usual blood-type compatibility problem resulting in shortages of certain types at various times. The third problem is the safety of the blood supply. This last issue has received much attention recently due to the contamination of donated blood with the human immunodeficiency virus (HIV). However, the three forms of hepatitis currently pose an even more serious viral contamination threat to the blood supply.

Unlike *ex vivo* expansion of stem and progenitor cells for transplantation, the large-scale production of fully mature blood cells for routine clinical use is less developed and represents a more distant goal. The large market would require systems of immense size, unless major improvements in culture productivity are attained. For example, the recent discovery of thrombopoietin [De Sauvage et al., 1994] may make the large-scale production of platelets feasible. At present, there are ongoing attempts in several laboratories to produce large numbers of neutrophils from CD34-selected cell populations. Thus, large-scale production of mature cells may soon become technically feasible, although the economic considerations are still unknown.

19.3 The History of Hematopoietic Cell Culture Development

As outlined above, there are many compelling scientific and clinical reasons for undertaking the development of efficient *ex vivo* hematopoietic systems. Such achievement requires the use of *in vivo* mimicry, sophisticated cell culture technology, and the development of clinically acceptable cell cultivation devices. The foundations for these developments lie in the BM cell culture methods which have been developed over the past 20 years. The history of BM culture will therefore be described briefly, as it provides the backdrop for tissue engineering of the hematopoietic system. More complete reviews have been published previously [Dexter et al., 1984; Eaves et al., 1991; Greenberger, 1984].

The Murine System

In the mid-1970s, Dexter and co-workers were successful in developing a culture system in which murine hematopoiesis could be maintained for several months [Dexter et al., 1977]. The key feature of this system was the establishment of a BM-derived stromal layer during the first 3 weeks of culture which was then recharged with fresh BM cells. One to 2 weeks after the cultures were recharged, active sites of hematopoiesis appeared. These sites are often described as cobblestone regions, which are the result of primitive cell proliferation (and accumulation) underneath the stromal layer. Traditionally, the cultures are fed by replacement of one-half of the medium either once or twice weekly. In these so-called Dexter cultures, myelopoiesis proceeds to the exclusion of lymphopoiesis. The selection of a proper lot of serum for long-term BM cultures (LTBMCs) was found to be very important. In fact, when using select lots of serum, one-step LTBMCs were successfully performed without the recharging step at week 3 [Dexter et al., 1984]. It is thought that good serum allows rapid development of stroma before the primitive cells are depleted, and once the stroma is developed, the culture is maintained from the remaining original primitive cells without need for recharging. The importance of stroma has often been demonstrated in these Dexter cultures, because the culture outcome was often correlated with stromal development.

The Human System

The adaptation of one-step LTBMC for human cells was first reported in 1980 [Gartner and Kaplan, 1980]. A mixture of fetal bovine serum and horse serum was found to be required for human LTBMC, and a number of other medium additives such as sodium pyruvate, amino acids, vitamins, and antioxidants were found to be beneficial [Gartner and Kaplan, 1980; Greenberg et al., 1981; Meagher et al., 1988]. Otherwise, the culture protocol has remained essentially the same as that used for murine culture. Unfortunately, human LTBMCs have never attained the productivity or longevity which is observed in cultures of other species [Dexter et al., 1984; Greenberger et al., 1986]. The exponentially decreasing numbers of total and progenitor cells with time in human LTBMC [Eastment and Ruscetti, 1984; Eaves et al., 1991] renders the cultures unsuitable for cell expansion and indicates that primitive stem cells are lost over time. The discovery of hematopoietic GFs was an important development in human hematopoietic cell culture, because addition of GFs to human LTBMC greatly enhanced cell output. However, GFs did not prolong the longevity of the cultures, indicating that primitive cell maintenance was not improved [Coutinho et al., 1990; Lemoli et al., 1992]. Furthermore, although the total number of progenitors obtained was increased by GFs, it was still less than the number used to initiate the culture. Therefore, a net expansion in progenitor cell numbers was not obtained. The increased cell densities that were stimulated by GF addition were not well supported by the relatively static culture conditions.

The disappointing results from human LTBMCs led to the development of other culture strategies. The development of an increasing number of recombinant GFs was soon joined by the discovery of the CD34 antigen (see above). As protocols for the selection of CD34$^+$ cells became available, it was thought that the low cell numbers generated by enrichment could be expanded in GF-supplemented cultures without the impediment of numerous mature cells in the system. Because the enrichment procedure results in a cell population depleted of stromal cells, CD34$^+$ cell cultures are often called suspension cultures, due to the lack of an adherent stromal layer. A number of groups have reported experiments in which CD34$^+$ cells were incubated with high doses of up to seven recombinant GFs in suspension culture [Brandt et al., 1992; Haylock et al., 1992]. Although 500- to 1000-fold cell expansion numbers are often obtained, the magnitude of CFU-GM expansion is usually less than 10-fold, suggesting that differentiation, accompanied by depletion of primitive cells, is occurring in these systems. In fact, when LTC-IC have been measured, the numbers obtained after static culture of enriched cells have always been significantly below the input value [Sutherland et al., 1991b, 1993; Verfaillie, 1992]. A further consideration in CD34$^+$ cell culture is the loss of cells during the enrichment procedure. It is not uncommon to experience 70 to 80% loss of progenitors with most CD34$^+$ cell purification protocols [Traycoff et al., 1994], and this can be very significant when trying to maximize the final cell number obtained (such as in clinical applications, see below). Nevertheless, cultures of purified CD34$^+$ cells, and especially the smaller subsets (e.g., CD33$^-$, CD38$^-$), have yielded valuable information on the biology of hematopoietic stem cells.

An alternative approach has also been taken to improve human hematopoietic cell culture. Most of these advances have come from the realization that traditional culture protocols are highly nonphysiologic and that these deficiencies can be corrected by *in vivo* mimicry. Therefore, these techniques do not involve cell purification or high-dose cytokine stimulation. Because these cultures attain fairly high densities, it was thought that the tradition of changing one-half of the culture medium either once or twice weekly was inadequate. When Dexter-type cultures were performed with more frequent medium exchanges, progenitor cell production was supported for at least 20 weeks [Schwartz et al., 1991b]. This increase in culture longevity indicates that primitive cells were maintained for a longer period, and this was accompanied by an increase in progenitor cell yield. Although the precise mechanisms of increased medium exchange are unknown, the increased feeding rate enhances stromal cell secretion of GFs [Caldwell et al., 1991].

As previously noted, recombinant GFs can significantly improve culture productivity, but GF-stimulated cell proliferation exacerbates the problems of nutrient depletion because cell proliferation and the consumption of metabolites increases manyfold. Therefore, increased feeding protocols also benefit GF-stimulated cultures. Cultures supplemented with IL-3/GM-CSF/Epo and fed with 50% daily medium exchanges were found to result in significant cell and progenitor expansion while maintaining culture longevity [Schwartz et al., 1991a]. Optimization of these manually fed cultures has been published for both BM [Koller et al., 1996] and cord blood [Koller et al., 1998b].

Tissue Engineering Challenges

Although increased manual feeding significantly enhanced the productivity and longevity of hematopoietic cultures, the labor required to feed each culture is a daunting task. In addition, the cultures are subjected to physical disruption and large discontinuous changes in culture conditions and may be exposed to contamination at each feeding. Thee complications frustrate the optimization of the culture environment for production of hematopoietic cells and limit the clinical usefulness of the cultures. A perfusion system, if properly designed and constructed, would eliminate many of the problems currently associated with these cultures.

The success of this manual frequently fed culture approach led to development of continuously perfused bioreactors for human cord blood [Koller et al., 1993a, 1998b], BM [Palsson et al., 1993], and mobilized peripheral blood [Sandstrom et al., 1995] cell culture. Human BM MNC cultures have been performed in spinner flasks in a fed-batch mode as well [Zandstra et al., 1994]. Slow single-pass medium perfusion and internal oxygenation have given the best results to date, yielding cell densities in excess of 10^7 per ml accompanied by significant progenitor and primitive cell expansion [Koller et al., 1993b]. These systems have also been amenable to scale-up, first by a factor of 10, and then by a further factor of 7.5 [Koller et al., 1998b]. When an appropriate culture substrate is provided [Koller et al., 1998c], perfusion bioreactors support the development and maintenance of accessory cell populations, resulting in significant endogenous growth factor production which likely contributes to culture success [Koller et al., 1995a, 1997]. Importantly, stromal-containing cultures appear to generate greater numbers of primitive cells from a smaller initial cell sample, as measured by *in vitro* [Koller et al., 1995b; Sandstrom et al., 1995] and *in vivo* assays [Knobel et al., 1994], as compared with CD34-enriched cell cultures.

19.4 Challenges for Scale-Up

To gauge the scale-up challenges, one first needs to state the requirements for clinically useful systems. The need to accommodate stroma that supports active hematopoiesis represents perhaps the most important consideration for the selection of a bioreactor system.

Bioreactors and Stroma

If stroma is required, the choices are limited to systems that can support the growth of adherent cells. This requirement may be eliminated in future systems if the precise GF requirements become known and if the microenvironment that the stroma provides is not needed for hematopoietic stem and progenitor cell expansion.

Currently, there are at least three culture systems that may be used for adherent cell growth. Fluidized bed bioreactors with macroporous bead carriers provide one option. Undoubtedly, significant effort will be required to develop the suitable bead chemistry and geometry, since the currently available systems are designed for homogeneous cell cultures. Beads for hematopoietic culture probably should allow for the formation of functional colonies comprised of a mixed cell population within each bead. Cell sampling from fluidized beds would be relatively easy, but final cell harvesting may require stressful procedures, such as prolonged treatment with collagenase and/or trypsin.

Flatbed bioreactors are a second type of system which can support stromal development. Such units can be readily designed to carry the required cell number, and, further, they can allow for direct microscopic observation of the cell culture. Flatbed bioreactors provide perhaps the most straightforward scale-up and automation of LTBMC. In fact, such automated systems have been developed and used in human clinical trials for the treatment of cancer [Mandalam et al., 1998].

Finally, membrane-based systems, such as hollow fiber units, could be used to carry out hematopoietic cell cultures of moderate size. Special design of the hollow fiber bed geometry with respect to axial length and radial fiber spacing should eliminate all undesirable spatial gradients. Such units have been made already and have proved effective for their use for *in vivo* NMR analysis of metabolic behavior of homogeneous cell cultures [Mancuso et al., 1990]. However, hematopoietic cell observation and harvesting may prove to be troublesome with this approach, as one report has suggested [Sardonini and Wu, 1993].

It is possible that the function of accessory cells may be obtained by the use of spheroids without classical adherent cell growth. This approach to the growth of liver cells in culture has met with some success (see Chapter 20). In fact, there have been reports of functional heterogeneous cell aggregates within BM aspirates [Blazsek et al., 1990; Funk et al., 1994]. If successfully developed, suspension cultures containing these aggregates could be carried out in a variety of devices, including the rotating wall vessels that have been developed by NASA [Schwarz et al., 1992].

Alternatives

The precise arrangement of future large-scale systems will be significantly influenced by continuing advances in the understanding of the molecular and microenvironmental regulation of the hematopoietic process. Currently, the proximity of a supporting stromal layer is believed to be important. It is thought to function through the provision of both soluble and membrane-bound GFs and by providing a suitable microenvironment. The characterization of the microenvironment is uncertain at present, but its chemistry and local geometry are both thought to play a role. If the proximity of stroma is found to be unimportant, one could possibly design culture systems in which the stroma and BM cells are separated [Verfaillie, 1992], resulting in the ability to control each function separately. Finally, if the GF requirements can be defined and artificially supplied, and the stromal microenvironment is found to be unimportant, large-scale hematopoietic suspension cultures would become possible.

Production of Mature Cells

Culture systems for generic allogeneic BMT, or for the large-scale production of mature cells, will pose more serious scale-up challenges. The number of cells required for these applications, in particular the latter, may be significantly higher than that for autologous BMT. Of the three alternatives discussed above, the fluidized bed system is the most readily scalable. The flatbed systems can be scaled by a simple stacking approach, whereas hollow fiber units are known for their shortcomings with respect to large-scale use.

19.5 Recapitulation

Rapid advances in our understanding of hematopoietic cell biology and the molecular control of hematopoietic cell replication, differentiation, and apoptosis are providing some of the basic information that is needed to reconstitute human hematopoiesis *ex vivo*. Compelling clinical applications provide a significant impetus for developing systems that produce clinically useful cell populations in clinically meaningful numbers. Use of *in vivo* mimicry and the bioreactor technologies that were developed in the 1980s are leading to the development of perfusion-based bioreactor systems that will meet some of the clinical needs. Further tissue engineering of human hematopoiesis is likely to continue to grow in scope and sophistication and lead to definition of basic structure-function relationships and the enablement of many needed clinical procedures.

Defining Terms

Colony-forming assay: Assay carried out in semisolid medium under GF stimulation. Progenitor cells divide, and progeny are held in place so that a microscopically identifiable colony results after 2 weeks.

Differentiation: The irreversible progression of a cell or cell population to a more mature state.

Engraftment: The attainment of a safe number of circulating mature blood cells after a BMT.

Flow cytometry: Technique for cell analysis using fluorescently conjugated monoclonal antibodies which identify certain cell types. More sophisticated instruments are capable of sorting cells into different populations as they are analyzed.

Graft-versus-host disease: The immunologic response of transplanted cells against the tissue of their new host. This response is often a severe consequence of allogeneic BMT and can lead to death (acute GVHD) or long-term disability (chronic GVHD).

Hematopoiesis: The regulated production of mature blood cells through a scheme of multilineage proliferation and differentiation.

Lineage: Refers to cells at all stages of differentiation leading to a particular mature cell type, i.e., one branch on the lineage diagram shown in Fig. 19.1.

Long-term culture-initiating cell: Cell that is measured by a 7–18 week *in vitro* assay. LTC-IC are thought to be very primitive, and the population contains stem cells. However, the population is heterogeneous, so not every LTC-IC is a stem cell.

Microenvironment: Refers to the environment surrounding a given cell *in vivo*.

Mononuclear cell: Refers to the cell population obtained after density centrifugation of whole BM. This population excludes cells without a nucleus (erythrocytes) and polymorphonuclear cells (granulocytes).

Progenitor cells: Cells that are intermediate in the development pathway, more mature than stem cells but not yet mature cells. This is the cell type measured in the colony-forming assay.

Self-renewal: Generation of a daughter cell with identical characteristics as the original cell. Most often used to refer to stem cell division, which results in the formation of new stem cells.

Stem cells: Cells with potentially unlimited proliferative and lineage potential.

Stromal cells: Heterogeneous mixture of support or accessory cells of the BM. Also refers to the adherent layer which forms in BM cultures.

References

Aizawa S, Tavassoli M. 1987. In vitro homing of hemopoietic stem cells is mediated by a recognition system with galactosyl and mannosyl specificities. Proc Natl Acad Sci USA 84:4485.

Ambrus JL Jr., Pippin J, Joseph A, Xu C, Blumenthal D, Tamayo A, Claypool K, McCourt D, Srikiatchatochorn A, and Ford RJ. 1993. Identification of a cDNA for a human high-molecular weight B-cell growth factor. Proc Natl Acad Sci USA 90:6330–6334.

Armstrong RD, Koller MR, Paul LA, et al. 1993. Clinical scale production of stem and hematopoietic cells ex vivo. Blood 82:296a.

Berenson RJ, Bensinger WI, Hill RS, et al. 1991. Engraftment after infusion of CD34+ marrow cells in patients with breast cancer or neuroblastoma. Blood 77:1717.

Blazsek I, Misset J-L, Benavides M, et al. 1990. Hematon, a multicellular functional unit in normal human bone marrow: Structural organization, hemopoietic activity, and its relationship to myelodysplasia and myeloid leukemias. Exp Hematol 18:259.

Bodine DM, Karlsson S, Nienhuis AW. 1989. Combination of interleukins 3 and 6 preserves stem cell function in culture and enhances retrovirus-mediated gene transfer into hematopoietic stem cells. Proc Natl Acad Sci USA 86:8897.

Boggs DR, Boggs SS, Saxe DF, et al. 1982. Hematopoietic stem cells with high proliferative potential. J Clin Invest 70:242.

Brandt JE, Briddell RA, Srour EF, Leemhuis TB, and Hoffman R. 1992. Role of *c-kit* ligand in the expansion of human hematopoietic progenitor cells. Blood 79:634–641.

Brandt JE, Srour EF, Van Besien K, et al. 1990. Cytokine-dependent long-term culture of highly enriched precursors of hematopoietic progenitor cells from human bone marrow. J Clin Invest 86:932.

Brott DA, Koller MR, Rummel SA, Palsson BO. 1995. Flow cytometric analysis of cells obtained from human bone marrow cultures. In M Al-Rubeai, AN Emery (eds) Flow Cytometry Applications in Cell Culture, pp 121–146, Marcel Dekker, New York.

Caldwell J, Palsson BØ, Locey B, et al. 1991. Culture perfusion schedules influence the metabolic activity and granulocyte-macrophage colony-stimulating factor production rates of human bone marrow stromal cells. J Cell Physiol 147:344.

Campbell AD, Long MW, Wicha MS. 1987. Haemonectin, a bone marrow adhesion protein specific for cells of granulocyte lineage. Nature 329:744.

Center DM, Kornfeld H, Cruikshand WW. 1997. Interleukin-16. Int J Biochem Cell Biol 29:1231–1234.

Civin CI, Gore SD. 1993. Antigenic analysis of hematopoiesis: A review. J Hematother 2:137.

Civin CI, Strauss LC, Brovall C, et al. 1984. Antigenic analysis of hematopoiesis: III. A hematopoietic progenitor cell surface antigen defined by a monoclonal antibody raised against KG-Ia cells. J Immunol 133:157.

Coulombel L, Vuillet MH, Leroy C, et al. 1988. Lineage- and stage-specific adhesion of human hemato-poietic progenitor cells to extracellular matrices from marrow fibroblasts. Blood 71:329.

Coutinho LH, Will A, Radford J, et al. 1990. Effects of recombinant human granulocyte colony-stimu-lating factor (CSF), human granulocyte macrophage-CSF, and gibbon interleukin-3 on hemato-poiesis in human long-term bone marrow culture. Blood 75:2118.

Cronkite EP. 1988. Analytical review of structure and regulation of hemopoiesis. Blood Cells 14:313.

De Sauvage FJ, Hass PE, Spencer SD, et al. 1994. Stimulation of megakaryocytopoiesis and thrombopoiesis by the c-Mpl ligand. Nature 369:533.

Dexter TM, Allen TD, Lajtha LG. 1977. Conditions controlling the proliferation of haemopoietic stem cells *in vitro*. J Cell Physiol 91:335.

Dexter TM, Spooncer E, Simmons P, et al. 1984. Long-term marrow culture: An overview of techniques and experience. In DG Wright, JS Greenberger (eds), Long-Term Bone Marrow Culture, pp 57–96, New York, Alan R. Liss.

Dinarello CA, Rosenwasser LJ, Wolff SM. 1981. Demonstrating of a circulating suppressor factor of thymocyte proliferation during endotoxin fever in humans. J Immunol 127:2517.

Donahue RE, Yang Y-C, Clark SC. 1990. Human P40 T-cell growth factor (interleukin 9) supports erythroid colony formation. Blood 75:2271.

Du XX, Williams DA. 1994. Interleukin-11: A multifunctional growth factor derived from the hemato-poietic microenvironment. Blood 83:2023.

Eastment CE, Ruscetti FW. 1984. Evaluation of hematopoiesis in long-term bone marrow culture: Com-parison of species differences. In DG Wright, JS Greenberger (eds), Long-Term Bone Marrow Culture, pp 97–118, New York, Alan R. Liss.

Eaves CJ, Cashman JD, Eaves AC. 1991. Methodology of long-term culture of human hemopoietic cells. J Tiss Cult Meth 13:55.

Funk PE, Kincade PW, Witte PL. 1994. Native associations of early hematopoietic stem cells and stromal cells isolated in bone marrow cell aggregates. Blood 83:361.

Gartner S, Kaplan HS. 1980. Long-term culture of human bone marrow cells. Proc Natl Acad Sci USA 77:4756.

Gluckman E, Broxmeyer HE, Auerback AD, et al. 1989. Hematopoietic reconstitution in a patient with Fanconi's anemia by means of umbilical-cord blood from an HLA-identical sibling. NE J Med 321:1174.

Gordon MY, Riley GP, Watt SM, et al. 1987. Compartmentalization of a haematopoietic growth factor (GM-CSF) by glycosaminoglycans in the bone marrow microenvironment. Nature 326:403.

Grabstein KH, Eisenman J, Shanebeck K, Rauch C, Srinivasan S, Fung V, Beers C, Richardson J, Schoen-born MA, Ahdieh M. 1994. Cloning of a T cell growth factor that interacts with the beta chain of the interleukin-2 receptor. Science 264:965–968.

Graham GJ, Wright EG, Hewick R, et al. 1990. Identification and characterization of an inhibitor of haemopoietic stem cell proliferation. Nature 344:442.

Greenberg HM, Newburger PE, Parker LM, et al. 1981. Human granulocytes generated in continuous bone marrow culture are physiologically normal. Blood 58:724.

Greenberger JS. 1984. Long-term hematopoietic cultures. In DW Golde (ed), Hematopoiesis, pp 203–242, New York, Churchill Livingstone.

Greenberger JS, Fitzgerald TJ, Rothstein L, et al. 1986. Long-term culture of human granulocytes and granulocyte progenitor cells. In Transfusion Medicine: Recent Technological Advances, pp 159–185, New York, Alan R. Liss.

Haylock DN, To LB, Dowse TL, et al. 1992. Ex vivo expansion and maturation of peripheral blood CD34[+] cells into the myeloid lineage. Blood 80:1405.

Herbert CA, Baker JB. 1993. Interleukin-8: A review. Cancer Invest 11:743.

Hoffman R, Benz EJ Jr, Shattil SJ, et al. 1991. Hematology: Basic Principles and Practice, New York, Churchill Livingstone.

Horowitz MM, Rowlings PA. 1997. An update from the International Bone Marrow Transplant Registry and the Autologous Blood and Marrow Transplant Registry on current activity in hematopoietic stem cell transplantation. Curr Opin Hematol 4:359–400.

Ihle JN, Pepersack L, Rebar L. 1981. Regulation of T cell differentiation: In vitro induction of 20 alpha-hydroxysteroid dehydrogenase in splenic lymphocytes is mediated by a unique lymphokine. J Immunol 126:2184.

Kansas GS, Muirhead MJ, Dailey MO. 1990. Expression of the CD11/CD18, leukocyte adhesion molecule 1, and CD44 adhesion molecules during normal myeloid and erythroid differentiation in humans. Blood 76:2483.

Kishimoto T. 1989. The biology of interleukin-6. Blood 74:1.

Knobel KM, McNally MA, Berson AE, Rood D, Chen K, Kilinski L, Tran K, Okarma TB, Lebkowski JS. 1994. Long-term reconstitution of mice after ex vivo expansion of bone marrow cells: Differential activity of cultured bone marrow and enriched stem cell populations. Exp Hematol 22:1227–1235.

Koller MR, Bender JG, Papoutsakis ET, et al. 1992a. Effects of synergistic cytokine combinations, low oxygen, and irradiated stroma on the expansion of human cord blood progenitors. Blood 80:403.

Koller MR, Bender JG, Papoutsakis ET, et al. 1992b. Beneficial effects of reduced oxygen tension and perfusion in long-term hematopoietic cultures. Ann NY Acad Sci 665:105.

Koller MR, Bender JG, Miller WM, et al. 1993a. Expansion of human hematopoietic progenitors in a perfusion bioreactor system with IL-3, IL-6, and stem cell factor. Biotechnology 11:358.

Koller MR, Emerson SG, Palsson BØ. 1993b. Large-scale expansion of human stem and progenitor cells from bone marrow mononuclear cells in continuous perfusion culture. Blood 82:378.

Koller MR, Bradley MS, Palsson BØ. 1995. Growth factor consumption and production in perfusion cultures of human bone marrow correlates with specific cell production. Exp Hematol 23:1275.

Koller MR, Manchel I, Palsson BO. 1997. Importance of parenchymal:stromal cell ratio for the ex vivo reconstitution of human hematopoiesis. Stem Cells 15:305–313.

Koller MR, Manchel I, Smith AK. 1998a. Quantitative long-term culture-initiating cell assays require accessory cell depletion that can be achieved by CD34-enrichment or 5-fluorouracil exposure. Blood 91:4056.

Koller MR, Manchel I, Maher RJ, Goltry KL, Armstrong RD, Smith AK. 1998b. Clinical-scale human umbilical cord blood cell expansion in a novel automated perfusion culture system. Bone Marrow Transplant 21:653.

Koller MR, Manchel I, Palsson MA, Maher RJ, Palsson, BØ. 1996. Different measures of human hematopoietic cell culture performance are optimized under vastly different conditions. Biotechnol Bioeng 50:505–513.

Koller MR, Palsson MA, Manchel I, Palsson BØ. 1995b. LTC-IC expansion is dependent on frequent medium exchange combined with stromal and other accessory cell effects. Blood 86:1784–1793.

Koller MR, Palsson MA, Manchel I, Maher RJ, Palsson BØ. 1998c. Tissue culture surface characteristics influence the expansion of human bone marrow cells. Biomaterials (in press).

Krantz SB. 1991. Erythropoietin. Blood 77:419.

Lajtha LG. 1979. Stem cell concepts. Differentiation 14:23.

Lemoli RM, Tafuri A, Strife A, et al. 1992. Proliferation of human hematopoietic progenitors in long-term bone marrow cultures in gas permeable plastic bags is enhanced by colony-stimulating factors. Exp Hematol 20:569.

Lewinsohn DM, Nagler A, Ginzton N, et al. 1990. Hematopoietic progenitor cell expression of the H-CAM (CD44) homing-associated adhesion molecule. Blood 75:589.

Long MW. 1992. Blood cell cytoadhesion molecules. Exp Hematol 20:288

Long MW, Dixit VM. 1990. Thrombospondin functions as a cytoadhesion molecule for human hematopoietic progenitor cells. Blood 75:2311.

Lyman SD, James L, Johnson L, Brasel K, de Vries P, Escobar SS, Downey H, Splett RR, Beckmann MP, McKenna HJ. 1994. Cloning of human homologue of the murine flt3 ligand: A growth factor for early hematopoietic progenitor cells. Blood 83:2795–2801.

Mancuso A, Fernandez EJ, Blanch HW, et al. 1990. A nuclear magnetic resonance technique for determining hybridoma cell concentration in hollow fiber bioreactors. Biotechnology 8:1282.

Mandalam R, Koller MR, Smith AK. 1998. Ex vivo hematopoietic cell expansion for bone marrow transplantation. In R Nordon (ed), Ex Vivo Cell Therapy. Landes Bioscience, Austin, TX.

Meagher RC, Salvado AJ, Wright DG. 1988. An analysis of the multilineage production of human hematopoietic progenitors in long-term bone marrow culture: Evidence that reactive oxygen intermediates derived from mature phagocytic cells have a role in limiting progenitor cell self-renewal. Blood 72:273.

Metcalf D. 1985. The granulocyte-macrophage colony-stimulating factors. Science 229:16.

Metcalf D. 1991. The leukemia inhibitory factor (LIF). Int J Cell Cloning 9:95.

Metcalf D. 1993. Hematopoietic regulators: Redundancy or subtlety? Blood 82:3515.

Minguell JJ, Tavassoli M. 1989. Proteoglycan synthesis by hematopoietic progenitor cells. Blood 73:1821.

Minty A, Chalon P, Derocq JM, et al. 1993. Interleukin-13 is a new human lymphokine regulating inflammatory and immune responses. Nature 362:248.

Mulligan RC. 1993. The basic science of gene therapy. Science 260:926–932.

Palsson BØ, Paek S-H, Schwartz RM, et al. 1993. Expansion of human bone marrow progenitor cells in a high cell density continuous perfusion system. Biotechnology 11:368.

Patel VP, Ciechanover A, Platt O, et al. 1985. Mammalian reticulocytes lose adhesion to fibronectin during maturation to erythrocytes. Proc Natl Acad Sci USA 82:440.

Pennica D, Nedwin GE, Hayflick JS, et al. 1984. Human tumor necrosis factor: Precursor structure, expression and homology to lymphotoxin. Nature 312:724.

Roberts R, Gallagher J, Spooncer E, et al. 1988. Heparan sulphate bound growth factors: A mechanism for stromal cell mediated haemopoiesis. Nature 332:376.

Sandstrom CE, Bender JG, Papoutsakis ET, Miller WM. 1995. Effects of CD34+ cell selection and perfusion on ex vivo expansion of peripheral blood mononuclear cells. Blood 86:958–970.

Sardonini CA, Wu Y-J. 1993. Expansion and differentiation of human hematopoietic cells from static cultures through small scale bioreactors. Biotechnol Prog 9:131.

Schneider JG, Crown J, Shapiro F, et al. 1992. Ex vivo cytokine expansion of CD34-positive hematopoietic progenitors in bone marrow, placental cord blood, and cyclophosphamide and G-CSF mobilized peripheral blood. Blood 80:268a.

Schwartz RM, Emerson SG, Clarke MF, et al. 1991a. In vitro myelopoiesis stimulated by rapid medium exchange and supplementation with hematopoietic growth factors. Blood 78:3155.

Schwartz RM, Palsson BØ, Emerson SG. 1991b. Rapid medium perfusion rate significantly increases the productivity and longevity of human bone marrow cultures. Proc Natl Acad Sci USA 88:6760.

Schwarz RP, Goodwin TJ, Wolf DA. 1992. Cell culture for three-dimensional modeling in rotating wall vessels: An application of simulated microgravity. J Tiss Cult Meth 14:51.

Smith KA. 1988. Interleukin-2: Inception, impact, and implications. Science 240:1169.

Spangrude GJ, Heimfeld S, Weissman IL. 1988. Purification and characterization of mouse hematopoietic stem cells. Science 241:58.

Spooncer E, Gallagher JT, Krizsa F, et al. 1983. Regulation of haemopoiesis in long-term bone marrow cultures: IV. Glycosaminoglycan synthesis and the stimulation of haemopoiesis by β-D-xylosides. J Cell Biol 96:510.

Sporn MB, Roberts AB. 1989. Transforming growth factor-β: Multiple actions and potential clinical applications. JAMA 262:938.

Stroncek DF, Holland PV, Bartch G, et al. 1993. Experiences of the first 493 unrelated marrow donors in the national marrow donor program. Blood 81:1940.

Sutherland HJ, Eaves AC, Eaves CJ. 1991a. Quantitative assays for human hemopoietic progenitor cells. In AP Gee (ed), Bone Marrow Processing and Purging, pp 155–167, Boca Raton, FL, CRC Press.

Sutherland HJ, Eaves CJ, Lansdorp PM, et al. 1991b. Differential regulation of primitive human hematopoietic stem cells in long-term cultures maintained on genetically engineered murine stromal cells. Blood 78:666.

Sutherland HJ, Hogge DE, Cook D, et al. 1993. Alternative mechanisms with and without steel factor support primitive human hematopoiesis. Blood 81:1465.

Tavassoli M, Hardy CL. 1990. Molecular basis of homing of intravenously transplanted stem cells to the marrow. Blood 76:1059.

Toksoz D, Zsebo KM, Smith KA, et al. 1992. Support of human hematopoiesis in long-term bone marrow cultures by murine stromal cells selectively expressing the membrane-bound and secreted forms of the human homolog of the steel gene product, stem cell factor. Proc Natl Acad Sci USA 89:7350.

Traycoff CM, Abboud CM, Abboud MR, Laver J, et al. 1994. Evaluation of the in vitro behavior of phenotyically defined populations of umbilical cord blood hematopoietic progenitor cells. Exp Hematol 22:215.

Tushinski RJ, McAlister IB, Williams DE, et al. 1991. The effects of interleukin 7 (IL-7) on human bone marrow in vitro. Exp Hematol 19:749.

Ushio S, Namba M, Okura T, Hattori K, Hukada Y, Akita K, Tanabe F, Konishi K, Micallef M, Fujii M, Torigoe K, Tanimoto T, Fukuda S, Ikeda M, Okamura H, Kurimoto M. 1996. Cloning of the cDNA for human IFN-gamma-inducing factor, espression in *Escherichia coli*, and studies on the biologic activities of the protein. J Immunol 156:4274–4279.

Verfaillie CM. 1992. Direct contact between human primitive hematopoietic progenitors and bone marrow stroma is not required for long-term in vitro hematopoiesis. Blood 79:2821.

Virelizier JL, Arenzana-Seisdedos F. 1985. Immunological functions of macrophages and their regulation by interferons. Med Biol 63:149–159.

Wagner JE, Broxmeyer HE, Byrd RL, et al. 1992. Transplantation of umbilical cord blood after myeloablative therapy: Analysis of engraftment. Blood 79:1874.

Weinstein R, Riordan MA, Wenc K, et al. 1989. Dual role of fibronectin in hematopoietic differentiation. Blood 73:111.

Wight TN, Kinsella MG, Keating A, et al. 1986. Proteoglycans in human long-term bone marrow cultures: Biochemical and ultrastructural analyses. Blood 67:1333.

Wolf SF, Temple PA, Kobayashi M, et al. 1991. Cloning of cDNA for natural killer cell stimulatory factor, a heterodimeric cytokine with multiple biologic effects on T and natural killer cells. J Immunol 146:3074.

Yamakazi K, Roberts RA, Spooncer E, et al. 1989. Cellular interactions between 3T3 cells and interleukin-3 dependent multipotent haemopoietic cells: A model system for stromal-cell-mediated haemopoiesis. J Cell Physiol 139:301.

Yao Z, Painter SL, Fanslow WC, Ulrich D, Macduff BM, Spriggs MK, and Armitage RJ. 1995. Human IL-17: A novel cytokine derived from T cells. J Immunol 155:5483-5486.

Yokota T, Arai N, de Vries JE, et al. 1988. Molecular biology of interleukin 4 and interleukin-5 genes and biology of their products that stimulate B cells, T cells and hemopoietic cells. Immunol Rev 102:137.

Zandstra PW, Eaves CJ, Piret JM. 1994. Expansion of hematopoietic progenitor cell populations in stirred suspension bioreactors of normal human bone marrow cells. Biotechnology 12:909–914.

Zipori D. 1989. Stromal cells from the bone marrow: Evidence for a restrictive role in regulation of hemopoiesis. Eur J Haematol 42:225.

Zlotnik A. Moore KW. 1991. Interleukin 10. Cytokine 3:366.

Zsebo KM, Wypych J, McNiece IK, et al. 1990. Identification, purification, and biological characterization of hematopoietic stem cell factor from buffalo rat liver-conditioned medium. Cell 63:195.

Zuckerman KS, Wicha MS. 1983. Extracellular matrix production by the adherent cells of long-term murine bone marrow cultures. Blood 61:540.

Further Information

The American Society of Hematology (ASH) is the premier organization dealing with both the experimental and clinical aspects of hematopoiesis. The society journal, *BLOOD*, is published twice per month, and can be obtained through ASH, 1200 19th Street NW, Suite 300, Washington, DC 20036 (phone: 202-857-1118). The International Society of Experimental Hematology (ISEH) publishes *Experimental Hematology* monthly.

20
Tissue Engineering of the Liver

Tao Ho Kim
Harvard University and Boston Children's Hospital

Joseph P. Vacanti
Harvard University and Boston Children's Hospital

Liver transplantation has been established as a curative treatment for end-stage adult and pediatric liver disease [Starlz et al., 1989], and over recent years, many innovative advances have been made in transplantation surgery. Unfortunately, a fundamental problem of liver transplantation has been severe donor shortage, and no clinical therapeutic bridge exists to abate the progression of liver failure (Table 20.1). As the demand for liver transplantation surgery increases, still fewer than 3500 donors are available annually for the approximately 25,000 patients who die from chronic liver disease [National Vital Statistic System, 1991, 1992]. Currently, cadaveric and living-related donors are the only available sources. Xenograft [Starlz et al., 1993] and split liver transplantation [Merio and Campbell, 1991] are under experimental and clinical evaluation. The research effort to engineer a functional liver tissue has been vigorous, since tissue engineering of the liver offers, in theory, an efficient use of limited organ availability.

Whereas other experimental hepatic support systems such as extracorporeal bioreactors and hemoperfusion devices [Yarmusch et al., 1992] attempt to temporarily support the metabolic functions of liver, transplantation of hepatocyte systems is a possible temporary or permanent alternative therapy to liver transplantation for treatment of liver failure. An experimental model system of hepatocellular transplantation should provide optimal cell survival, proliferation, and maintenance of sufficient functional hepatocyte mass to replace liver function. Direct hepatocellular injection or infusion into various organs or tissues and a complex hepatocyte delivery system utilizing polymer matrices have been two major areas of research interest. Just as the liver is one of the most sophisticated organs in the human body, the science of hepatocyte or liver tissue construction has proved to be equally complex.

20.1 Background

The causes of end-stage liver disease are many, including alcoholic or viral cirrhosis, biliary atresia, inborn errors of metabolism, and sclerosing cholangitis. With chronic and progressive liver injury, hepatic necrosis occurs followed by fatty infiltration and inflammation. Scar tissue and nodular regeneration replace the normal liver architecture and increase the microcirculatory resistance, which results in portal hypertension; the liver is further atrophied as important factors in the portal blood which regulate liver growth and maintenance are shunted away from the liver. Currently, end-stage liver disease must be present to be considered for orthotopic liver transplantation therapy, but a significant difference exists between alcohol- or viral-induced liver injury and congenital liver diseases such as isolated gene defects and biliary atresia. With alcohol- or viral-induced chronic hepatic injury, the degree of liver injury is unknown until metabolic functions are severely impaired and signs of progressive irreversible hepatic failure including portal hypertension, coagulopathy, progressive jaundice, and hepatic encephalopathy have developed. In congenital liver diseases, normal hepatic metabolic functions exist until dangerous toxins build up and destroy the liver parenchyma. Hepatocellular transplantation could potentially *prevent* hepatic injury and preserve host hepatic function for congenital inborn errors of liver metabolism.

TABLE 20.1   UNOS Liver Transplantation Data Summary from 1989 to 1993 in the United States: Total Number of Liver Transplant Candidates and Deaths Reported per Year While on Transplant Waiting List

Year	No. of Patients	No. of Deaths Reported
1989	3096	39
1990	4008	45
1991	4866	67
1992	5785	104
1993	7040	141

Source: United Network for Organ Sharing and the Organ Procurement and Transplantation Network. Data as of January 12, 1994.

As liver transplantation emerged as an important therapeutic modality, research activity intensified to improve or understand many areas of liver transplantation such as immunological tolerance, preservation techniques, and the mechanism of healing after acute and chronic liver injury. Liver growth and regulation, in particular, have been better understood: For example, after partial hepatectomy, several *mitogens*—epidermal growth factor, alpha fibroblastic growth factor, hepatocyte growth factor, and transforming growth factor-alpha—are produced early after injury to stimulate liver regeneration. Comitogens—including insulin, glucagon, estrogen, norepinephrine, and vasopressin—also aid with liver regeneration [Michalopoulos, 1993]. These stimulation factors help govern the intricate regulatory process of liver growth and regeneration, but much about what controls these factors is still unknown. *In vitro* and *in vivo* experiments with mitogens such as hepatocyte growth factor, epidermal growth factor, and insulin have yielded only moderate improvement in hepatic proliferation.

The importance of hepatocyte proliferation and hepatic regeneration becomes evident when one considers the difficulty in delivering large numbers of hepatocytes in hepatocyte replacement systems. The potential advantage of hepatocyte cellular transplantation is to take a small number of hepatocytes and proliferate these cells, *in vitro* or *in vivo*, to create functional liver equivalents for replacement therapy. Without hepatocyte regeneration, delivery of a very large number of hepatocytes is required. Asonuma and co-workers [1992] have determined that approximately 12% of the liver by heterotopic liver transplantation can significantly correct hyperbilirubinemia in the Gunn rat, which is deficient in uridine diphosphate glucuronyl tranferase. Although long-term efficacy remains unclear, 10–12% of the liver is an approximate critical hepatocellular mass thought necessary to replace the metabolic functions of the liver. The inability to mimic normal liver growth and regeneration in *in vitro* and *in vivo* systems has been one significant obstacle for hepatocyte tissue construction thus far.

20.2   Hepatocyte Transplantation Systems

Hepatocyte transplant systems offer the possibilities of creating many functional liver equivalents, storing hepatocytes by cryopreservation for later application [Yarmush et al., 1992], and using autologous cells for gene therapy [Jauregui and Gann, 1991]. The two systems discussed below differ in the amount of hepatocytes delivered, use of implantation devices, and implantation sites and techniques. Yet, in both systems, one significant roadblock in proving the efficacy of hepatocyte transplantation has been in the lack of a definitive, reproducible isolated liver defect model. Previous studies using syngeneic rat models such as the jaundice Gunn rat, the analbuminemic Nagase rat, or acute and chronic liver injury rat models have attributed significant correction of their deficit from hepatocyte transplantation. However, either inconsistencies or variation of animal strains and lack of consistent reproducible results have made accurate scientific interpretations and conclusions difficult. For instance, a study assessing hepatocyte delivery with microcarrier beads reported significant decrease in bilirubin in the hyperbilirubinemic

Gunn rat and elevation of albumin in the Nagase analbuminemic rat after intraperitoneal implantation [Demetriou et al., 1986]. Other studies have not demonstrated significant hepatocyte survival with intraperitoneal injection of hepatocytes with or without microcarriers; histology showed predominant cell necrosis and granuloma formation after 3 days [Henne-Bruns et al., 1991]. In *allogeneic* models, the possibility of immunological rejection further complicates the evaluation of the hepatocyte transplant system. Clearly, determining the efficacy of hepatocyte transplantation in liver metabolic-deficient models requires significant chemical results, and histologic correlation without confounding variables.

Hepatocellular Injection Model

Hepatocytes require an extracellular matrix for growth and differentiation, and the concept of utilizing existing *stromal* tissue as a vascular extracellular matrix is inviting. Isolated hepatocytes have been injected directly into the spleen or liver or in the portal or splenic vein. Several studies have reported significant but temporary correction of acute and metabolic liver defects in rat models as a result of intrahepatic, intraportal [Matas et al., 1976], or intrasplenic injections [Vroemen et al., 1985]. However, elucidating the efficacy of hepatocellular injection transplantation has been difficult for three significant reasons: (1) Differentiation of donor transplanted hepatocytes from host liver parenchyma has not been well established in an animal liver defect model, (2) how much hepatocyte mass needed to inject for partial or total liver function replacement has not been determined [Onodera et al., 1992], and (3) establishing a definitive animal liver defect model to prove efficacy of hepatocyte injection has been difficult.

Transgenic animal strains have been developed and offer a reproducible model in differentiating host from transplanted hepatocytes. Using transgenic mouse lines, donor hepatocytes injected into the spleen were histologically shown to migrate to the host liver, survive, and maintain function [Ponder et al., 1991]. Recently, a transgenic liver model in a mouse was used to evaluate the replicative potential of adult mouse hepatocytes. Normal adult mouse hepatocytes from two established transgenic lines were injected into the spleen of an Alb-uPA transgenic mouse that had an endogenous defect in hepatic growth potential and function (see Fig. 20.1). The adult mouse hepatocytes were shown to translocate to the liver and undergo up to 12 cell doublings; however, function of the transplanted hepatocytes was not fully reported [Rhim et al., 1994]. Rhim's study suggests that a hepatocyte has the potential to replicate manyfold so long as the structural and chemical milieu is optimal for survival and regeneration. If a small number of transplanted hepatocytes survive and proliferate manyfold in the native liver, sufficient hepatocyte mass to replace liver function would be accomplished, ameliorating the need to deliver a large quantity of donor hepatocytes.

Although many questions about hepatocyte injection therapy remain, the transgenic liver model has been used to test the safety and efficacy of *ex vivo* gene therapy for metabolic liver diseases. The Watanabe heritable hyperlipidemic rabbit, a strain deficient in low density lipoprotiens (LDL) receptors, has been used to evaluate the possible application of a gene therapy by hepatocyte injection. *Autologous* hepatocytes were obtained from a liver segment, genetically modified *ex vivo*, and infused into the inferior mesenteric vein through a catheter placed intraoperatively without postoperative sequelae to the rabbit. Decreased levels of LDL have been reported out to 6 months [Wilson et al., 1992]. Larger animal models have shown engraftment of the genetically altered hepatocytes for as long as 1.5 years. The first clinical application of hepatocellular injection has been performed on a patient diagnosed with homozygous familial hyper-cholesterolemia. The patient has had decreased levels of cholesterol and has maintained expression of the transfected gene after 18 months [Grossman et al., 1994]. This is an important step forward as we await long-term results.

Hepatocyte Transplantation on Polymer Matrices

Since the practical application of implanting few hepatocytes to proliferate and replace function is not yet possible, hepatocyte tissue construction, using polymer as a scaffold, relies on transplanting a large number of hepatocytes to allow survival of enough hepatocyte mass to replace function. The large surface

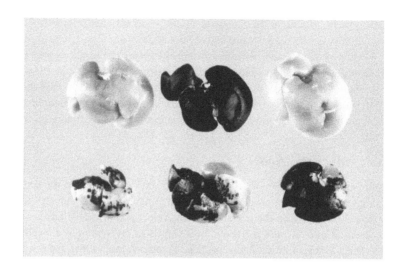

FIGURE 20.1   Control and transgenic liver specimens: a nontransgenic (normal mouse) control with normal liver color (top, left); a *transgenic (MT-lacZ)* liver with normal function which is stained in blue and served as a positive control (top, center); a *notransgenic* control transplanted with *transgenic MIT-lacZ* hepatocytes (top, right); and three livers with a different *transgene Alb-uPA* transplanted with *transgenic (MT-lacZ)* hepatocytes. A deficiency in hepatic growth potential and function is induced by the *Alb-uPA transgene*, resulting in a chronic stimulus for liver growth. The liver with *Alb-uPA transgene* has the same color as the *nontransgenic* control liver but is partially replaced by the blue-stained *transgencic (MT-lacZ)* normal functioning hepatocytes, showing the regenerative response of normal hepatocytes in a mouse liver with a chronic stimulus for live growth. (Rhim, Sandgren, and Brinster, University of Pennsylvania. Reprinted with permission from American Association for the Advancement of Science.)

area of the polymer accommodates hepatocyte attachment in large numbers so that many cells may survive initially by diffusion of oxygen and other vital nutrients (see Fig. 20.2). The polymer scaffold is constructed with a high porosity to allow vascular ingrowth, and vascularization of surviving cells then can provide permanent nutritional access [Cima et al., 1991]. The cell-polymer system has been used in several other tissue-engineering applications such as cartilage, bone, intestine, and urologic tissue construction [Langer and Vacanti, 1993]. Hepatocytes adhere to the polymer matrix for growth and differentiation as well as locate into the interstices of the polymer. The polymer-hepatocyte interface can be manipulated with surface proteins such as laminin, fibronectin, and growth factors to improve adherence, viability, function, or growth [Mooney et al., 1992]. Hepatocyte proliferation by attaching mitogenic factors like hepatocyte growth factor, epidermal growth factor, or transforming growth factor-alpha is under current investigation.

Synthetic polymer matrices, both degradable and nondegradable, have been evaluated for hepatocyte-polymer construction. As degradable polymers were being studied and evaluated for tissue engineering, a nondegradable polymer, polyvinyl (PVA), was used for *in vitro* and *in vivo* systems. The polyvinyl alcohol sponge offered one significant advantage: a uniform, noncollapsible structure which allowed quantification of hepatocyte engraftment [Uyama et al., 1993]. *In vitro* and *in vivo* studies have demonstrated hepatocyte survival on the polyvinyl alcohol scaffold. However, the polyvinyl alcohol sponge will not degrade and could act as a nidus for infection and chronic inflammation. A degradable polymer conceptually serves as a better implantable scaffold for hepatocyte-polymer transplantation, since the polymer dissolves to leave only tissue. Polyglycolic acid (PGA), polyactic acid (PLA), and copolymer hybrids have been employed in several animal models of liver insufficiency (see Fig. 20.3). Histologic analyses have shown similar survival of hepatocytes when compared to studies with polyvinyl alcohol.

The experimental design for the hepatocyte-polymer model has been standardized as follows: (1) an end-to-side portacaval shunt is performed to provide hepatotrophic stimulation to the graft, (2) hepatocytes

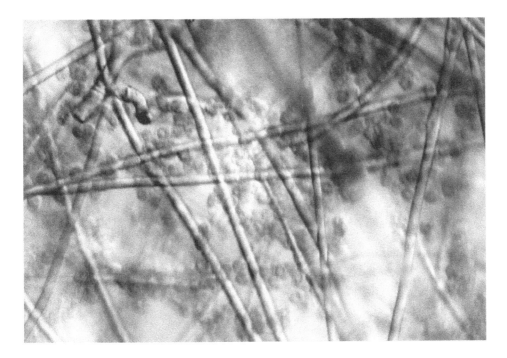

FIGURE 20.2   Hepatocytes are seen adhering to polyglycolic acid polymer in culture [Mooney, unpublished data].

are isolated and seeded onto degradable polyglycolic acid polymer, (3) the hepatocyte-polymer construct is implanted into the abdominal cavity on vascular beds of small intestinal mesentery and omentum, (4) pertinent chemical studies are obtained and analyzed at periodic intervals, and (5) histologic analysis in the specimens is performed at progressive time points. Early studies have shown that a large percentage of hepatocytes perish from hypoxia within 6–24 hours after implantation. To improve hepatocyte survival, implantation of hepatocytes onto large vascular surface areas for engraftment and exposing the hepatocytes to hepatotrophic factors were two important maneuvers. The small intestinal mesentery and omentum have offered large vascular surface areas. Hepatocyte survival has been reported at other sites such as the peritoneum [Demetriou et al., 1991], renal capsule [Ricordi et al., 1989], lung [Sandbichler et al., 1992], and pancreas [Vroemen et al., 1988], but these sites do not provide enough vascular surface area to allow survival of a large number of hepatocytes.

The concept of hepatotrophic factors originated when atrophy and liver insufficiency was observed with heterotopic liver transplantation. Later studies have confirmed that important factors regulating liver growth and maintenance existed in the portal blood [Jaffe et al., 1991]. Thus, when a portacaval shunt to redirect hepatotrophic factors from the host liver to the hepatocyte-polymer construct was performed, survival of heterotopically transplanted hepatocytes significantly improved [Uyama et al., 1993]; consequently, portacaval shunts were instituted in all experimental models. Studies thus far have shown survival of functional hepatocytes over 6 months in rat and dog models (unpublished data); replacement of liver function has been of shorter duration.

A study using the Dalmatian dog model of hyperuricosuria typifies the current status of the hepatocyte-polymer system. The hepatocyte membrane of the Dalmatian dog has a defect in the uptake of uric acid, which results in hyperuricemia and hyperuricosuria [Giesecke and Tiemeyer, 1984]. The study has shown a significant but temporary correction of the liver uric acid metabolic defect after implantation of normal beagle hepatocytes, which have normal uric acid metabolism, on degradable polyglycolic acid polymer [Takeda et al., 1994]. Cyclosporine was administered for immunosuppression. The results of the Dalmatian dog study suggest that (1) successful engraftment of the hepatocyte-polymer construct occurred,

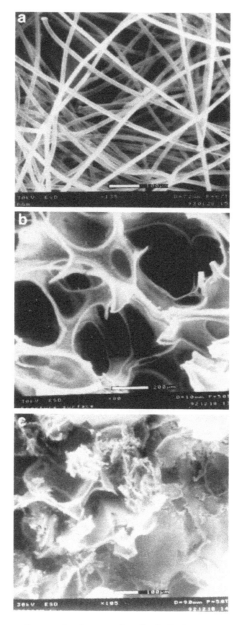

FIGURE 20.3 Scanning electron microscopic photographs of polyglyclic acid (a), polyvinyl alcohol (b), and poly-lactic acid (c) demonstrate the high porosity of these polymers. (Mooney. Reprinted with permission from W.B. Saunders Company.)

(2) maintenance of functional hepatocytes under current conditions was temporary, and (3) loss of critical hepatocyte mass to replace the liver uric acid metabolism defect occurred at 5–6 weeks after hepatocyte-polymer transplantation. The temporary effect could be attributed to suboptimal immunosuppression or suboptimal regulation of growth factors and hormones involved with hepatic growth, regeneration, and maintenance, or both.

Coculture of hepatocytes with pancreatic islet cells also has been under investigation to aid in hepatocyte survival, growth, and maintenance. Trophic factors from islet cells have been shown to improve hepatocyte survival [Ricordi et al., 1988], and cotransplantation of hepatocytes with islet cells on a polymer matrix has been shown to improve hepatocyte survival as well [Kaufmann et al., 1994]. Coculture with other cell types such as the biliary epithelial cell also may improve hepatocyte survival. Other studies with biliary epithelial cells have shown ductular formation in *in vitro* and *in vivo* models [Sirica et al., 1990], and vestiges of ductular formation in hepatocyte-polymer tissue have been histologically observed [Hansen and Vacanti, 1992]. A distinct advantage of the cell-polymer engineered construct is that one can manipulate the polymer to direct function. Thus far, diseases involving the biliary system, primarily biliary atresia, are not amenable to hepatocyte transplantation. An attempt to develop a biliary drainage system with biliary epithelial cells, hepatocytes, and polymer has been initiated. In the future, the potential construction of a branching polymer network could serve as the structural cues for the development of an interconnecting ductular system.

Ex vivo gene therapy with the hepatocyte-polymer system is also an exciting potential application as demonstrated by the recent clinical trial with hepatocyte injection therapy. Genetically altered hepatocytes transplanted on polymer constructs have been studied with encouraging results [Fontaine et al., 1993].

20.3 Conclusion

Studies in hepatocyte transplantation through tissue engineering methods have made important advances in recent years. The research in the hepatocellular injection and the research in the hepatocyte-polymer construct models have complemented each other in understanding the difficulties as well as the possibilities of liver replacement therapy. In order to make further advances with hepatocyte replacement systems, the process of liver development, growth, and maintenance needs to be better understood. Currently, the amount of hepatocyte engraftment, proliferation, and the duration of hepatocyte survival remain undetermined in both systems. The amount of functional hepatocyte engraftment necessary may vary for different hepatic diseases. For instance, isolated gene defects of the liver may require a small number of functional transplanted hepatocytes to replace function, whereas end-stage liver disease may require a large amount of hepatocyte engraftment.

Current hepatic replacement models have both advantages and disadvantages. For hepatocellular injection, the application of *ex vivo* gene therapy for an isolated gene defect of liver metabolism is promising. However, the small amount of hepatocyte delivery and significant potential complications for patients with portal hypertension may preclude application of the hepatocellular injection method for end-stage liver disease. A significant amount of intrapulmonary shunting of hepatocytes was observed in rats with portal hypertension after intrasplenic injection of hepatocytes, which resulted in increased portal pressures, pulmonary hypertension, pulmonary infarction, and reduced pulmonary compliance [Gupta et al., 1993]. With the hepatocyte-polymer system, delivery of a large number of hepatocytes is possible. In patients with portal hypertension, portal blood-containing hepatotrophic factors are shunted away from the liver, obviating the need for a portacaval shunt. Thus, patients with end-stage liver disease and portal hypertension may need only transplantation of the hepatocyte-polymer construct. However, an end-to-side portacaval shunt operation is needed in congenital liver diseases with normal portal pressures to deliver hepatotrophic factors to the heterotopically place hepatocytes. In the future, each hepatocyte transplant system could have specific and different clinical applications. More important, both offer the hope of increasing therapeutic options for patients requiring liver replacement therapy. Approximately 260,000 patients out of 634,000 patients hospitalized for liver diseases have liver diseases which could have been considered for hepatic transplantation. The total acute care nonfederal hospital cost for liver diseases in 1992, which does not include equally substantial outpatient costs, exceeded $9.2 billion [HCIA Inc., 1992].

Defining Terms

Allogeneic: Pertaining to different genetic compositions within the same species.

Cadaveric: Related to a dead body. In transplantation, *cadaveric* is related to a person who has been declared brain dead; organs should be removed prior to cardiac arrest to prevent injury to the organs.

Heterotopic: Related to a region or place where an organ or tissue is not present in normal conditions.

Mitogens: Substances that stimulate mitosis or growth.

Orthotopic: Related to a region or place where an organ or tissue is present in normal conditions.

Portacaval shunt: A surgical procedure to partially or completely anastomose the portal vein to the inferior vena cava to divert portal blood flow from the liver to the systemic circulation.

Stroma: The structure or framework of an organ or gland usually composed of connective tissue.

Transgenic: Referred to introduction of a foreign gene into a recipient which can be used to identify genetic elements and examine gene expression.

Xenograft: A graft transferred from one animal species to another species.

References

Asonuma K, Gilber JC, Stein JE, et al. 1992. Quantitation of transplanted hepatic mass necessary to cure the Gunn rat model of hyperbilirubinemia. J Pediatr Surg 27(30):298.

Asonuma K, Vacanti JP. 1992. Cell transplantation as replacement therapy for the future. Pediatr Transplantation 4(2):249.

Cima L, Vacanti JP, Vacant C, et al. 1991. Tissue engineering by cell transplantation using degradable polymer substrates. J Biomech Eng 113:143.

Demetriou AA, Felcher A, Moscioni AD. 1991. Hepatocyte transplantation. A potential treatment for liver disease. Dig Dis Sci 12(9):1320.

Demetriou AA, Whiting JF, Feldman D, et al. 1986. Replacement of liver function in rats by transplantation of microcarrier-attached hepatocytes. Science 233:1190.

Fontaine MJ, Hansen, LK, Thompson S, et al. 1993. Transplantation of genetically altered hepatocytes using cell-polymer constructs leads to sustained human growth hormone secretion in vivo. Transplant Proc 25(1):1002.

Giesecke D, Tiemeyer W. 1984. Defect of uric acid in Dalmatian dog liver. Experientia 40:1415.

Grossman M, Roper SE, Kozarsky K, et al. 1994. Successful ex vivo gene therapy directed to liver in a patient with familial hypercholesterolemia. Nat Genet 6:335.

Gupta S, Yereni PR, Vemuru RP, et al. 1993. Studies on the safety of intrasplenic hepatocyte transplantation: Relevance to ex vivo gene therapy and liver repopulation in acute hepatic failure. Hum Gene Ther 4(3):249.

Hansen LK, Vacanti JP. 1992. Hepatocyte transplantation using artificial biodegradable polymers. In MA Hoffman (ed), Current Controversies in Biliary Atresia. The Medical Intelligence Unit Series pp 96–106, (CRC Press), Austin, R.G. Landes.

HCIA Inc. 1992. Survey of costs in non-federal, acute care hospitals in the United States prepared for the American Liver Foundation, Baltimore.

Henne-Bruns D, Kruger U, Sumpelman D, et al. 1991. Intraperitoneal hepatocyte transplantation: Morphological results. Virchows Arch A, Pathol Anat Histopathol 419(1):45.

Jaffe V, Darby H, Bishop A, et al. 1991. The growth of liver cells in the pancreas after intrasplenic implantation: The effects of portal perfusion. Int J Exp Pathol 72(3):289.

Jauregui HO, Gann KL. 1991. Mammalian hepatocytes as a foundation for treatment in human liver failure [Review]. J Cell Biochem 45(4):359.

Kaufmann P-M, Sano K, Uyama S, et al. 1994. Heterotopic hepatocyte transplantation using three dimensional polymers. Evaluation of the stimulatory effects by portacaval shunt or islet cell co-transplantation. Second International Congress of the Cell Transplant Society, Minneapolis.

Langer R, Vacanti J. 1993. Tissue Eng Sci 260:920.

Matas AJ, Sutherland DER, Steffes MW, et al. 1976. Hepatocellular transplantation for metabolic deficiencies: Decrease of plasma bilirubin in Gunn rats. Science 192:892.

Merion RM, Campbell DA Jr. 1991. Split liver transplantation: One plus one doesn't always equal two. Hepatology 14(3):572.

Michalopoulos G. 1993. HGF and liver regeneration. Gasterol Jpn 28(suppl 4):36.

Mooney DJ, Hansen LK, Vacanti JP, et al. 1992. Switching from differentiation to growth in hepatocytes: Control by extracellular matrix. J Cell Physiol 151:497.

National Vital Statistic System. 1991, 1992. Data derived from National Center for Health Statistics.

Onodera K, Ebata H, Sawa M, et al. 1992. Comparative effects of hepatocellular transplantation in the spleen, portal vein, or peritoneal cavity in congenitally ascorbic acid biosynthetic enzyme-deficient rats. Transplant Proc 24(6):3006.

Ponder KP, Gupta S, Leland F, et al. 1991. Mouse hepatocytes migrate to liver parenchyma and function indefinitely after intrasplenic transplantation. Proc Natl Acad Sci USA 88(4):1217.

Rhim JA, Sandgren EP, Degen JL, et al. 1994. Replacement of diseased mouse liver by hepatic cell transplantation. Science 263:1149.

Ricordi C, Lacy PE, Callery MP, et al. 1989. Trophic factors from pancreatic islets in combined hepatocyte-islet allografts enhance hepatocellular survival. Surgery 105:218.

Sandbichler P, Then P, Vogel W, et al. 1992. Hepatocellular transplantation into the lung for temporary support of acute liver failure in the rat. Gastroenterology 102(2):605.

Sirica AE, Mathis GA, Sano N, et al. 1990. Isolation, culture, and transplantation of intrahepatic biliary epithelial cells and oval cells. Pathobiology 58:44.

Starzl TE, Demetris AJ, Van Thiel D. 1989. Chronic liver failure: Orthotopic liver transplantation. N Engl J Med 321:1014.

Takeda T, Kim TH, Lee SK, et al. 1994. Hepatocyte transplantation in biodegradable polymer scaffolds using the Dalmatian dog model of hyperuricosuria. Fifteenth Congress of the Transplantation Society, Kyoto Japan. Submitted.

Uyama S, Takeda T, Vacanti JP. 1993. Delivery of whole liver equivalent hepatic mass using polymer devices and hetertrophic stimulation. Transplantation 55(4):932.

Uyama S, Takeda T, Vacanti JP. In press. Hepatocyte transplantation equivalent to whole liver mass using cell-polymer devices. Polymer Preprints.

Vacanti JP, Morse MA, Saltzman WM, et al. 1988. Selective cell transplantation using bioabsorbable artificial polymers as matrices. J Pediatr Surg 23(1):3.

Vroemen JPAM, Blanckaert N, Buurman WA, et al. 1985. Treatment of enzyme deficiency by hepatocyte transplantation in rats. J Surg Res 39:267.

Vroemen JPAM, Buurman WA, van der Linden CJ, et al. 1988. Transplantation of isolated hepatocytes into the pancreas. Eur Surg Res 20:1.

Wilson JM, Grossman M, Raper SE, et al. 1992. Ex vivo gene therapy of familial hypercholesterolemia. Human Gene Ther 3(2):179.

Yarmush ML, Toner M, Dunn JCY, et al. 1992. Hepatic tissue engineering: Development of critical technologies. Ann NY Acad Sci 665:238.

21

Tissue Engineering in the Nervous System

Ravi Bellamkonda
Lausanne University Medical School

Patrick Aebischer
Lausanne University Medical School

Tissue engineering in the nervous system facilitates the controlled application and/or organization of neural cells to perform appropriate diagnostic, palliative, or therapeutic tasks. As the word *tissue* implies, tissue engineering in general involves cellular components and their organization. Any cell, given its broad genetic program, expresses a particular phenotype in a manner that is dependent on its environment. The extracellular environment consists of cells, humoral factors, and the extracellular matrix. Research in genetic engineering and the intense focus on growth factors and extracellular matrix biology have made it possible to manipulate both the cell's genetic program and its phenotypic expression.

In the nervous system, degeneration or injury to neurons or glia and/or an aberrant extracellular environment can cause a wide variety of ailments. Diseases such as Parkinson's may required the replacement of diminished levels of a particular neurochemical, e.g., dopamine. Other pathologies such as injured nerves or reconnection of served neural pathways may require regeneration of nervous tissue.

Tissue engineering efforts in the nervous system have currently been addressing the following goals:

1. Functional replacement of a missing neuroactive component
2. Rescue or regeneration of damaged neural tissue
3. Human-machine interfaces: neural coupling elements

21.1 Delivery of Neuroactive Molecules to the Nervous System

Deficiency of specific neuroactive molecules has been implicated in several neurologic disorders. These factors may be neurotransmitters, neurotrophic agents, or enzymes. For example, part of the basal ganglia circuitry that plays a role in motor control consists of striatal neurons receiving dopaminergic input from

Table 21.1 *Engineering* Solutions for Parkinson's Disease

Mode of Delivery	Rodents	Monkey	Human	Reference
Infusion	Rat striatum			Hargraves et al., 1987
		Cerebroventricular		De Yebenes et al., 1988
			Systemic	Hardie et al., 1984
Polymer slow release	Rat striatum (EVA rods)			Winn et al., 1989
	Rat subcutaneous (EVA rods)			Sabel et al., 1990
	Rat striatum (Si pellet)			Becker et al., 1990
	Rat striatum (liposomes)			During et al., 1992
Cell transplantation				
Fetal				
Substantia nigra	Rat striatum			Björklund et al., 1980
				Freund et al., 1985
Ventral mesencephalon	Rat striatum			Bolam et al., 1987
Human DA neurons			Putamen	Lindvall et al., 1990
Autologous primary				
Genetically altered skin fibroblasts	Rat striatum			Chen et al., 1991
Genetically altered skin fibroblasts with myoblasts	Rat striatum			Jiao et al., 1993
Encapsulated xenogeneic tissue				
Bovine adrenal chromaffin cells	Striatum (microcapsules)			Aebischer et al., 1991
PC12 cells	Rat striatum (microcapsules)			Winn et al., 1991
	Rat striatum (macrocapsule)			Aebischer et al., 1988
		Striatum (macrocapsule)		Aebischer et al., 1994
Mouse mesencephalon	Rat parietal cortex (macrocapsule)			Aebischer et al., 1988

the mesencephalic substantia nigra neurons. It has been shown that a lesioned nigrostriatal dopaminergic pathway is responsible for Parkinson's disease [Ehringer and Hornykiewicz, 1960]. In chronic cancer patients, the delivery of antinociceptive neurotransmitters such as enkephalins, endorphins, catecholamines, neuropeptide Y, neurotensin, and somatostatin to the cerebrospinal fluid may improve the treatment of severe pain [Akil et al., 1984; Joseph et al., in press]. Neurotrophic factors may play a role in the treatment of several neurodegenerative disorders. For example, local delivery of nerve growth factor (NGF) [Hefti et al., 1984; Williams et al., 1986] and/or brain-derived growth factor (BDNF) may be useful in the treatment of Alzheimer's disease [Anderson et al., 1990, Knüsel et al., 1991]. BDNF [Hyman et al., 1991; Knüsel et al., 1991] and glial cell line-derived nerve growth factor (GDNF) may be beneficial in Parkinson's disease [Lin et al., 1993]. Other neurotrophins such as ciliary neurotrophic factor (CNTF) [Oppenheim et al., 1991; Sendtner et al., 1990], BDNF [Yan et al., 1992], neurotrophin-3 (NT-3), neurotrophin-4 (NT-4/5) [Hughes et al., 1993], and GDNF [Zurn et al., 1994] also could have an impact on amyotrophic lateral sclerosis (ALS) or Lou Gehrig disease.

Therefore, augmentation or replacement of any of the above-mentioned factors in the nervous system would be a viable therapeutic strategy for the treatment of the pathologies listed above. There are several issues that ought to be considered in engineering a system to deliver these factors. The stability of the factors, the dosage required, the solubility, the target tissue, and possible side effects all are factors that influence the choice of the delivery mode. Pumps, slow-release polymer systems, and cells from various sources that secrete the compound of interest are the main modes by which these factors can be delivered. Table 21.1 lists all the means employed to deliver dopamine to alleviate the symptoms of Parkinson's disease.

Pumps

Pumps are used to deliver opiates epidurally to relieve severe pain [Ahlgren et al., 1987]. Pumps also have been used to deliver neurotrophic factors such as NGF intraventricularly as a prelude or supplement to transplantation of chromaffin cells for Parkinson's disease [Olson et al., 1991] or as a potential therapy for Alzheimer's disease [Olson et al., 1992]. Pumps also have been used to experimentally deliver dopamine or dopamine receptor agonists in Parkinson's disease models [DeYebenes et al., 1988; Hargraves et al., 1987]. While pumps have been employed successfully in these instances, they may need to be refilled every 4 weeks, and this may be a limitation. Other potential drawbacks include susceptibility to "dumping" of neuroactive substance due to presence of a large reservoir of neuroactive element, infections, and diffusion limitations. Also, some factors such as dopamine and ciliary neurotrophic factor (CNTF) are very unstable chemically and have short half-life periods, rendering their delivery by such devices difficult. Some of these problems may be eliminated by well designed slow-release polymer systems.

Slow-Release Polymer Systems

Slow-release polymer systems essentially trap the molecule of interest in a polymer matrix and release it slowly by diffusion over a period of time. Proper design of the shape and composition of the polymer matrix may achieve stabilization of the bioactive molecule and facilitate a steady, sustained release over a period of time. For instance, it has been shown that the dopamine precursor L-dopa may be effective in alleviating some motor symptoms of Parkinson's disease [Birkmayer, 1969], fluctuations in the plasma levels of L-dopa due to traditional, periodic oral administration and difficulties in converting L-dopa to dopamine may cause the clinical response to fluctuate as well [Albani et al., 1986; Hardie et al., 1984; Muenter et al., 1977; Shoulson et al., 1975]. It has been demonstrated that a slow-release ethylene vinyl acetate polymer system loaded with L-dopa can sustain elevated plasma levels of L-dopa for at least 225 days when implanted subcutaneously in rats [Sabel et al., 1990]. Dopamine can only be released directly in the CNS, since it does not pass the blood-brain barrier. It has been demonstrated that experimental parkinsonism in rats can be alleviated by intrastriatal implantation of dopamine-releasing ethylene vinyl acetate rods [Winn et al., 1989]. Silicone elastomer as well as resorbable polyester pellets loaded with dopamine also have been implanted intrastriatally and shown to induce a behavioral recovery in parkinsonian rats [Becker et al., 1990; McRae et al., 1991].

Slow-release systems also may be employed to deliver trophic factors to the brain either to avoid side affects that may come about due to systemic administration or to overcome the blood-brain barrier, getting the factor delivered to the brain directly [During et al., 1992; Hoffman et al, 1990]. Therefore, polymeric systems with the molecule of interest trapped inside may be able to achieve many of the goals of an ideal delivery system, including targeted local delivery and zero-order continuos release [Langer, 1981; Langer et al., 1976]. However, some of the disadvantages of this system are the finite amounts of loaded neuroactive molecules and difficulties in shutting off release or adjusting rate of release once the polymer is implanted. Also, for the long-term release in humans, the device size may become a limiting factor. Some of these limitations may be overcome by the transplantation of cells that release neuroactive factors to the target site.

Cell Transplantation

Advances in molecular biology and gene transfer techniques have given rise to a rich array of cellular sources, which have been engineered to secrete a wide range of neurologic compounds. These include cells that release neurotransmitters, neurotrophic factors, and enzymes. Transplantation of these cells leads to functional replacement or augmentation of the original source of these compounds in the host. They can deliver neuroactive molecules as long as they survive, provided they maintain their phenotype and/or transgene expression, in the case of gene therapy. Some of the disadvantages of the slow-release systems, such as the presence of a large reservoir for long-term release or reloading of an exhausted reservoir, can thus be overcome. Some of the tissues transplanted so far may be classified in the following manner.

Transplantation of Autologous Primary Cells

This technique involves the procurement of primary cells from the host, expanding them if necessary to generate requisite amounts of tissue, engineering them if so required by using gene transfer techniques, and then transplanting them back into the "donor" at the appropriate site. For instance, autologous Schwann cells have been isolated and transplanted experimentally into the brain and have been shown to enhance retinal nerve regeneration, presumably by the release of factors that influence regeneration [Morrissey et al., 1991]. Schwann cells also express various neurologically relevant molecules [Bunge and Bunge, 1983; Muir et al., 1989]. Autologous Schwann cells also can work as nerve bridges to help reconstruction of rat sciatic nerve after axotomy [Guénard et al., 1992]. Primary skin fibroblasts also have been genetically engineered to secrete L-dopa and transplanted successfully into the autologous host's striatum in an experimental model of Parkinson's disease in rats [Chen et al., 1991]. The same group also has reported that nerve growth factor, tyrosine hydroxylase, glutamic acid decarboxylase, and choline acetyltransferase genes may be introduced successfully and expressed in primary fibroblasts [Gage et al., 1991]. More recently, muscle cells have been engineered to express tyrosine hydroxylase and transplanted successfully in a rat model of Parkinson's disease [Jiao et al., 1993].

Thus nonneural cells such as a fibroblast or muscle cells may be selected, in part, for the ease with which they can be engineered genetically and made neurologically relevant. It is therefore possible to engineer cells to suit particular pathologies as a step toward being able to engineer biomimetic tissues and then place them in appropriate locations and contexts *in vivo*. However, it may not always be technically possible to procure sufficient amounts of autologous tissue. Other sources of tissues have therefore been explored, and these include fetal tissue, used usually in conjunction with immunosuppression.

Fetal Tissue Transplantation

One of the important advantages of fetal tissue is its ability to survive and integrate into the host adult brain. Transplantation of fetal neural tissue allografts might be useful in treating Parkinson's disease [Lindvall et al., 1990]. While promising results have been reported using neural fetal tissue disease [Björklund, 1991; Björklund et al., 1980], availability of donor tissue and potential ethical issues involved with the technique may be potential shortcomings. One promising strategy to obtain allogeneic fetal tissue in large quantities is to isolate neural stem cells and have them proliferate *in vitro*. It has been demonstrated recently that CNS progenitor cells may be selected using epidermal growth factor (EGF). The cells thus selected have been shown to proliferate *in vitro* under appropriate culture conditions. With time and appropriate culture conditions, they differentiate into mature CNS neurons and glia [Reynolds et al., 1992; Vescovi et al., 1993]. When optimized, this technique could be useful to select and expand fetal neurons of interest *in vitro* and then transplant them. Transplantation of xenogeneic fetal tissue with immunosuppression using cyclosporin A is another alternative to using fetal tissue [Wictorin et al., 1992], and this approach might yield more abundant amounts of tissue for transplantation and overcome some of the possible ethical dilemmas in using human fetal tissue. However, immunosuppression may not be sufficient to prevent long-term rejection and may have other undesirable side effects.

Transplantation of Encapsulated Xenogeneic Tissue

Polymeric encapsulation of xenogeneic cells might be a viable strategy to transplant cells across species in the absence of systemic immunosuppression [Aebischer et al., 1988; Tresco et al., 1992]. Typically, the capsules have pores large enough for nutrients to reach the transplanted tissue and let the neuroactive factors out, but the pores are too small to let the molecules and the cells of the immune system reach the transplanted tissue (Fig. 21.1). At the same time, this strategy retains all the advantages of using cells as controlled, local manufacturers of the neuroactive molecules. The use of encapsulation also eliminates the restriction of having to use postmitotic tissue for transplantation to avoid tumor formation. The physical restriction of the polymeric capsule prevents escape of the encapsulated tissue. Should the capsule break, the transplanted cells are rejected and eliminated by the host immune system. However, no integration of the transplanted tissue into the host is possible with this technique.

Some of the tissue engineering issues involved in optimizing the encapsulation technique are (1) the type and configuration of the encapsulating membrane, (2) the various cells to be used for encapsulation, and (3) the matrix in which the cells are immobilized.

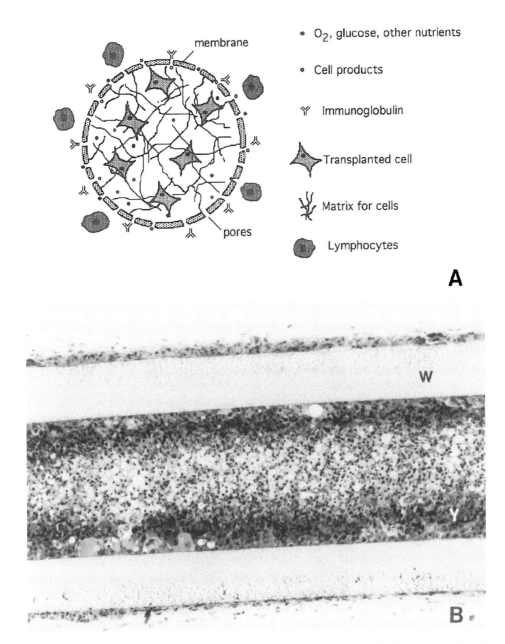

FIGURE 21.1 (A)Schematic illustration of the concept of immunoisolation involved in the transplantation of xenogenic tissue encapsulated in semipermeable polymer membranes. (B) Light micrograph of a longitudinal section shown baby hamster kidney cells encapsulated in a polyacryolonitrile-vinylchloride membrane and transplanted in an axotomized rat pup after 2 weeks *in vivo*. W denotes the capsule's polymeric wall, and Y shows the cells.

Type and Configuration of the Encapsulating Membrane. One important factor determining the size of the device is oxygen diffusion and availability to the encapsulated cells. This consideration influences the device design and encourages situations where the distances between the oxygen source, usually a capillary, and the inner core of transplanted tissue are kept as minimal as possible. The size and configuration of the device also influence the kinetics of release of the neuroactive molecules, the "response time" being slower in larger capsules with thicker membrane walls.

The capsule membrane may be a water-soluble system stabilized by ionic or hydrogen bonds formed between two weak polyelectrolytes—typically an acidic polysaccharide, such as alginic acid or modified cellulose, and a cationic polyaminoacid, such as polylysine or polyornithine [Goosen et al., 1985; Lim and Sun, 1980; Winn et al., 1991]. Gelation of the charged polyelectrolytes is caused by ionic cross-linking in the presence of di- or multivalent counterions. However, the stability and mechanical strength of these systems are questionable in the physiologic ionic environments. The major advantage of using these systems is that they obviate the need of organic solvent use in the making of the capsules and might be less cytotoxic in the manufacturing process.

The capsule membrane also may be a thermoplastic, yielding a more mechanically and chemically stable membrane. This technique involves loading of cells of interest in a preformed hollow fiber and then sealing the ends either by heat or with an appropriate glue. The hollow fibers are typically fabricated by a dry jet wet-spinning technique involving a phase-inversion process [Aebischer et al., 1991]. The use of thermoplastic membranes allows the manipulation of membrane structure, porosity, thickness, and permeability by appropriate variation of polymer solution flow rates, viscosity of the polymer solution, the nonsolvent used, etc.

Long-term cross-species transplants of dopaminergic xenogeneic tissues and functional efficacy in the brain have been reported [Aebischer et al., 1991, 1994] using the preceding system. PC12 cells, a catecholaminergic cell line derived from a rat pheochromocytoma, ameliorated experimental Parkinson's disease when encapsulated within thermoplastic PAN/PVC capsules and implanted in the striatum of adult guinea pigs [Aebischer et al., 1991].

The Choice of Cells and Tissues for Encapsulation.   Three main types of cells can be used for encapsulation. Cells may be postmitotic, cell lines that differentiate under specific conditions, or slow-dividing cells. The latter two types of cells lend themselves to genetic manipulation.

Postmitotic Cells.   Primary xenogeneic tissue may be encapsulated and transplanted across species. For instance, chromaffin cells release various antinociceptive substances such as enkephalins, catecholamines, and somatostatin. Allografts of adrenal chromaffin cells have been shown to alleviate pain when transplanted in the subarachnoid space in rodent models and terminal cancer patients [Sagen et al., 1993]. Transplantation of encapsulated xenogeneic chromaffin cells may provide a long-term source of pain-reducing neuroactive substances [Sagen et al., 1993]. In our laboratory, clinical trials are currently under way using the transplantation of encapsulated bovine chromaffin tissue into human cerebrospinal fluid as a strategy to alleviate chronic pain in terminal cancer patients [Aebischer et al., 1994]. This may circumvent the problem of the limited availability of human adrenal tissue in grafting procedures of chromaffin tissue.

Cell Lines that Differentiate under Specific Conditions.   Postmitotic cells are attractive for transplantation applications because the possibility of tumor formation, loss of phenotypic expression, is potentially lower. Also, when encapsulated, there is less debris accumulation inside the capsule due to turnover of dividing cells. However, the disadvantage is that the amount of postmitotic tissue is usually too limited in quantity for general clinical applications. Therefore, the use of cells that are mitotic and then are rendered postmitotic under specific conditions is attractive for transplantation applications.

Under appropriate culture conditions, primary myoblasts undergo cell division for at least 50 passages. Fusion into resting myoblasts can be obtained by controlling the culture conditions. Alternatively, a transformed myoblast cell line C_2C_{12} derived from a C_2H mouse thigh differentiates and forms myotubes when cultured under low serum conditions [Yaffe and Saxel, 1977]. Therefore, these cells could be genetically altered, expanded *in vitro* and then made postmitotic by varying the culture conditions. They can then be transplanted with the attendant advantages of using postmitotic tissue. Since myoblasts can be altered genetically, they have the potential to be a rich source for augmentation of tissue function via cell transplantation.

Slow-Dividing Cells.   Slow-dividing cells that reach a steady state in a capsule either due to contact inhibition or due to the encapsulation matrix are an attractive source of cells for transplantation. Potentially, their division can result in a self-renewing supply of cells inside the capsule. Dividing cells are also easier to transfect reliably with retroviral methods and therefore lend themselves to genetic manipulation. It is therefore possible to envisage the transplantation of various genetically engineered cells for the treatment of several neurologic disorders. This technique allows access to an ever-expanding source of xenogeneic tissues that have been engineered to produce the required factor of interest. For instance, Horellou and Mallet [1989] have retrovirally transferred the human TH cDNA into mouse anterior pituitary AtT-20 cell line, potentially resulting in a plentiful supply of dopamine-secreting cells that can then be encapsulated and transplanted into the striatum.

Another promising area for the use of such techniques is in the treatment of some neurodegenerative disorders where a lack of neurotrophic factors is believed to be part of the pathophysiology. Neurotrophic factors are soluble proteins that are required for the survival of neurons. These factors often exert a trophic effect; i.e., they have the capability of attracting growing axons. The "target" hypothesis describes the dependence of connected neurons on a trophic factor that is retrogradely transported along the axons after release from the target neurons. In the absence of the trophic factors, the neurons shrink and die, presumably to avoid potential misconnections. Experimentally, fibroblast lines have been used in CNS transplantation studies because of their convenience for gene transfer techniques [Gage et al., 1991]. The transplantation of encapsulated genetically engineered fibroblasts to produce NGF has been shown to prevent lesion-induced loss of septal ChaT expression following a fimbria-fornix lesion [Hoffman et al., 1993]. The fimbria-fornix lesion is characterized by deficits in learning and memory resembling those of Alzheimer's disease.

Matrices for Encapsulation. The physical, chemical, and biologic properties of the matrix in which the cells have been immobilized may play an important role in determining the transplanted cell's state and function. Broadly, matrices can be classified into the following types: cross-linked polyelectrolytes, collagen in solution or as porous beads, naturally occurring extracellular matrix derivatives such as Matrigel, fibrin clots, and biosynthetic hydrogels with appropriate biologic cues bound to them to elicit a specific response from the cells of interest. The matrix has several functions: It can prevent the formation of large cell aggregates that lead to the development of central necrosis as a consequence of insufficient oxygen and nutrient access; it may allow anchorage-dependent cells to attach and spread on the matrix substrate; and it may induce differentiation of a cell line and therefore slow or stop its division rate.

Negatively charged polyeletrolytes such as alginate have been used successfully for the immobilization of adrenal chromaffin cells [Aebischer et al., 1991]. Positively charged substrates, such as those provided by the amine groups of chitosan, allow attachment and spreading of fibroblasts [Zielinski et al., in press]. Biologically derived Matrigel induces differentiation of various cell lines such as Chinese hamster ovary (CHO) cells, astrocyte lines, or fibroblast lines (unpublished observations). Spongy collagen matrices, as well as fibrin matrices, seem to possess similar qualities. Our laboratory is currently evaluating the use of biosynthetic hydrogel matrices with biologically relevant peptides covalently bound to the polymer backbone. It is hypothesized that these matrices may elicit a specific designed response from the encapsulated cells.

21.2 Tissue Reconstruction: Nerve Regeneration

Most of the techniques described above were attempts at identifying the missing molecules of various neuropathologies, finding an appropriate source for these molecules and, if necessary, designing a cellular source via genetic engineering, and ultimately, choosing an optimal mode of delivery of the molecules, be it chemical or cellular. This approach, however, falls short of replacing the physical neuroanatomic synaptic circuits in the brain, which, in turn, may play an important role in the physiologic feedback regulating mechanisms of the system. Attempts to duplicate *in vivo* predisease neuronal structure have been made. For instance, the bridging of the nigrostriatal pathway, which when disrupted may cause Parkinson's disease, and the septohippocampal pathway, which may serve as a model for Alzheimer's disease, has attracted some attention. Wictorin and colleagues [1992] have reported long-distance directed axonal growth from human dopaminergic mesencephalic neuroblasts implanted along the nigrostriatal pathway in 6-hydroxydopamine-lesioned rats. In this section we shall examine the use of synthetic

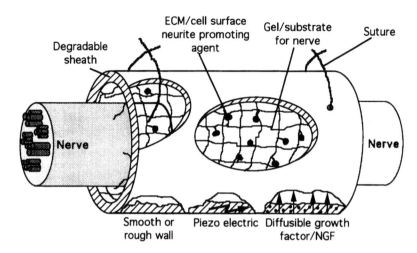

FIGURE 21.2   Schematic illustration of a nerve guidance channel and some of the possible strategies for influencing nerve regeneration.

guidance channels and extracellular matrix cues to guide axons to their appropriate targets. Thus a combination of all these techniques may render the complete physical and synaptic reconstruction of a degenerated pathway feasible.

The promotion of nerve regeneration is an important candidate task for tissue reconstruction in the nervous system. Synthetic nerve guidance channels (NGCs) have been used to study the underlying mechanisms of mammalian peripheral nerve regeneration after nerve injury and enhance the regeneration process. Guidance channels may simplify end-to-end repair and may be useful in repairing long nerve gaps. The guidance channel reduces tension at the suture line, protects the regenerating nerve from infiltrating scar tissue, and directs the sprouting axons toward their distal targets. The properties of the guidance channel can be modified to optimize the regeneration process. Nerve guidance channels also may be used to create a controlled environment in the regenerating site. In the peripheral nervous system, NGCs can influence the extent of nerve gap that can be bridged and the quality of regeneration. The channel properties, the matrix filling the NGC, the cells seeded within the channel lumen, and polymer-induced welding of axons all can be strategies used to optimize and enhance nerve regeneration and effect nervous tissue reconstruction (see Fig. 21.2 for a schematic). Table 21.2 lists some of the kinds of nerve guidance channels used so far.

The Active Use of Channel Properties

In the past, biocompatability of a biomaterial was evaluated by the degree of its passivity or lack of "reaction" when implanted into the body. However, the recognition that the response of the host tissue is related to the mechanical, chemical, and structural properties of the implanted biomaterial has led to the design of materials that promote a beneficial response from the host. In the context of a synthetic nerve guidance channel, this may translate to manipulation of its microstructural properties, permeability, electrical properties, and the loading of its channel wall with neuroactive components that might then be released locally into the regenerating environment. The strategy here is to engineer a tailored response from the host and take advantage of the natural repair processes.

Surface Microgeometry

The morphology of regenerating peripheral nerves is modulated by the surface microgeometry of polymeric guidance channels [Aebischer et al., 1990]. Channels with smooth inner walls give rise to organized, longitudinal fibrin matrices, resulting in discrete free-floating nerve cables with numerous myelinated axons. The rough inner surface channels, however, give rise to an unorganized fibrin matrix with nerve

TABLE 21.2 Nerve Guidance Channels

I. The Channel Wall	
1. *Passive polymeric channels*	
Silicone elastomer	Lundborg et al., 1982
Polyvinyl chloride	Scaravalli, 1984
Polyethylene	Madison et al., 1988
2. *Permeable polymer channels*	
Acrylonitrile vinychloride copolymer	Uzman and Villegas, 1983
Collagen	Archibald et al., 1991
Expanded polytetrafluroethylene	Young et al., 1984
3. *Resorbable polymer channels*	
Polyglycolic acid	Molander et al., 1989
Poly-L-lactic acid	Nyilas et al., 1983
Collagen	Archibald et al., 1991
4. *Electrically shaped polymer channels*	
Silicone channels with electrode cuffs	Kerns and Freeman, 1986; Kerns et al., 1991
Polyvinylidenefluoride (piezoelectric)	Aebischer et al., 1987
Polytetrofluoroethylene (electret)	Valentini et al., 1989
5. *Polymer channels releasing trophic factors*	
Ethylene vinylacetate copolymer	Aebischer et al., 1989
II. Intrachannel, luminal matrices	
1. Fibrin matrix	Williams et al., 1987
2. Collagen-glycosaminoglycan template	Yannas et al., 1985
3. Matrigel	Valentini et al., 1987
III. Cell seeded lumens for trophic support	
1. Schwann cell-seeded lumens (PNS)	Guénard et al., 1992
2. Schwann cell-seeded lumens (CNS)	Guénard et al., 1993; Kromer and Cornbrooks, 1985, 1987; Smith and Stevenson, 1988

fascicles scattered in a loose connective tissue filling the entire channel's lumen. Thus the physical textural properties and porosity of the channel can influence nervous tissue behavior and may be used to elicit a desirable reaction from the host tissue.

Molecular Weight Cutoff

The molecular weight cutoff of the NGCs influences peripheral nerve regeneration in rodent models [Aebischer et al., 1989]. The molecular weight cutoff may influence nerve regeneration possibly by controlling the exchange of molecules between the channel lumen and the external wound-healing environment. This may be important because the external environment consists of humoral factors that can play a role in augmenting regenerative processes in the absence of a distal stump.

Electrical Properties

In vivo regeneration following transection injury in the peripheral nervous system has been reported to be enhanced by galvantropic currents produced in silicone channels fitted with electrode cuffs [Kerns and Freeman, 1986; Kerns et al., 1991]. Polytetrafluoroethylene (PTFE) "electret" tubes show more myelinated axons compared with uncharged tubes in peripheral nerves [Valentini et al., 1989]. Dynamically active piezoelectric polymer channels also have been shown to enhance nerve regeneration in the sciatic nerves of adult mice and rats [Aebischer et al., 1987; Fine et al., 1991].

Release of Bioactive Factors from the Channel Wall

Polymer guidance channels can be loaded with various factors to study and enhance nerve regeneration. Basic fibroblast growth factor released from an ethylene-vinyl acetate copolymer guidance channel facilitates peripheral nerve regeneration across long nerve gaps after a rat sciatic nerve lesion [Aebischer et al., 1989]. The possible influence of interleukin-1 (IL-1) on nerve regeneration also was studied by the release of IL-1 receptor antagonist (IL-1ra) from the wall of an EVA copolymer channel [Guénard et al., 1991]. It is conceivable that the release of appropriate neurotrophic factors from the channel wall may enhance specifically subsets of axons, e.g., ciliary neurotrophic factor on motor neurons and nerve growth factor on sensory neurons.

Resorbable Channel Wall

Bioresorbable nerve guidance channels are attractive because once regeneration is completed, the channel disappears without further surgical intervention. Mice sciatic nerves have been bridged with poly-L-lactic acid channels [Nyilas et al., 1983] and polyester guidance channels [Henry et al., 1985]. Rabbit tibial nerves also have been bridged with guidance channels fabricated from polyglycolic acid [Molander et al., 1989]. Resorbable guidance channels need to retain their mechanical integrity over 4 to 12 weeks. At the same time, their degradation products should not interfere with the regenerative processes of the nerve. These issues remain the challenging aspects in the development of bioresorbable nerve guidance channels for extensive use in animals and humans.

Intraluminal Matrices for Optimal Organization of Regeneration Microenvironment

The physical support structure of the regenerating environment may play an important role in determining the extent of regeneration. An oriented fibrin matrix placed in the lumen of silicone guidance channels accelerates the early phases of peripheral nerve regeneration [Williams et al., 1987].

Silicone channels filled with a collagen-glycosaminoglycan template bridged a 15-mm nerve gap in rats, whereas no regeneration was observed in unfilled tubes [Yannas et al., 1985]. However, even matrices known to promote neuritic sprouting *in vitro* may impede peripheral nerve regeneration in semipermeable guidance channels if the optimal physical conditions are not ensured [Madison et al., 1988; Valentini et al., 1987]. Therefore, the structural, chemical, and biologic aspects of the matrix design may all play a role in determining the fate of the regenerating nerve. The importance of the effect of the physical environment on regeneration, mediated by its influence on fibroblast and Schwann cell behavior, has been demonstrated in several studies and has been reviewed by Schwartz [1987] and Fawcett and Keynes [1990]. Thus the choice of a hydrogel with physical, chemical, and biologic cues conducive to nerve regeneration may enhance nerve regeneration. This strategy is currently being explored [Belamkonda et al., in press]. Neurite-promoting oligopeptides from the basement membrane protein laminin (LN) were covalently coupled to agarose hydrogels. Agarose gels derivatized with LN oligopeptides specifically enhance neurite extension from cells that have receptors to the LN peptides *in vitro* [Bellamkonda et al., in press]. Preliminary results show that the presence of an agarose gel carrying the LN peptide CDPGYIGSR inside the lumen of a synthetic guidance channel enhances the regeneration of transected peripheral nerves (Fig. 21.3) in rats. Thus it is feasible to tailor the intraluminal matrices with more potent neurite-promoting molecules such as the cell adhesion molecules (CAMs) L1, N-CAM, or tenascin and "engineer" a desired response from the regenerating neural elements.

Cell-Seeded Lumens for Trophic Support

Cells secreting various growth factors may play an important role in organizing the regeneration environment, e.g., Schwann cells in the peripheral and central nervous system. It has been reported that regenerating axons do not elongate through acellular nerve grafts if Schwann cell migration was impeded [Hall et al., 1986]. Syngeneic Schwann cells derived from adult nerves and seeded in semipermeable guidance channels enhance peripheral nerve regeneration [Guénard et al., 1992]. Schwann cells in the preceding study orient themselves along the axis of the guidance channel, besides secreting various neurotrophic factors. Schwann cells could play a role in organizing the fibirin cable formed during the initial phases of nerve regeneration. Schwann cells may be effective in inducing regeneration in the CNS, too [Kromer and Cornbrook, 1985, 1987; Smith and Stevenson, 1988]. The use of tailored intraluminal matrices and presenting exogeneic Schwann cells to the regeneration environment in a controlled matter

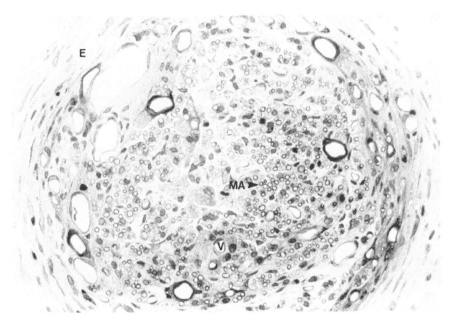

FIGURE 21.3 Light micrograph of a cross-sectional cut of a sural nerve regenerating through a polymer guidance channel 4 weeks after transection. The nerve guidance channel had been filled with a CDPGYIGSR derivatized agarose gel. E is the epineurium; V shows neovascularization; and MA is myelinated axon.

are strategies aimed at engineering the desired tissue response by creating the optimal substrate, trophic, and cellular environments around the regenerating nerves.

CNS glial cells have a secretory capacity that can modulate neuronal function. Astrocytes release proteins that enhance neuronal survival and induce neuronal growth and differentiation. When a silicone channel was seeded with astrocytes of different ages, ranging from P9 to P69 (postnatal), it was observed that while P9 astrocytes did not interfere with peripheral nerve regeneration, adult astrocytes downregulate axonal growth [Kalderon, 1988]. However, the presence of Schwann cells reverses the inhibition of PNS regeneration due to adult astrocytes [Guénard et al., 1994]. Thus the cellular environment in the site of injury may play an important role in determining the extent of regeneration. Knowledge of these factors also may be employed in designing optimal environments for nerve regeneration.

Polyethyleneglycol-Induced Axon Fusion

Rapid morphologic fusion of severed myelinated axons may be achieved by the application of polyethylene glycol (PEG) to the closely apposed ends of invertebrate-myelinated axons [Krause and Bittner, 1990]. Selection of appropriate PEG concentration and molecular mass, tight apposition, and careful alignment of the cut ends of the nerve may facilitate the direct fusion of axons. However, this technique is only applicable when the two ends of the severed nerve are closely apposed to each other, before the onset of wallerian degeneration.

CNS Nerve Regeneration

Most of the preceding studies have been conducted in the peripheral nervous system (PNS). In the CNS, however, endogenous components express poor support for axonal elongation. Significant regeneration may, however, occur with supporting substrates. Entubulation with a semipermeable acrylic copolymer tube allows bridging of a transected rabbit optic nerve with a cable containing myelinated axons [Aebischer et al., 1988]. Cholinergic nerve regeneration into basal lamina tubes containing Schwann cells has been reported in a transected septohippocampal model in rats [Kromer and Cornbrooks, 1985].

Thus the appropriate combination of physical guidance, matrices, and growth factors can create the right environmental cues and may be effective in inducing regeneration in the CNS. Therefore, both in the PNS and CNS, manipulation of the natural regenerative capacities of the host either by guidance factor or stimulation by electrical or trophic factors or structural components of the regenerating microenvironment can significantly enhance regeneration and help the reconstruction of severed or damaged neural tissue.

21.3 *In Vitro* Neural Circuits and Biosensors

The electrochemical and chemoelectrical transduction properties of neuronal cells can form the basis of a cell-based biosensing unit. The unique information-processing capabilities of neuronal cells through synaptic modulation may form the basis of designing simple neuronal circuits in vitro. Both the preceding applications necessitate controlled neuronal cell attachment, tightly coupled to the substrate and a sensitive substrate to monitor changes in the cell's electrical activity.

The use of bioactive material systems tailored to control neuronal cell attachment on the surface and still amenable to the incorporation of electrical sensing elements like a field effect transistor (FET) could be one feasible design. Therefore, composite material systems, which might incorporate covalently patterned bioactive peptides on their surface to control cell attachment and neurite extension, may be a step toward the fulfillment of the preceding goal. Oligopeptides derived from larger extracellular proteins like laminin have been shown to mediate specific cell attachment via cell surface receptors [Graf et al., 1987; Iwamoto et al., 1987; Kleinman et al., 1988]. Cell culture on polymeric membranes modified with the preceding bioactive peptidic components may give rise to a system where neuronal cell attachment and neuritic process outgrowth may be controlled. This control may help in designing microelectronic leads to complete the cell-electronic junction. Preliminary recordings from a FET-based neuron-silicon junction using leech Retzius cells [Fromherz et al., 1991] have been reported. Though there are many problems, such as attaining optimal coupling, this could form the basis of a "neural chip." A neural chip could potentially link neurons to external electronics for applications in neuronal cell-based biosensors, neural circuits, and limb prosthesis. Polymer surface modification and intelligent use of extracellular matrix components through selective binding could help attain this goal.

Studies in our laboratory have been trying to understand the underlying mechanisms involving protein adsorption onto polymeric substrates and their role in influencing and controlling nerve cell attachment [Ranieri et al., 1993]. Controlled neuronal cell attachment within a tolerance range of 20 μm may be achieved either nonspecifically monoamine surfaces or specifically via oligopeptides derived from ECM proteins like laminin and fibronectin [Fig. 21.4], mediated by integrin cell surface receptors [Ranieri et al., in press]. Molecular control of neuronal cell attachment and interfacing neuronal cells with electrodes may find applications in the design and fabrication of high-sensitivity neuron-based biosensors with applications in detection of low level neurotransmitters.

Studies are also currently in progress involving polymeric hydrogels and controlling neuronal cell behavior in a three-dimensional (3D) tissue culture environs as a step toward building 3D neuronal tissues [Bellamkonda et al., in press]. The choice of an appropriate hydrogel chemistry and structure, combined with the possibility of the gel serving as a carrier for ECM proteins or their peptidic analogues, can enable one to enhance regeneration when seeded in a nerve guidance channel. Also, the use of appropriate hydrogel chemistries in combination with the chemical modification of the polymer backbone by laser-directed photochemistry may be feasible in controlling the direction and differentiation of neuronal cells in three dimensions. Covalent binding of bioactive components like the laminin oligopeptides to the hydrogel backbone gives a specific character to the gel so that it elicits specific responses from anchorage-dependent neuronal cells [Bellamkonda et al., in press] (Fig. 21.5). Such a system could be useful in reorganizing nerves in 3D either for bridging different regions of the brain with nerve cables or for the 3D organization of nerves for optimal coupling with external electronics in the design of artificial limb prostheses. In either case, development of such systems presents an interesting challenge for tissue engineering.

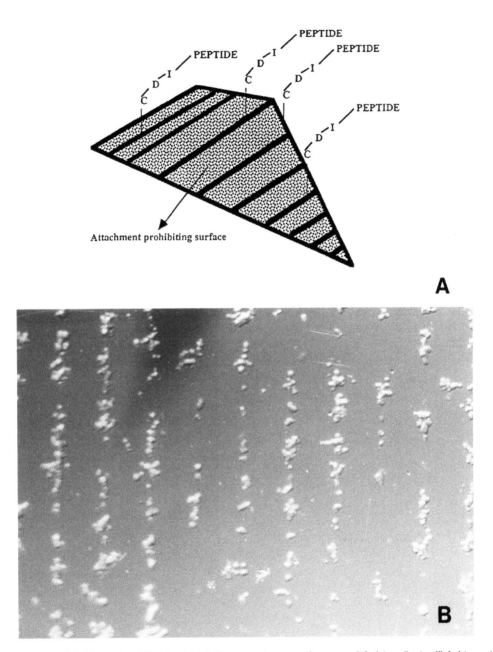

FIGURE 21.4 (A) Schematic of fluorinated ethylene propylene membrane modified in a "striped" fashion with bioactive oligopeptides using carbonyldiimidazole homobifunctional linking agent. (B) Light micrograph of Ng108-15 cells "striping" on FEP membrane surfaces selectively modified with CDPGYIGSR oligopeptide.

21.4 Conclusion

Advances in gene transfer techniques and molecular and cell biology offer potent tools in the functional replacement of various tissues of the nervous system. Each of these cells' functions can be optimized with the design and selection of its optimal extracellular environment. Substrates that support neuronal differentiation in two and three dimensions may play an important role in taking advantage of the advances in molecular and cell biology. Thus research aimed at tailoring extracellular matrices with the

Neuron   Hydrogel backbone

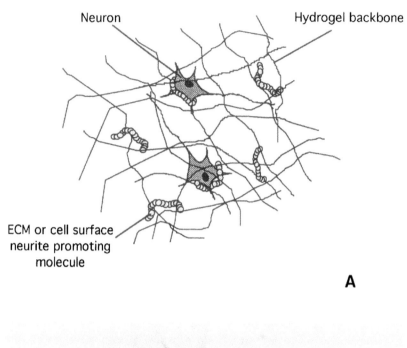

ECM or cell surface
neurite promoting
molecule

A

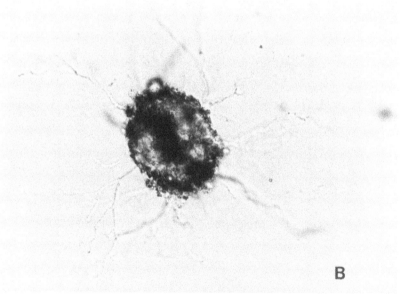

B

FIGURE 21.5   (A) Schematic of hydrogel derivatized with bioactive peptides with an anchorage-dependent neuron suspended in 3D. (B) Light micrograph of a E14 chick superior cervical ganglion suspended in 3D and extending neurites in an agarose gel derivatized with the laminin oligopeptide CDPGYIGSR.

appropriate physical, chemical, and biologic cues may be important in optimizing the function of transplanted cells, inducing nerve regeneration, or in the construction of neuronal tissues in two and three dimensions in a controlled fashion. Controlled design and fabrication of polymer hydrogels and polymer scaffolds on a scale that is relevant for single cells also may be important. This would presumably control the degree and the molecular location of permissive, attractive, and repulsive regions of the substrate and in turn control cellular and tissue response *in vitro* and *in vivo*.

   Biologic molecules like laminin, collagen, fibronectin, and tenascin may provide attractive and per-missive pathways for axons to grow. On the other hand, some sulfated proteoglycans have been shown to inhibit or repulse neurites [Snow and Letourneau, 1992]. The use of these molecules coupled with a clearer understanding of protein-mediated material-cell interaction may pave the way for neural tissue engineering, molecule by molecule, in three dimensions. Thus it is possible to tailor the genetic material of a cell to make it neurologically relevant and to control its expression by optimizing its extracellular environment. All the preceding factors make tissue engineering in the nervous system an exciting and challenging endeavor.

Acknowledgments

We wish to than Mr. Nicolas Boche for the illustrations.

References

Aebischer P, Goddard M, Signore A, Timpson R. 1994. Functional recovery in MPTP lesioned primates transplanted with polymer encapsulated PC12 cells. Exp Neurol 26:1.

Aebischer P, Buchser E, Joseph JN. 1994. Transplantation in humans of encapsulated xenogeneic cells without immunosuppression. Transplantation 58:1275.

Aebischer P, Guénard V, Brace S. 1989a. Peripheral nerve regeneration through blind-ended semipermeable guidance channels: Effect of the molecular weight cutoff. J Neurosci 9:3590.

Aebischer P, Salessiotis AN, Winn SR. 1989b. Basic fibroblast growth factor released from synthetic guidance channels facilitates peripheral nerve regeneration across long nerve gaps. J Neurosci Res 28:282.

Aebischer P, Guénard V, Valentini RF. 1990. The morphology of regenerating peripheral nerves is modulated by the surface microgeometry of polymeric guidance channels. Brain Res 531:211.

Aebischer P, Tresco PA, Winn SR, et al. 1991a. Long-term cross-species brain transplantation of a polymer-encapsulated dopamine-secreting cell line. Exp Neurol 111:269.

Aebischer P, Tresco PA, Sagen J, Winn SR. 1991b. Transplantation of microencapsulated bovine chromaffin cells reduces lesion-induced rotational asymmetry in rats. Brain Res 560:43.

Aebischer P, Wahlberg L, Tresco PA, Winn SR. 1991c. Macroencapsulation of dopamine secreting cells by coextrusion with an organic polymer solution. Biomaterials 12:50.

Aebischer P, Valentini RF, Dario P, et al. 1987. Piezoelectric guidance channels enhance regeneration in the mouse sciatic nerve after axotomy. Brain Res 436:165.

Aebischer P, Winn SR, Galletti PM. 1988a. Transplantation of neural tissue in polymer capsules. Brain Res 448:364.

Aebischer P, Valentini RF, Winn SR, Galletti PM. 1988b. The use of a semipermeable tube as a guidance channel for a transected rabbit optic nerve. Brain Res 78:599.

Ahlgren FI, Ahlgren MB. 1987. Epidural administration of opiates by a new device. Pain 31:353.

Akil H, Watson SJ, Young E, et al. 1984. Endogenous opioids: biology and function. Annu Rev Neurosci 7:223.

Albani C, Asper R, Hacisalihzade SS, Baumgartner F. 1986. Individual levodopa therapy in Parkinson's disease. In Advances in Neurology: Parkinson's Disease, pp 497–501. New York, Raven Press.

Anderson RF, Alterman AL, Barde YA, Lindsay RM. 1990. Brain-derived neurotrophic factor increases survival and differentiation of septal cholinergic neurons in culture. Neuron 5:297.

Archibald SJ, Krarup C, Shefner J, et al. 1991. A collagen-based nerve guide conduit for peripheral nerve repair: An electrophysiological study of nerve regeneration in rodents and nonhuman primates. J Comp Neurol 306–685.

Becker JB, Robinson TE, Barton P, et al. 1990. Sustained behavioral recovery from unilateral nigrostriatal damage produced by the controlled release of dopamine from a silicone polymer pellet placed into the denervated striatum. Brain Res 508:60.

Bellamkonda R, Ranieri JP, Aebischer P. In press. Laminin oligopeptide derivatized agarose gels allow three-dimensional neurite outgrowth in vitro. J Neurosci Res.

Bellamkonda R, Ranieri JP, Bouche N, Aebischer P. In press. A hydrogel-based three-dimensional matrix for neural cells. J Biomed Nat Res.

Birkmayer W. 1969. Experimentalle Ergebnisse uber die Kombinationsbehandlung des Parkinsonsyndroms mit 1-dopa und einem Decarboxylasehemmer. Wien Klin Wochenschr 81:677.

Björklund A. 1991. Neural transplantation—An experimental tool with clinical possibilities. TINS 14:319.

Björklund A, Dunnett SB, Stenevi U, et al. 1980. Reinnervation of the denervated striatum by substantia nigra transplants: Functional consequences as revealed by pharmacological and sensorimotor testing. Brain Res 199:307.

Bolam JP, Freund TF, Björklund A, et al. 1987. Synaptic input and local output of dopaminergic neurons in grafts that functionally reinnervate the host neostriatum. Exp Brain Res 68:131.

Bunge RP, Bunge MB. 1983. Interrelationship between Schwann cell function and extracellular matrix production. TINS 6:499.

Chen LS, Ray J, Fisher LJ, et al. 1991. Cellular replacement therapy for neurologic disorders: Potential of genetically engineered cells. J Cell Biochem 45:252.

De Yebenes JG, Fahn S, Jackson-Lewis V, et al. 1988. Continuous intracerebroventricular infusion of dopamine and dopamine agonists through a totally implanted drug delivery system in animal models of Parkinson's disease. J Neural Transplant 27:141.

During MJ, Freese A, Deutch AY, et al. 1992. Biochemical and behavioral recovery in a rodent model of Parkinson's disease following stereotactic implantation of dopamine-containing liposomes. Exp Neurol 115:193.

Ehringer H, Hornykiewicz O. 1960. Vetreilung von Noradrenalin und Dopamin (3-Hydroxtyramin) im Gehirn des Menschen und ihr Verhalten bei Erkrankungen des extrapyramidalen Systems. Klin Ther Wochenschr 38:1236.

Fawcett JW, Keynes RJ. 1990. Peripheral nerve regeneration. Annu Rev Neurosci 13:43.

Fine EG, Valentini RF, Bellamkonda R, Aebischer P. 1991. Improved nerve regeneration through piezoelectric vinylidenefluoride-trifluoroethylene copolymer guidance channels. Biomaterials 12:775.

Fromherz P, Offenhausser A, Vetter T, Weis J. 1991. A neuron-silicon junction: A Retzius cell of the leech on an insulated-gate field-effect transistor. Science 252:1290.

Gage FH, Kawaja MD, Fisher LJ. 1991. Genetically modified cells: Applications for intracerebral grafting. TINS 14:328.

Goosen MFA, Shea GM, Gharapetian HM, et al. 1985. Optimization of microencapsualtion parameters: Semipermeable microcapsules as a bioartificial pancreas. Biotech Bioeng 27:146.

Graf J, Ogle RC, Robey FA, et al. 1987. A pentrapeptide from the laminin B1 chain mediates cell adhesion and binds the 67,000 laminin receptor. Biochemistry 26:6896.

Guénard V, Aebischer P, Bunge R. 1994. The astrocyte inhibition of peripheral nerve regeneration is reversed by Schwann cells. Exp Neurol 126:44.

Guénard V, Dinarello CA, Weston PJ, Aebischer P. 1991. Peripheral nerve regeneration is impeded by interleukin 1 receptor antagonist released from a polymeric guidance channel. J Neurosci Res 29:396.

Guénard V, Kleitman N, Morrissey TK, et al. 1992. Syngeneic Schwann cells derived from adult nerves seeded in semipermeable guidance channels enhance peripheral nerve regeneration. J Neurosci 2:3310.

Guénard V, Xu XM, Bunge MB. 1993. The use of Schwann cell transplantation to foster central nervous system repair. Semin Neurosci 5:401.

Hall SM. 1986. The effect of inhibiting Schwann cells mitosis on the re-innervation of acellular autografts in the peripheral nervous system of the mouse. Neuropathol Appl Neurobiol 12:27.

Hardie RJ, Lees AJ, Stern GM. 1984. On-off fluctuations in Parkinson's disease: A clinical and neuropharmacological study. Brain 107:487.

Hargraves R, Freed WJ. 1987. Chronic intrastriatal dopamine infusions in rats with unilateral lesions of the substantia nigra. Life Sci 40:959.

Hefti F, Dravid A, Hartikka J. 1984. Chronic intraventricular injections of nerve growth factor elevate hippocampal choline acetyltransferase activity in adult rats with partial septo-hippocampal lesions. Brain Res 293:305.

Henry EW, Chiu TH, Nyilas E, et al. 1985. Nerve regeneration through biodegradable polyester tubes. Exp Neurol 90:652.

Hoffman D, Breakefield XO, Short MP, Aebischer P. 1993. Transplantation of a polymer-encapsulated cell line genetically engineered to release NGF. Exp Neurol 122:100.

Hoffman D, Wahlberg L, Aebischer P. 1990. NGF released from a polymer matrix prevents loss of ChaT expression in basal forebrain neurons following a fimbria-fornix lesion. Exp Neurol 110:39.

Horellou P, Guilbert B, Leviel V, Mallet J. 1989. Retroviral transfer of a human tyrosine hydroxylase cDNA in various cell lines: Regulated release of dopamine in mouse anterior pituitary AtT-20 cells. Proc Natl Acad Sci USA 86:7233.

Hughes RA, Sendtner M, Thoenen H. 1993. Members of several gene families influence survival of rat motoneurons in vitro and in vivo. J Neurosci Res 36:663.

Hyman C, Hofer M, Barde YA, et al. 1991. BDNF is a neurotrophic factor for dopaminergic neurons of the substantia nigra. Nature 350:230.

Iwamoto Y, Robey FA, Graf J, et al. 1987. YIGSR, a synthetic laminin pentapeptide, inhibits experimental metastasis formation. Science 238:1132.

Jiao S, Gurevich V, Wolff JA. 1993. Long-term correction of rat model of Parkinson's disease by gene therapy. Nature 362:450.

Joseph JM, Goddard MB, Mills J, et al. 1994. Transplantation of encapsulated bovine chromaffin cells in the sheep subarachnoid space: a preclinical study for the treatment of cancer pain. Cell Transplant 3:355.

Kalderon N. 1988. Differentiating astroglia in nervous tissue histogenesis regeneration: studies in a model system of regenerating peripheral nerve. J Neurosci Res 21:501.

Kerns JM, Fakhouri AJ, Weinrib HP, Freeman JA. 1991. Electrical stimulation of nerve regeneration in the rat: The early effects evaluated by a vibrating probe and electron microscopy. J Neurosci 40:93.

Kleinman H, Ogle RC, Cannon FB, et al. 1988. Laminin receptors for neurite formation. Proc Natl Acad Sci USA 85:1282.

Knüsel B, Winslow JW, Rosenthal A, et al. 1991. Promotion of central cholinergic and dopaminergic neuron differentiation by brain derived neurotrophic factor but not neurotrophin-3. Proc Natl Acad Sci USA 88:961.

Krause TL, Bittner GD. 1990. Rapid morphological fusion of severed myelinated axons by polyethylene glycol. Proc Natl Acad Sci USA 87:1471.

Kromer LF, Cornbrooks CJ. 1985. Transplants of Schwann cell culture cultures promote axonal regeneration in adult mammalian brain. Proc Natl Acad Sci USA 82:6330.

Kromer LF, Cornbrooks CJ. 1987. Identification of trophic factors and transplanted cellular environments that promote CNS axonal regeneration. Ann NY Acad Sci 495:207.

Langer R. 1981. Polymers for sustained release of macromolecules: Their use in a single-step method for immunization. In JJ Langone, J Van Vunakis (eds), Methods of Enzymology, pp 57–75. San Diego, Academic Press.

Langer R, Folkman J. 1976. Polymers for sustained release of proteins and other macromolecules. Nature 263:797.

Lim F, Sun AM. 1980. Microencapsulated islets as bioartificial endocrine pancreas. Science 210:908.

Lin HL-F, Doherty DH, Lile JD, et al. 1993. GDNF: A glial derived neurotrophic factor for midbrain dopaminergic neurons. Science 260:1130.

Lindvall O. 1991. Prospects of transplantation in human neurodegenerative diseases. TINS 14:376.

Lindvall O, Brundin P, Widner H, et al. 1990. Grafts of fetal dopamine neurons survive and improve motor function in Parkinson's disease. Science 247:574.

Lundborg G, Dahlin LB, Danielsen N, et al. 1982. Nerve regeneration in silicone chambers: Influence of gap length and of distal stump components. Exp Neurol 76:361.

Madison RD, Da Silva CF, Dikkes P. 1988. Entubulation repair with protein additives increases the maximum nerve gap distance successfully bridged with tubular prosthesis. Brain Res 447:325.

McRae A, Hjorth S, Mason DW, et al. 1991. Microencapsulated dopamine (DA)-induced restitution of function in 6-OHDA denervated rat striatum in vivo: Comparison between two microsphere excipients. J Neural Transplant Plast 2:165.

Molander H, Olsson Y, Engkvist O, et al. 1989. Regeneration of peripheral nerve through a polygalactin tube. Muscle Nerve 5:54.

Morrissey TK, Kleitman N, Bunge RP. 1991. Isolation and functional characterization of Schwann cells derived from adult nerve. J Neurosci 11:2433.

Muenter MD, Sharpless NS, Tyce SM, Darley FL. 1977. Patterns of dystonia (I-D-I) and (D-I-D) in response to 1-dopa therapy for Parkinson's disease. Mayo Clin Proc 52:163.

Muir D, Gennrich C, Varon S, Manthorpe M. 1989. Rat sciatic nerve Schwann cell microcultures: Responses to mitogens and production of trophic and neurite-promoting factors. Neurochem Res 14:1003.

Nyilas E, Chiu TH, Sidman RL, et al. 1983. Peripheral nerve repair with bioresorbable prosthesis. Trans Am Soc Artif Intern Organs 29:307.

Olson L, Backlund EO, Ebendal T, et al. 1991. Intraputaminal infusion of nerve growth factor to support adrenal medullary autografts in Parkinson's disease: One year follow-up of first clinical trial. Arch Neurol 48:373.

Olson L, Nordberg A, Von-Holst H, et al. 1992. Nerve growth factor affects ^{11}C-nicotine binding, blood flow, EEG, and verbal episodic memory in an Alzheimer patient (case report). J Neural Transm Park Dis Dement Sect 4:79.

Oppenheim RW, Prevette D, Yin QW, et al. 1991. Control of embryonic motoneuron survival in vivo by ciliary neurotrophic factor. Science 251:1616.

Ranieri JP, Bellamkonda R, Bekos E, et al. 1994. Spatial control of neural cell attachment via patterned laminin oligopeptide chemistries. Int J Dev Neurosci 12:725.

Ranieri JP, Bellamkonda R, Jacob J, et al. 1993. Selective neuronal cell attachment to a covalently patterned monoamine of fluorinated ethylene propylene films. J Biomed Mater Res 27:917.

Reynolds BA, Tetzlaff W, Weiss S. 1992. A multipotent EGF_responsive striatal embryonic progenitor cell produces neurons and astrocytes. J Neurosci 12:4565.

Sabel BA, Dominiak P, Hauser W, et al. 1990. Levodopa delivery from controlled release polymer matrix: Delivery of more than 600 days in vitro and 225 days elevated plasma levels after subcutaneous implantation in rats. J Pharmacol Exp Ther 255:914.

Sagen J, Pappas GD, Winnie AP. 1993a. Alleviation of pain in cancer patients by adrenal medullary transplants in the spinal subarachnoid space. Cell Transplant 2:259.

Sagen J, Wang H, Tresco PA, Aebischer P. 1993b. Transplants of immunologically isolated xenogeneic chromaffin cells provide a long-term source of pain-reducing neuroactive substances. J Neurosci 13:2415.

Scaravalli F. 1984. Regeneration of peineurium across a surgically induced gap in a nerve encased in a plastic tube. J Anat 139:411.

Schwartz M. 1987. Molecular and cellular aspects of nerve regeneration. CRC Crit Rev Biochem 22:89.

Sendtner M, Kreutzberg GW, Thoenen H. 1990. Ciliary neurotrophic factor prevents the degeneration of motor neurons after axotomy. Nature 345:440.

Shoulson I, Claubiger GA, Chase TN. 1975. On-off response. Neurology 25:144.

Smith GV, Stevenson JA. 1988. Peripheral nerve grafts lacking viable Schwann cells fail to support central nervous system axonal regeneration. Exp Brain Res 69:299.

Snow DM, Letourneau PC. 1992. Neurite outgrowth on a step gradient of chondroitin sulfate proteoglycan (CS-PG). J Neurobiol 23:322.

Tresco PA, Winn SR, Aebischer P. 1992. Polymer encapsulated neurotransmitter secreting cells; potential treatment for Parkinson's disease. ASAIO J 38:17.

Uzman BG, Villegas GM. 1983. Mouse sciatic nerve regeneration through semipermeable tubes: A quantitative model. J Neurosci Res 9:325.

Valentini RF, Aebischer P, Winn SR, Galletti PM. 1987. Collagen- and laminin-containing gels impede peripheral nerve regeneration through semipermeable nerve guidance channels. Exp Neurol 98:350.

Valentini RF, Sabatini AM, Dario P, Aebischer P. 1989. Polymer electret guidance channels enhance peripheral nerve regeneration in mice. Brain Res 48:300.

Vescovi AL, Reynolds BA, Fraser DD, Weiss S. 1993. BFGF regulates the proliferative fate of unipotent (neuronal) and bipotent (neuronal/astroglial) EGF-generated CNS progenitor cells. Neuron 11:951.

Wictorin K, Brundin P, Sauer H, et al. 1992. Long distance directed axonal growth from human dopaminergic mesencephalic neuroblasts implanted along the nigrostriatal pathway in 6-hydroxydopamine lesioned rats. J Comp Neurol 323:475.

Williams LR, Danielsen N, Muller H, Varon S. 1987. Exogenous matrix precursors promote functional nerve regeneration across a 15-mm gap within a silicone chamber in the rat. J Comp Neurol 264:284.

Williams LR, Varon S, Peterson GM, et al. 1986. Continuous infusion of nerve growth factor prevents basal forebrain neuronal death after fimbria-fornix transection. Proc Natl Acad Sci USA 83:9231.

Winn SR, Tresco PA, Zielinski B, et al. 1991. Behavioral recovery following intrastriatal implantation of microencapsulated PC12 cells. Exp Neurol 113:322.

Winn SR, Wahlberg L, Tresco PA, Aebischer P. 1989. An encapsulated dopamine-releasing polymer alleviates experimental parkinsonism in rats. Exp Neurol 105:244.

Yaffe D, Saxel O. 1977. Serial passaging and differentiation of myogenic cells isolated from dystrophic mouse muscle. Nature 270:725.

Yan Q, Elliott J, Snider WD. 1992. Brain-derived neurotrophic factor rescues spinal motor neurons from axotomy-induced cell death. Nature 360:753.

Yannas EV, Orgill DP, Silver J, et al. 1985. Polymeric template facilitates regeneration of sciatic nerve across 15 mm gap. Trans Soc Biomater 11:146.

Young BL, Begovac P, Stuart D, Glasgow GE. 1984. An effective sleeving technique for nerve repair. J Neurosci Methods 10:51.

Zielinski B, Aebischer P. 1994. Encapsulation of mammalian cells in chitosan-based microcapsules: Effect of cell anchorage dependence. Biomaterials.

Zurn AD, Baetge EE, Hammang JP, et al. 1994. Glial cell line-derived neurotrophic factor (GDNF): A new neurotrophic factor for motoneurones. Neuroreport 6:113.

22

Tissue Engineering of Skeletal Muscle

Susan V. Brooks
University of Michigan

John A. Faulkner
University of Michigan

22.1 Introduction

Contractions of skeletal muscles generate the stability and power for all movement. Consequently, any impairment in skeletal muscle function results in at least some degree of instability or immobility. Muscle function can be impaired as a result of injury, disease, or old age. The goal of tissue engineering is to restore the structural and functional properties of muscles to permit the greatest recovery of normal movement. Impaired movement at all ages, but particularly in the elderly, increases the risk of severe injury, reduces participation in the activities of daily living, and has an impact on the quality of life.

Contraction is defined as the activation of muscle fibers with a tendency of the fibers to shorten. Contraction occurs when an increase in the cytosolic calcium concentration triggers a series of molecular events that includes the binding of calcium to the muscle regulatory proteins, the formation of strong interactions between the myosin cross-bridges and the actin filaments, and the generation of the cross-bridge driving stroke. *In vivo*, muscles perform three types of contractions depending on the interaction between the magnitude of the force developed by the muscle and the external load placed on the muscle. When the force developed by the muscle is greater than the load on the muscle, the fibers shorten during the contraction. When the force developed by the muscle is equal to the load, or if the load is immovable, the overall length of the muscle remains the same. If the force developed by the muscle is less than the load placed on the muscle, the muscle is stretched during the contraction. The types of contractions are termed miometric, isometric, and pliometric, respectively. Most normal body movements require varying proportions of each type of contraction.

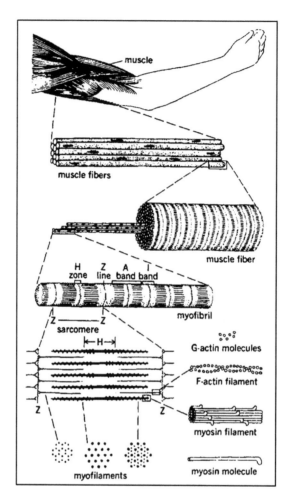

FIGURE 22.1 Levels of anatomical organization within a skeletal muscle. (From Bloom, W. and Fawcett, D.W., 1968. *A Textbook of Histology,* 9th ed., W.B. Saunders, Philadelphia. With permission.)

22.2   Skeletal Muscle Structure

Each of the 660 skeletal muscles in the human body is composed of hundreds to hundreds of thousands of single muscle fibers (Fig. 22.1). The plasma membrane of a muscle fiber is termed the sarcolemma. Contractile, structural, metabolic, regulatory, and cytosolic proteins, as well as many myonuclei and other cytosolic organelles, are contained within the sarcolemma of each fiber (Fig. 22.2). The contractile proteins myosin and actin are incorporated into thick and thin myofilaments, respectively, which are arrayed in longitudinally repeated banding patterns termed sarcomeres (Fig. 22.1). Sarcomeres in series form myofibrils, and many parallel myofibrils exist within each fiber. The number of myofibrils arranged in parallel determines the cross-sectional area (CSA) of single fibers, and consequently, the force generating capability of the fiber. During a contraction, the change in the length of a sarcomere occurs as thick and thin filaments slide past each other, but the overall length of each actin and myosin filament does not change. An additional membrane, referred to as the basement membrane or the basal lamina, surrounds the sarcolemma of each fiber (Fig. 22.2).

In mammals, the number of fibers in a given muscle is determined at birth and changes little throughout the life span except in cases of injury or disease. In contrast, the number of myofibrils can change dramatically, increasing with normal growth or hypertrophy induced by strength training and decreasing

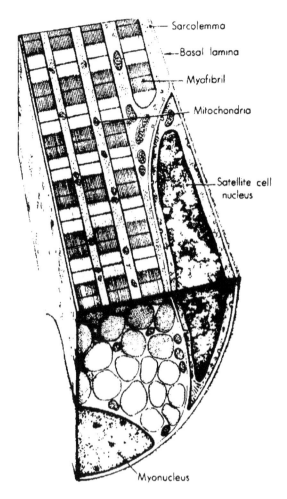

Sarcolemma

Basal lamina

Myofibril

Mitochondria

Satellite cell nucleus

Myonucleus

FIGURE 22.2   Drawing of a muscle fiber-satellite cell complex. Note that the satellite cell is located between the muscle fiber sarcolemma and the basal lamina. (From Carlson and Faulkner, 1983. With permission.)

with atrophy associated with immobilization, inactivity, injury, disease, or old age. A single muscle fiber is innervated by a single branch of a motor nerve. A motor unit is composed of a single motor nerve, its branches, and the muscle fibers innervated by the branches. The motor unit is the smallest group of fibers within a muscle that can be activated volitionally. Activation of a motor unit occurs when action potentials emanating from the motor cortex depolarize the cell bodies of motor nerves. The depolarization generates an action potential in the motor nerve that is transmitted to each muscle fiber in the motor unit, and each of the fibers contracts more or less simultaneously. Motor units range from small slow units to large fast units dependent on the CSA of the motor nerve.

22.3   Skeletal Muscle Function

Skeletal muscles may contract singly or in groups, working synergistically. On either side of limbs, muscles contract against one another or antagonistically. The force or power developed during a contraction depends on the frequency of stimulation of the motor units, the total number of motor units, and the size of the motor units recruited. The frequency of stimulation, particularly for the generation of power, is normally on the order of the frequency-power relationship. Consequently, the total number of motor units recruited is the major determinant of the force or power developed.

Motor units are classified into three general categories based on their functional properties [Burke et al., 1973]. Slow (S) units have the smallest single muscle fiber CSAs, the fewest muscle fibers per motor unit, and the lowest velocity of shortening. The cell bodies of the S units are the most easily depolarized to threshold [Henneman, 1965]. Consequently, S units are the most frequently recruited during tasks that require low force or power but highly precise movements. Fast-fatigable (FF) units are composed of the largest fibers, have the most fibers per unit, and have the highest velocities of shortening. The FF units are the last to be recruited and are recruited for high force and power movements. The fast fatigue-resistant (FR) units are intermediate in terms of the CSAs of their fibers, the number of fibers per motor unit, the velocity of shortening, and the frequency of recruitment. The force normalized per unit CSA is ~280 kN/m^2 for each type of fiber, but the maximum normalized power (W/kg) developed by FF units is as much as fourfold greater than that of the S units due to a fourfold higher velocity of shortening for FF units. Motor units may also be identified by histochemical techniques as Type I (S), IIA (FR), and IIB (FF). Classifications based on histochemical and functional characteristics are usually in good agreement with one another, but differences do exist, particularly following experimental interventions. Consequently, in a given experiment, the validity of this interpretation should be verified.

22.4 Injury and Repair of Skeletal Muscle

Injury to skeletal muscles may occur as a result of disease, such as dystrophy; exposure to myotoxic agents, such as bupivacaine or lidocaine; sharp or blunt trauma, such as punctures or contusions; ischemia, such as that which occurs with transplantation; exposure to excessively hot or cold temperatures; and con-tractions of the muscles. Pliometric contractions are much more likely to injure muscle fibers than are isometric or miometric contractions [McCully and Faulkner, 1985]. Regardless of the factors responsible, the manner in which the injuries are manifested appears to be the same, varying only in severity. In addition, the processes of fiber repair and regeneration appear to follow a common pathway regardless of the nature of the injurious event [Carlson and Faulkner, 1983].

Injury of Skeletal Muscle

The injury may involve either some or all of the fibers within a muscle [McCully and Faulkner, 1985]. In an individual fiber, focal injuries, localized to a few sarcomeres in series or in parallel (Fig. 22.3), as well as more widespread injuries, spreading across the entire cross section of the fiber, are observed using electron microscopic techniques [Macpherson et al., 1997]. Although the data are highly variable, many injuries also give rise to increases in serum levels of muscle enzymes, particularly creatine kinase, leading to the conclusion that sarcolemmal integrity is impaired [McNeil and Khakee, 1992; Newham et al., 1983]. This conclusion is further supported by an influx of circulating proteins, such as serum albumin [McNeil and Khakee, 1992], and of calcium [Jones et al., 1984]. An increase in intracellular calcium concentration may activate a variety of proteolytic enzymes leading to further degradation of sarcoplasmic proteins.

In cases when the damage involves a large proportion of the sarcomeres within a fiber, the fiber becomes necrotic. If blood flow is impaired, fibers remain as a necrotic mass of noncontractile tissue [Carlson and Faulkner, 1983]. In contrast, in the presence of an adequate blood supply, the injured fibers are infiltrated by monocytes and macrophages [McCully and Faulkner, 1985]. The phagocytic cells remove the disrupted myofilaments, other cytosolic structures, and the damaged sarcolemma (Fig. 22.4). The most severe injuries result in the complete degeneration of the muscle fiber, leaving only the empty basal lamina. The basal lamina appears to be highly resistant to any type of injury and generally remains intact [Carlson and Faulkner, 1983].

An additional indirect measure of injury is the subjective report by human beings of delayed onset muscle soreness, common following intense or novel exercise [Newham et al., 1983]. Because of the focal nature of the morphological damage, the variability of serum enzyme levels and the subjectivity of reports

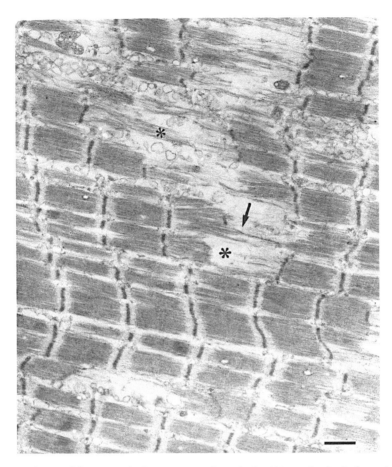

FIGURE 22.3 Focal areas of damage to single sarcomeres after a single 40% stretch of a single maximally activated rat skeletal muscle fiber (average sarcomere length 2.6 μm). Two types of damage are observed in this electron micrograph. The arrow indicates Z-line streaming and asterisks show disruption of the thick and thin filaments in the region of overlap, the A-band. A third type of damage, the displacement of thick filaments to one Z-line is not shown. Note that with the return of the relaxed fiber to an average sarcomere length of 2.6 μm, the sarcomeres indicated by asterisks are at 5.1 and 3.8 μm while sarcomeres in series are shortened to ~1.8 μm. Scale bar is 1.0 μm. (Modified from Macpherson et al., 1997. With permission.)

of soreness, the most quantitative and reproducible measure of the totality of a muscle injury is the decrease in the ability of the muscle to develop force [McCully and Faulkner, 1985; Newham et al., 1983].

Repair of Injured Skeletal Muscles

Under circumstances when the injury involves only minor disruptions of the thick or thin filaments of single sarcomeres, the damaged molecules are likely replaced by newly synthesized molecules available in the cytoplasmic pool [Russell et al., 1992]. In addition, contraction-induced disruptions of the sarcolemma are often transient and repaired spontaneously, allowing survival of the fiber [McNeil and Khakee, 1992]. Following more severe injuries, complete regeneration of the entire muscle fiber will occur.

Satellite Cell Activation

A key element in the initiation of muscle fiber regeneration following a wide variety of injuries is the activation of satellite cells [Carlson and Faulkner, 1983]. Satellite cells are quiescent myogenic stem cells located between the basal lamina and the sarcolemma (Fig. 22.2). Upon activation, satellite cells divide

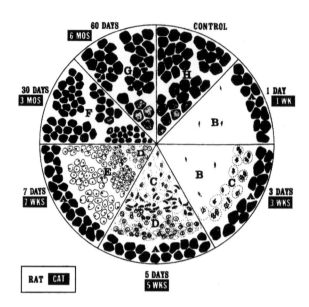

FIGURE 22.4   Schematic representation of the cellular responses during the processes of degeneration and regeneration following transplantation of extensor digitorum longus muscles in rats and cats. The diagram is divided into segments that represent the histological appearance of the muscle cross section at various times after transplantation. The times given in days refer to rat muscles and those given in weeks refer to the larger cat muscles. The letters indicate groups of muscle fibers with similar histological appearances. A: surviving fibers, B: fibers in a state of ischemic necrosis, C: fibers invaded by phagocytic cells, D: myoblasts and early myotubes, E: early myofibers, F: immature regenerating fibers, G: mature regenerated fibers, H: normal control muscle fibers [Carlson and Faulkner, 1983]. (From Mauro, A. 1979. *Muscle Regeneration*, pp. 493-507, Raven Press, New York. With permission.)

mitotically to give rise to myoblasts. The myoblasts can then fuse with existing muscle fibers, acting as a source of new myonuclei. This is the process by which a muscle fiber increases the total number of myonuclei in fibers that are increasing in size [Moss and Leblond, 1971] and may be necessary to repair local injuries. Alternatively, the myoblasts can fuse with each other to form multinucleated myotubes inside the remaining basal lamina of the degenerated fibers [Carlson and Faulkner, 1983]. The myotubes then begin to produce muscle specific proteins and ultimately differentiate completely into adult fast or slow muscle fibers [Carlson and Faulkner, 1983]. Recent evidence also suggests that in addition to the activation of resident satellite cells, regenerating muscle may recruit undifferentiated myogenic precursor cells from other sources [Ferrari et al., 1998]

Following a closed contusion injury, mitotic activation of satellite cells has been observed within the first day after the injury and is correlated in time with the appearance of phagocytes and newly formed capillaries [Hurme and Kalimo, 1992]. Similarly, DNA synthesis by the satellite cells is observed within the first day following crush injuries [Bischoff, 1986] and exercise-induced injuries [Darr and Schultz, 1987] in rats. These observations are consistent with the hypothesis that the factors that activate satellite cells may be endogenous to the injured tissue itself or synthesized and secreted by platelets at the wound site, infiltrating neutrophils, and macrophages [reviewed in Husmann et al., 1996]. The primary candidates for the factors that activate and regulate satellite cell function include the fibroblast growth factors (FGFs), platelet-derived growth factor (PDGF), transforming growth factor beta (TGF-β), and insulin-like growth factors I and II (IGF-I, II).

The effects of these factors on muscle satellite cell proliferation and differentiation have been studied extensively in cell culture [reviewed in Florini and Magri, 1989]. FGF is a powerful mitogen for myogenic cells from adult rat skeletal muscle, but a potent inhibitor of terminal differentiation, i.e., myoblast fusion and expression of the skeletal muscle phenotype. PDGF also shows a strong stimulating effect on proliferation and inhibitory effect on differentiation of satellite cells [Jin et al., 1990]. Similarly, the presence of TGF-β prevents myotube formation as well as muscle-specific protein synthesis by rat embryo myoblasts and by adult rat satellite cells. In contrast to the previously mentioned growth factors, all of which inhibit myoblast differention, IGFs stimulate both proliferation and differentiation of myogenic cells [Ewton and Florini, 1980]. Despite our extensive knowledge of the actions of many individual growth factors *in vitro* and *in vivo*, the interactions between different growth factors have been less thoroughly investigated [Rosenthal et al., 1991]. A better understanding of the interactions between growth factors and the mechanisms that guide satellite cells through the regeneration process is necessary.

Myogenic Regulatory Factors

The conversion of pluripotent embryonic stem cells to differentiated muscle cells involves the commitment of these cells to the myogenic lineage and the subsequent proliferation, differentiation, and fusion to form multinucleated myotubes and ultimately mature muscle cells. New muscle cell formation from muscle satellite cells resembles embryonic development in the sense that in regenerating muscle cells embryonic isoforms of the muscle proteins are expressed [Whalen et al., 1985]. The conversion of stem cells to mature fibers, in both developing muscle and regenerating muscle, is directed by a group of related regulatory factors. These so-called muscle regulatory factors (MRFs) are part of a superfamily of basic helix-loop-helix DNA binding proteins that interact to regulate the transcription of skeletal muscle genes [reviewed in Weintraub et al., 1991]. MyoD was the first MRF identified followed by three other related genes including myogenin, MRF4 (also called herculin or Myf-6), and Myf-5 [Weintraub et al., 1991].

The observations that each of the MRFs has the ability to independently convert cultured fibroblasts into myogenic cells led to the original conclusion that functionally the MRFs were largely redundant. Subsequent gene targeting experiments, in which null mutations were introduced in each of the MRF genes, support separate and distinct roles in myogenesis for each MRFs [reviewed in Rudnicki and Jaenisch, 1995]. For example, mice that lack either Myf-5 or MyoD apparently have normal skeletal muscle but deletion of both genes results in the complete absence of skeletal myoblasts [Rudnicki et al., 1992; 1993; Braun et al., 1992]. While these observations suggest that Myf-5 and MyoD do have overlapping functions, characterization of the temporal-spatial patterns of myogenesis in Myf-5- and MyoD-deficient mouse embryos support the hypothesis that during normal development Myf-5 and MyoD primarily regulate epaxial (paraspinal and intercostal) and hypaxial (limb and abdominal wall) muscle development, respectively [Kablar et al., 1997]. In mice lacking myogenin, the number of myoblasts is not different from that of control mice, but skeletal muscles in myogenin-deficient mice display a marked reduction in the number of mature muscle fibers [Hasty et al., 1993; Nabeshima et al., 1993].

In summary, the MRF family can be divided into two functional groups. MyoD and Myf-5 are referred to as primary factors and are required for the determination of skeletal myoblasts whereas myogenin and MRF4 are secondary factors that act later and are necessary for differentiation of myoblasts into myotubes. How the MRFs control the series of events required for myoblast determination and differentiation are important questions for the future. In addition, the roles played by this family of proteins in regeneration, adaptation, and changes in skeletal muscle with aging are areas of active investigation [Jacobs-El et al., 1995; Marsh et al., 1997; Megeney et al., 1996].

22.5 Reconstructive Surgery of Whole Skeletal Muscles

When an injury or impairment is so severe that the total replacement of the muscle is required, a whole donor muscle must be transposed or transplanted into the recipient site [Faulkner et al., 1994a]. One of the most versatile muscles for transpositions is the latissimus dorsi (LTD) muscle. LTD transfers have been used in breast reconstruction [Moelleken et al., 1989], to restore elbow flexion, and to function as a heart assist pump [Carpentier and Chachques, 1985]. Thompson [1974] popularized the use of small free standard grafts to treat patients with partial facial paralysis. The transplantation of large skeletal muscles in dogs with immediate restoration of blood flow through the anastomosis of the artery and vein provided an operative technique with numerous applications [Tamai et al., 1970]. Coupled with cross-face nerve grafts, large skeletal muscles are transplanted with microneurovascular repair to correct deficits in the face [Harii et al., 1976] and adapted for reconstructive operations to treat impairments in function of the limbs, anal and urinary sphincters, and even the heart [Freilinger and Deutinger, 1992].

Transposition and transplantation of muscles invariably results in structural and functional deficits [Guelinckx et al., 1992]. The deficits are of the greatest magnitude during the first month and then a gradual recovery results in the stabilization of structural and functional variables between 90 and 120 days [Guelinckx et al., 1992]. In stabilized vascularized grafts ranging from 1 to 3 g in rats to 90 g in dogs, the major deficits are a ~30% decrease in muscle mass and in most grafts a ~40% decrease in maximum force [Faulkner et al., 1994a]. The decrease in power is more complex since it depends on both the average shortening force and the velocity of shortening. As a consequence, the deficit in maximum power may be either greater or less than the deficit in maximum force [Kadhiresan et al., 1993]. Tenotomy and repair are major factors responsible for the deficits [Guelinckx et al., 1988]. When a muscle is transplanted to act synergistically with other muscles, the action of the synergistic muscles may contribute to the deficits observed [Miller et al., 1994]. Although the data are limited, skeletal muscle grafts appear to respond to training stimuli in a manner not different from that of control muscles [Faulkner et al., 1994a]. The training stimuli include traditional methods of endurance and strength training [Faulkner et al., 1994b], as well as chronic electrical stimulation [Pette and Vrbova, 1992]. In spite of the deficits, transposed and transplanted muscles develop sufficient force and power to function effectively to maintain posture and patent sphincters and to move limbs or drive assist devices in parallel or in series with the heart [Faulkner et al., 1994a].

22.6   Myoblast Transfer and Gene Therapy

Myoblast transfer and gene therapy are aimed at delivering exogenous genetic constructs to skeletal muscle cells. The implications of myoblast and gene therapy hold great promise for skeletal muscle research and for those afflicted with inherited myopathies such as Duchenne and Becker muscular dystrophy (DMD and BMD). Myoblast transfer is a cell-mediated technique designed to treat inherited myopathies by intramuscular injection of myoblasts containing a normal functional genome. The goal is to correct for a defective or missing gene in the myopathic tissue through the fusion of normal myoblasts with growing or regenerating diseased cells. Gene therapy presents a more complex and flexible approach, whereby genetically engineered DNA constructs are delivered to a host cell to specifically direct production of a desired protein. By re-engineering the coding sequence of the gene and its regulatory regions, the function, the quantity of expression, and the protein itself can be altered. For many years, cells have been genetically altered to induce the production of a variety of useful proteins, such as human growth hormone and interferon.

As a focus in skeletal muscle tissue engineering, DMD is an X-linked recessive disorder characterized by progressive muscle degeneration resulting in debilitating muscle weakness and death in the second or third decade of life as a result of respiratory failure [Emery, 1988]. DMD and the milder BMD are due to genetic defects that lead to the absence or marked deficiency in the expression or functional stability of the protein dystrophin [Bonilla et al., 1988; Hoffman et al., 1988]. Similarly, a mutation in the dystrophin gene leads to the complete absence of the protein in muscle and brain tissues of the *mdx* mouse [Bulfield et al., 1984; Sicinski et al., 1989]. The homology of the genetic defects in DMD patients and *mdx* mice support the use of *mdx* mice as a model of dystrophin deficiency to explore the processes of the dystrophic disease and test proposed therapies or cures.

Myoblast Transfer Therapy

The concept of myoblast transfer is based on the role satellite cells play in muscle fiber growth and repair [Carlson and Faulkner, 1983]. As a therapy for DMD, the idea is to obtain satellite cells containing a functional dystrophin gene from a healthy compatible donor, have the cells multiply in culture, and then inject the "normal" myoblasts into the muscles of the patient. The objective is for the injected myoblasts to fuse with growing or regenerating muscle fibers to form a mosaic fiber in which the cytoplasm will contain normal myoblast nuclei capable of producing a functional form of dystrophin.

Experiments involving *mdx* mice have had varying success. Several investigators have reported that implantation of healthy myoblasts into muscles of *mdx* mice led to the production of considerable quantities of dystrophin [Morgan et al., 1990; Partridge et al., 1989]. Others found that myoblasts injected into limb muscles of *mdx* and control host mice showed a "rapid and massive" die off shortly after injection [Fan et al., 1996] with large and permanent decreases in muscle mass and maximum force [Wernig et al., 1995]. The successful transfer and fusion of donor myoblasts may be enhanced by x-ray irradiation of *mdx* muscles prior to myoblast injection to prevent the proliferation of myoblasts endogenous to the host and encourage the growth of donor myoblasts [Morgan et al., 1990].

In contrast to the studies with mice, delivery of myoblasts to DMD patients has shown very low levels of fusion efficiency, transient expression of dystrophin, and immune rejection [Gussoni et al., 1992; Karpati et al., 1993; Mendell et al., 1995; Morgan, 1994]. The use of X-ray irradiation in an attempt to enhance transfer efficiency is not applicable to DMD boys due to substantial health risks. Furthermore, immunosuppression may be necessary to circumvent immune rejection, which carries risks of its own. A better understanding of the factors that govern the survival, fusion, and expression of donor myoblasts is required before the viability of myoblast transfer as a treatment of DMD can be evaluated.

Gene Therapy

The aim of gene therapy for DMD is to transfer a functional dystrophin gene directly into the skeletal muscle. The challenge behind gene therapy is not only obtaining a functional genetic construct of the dystrophin gene and regulatory region but the effective delivery of the gene to the cell's genetic machinery. Methods to transfer genetic material into a muscle cell include direct injection and the use of retroviral and adenoviral vectors. Each of these strategies presents highly technical difficulties that to date remain unresolved.

Transgenic Mice

To explore the feasibility of gene therapy for DMD, Cox and colleagues [1993] examined the introduction of an exogenous dystrophin gene into the germ line of *mdx* mice to produce transgenic animals. The transgenic *mdx* mice expressed nearly 50 times the level of endogenous dystrophin found in muscles of control C57BL/10 mice and displayed the complete absence of any morphological, immunohistological, or functional symptoms of the murine muscular dystrophy with no deleterious side effects. Although transgenic technology does not provide an appropriate means for treating humans, these results demonstrated the efficacy of gene therapy to correct pathological genetic defects such as DMD.

Direct Intramuscular Injection

The straightforward gene delivery method of direct injection of plasmid DNA into skeletal and heart muscles [Lin et al., 1990; Wolff et al., 1990] has been proposed as a treatment for DMD and BMD. The idea is that dystrophic cells will incorporate the genetic constructs, whereby the genes will use the cell's internal machinery to produce the protein dystrophin. The advantages of direct injection of DNA as a gene delivery system are its simplicity, and it presents no chance of viral infection or the potential of cancer development that can occur with viral vectors [Morgan, 1994]. Although this approach is appealing in principle, direct intramuscular injection of human dystrophin plasmid DNA into the quadriceps muscles of *mdx* mice led to the expression of human dystrophin in only 1% to 3% of the muscle fibers [Acsadi et al., 1991]. In order for this method to be clinically effective, a much larger number of transfected myofibers must be achieved.

Retrovirus-Mediated Gene Transfer

Retroviruses reverse the normal process by which DNA is transcribed into RNA. A single-stranded viral RNA genome enters a host cell and a double helix comprised of two DNA copies of the viral RNA is created by the enzyme reverse transcriptase. Catalyzed by a viral enzyme, the DNA copy then integrates into a host cell chromosome where transcription, via the host cell RNA polymerase, produces large quantities of viral RNA molecules identical to the infecting genome [Alberts et al., 1989]. Eventually, new viruses emerge and bud from the plasma membrane ready to infect other cells. Consequently, retroviral vectors used for gene therapy are, by design, rendered replication defective. Once they infect the cell and integrate into the genome, they cannot make functional retroviruses to infect other cells. After the infective process is completed, cells are permanently altered with the presence of the viral DNA that causes the synthesis of proteins not originally endogenous to the host cell.

A primary obstacle to the efficiency of a retroviral gene delivery system is its dependence on host cell division. The requirement that a cell must be mitotically active for the virus to be incorporated into the host cell genetic machinery [Morgan, 1994] presents a problem for skeletal muscle tissue engineering since skeletal muscle is in a post-mitotic state. Nonetheless, as described above, recovery from injury in skeletal muscle involves the proliferation of myogenic precursor cells and either the incorporation of these cells into existing muscle fibers or the fusion of these cells with each other to form new fibers. Furthermore, since degeneration and regeneration of muscle cells are ongoing in DMD patients, viral transfection of myoblasts may be an effective route for gene delivery to skeletal muscle for treatment of DMD.

Another limitation of the retroviral gene delivery system is the small carrying capacity of the retroviruses of approximately 7 kilobases. This size limitation precludes the delivery of a full-length dystrophin construct of 12 to 14 kilobases [Dunckley et al., 1993; Morgan, 1994]. A 6.3 kilobase dystrophin construct, containing a large in-frame deletion resulting in the absence of ~40% of the central domain of the protein, has received a great deal of attention since its discovery in a BMD patient expressing a very mild phenotype. A single injection of retrovirus containing the Becker dystrophin minigene into the quadriceps or tibialis anterior muscle of *mdx* mice led to the sarcolemmal expression of dystrophin in an average of 6% of the myofibers [Dunckley et al., 1993]. Restoration of the 43-kDa dystrophin-associated glycoprotein was also observed and expression of the recombinant dystrophin was maintained for up to 9 months. Transduction of the minigene was significantly enhanced when muscles were pretreated with an intramuscular injection of the myotoxic agent bupivacaine to experimentally induce muscle regeneration.

Adenovirus-Mediated Gene Transfer

Adenoviruses have many characteristics that make the adenovirus-mediated gene transfer the most promising technology for gene therapy of skeletal muscle. The primary advantages are the stability of the viruses allowing them to be prepared in large amounts and the ability of adenoviral vectors to infect nondividing or slowly proliferating cells. In addition, adenoviral vectors have the potential to be used for systemic delivery of exogenous DNA. Through the use of tissue-specific promoters, specific tissues such as skeletal muscle may be targeted for transfection via intravenous injection.

Initial studies using adenoviral vectors containing the Becker dystrophin minigene driven by the Rous Sarcoma Virus promoter demonstrated that after a single intramuscular injection in newborn *mdx* mice, 50% of muscle fibers contained dystrophin [Ragot et al., 1993]. The truncated dystrophin was correctly localized to the sarcolemmal membrane and appeared to protect myofibers from the degeneration process characteristic of *mdx* muscles [Vincent et al., 1993]. Six months after a single injection, expression of the minigene was still observed in the treated muscle. More recently, these same investigators demonstrated that the injection of the adenoviral vector containing the dystrophin minigene into limb muscles of newborn *mdx* mice provided protection from the fiber damage and force deficit associated with a protocol of pliometric contractions that was administered at 4 months of age [Deconinck et al., 1996].

Despite the promise of adenovirus-mediated gene therapy, a number of limitations to its usefulness remain to be resolved. One major drawback of the system is the relatively brief duration of transgene expression observed following injection of adenoviral vectors into adult immunocompetent animals [Kass-Eisler et al., 1994]. The lack of long-term exogenous gene expression is likely the result of low level expression of endogenous viral proteins triggering an inflammatory response that attacks infected cells [Yang et al., 1994]. In addition to the difficulties resulting from the potent immune response triggered by adenovirus, direct cytotoxic effects of adenovirus injection on skeletal muscle have been reported [Petrof et al., 1995]. Current generation adenoviruses are also limited by their relatively small cloning capacity of ~8 kilobases. The development of adenoviral vectors with increased cloning capacity, the ability to evade host immune rejection, and no toxic effects are areas of active investigation [Kumar-Singh and Chamberlain, 1996; Petrof et al., 1996; Hauser et al., 1997].

Acknowledgments

The research in our laboratory and the preparation of this chapter was supported by grants from the United States Public Health Service, National Institute on Aging, AG-15434 (SVB) and AG-06157 (JAF), and the Nathan Shock Center for Basic Biology of Aging at the University of Michigan.

References

Acsadi, G., Dickson, G., Love, D.R., Jani, A., Walsh, F.S., Gurusinghe, A., Wolff, J.A., and Davies, K.E. 1991. Human dystrophin expression in *mdx* mice after intramuscular injection of DNA constructs. *Nature* 352:815-818.

Alberts, B., Bray, D., Lewis, J., Raff, M., Roberts, K., and Watson, J.D. 1989. *Molecular Biology of the Cell,* 2nd ed. Garland Publishing, New York, p. 254.

Bischoff, R. 1986. A satellite cell mitogen from crushed adult muscle. *Dev. Biol.* 115:140-147.

Bonilla, E., Samitt, C.E., Miranda, A.F., Hays, A.P., Salviati, G., DiMauro, S., Kunkel, L.M., Hoffman, E.P., and Rowland, L.P. 1988. Duchenne muscular dystrophy: deficiency of dystrophin at the muscle cell surface. *Cell* 54:447-452.

Braun, T., Rudnicki, M.A., Arnold, H.H., and Jaenisch, R. 1992. Targeted inactivation of the muscle regulatory gene Myf-5 results in abnormal rib development and perinatal death. *Cell* 71:369-382.

Bulfield, G., Siller, W.G., Wight, P.A.L., and Moore, K.J. 1984. X chromosome-linked muscular dystrophy (*mdx*) in the mouse. *Proc. Natl. Acad. Sci. U.S.A.* 81:1189-1192.

Burke, R.E., Levin, D.N., Tsairis, P. and Zajac, F.E., III. 1973. Physiological types and histochemical profiles in motor units of the cat gastrocnemius muscle. *J. Physiol. (Lond.)* 234:723-748.

Carlson, B.M. and Faulkner, J.A. 1983. The regeneration of skeletal muscle fibers following injury: a review. *Med. Sci. Sports Exer.* 15:187-198.

Carpentier, A. and Chachques, J.C. 1985. Myocardial substitution with a stimulated skeletal muscle: first successful clinical case. *Lancet* 1(8440):1267.

Cox, G.A., Cole, N.M., Matsumura, K., Phelps, S.F., Hauschka, S.D., Campbell, K.P., Faulkner, J.A., and Chamberlain, J.S. 1993. Overexpression of dystrophin in transgenic *mdx* mice eliminates dystrophic symptoms without toxicity. *Nature* 364:725-729.

Darr, K.C. and Schultz, E. 1987. Exercise-induced satellite cell activation in growing and mature skeletal muscle. *J. Appl. Physiol.* 63:1816-1821.

Deconinck, N., Ragot, T., Maréchal, G., Perricaudet, M., and Gillis, J.M. 1996. Functional protection of dystrophic mouse (*mdx*) muscles after adenovirus-mediated transfer of a dystrophin minigene. *Proc. Natl. Acad. Sci. U.S.A.* 93:3570-3574.

Dunckley, M.G., Wells, D.J., Walsh, F.S., and Dickson, G. 1993. Direct retroviral-mediated transfer of a dystrophin minigene into *mdx* mouse muscle *in vivo. Hum. Mol. Genet.* 2:717-723.

Emery, A.E.H. 1988. *Duchenne Muscular Dystrophy,* 2nd ed. Oxford University Press, New York.

Ewton, D.A. and Florini, J.R. 1980. Relative effects of the somatomedins, multiplication-stimulating activity, and growth hormone on myoblast and myotubes in culture. *Endocrinology* 106:577-583.

Fan, Y., Maley, M., Beilharz, M., and Grounds, M. 1996. Rapid death of injected myoblasts in myoblast transfer therapy. *Muscle Nerve* 19:853-860.

Faulkner, J.A., Carlson, B.M., and Kadhiresan, V.A. 1994a. Whole muscle transplantation: mechanisms responsible for functional deficits. *Biotech. Bioeng.* 43:757-763.

Faulkner, J.A., Green, H.J., and White, T.P. 1994b. Response and adaptation of skeletal muscle to changes in physical activity. In *Physical Activity Fitness and Health*, eds. C. Bouchard, R.J. Shephard, and T. Stephens, pp. 343-357. Human Kinetics Publishers, Champaign, IL.

Ferrari, G., Cusella-De Angelis, G., Coletta, M., Paolucci, E., Stornaiuolo, A., Cossu, G., and Mavilio, F. 1998. Muscle regeneration by bone marrow-derived myogenic progenitors. *Science* 279:1528-1530.

Florini, J.R. and Magri, K.A. 1989. Effects of growth factors on myogenic differentiation. *Am. J. Physiol.* 256 (*Cell Physiol.* 25):C701-C711.

Freilinger, G. and Deutinger, M. 1992. *Third Vienna Muscle Symposium*, Blackwell-MZV, Vienna, Austria.

Guelinckx, P.J., Faulkner, J.A., and Essig, D.A. 1988. Neurovascular-anastomosed muscle grafts in rabbits: functional deficits result from tendon repair. *Muscle Nerve* 11:745-751.

Guelinckx, P.J., Carlson, B.M., and Faulkner, J.A. 1992. Morphologic characteristics of muscles grafted in rabbits with neurovascular repair. *J. Recon. Microsurg.* 8:481-489.

Gussoni, E., Pavlath, G.K., Lancot, A.M., Sharma, K.R., Miller, R.G., Steinman, L., and Blau, H.M. 1992. Normal dystrophin transcrips detected in Duchenne muscular dystrophy patients after myoblast transplantation. *Nature* 356:435-438.

Harii, K., Ohmori, K., and Torii, S. 1976. Free gracilis muscle transplantation with microneurovascular anastomoses for the treatment of facial paralysis. *Plast. Recon. Surg.* 57:133-143.

Hasty, P., Bradley, A., Morris, J.H., Edmondson, J.M., Venuti, J.M., Olson, E.N., and Klein, W.H. 1993. Muscle deficiency and neonatal death in mice with a targeted mutation in the myogenin gene. *Nature* 364:501-506.

Hauser, M.A., Amalfitano, A., Kumar-Singh, R., Hauschka, S.D., and Chamberlain, J.S. 1997. Improved adenoviral vectors for gene therapy of Duchenne muscular dystrophy. *Neuromusc. Dis.* 7:277-283.

Henneman, E., Somjen, G., and Carpenter, D. 1965. Functional significance of cell size in spinal motor neurons. *J. Neurophysiol.* 28:560-580.

Hoffman, E.P., Fischbeck, R.H., Brown, R.H., Johnson, M., Medori, R., Loike, J.D., Harris, J.B., Waterson, R., Brooke, M., Specht, L., Kupsky, W., Chamberlain, J., Caskey, C.T., Shapiro, F., and Kunkel, L.M. 1988. Characterization of dystrophin in muscle-biopsy specimens from patients with Duchenne's or Becker's muscular dystrophy. *N. Engl. J. Med.* 318:1363-1368.

Hurme, T. and Kalimo, H. 1992. Activation of myogenic precursor cells after muscle injury. *Med. Sci. Sports Exer.* 24:197-205.

Husmann, I., Soulet, L., Gautron, J., Martelly, I., and Barritault, D. 1996. Growth factors in skeletal muscle regeneration. *Cytokine Growth Factor Rev.* 7:249-258.

Jacobs-El, J., Zhou, M.Y., and Russell, B. 1995. MRF4, Myf-5, and myogenin mRNAs in the adaptive responses of mature rat muscle. *Am. J. Physiol.* 268:C1045-C1052.

Jin, P., Rahm, M., Claesson-Wesh, L., Heldin, C.-H., and Sejerson, T. 1990. Expression of PDGF A chain and β-receptor genes during rat myoblast differentiation. *J. Cell Biol.* 110:1665-1672.

Jones, D.A., Jackson, M.J., McPhail, G., and Edwards, R.H.T. 1984. Experimental mouse muscle damage: the importance of external calcium. *Clin. Sci.* 66:317-322.

Kablar, B., Krastel, K., Ying, C., Asakura, A., Tapscott, S.J., and Rudnicki, M.A. 1997. MyoD and Myf-5 differentially regulate the development of limb versus trunk skeletal muscle. *Development* 124:4729-4738.

Kadhiresan, V.A., Guelinckx, P.J., and Faulkner, J.A. 1993. Tenotomy and repair of latissimus dorsi muscles in rats: implications for transposed muscle grafts. *J. Appl. Physiol.* 75:1294-1299.

Karpati, G., Ajdukovic, D., Arnold, D., Gledhill, R.B., Guttmann, R., Holland, P., Koch, P.A., Shoubridge, E., Spence, D., Vanasse, M., Watters, G.V., Abrahamowicz, M., Duff, C., and Worton, R.G. 1993. Myoblast transfer in Duchenne muscular dystrophy. *Ann. Neurol.* 34:8-17.

Kass-Eisler, A., Falck-Pedersen, E., Elfenbein, D.H., Alvira, M., Buttrick, P.M., and Leinwand, L.A. 1994. The impact of developmental stage, route of administration and the immune system on adenovirus-mediated gene transfer. *Gene Ther.* 1:395-402.

Kumar-Singh, R. and Chamberlain, J.S. 1996. Encapsidated adenovirus minichromosomes allow delivery and expression of a 14 kb dystrophin cDNA to muscle cells. *Hum. Mol. Genet.* 5:913-921.

Lin, H., Parmacek, M.S., Morle, G., Bolling, S., and Leiden, J.M. 1990. Expression of recombinant genes in myocardium *in vivo* after direct injection of DNA. *Circulation* 82:2217-2221.

Macpherson, P.C.D., Dennis, R.G., and Faulkner, J.A. 1997. Sarcomere dynamics and contraction-induced injury to maximally activated single muscle fibres from soleus muscles of rats. *J. Physiol. (Lond.)* 500:523-533.

Marsh, D.R., Criswell, D.S., Carson, J.A., and Booth, F.W. 1997. Myogenic regulatory factors during regeneration of skeletal muscle in young, adult, and old rats. *J. Appl. Physiol.* 83:1270-1275.

McCully, K.K. and Faulkner, J.A. 1985. Injury to skeletal muscle fibers of mice following lengthening contractions. *J. Appl. Physiol.* 59:119-126.

McNeil, P.L. and Khakee, R. 1992. Disruptions of muscle fiber plasma membranes. Role in exercise-induced damage. *Am. J. Pathol.* 140:1097-1109.

Megeney, L.A., Kablar, B., Garrett, K., Anderson, J.E., and Rudnicki, M.A. 1996. MyoD is required for myogenic stem cell function in adult skeletal muscle. *Genes Dev.* 10:1173-1183.

Mendell, J.R., Kissel, J.T., Amato, A.A., King, W., Signore, L., Prior, T.W., Sahenk, Z., Benson, S., McAndrew, P.E., Rice, R., Nagaraja, H., Stephens, R., Lantry L., Morris, G.E., and Burghes A.H.M. 1995. Myoblast transfer in the treatment of Duchenne's muscular dystrophy. *N. Engl. J. Med.* 333:832-838.

Miller, S.W., Hassett, C.A., White, T.P., and Faulkner, J.A. 1994. Recovery of medial gastrocnemius muscle grafts in rats: implications for the plantarflexor group. *J. Appl. Physiol.* 77:2773-2777.

Moelleken, B.R.W., Mathes, S.A., and Chang, N. 1989. Latissimus dorsi muscle-musculocutaneous flap in chest-wall reconstruction. *Surg. Clinics of North Am.* 69(5):977-990.

Morgan, J.E. 1994. Cell and gene therapy in Duchenne muscular dystrophy. *Hum. Gene Ther.* 5:165-173.

Morgan, J.E., Hoffman, E.P., and Partridge, T.A. 1990. Normal myogenic cells from newborn mice restore normal histology to degenerating muscles of the *mdx* mouse. *J. Cell. Biol.* 111:2437-2449.

Moss, F.P. and Leblond, C.P. 1971. Satellite cells as the source of nuclei in muscles of growing rats. *Anat. Rec.* 170:421-436.

Nabeshima, Y., Hanaoka, K., Hayasaka, M., Esumi E., Li, S., Nonaka, I., and Nabeshima, Y. 1993. Myogenin gene disruption results in perinatal lethality because of a severe muscle defect. *Nature* 364:532-535.

Newham, D.J., McPhail, G., Jones, D.A., and Edwards, R.H.T. 1983. Large delayed plasma creatine kinase changes after stepping exercise. *Muscle Nerve* 6:380-385.

Partridge, T.A., Morgan, J.E., Coulton, G.R., Hoffman, E.P., and Kunkel, L.M. 1989. Conversion of *mdx* myofibers from dystrophin-negative to -positive by injection of normal myoblasts. *Nature* 337:176-179.

Petrof, B.J., Acsadi, G., Jani, A., Bourdon, J., Matusiewicz, N., Yang, L., Lochmüller, H., and Karpati, G. 1995. Efficiency and functional consequences of adenovirus-mediated *in vivo* gene transfer to normal and dystrophic (*mdx*) mouse diaphragm. *Am. J. Respir. Cell Mol. Biol.* 13:508-517.

Petrof, B.J., Lochmüller, H., Massie, B., Yang, L., Macmillan, C., Zhao, J.-E., Nalbantoglu, J., and Karpati, G. 1996. Impairment of force generation after adenovirus-mediated gene transfer to muscle is alleviated by adenoviral gene inactivation and host $CD8^+$ T cell deficiency. *Hum. Gene Ther.* 7:1813-1826.

Pette, D. and Vrbova, G. 1992. Adaptation of mammalian skeletal muscle fibers to chronic electrical stimulation. *Rev. Physiol. Biochem. Pharmcol.*, 120:115-202.

Ragot, T., Vincent, N., Chafey, P., Vigne, E., Gilgenkrantz, H., Couton, D., Cartaud, J., Briand, P., Kaplan, J., Perricaudet, M., and Kahn, A. 1993. Efficient adenovirus-mediated transfer of a human minidystrophin gene to skeletal muscle of *mdx* mice. *Nature* 361:647-650.

Rosenthal, S.M., Brown, E.J., Brunetti, A., and Goldfine, J.D. 1991. Fibroblast growth factor inhibits insulin-like growth factor-II (IGF-II) gene expression and increases IGF-I receptor abundance in BC3H-1 muscle cells. *Mol. Endocrinol.* 5:678-684.

Rudnicki, M.A., Braun, T., Hinuma, S., and Jaenisch, R. 1992. Inactivation of MyoD in mice leads to up-regulation of the myogenic HLH gene Myf-5 and results in apparently normal muscle development. *Cell* 71:383-390.

Rudnicki, M.A. and Jaenisch, R. 1995. The MyoD family of transcription factors and skeletal myogenesis. *BioEssays* 17:203-209.

Rudnicki, M.A., Schnegelsberg, P.N.J., Stead, R.H., Braun, T., Arnold, H.H., and Jaenisch, R. 1993. MyoD or Myf-5 is required for the formation of skeletal muscle. *Cell* 75:1351-1359.

Russell, B., Dix, D.J., Haller, D.L., and Jacobs-El, J. 1992. Repair of injured skeletal muscle: a molecular approach. *Med. Sci. Sports Exer.* 24:189-196.

Sicinski, P., Geng, Y., Ryder-Cook, A.S., Barnard, E.A., Darlison, M.G., and Barnard, P.J. 1989. The molecular basis of muscular dystrophy in the *mdx* mouse: a point mutation. *Science* 244:1578-1580.

Tamai, S., Komatsu, S., Sakamoto, H., Sano, S., and Sasauchi, N. 1970. Free-muscle transplants in dogs with microsurgical neuro-vascular anastomoses. *Plast. Reconstr. Surg.* 46:219-225.

Thompson, N. 1974. A review of autogenous skeletal muscle grafts and their clinical applications. *Clin. Plast. Surg.* 1:349-403.

Vincent, N., Ragot, T., Gilgenkrantz, H., Couton, D., Chafey, P., Gregoire, A., Briand, P., Kaplan, J., Kahn, A., and Perricaudet, M. 1993. Long-term correction of mouse dystrophic degeneration by adenovirus-mediated transfer of a minidystrophin gene. *Nat. Genet.* 5:130-134.

Weintraub, H., Davis, R., Tapscott, S., Thayer, M., Krause, M., Benezra, R., Blackwell, T.K., Turner, D., Rupp, R., Hollenberg, S., Zhuang, Y., and Lassar, A. 1991. The *myoD* gene family: nodal point during specification of the muscle cell lineage. *Science* 251:761-766.

Wernig, A., Irintchev, A., and Lange, G. 1995. Functional effects of myoblast implantation into histoin-compatible mice with or without immunosuppression. *J. Physiol. (Lond.)* 484:493-504.

Whalen, R.G., Butler-Browne, G.S., Bugaisky, L.B., Harris, J.B., and Herliocoviez, D. 1985. Myosin isozyme transitions in developing and regenerating rat muscle. *Adv. Exp. Med. Biol.* 182:249-257.

Wolff, J.A., Malone, R.W., Williams, P., Chong, W., Acsadi, G., Jani, A., and Felgner, P.L. 1990. Direct gene transfer into mouse muscle *in vivo*. *Science* 247:1465-1468.

Yang, Y., Nunes, F.A., Berencsi, K., Gönczöl, E., Englelhardt, J.F., and Wilson, J.M. 1994. Inactivation of *E2a* in recombinant adenoviruses improves the prospect for gene therapy in cystic fibrosis. *Nat. Genet.* 7:362-369.

23

Tissue Engineering of Cartilage

L.E. Freed
Harvard University

G. Vunjak-Novakovic
Massachusetts Institute of Technology

23.1 Scope

This chapter reviews the current state of the art of articular cartilage tissue engineering, and focuses on a cell-polymer-bioreactor model system which can be used for controlled studies of chondrogenesis and the modulation of engineered cartilage by environmenal factors.

23.2 Cell-Based Approaches to Cartilage Tissue Engineering

Articular cartilage is an avascular tissue that contains only one cell type (the chondrocyte), and has a very limited capacity for self-repair. The chondrocytes are responsible for the synthesis and maintenance of their extracellular matrix (ECM), which is composed of a hydrated collagen network (~60% of the tissue dry weight, dw), a highly charged proteoglycan gel (PG, ~25% dw), and other proteins and glycoproteins (~15% dw).[1] Its high water content (70 to 80% of the tissue wet weight, ww) enables cartilage to withstand the compressive, tensile, and shear forces associated with joint loading. None of the methods conventionally used for cartilage repair (e.g., tissue auto- or allografts) can predictably restore a durable articular surface to an osteoarthrotic joint.[2] Cell-based therapies, i.e., implantation of cells or engineered cartilage, represent an alternative approach to articular cartilage repair.

Figure 23.1 shows the cell-polymer-bioreactor system for cartilage tissue engineering. Constructs based on chondrogenic cells and polymer scaffolds are cultured in bioreactors to form three-dimensional (3D) cartilaginous tissues. Engineered cartilage can be used either *in vivo*, to study articular cartilage repair, or *in vitro*, for controlled studies of cell and tissue-level responses to molecular, mechanical, and genetic manipulations.

Table 23.1 lists selected, representative examples of recent articular cartilage tissue engineering studies in which the stated research goals were either *in vivo* cartilage repair or *in vitro* studies of chondrogenesis. Several key parameters varied from study to study: (i) cell source and expansion in culture, (ii) scaffold material and structure, (iii) *in vitro* cultivation (conditions and duration), (iv) additional components (e.g., perichondrium), (v) experimental animal (species and age), (vi) surgical model (defect location

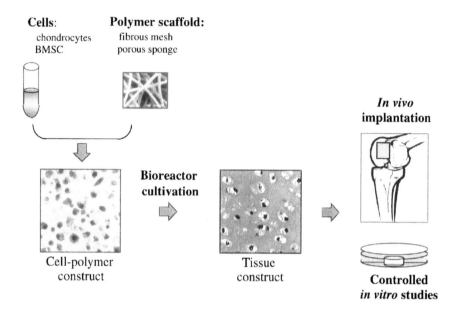

FIGURE 23.1 Cell-based approach to articular cartilage repair. Isolated cells, e.g., chondrocytes or bone marrow stromal cells (BMSC) are seeded onto three-dimensional scaffolds, e.g., polymers formed as fibrous meshes or porous sponges, to form cell-polymer constructs. Constructs are first cultured *in vitro*, e.g., in bioreactors, and then used either as implants or for *in vitro* research.

and dimensions), (vii) graft type (autograft or allograft), (viii) duration of *in vivo* implantation, and (viii) methods used to assess the resulting tissue (e.g., histological, biochemical, and/or mechanical).

In Vivo Cartilage Repair

Brittberg et al.[3] reported a new cell-based procedure for the repair of human knee injuries that could potentially eliminate the need for more than half a million arthroplastic procedures and joint replacements performed annually in the United States. Autologous articular cartilage was harvested from a minor load-bearing area on the distal femur, and component cells were isolated, expanded *in vitro*, and reimplanted back into the patient. In particular, after excising the damaged cartilage down to the subchondral bone, defects (1.65 to 6.5 cm²) were sutured closed with a periosteal flap creating a pocket into which the cultured cells were injected. Disabling symptoms (e.g., knee pain, swelling, locking) were markedly reduced over a follow-up period of up to 5 years. Femoral transplants were clinically graded as good or excellent in 88% of the cases, with 73% of the biopsy specimens resembling hyaline cartilage. In contrast, patellar transplants were graded as good or excellent in only 29% of the cases, with only 14% of the biopsies resembling hyaline cartilage. A therapy based on this technique was approved for clinical use by the Food and Drug Administration (FDA) in August, 1997 and is being marketed under the tradename Carticel®.[4] However, the original clinical study report has been criticized for not being a prospective controlled, randomized study and for its lack of a standard outcome analysis (i.e., for subjective evaluation with little quantitative biochemical or mechanical data).[5,6]

The Carticel® technique was also assessed in rabbits and dogs. In one study, cultured autologous chondrocytes were transplanted into patellar defects in conjunction with periosteal flaps and in some cases carbon fiber pads.[7] The repair tissue was characterized as hyaline-like and reported to develop *in vivo*, as assessed by an increasing degree of cellular columnarization. Histological scores were highest in defects treated with transplanted chondrocytes and periosteum, as compared to the combination of chondrocytes, carbon fibers, and periosteum or periosteum only. The finding that the use of carbon fibers did not improve long-term repair was attributed to scaffold-induced diffusional limitations.

Table 23.1 Representative Studies of Articular Cartilage Tissue Engineering

Cells (source, expansion) and other components	Scaffold		In Vitro Culture		Animal Model			Assessment	Results	Ref.
	Material	Dimensions	Conditions	Duration	Species, Age	Implant Site, Defect Size	Graft Type, Duration			
1 *In vivo* cartilage repair										
Articular chondrocyte (human, expanded 2-3 wks)	None				Human 14-48 yr old	Distal femur, patella 1.6-6.5 cm², full thickness	Autograft 16-66 mo	Arthroscopy clinical signs	Symptomatic relief Femur repair better than patella	[3]
Articular chondrocyte (rabbit, expanded 2 wks) and periosteum	None or carbon fibers		Static dish	Several hours	Rabbit 4 mo old	Patella 3 mm dia, full thickness	Autograft 2-12 mo	H (semiquantitative)	Cells plus periosteum better than cells on carbon meshes	[7]
Articular chondrocyte (dog, expanded 3 wks) and periosteum	None				Dog 2 yr-adult	Distal femur, 4 mm dia, full thickness	Autograft 1.5-18 mo	H (semiquantitative) IH (collagen types I, II)	Fibroblastic and chondrocytic cells, collagen II early repair better than late repair	[8, 9]
Precursor cells from bone marrow and periosteum; chondrocytes (rabbit, expanded); glue	None or collagen gel				Rabbit 3 mo-adult	Distal femur up to 3×6× 3 mm ± protease treatment	Autograft precursor cells Allograft chondrocytes 1 wk-1 yr	H (semiquantitative); TEM mechanics (microindentation)	Hyaline cartilage (surface), new bone (deep) Precursor cells better than chondrocytes Bone marrow better than periosteum Integration improved by protease treatment	[10, 11]
Precursor cells from bone marrow (goat, expanded)	Hyaluronic acid gel				Goat adult	Distal femur 4 mm dia, full thickness	Auto- and allografts 3 mo	H (quantitative) IH (collagen type II, KS, PG)	Autograft better than allograft	[13]
Precursor cells from bone marrow (embryonic and adult chick); chondrocytes (chick, expanded)	Hyaluronic acid gel				Chick 3 yr old	Proximal tibia 3 mm dia × 2 mm deep	Auto- and allografts 3 mo	H (semiquantitative) IH (collagen types I, II)	Autograft better than allograft Embryonic cells better than adult	[14]
Perichondral chondrocyte (rabbit, expanded 3 wks)	Poly(D,D,L,L) lactic acid	3.7 mm dia × 10 mm thick	Mixed vial	2 h	Rabbit 9-12 mo old	Distal femur 3.7 mm dia, 5 mm deep	Allograft 6 wks- 12 mo	H; amounts of GAG and collagen; IH (collagen types I, II); Confined compression modulus	Cell alignment determined by scaffold geometry Hyaline cartilage: collagen mainly type II GAG subnormal, mechanical properties normal	[15, 16]

Table 23.1 (continued) Representative Studies of Articular Cartilage Tissue Engineering

Cells (source, expansion, and other components)	Scaffold		In Vitro Culture		Animal Model			Assessment	Results	Ref.
	Material	Dimensions	Conditions	Duration	Species, Age	Implant Site, Defect Size	Graft Type, Duration			
Articular chondrocyte (3 wk old rats)	Collagen gel		Static dish	2 wks	Rat 8-9 wks old	Distal femur 1.5 mm dia × 1.5 mm deep	Auto- and allografts 2 wks– 12 mo	H (semiquantitative)	Slight inflammation that resolved by 8 wks 6-12 mo autografts and allografts comparable	[17]
Articular chondrocytes (2-8 mo old rabbits)	Fibrous PGA	10 mm dia × 2 mm thick	Static dish	3-4 wks	Rabbit 8 mo old	Distal femur 3 mm dia, full thickness	Allograft 1–6 mo	H (semiquantitative)	Fairly good repair at 6 mo	[18]
Muscle mesenchymal stem cell (expanded 3 wks)	Fibrous PGA	10 mm dia × 2 mm thick	Static dish	2.5 wks	Rabbit 8 mo old	Distal femur 3 mm dia, full thickness	Allograft 6 wks– 3 mo	H (qualitative)	Fairly good repair at 3 mo	[19]
Articular chondrocyte (1 mo old rabbits)	Collagen gel		Static dish	2 wks	Rabbit 6 mo old	Distal femur 4 mm dia × 4 mm deep	Allograft 1 day– 6 mo	H (semiquantitative)	Hyaline cartilage without endochondral ossification	[12]

2 *In vitro* chondrogenesis

Cells (source, expansion, and other components)	Material	Dimensions	Conditions	Duration	Species, Age	Implant Site, Defect Size	Graft Type, Duration	Assessment	Results	Ref.
Articular chondrocyte (bovine)	Agarose gel	16 mm dia × 1 mm thick	Static dish; compression chamber	10 wks 7 wks				H; SEM; GAG and DNA content Incorporation of ^{35}S and ^{3}H Mechanical properties	Development of mechanically functional matrix (25% of normal) after 7 wks Dynamic compression enhanced synthesis of GAG and collagen	[20, 21]
Articular chondrocyte (human, 5-42 yr old)	Alginate beads	Not reported	Static dish	30 days				H; TEM; IH (keratan sulfate) Amounts of DNA, aggrecan, GAG, Incorporation of ^{35}S and ^{3}H	Formation of cartilaginous matrix composed of two compartments with different rates of proteoglycan turnover	[23]
Articular chondrocyte (bovine)	Fibrous PGA; porous PLLA fibrous PGA	10 mm × (5-10) mm × (2-3) mm 10 mm dia × (1-5) mm thick	Static and mixed dishes Mixed dish	6-8 wks 6-8 wks				H; IH (type II collagen) amounts of GAG, DNA, collagen and undegraded PGA	PGA better than PLLA 1.2-3.5 mm thick cartilaginous constructs Mixing and high initial cellularity improved construct structures	[24, 25, 32, 34]
Articular chondrocyte (bovine; expanded up to P2)	Fibrous PGA and nylon; PLGA mesh porous collagen	2 mm thick	Perfused teflon bag Static dish	5 wks				H; GAG content incorporation of ^{35}S and ^{3}H	Scaffold materials affected GAG and collagen synthesis Perfused bag better than static dish	[26]

Cell type	Scaffold	Dimensions	Culture system	Duration	Analysis	Results	Ref.
Articular chondrocyte (human, 30-65 yr old)	PLGA and polydioxanon meshes coated with adhesion factors and agarose	Not reported	Perfused chamber	2 wks	H; TEM; IH (collagen types I and II)	Evidence of collagen fibrils and proteoglycan	[27]
Articular chondrocyte (rabbit)	Fibrous PGA	10 mm dia × 2 mm thick	Perfused cartridge (1.2 ml) Static dish	4 wks	H, IH (type II collagen, CS) amounts of GAG and collagen	2 mm thick constructs More tissue at edge than center	[28]
Articular chondrocyte (equine; young and adult)	Fibrous PGA	10 mm × 10 mm × 1 mm	Compression chamber (3.4 or 6.9 MPa; 5s on, 30s off)	5 wks	H; amounts of GAG and total collagen compressive stiffness	Cyclical loading promoted the production of GAG and collagen and increased compressive stiffness in constructs based on young cells	[29, 30]
Articular chondrocyte (human fetal)	None		Static dish	4 mo	H, TEM; IH (collagen types I, II, IX; CS, KS) amounts of GAG and total collagen	Fetal chondrocytes cultured without serum formed 1.5-2 mm thick layer of hyaline cartilage	[31]
Articular chondrocyte (bovine)	Fibrous PGA	10 mm dia × 5 mm thick	Static and mixed dishes Static and mixed flasks	8 wks	H; amounts of GAG, DNA, and total collagen	2.7-4.8 mm thick constructs Seeding and cultivation in mixed flasks yielded largest constructs and highest fractions of ECM	[33, 39]
Articular chondrocyte (bovine)	Fibrous PGA	5 mm × 5 mm × 2 mm 5 mm dia × 2 mm thick	Rotating vessel	1 wk–7 mo	H; TEM; IH (collagen types II, IX) amounts of DNA, GAG, and collagen Incorporation of ^{35}S and ^{3}H Mechanical properties	3-8 mm thick constructs After 6 wks ECM was continuously cartilaginous After 7 months, compressive stiffness became comparable to normal cartilage	[36, 37]
Articular chondrocyte (bovine)	Fibrous PGA	5 mm dia × 2 mm thick	Rotating vessel	6 wks	SEM; amounts of DNA, GAG and collagen (total and types II, IX and X); collagen pyridinium cross-links	Structure and composition of collagen network in 6 wk constructs comparable to native cartilage; collagen content and cross-linking subnormal	[38]

Table 23.1 (continued)   Representative Studies of Articular Cartilage Tissue Engineering

Cells (source, expansion) and other components	Scaffold		In Vitro Culture		Animal Model			Assessment	Results	Ref.
	Material	Dimensions	Conditions	Duration	Species, Age	Implant Site, Defect Size	Graft Type, Duration			
Articular chondrocyte (bovine)	Fibrous PGA	5 mm dia × 2 mm thick	Static and mixed flasks Rotating vessel	6 wks				H; amounts of DNA, GAG and collagen (total and type II); mechanical properties	Construct structure and function could be modulated by the conditions of flow and mixing. Mechanical parameters correlated with wet weight fractions of GAG, collagen and water	[39]
BMSC (chick embryo; bovine)	Fibrous PGA Porous PLGA	5 mm dia × 2 mm thick	Mixed dish	4 wks				H; IH (collagen types II and X) amounts of DNA, GAG and collagen	Selective cell expansion and the cultivation on 3-dimensional scaffolds resulted in the formation of cartilaginous tissues	[42–44]

* Review.

Note:
BMSC	bone marrow stromal cells
CS	chondroitin sulfate
ECM	extracellular matrix
GAG	glycosaminoglycan
H	histology
IH	immunohistochemistry
KS	keratan sulfate
PG	proteoglycan
PGA	polyglycolic acid
PLGA	polylactic–co–glycolic acid
PLLA	poly (L) lactic acid
SEM	scanning electron microscopy
TEM	transmission electron microscopy

In other studies, cultured autologous chondrocytes in conjunction with periosteal flaps were transplanted into femoral defects in dogs and compared to periosteal flaps alone and to untreated defects.[8,9] Three phases of healing were demonstrated: formation of repair tissue (at 1.5 months), remodeling (at 3 and 6 months), and degradation (at 12 and 18 months). Neither periosteum nor transplanted chondrocytes enhanced healing after 1 year, at which time hyaline-like repair tissue appeared to be displaced by fibrocartilage. The differences between results obtained in rabbit and dog studies were attributed to several variables including species, subject age, defect location, surgical technique, and postoperative animal activity. Low retention of implanted cells in the lesion and failure of immature repair tissue subjected to high mechanical forces were listed as possible causes of degradation.

The group of Caplan et al. pioneered the use of autologous mesenchymal stem cells in the repair of osteochondral defects.[10] Osteoprogenitor cells were selected from whole bone marrow based on their ability to adhere to Petri dishes and expanded in monolayer culture prior to implantation. Autologous precursor cells were delivered in collagen gels into defects that were in some cases pretreated with proteolytic enzymes. Other implants were based on either autologous precursor cells derived from periosteum or allogeneic chondrocytes derived from articular cartilage. The dimensions of defects were up to 3 mm wide, 6 mm long, and 3 mm deep, among the largest reported for repair studies in rabbits. Repair was assessed histologically and in some cases mechanically, e.g., relative compliance using a microindentation probe.[11]

Autologous precursor cells in collagen gels formed a cartilaginous surface zone while tissue at the base of the defect hypertrophied, calcified, and was replaced by host-derived vasculature, marrow, and bone.[10] It was postulated that the different biological milieus of the synovial fluid at the joint surface and the osseus recepticle in the underlying bone played key roles in architecturally appropriate precursor cell differentiation. Improved integration of the graft with the surrounding host tissue was reported following partial digestion at the defect site (e.g., with trypsin) prior to implantation; this finding was attributed to enhanced interdigitation of newly synthesized ECM molecules. However, progressive thinning of the cartilaginous surface zone was observed over 6 months, which was more pronounced with periosteally derived than with bone marrow-derived precursor cells. In contrast, allografted chondrocytes in collagen gels rapidly formed plugs of hyaline cartilage that filled the entire defect but failed to develop a region of subchondral bone at the base or to integrate with the surrounding host tissue even after 6 months. Similar results were obtained when chondrocytes were cultured *in vitro* in collagen gels prior to *in vivo* implantation[12] (as described below).

Nevo et al.[13,14] have explored the use of both chondrocytes and osteoprogenitor cells derived from bone marrow delivered in a hyaluronic acid gel. Autografts or allografts were used to repair tibial defects in goats and femoral defects in chicks. The autografts were superior to the allografts, which evoked a typical immune response and progressive arthrosis. In both animal models, autografted defects were repaired with a well-integrated tissue that resembed hyaline cartilage at the surface and bone at the base.

Amiel et al. qualitatively (i.e., histologically) and quantitatively (i.e., biochemically and mechanically) assessed osteochondral defects repaired with perichondral cells and porous polylactic acid in a rabbit allograft model.[15,16] After 6 weeks, the alignment of cells in the repair tissue followed the architecture of the scaffold. After 1 year, the repair tissue had variable histological appearance (only 50% of the subchondral bone reformed) and biochemical composition (dry weight fractions of GAG were 55% those of the host cartilage), but mechanical properties (i.e., modulus and permeability in radially confined compression) were comparable to those measured for the host cartilage. In this case, mechanical testing appeared to be less sensitive than histological and biochemical assessments; this finding was attributed to difficulties in mechanical measurements and the derivation of intrinsic parameters, due to the geometry and the non-homogeneous nature of the repair tissue, respectively.

Noguchi et al.[17] compared autologous and allogenic repair using chondrocytes cultured in collagen gels prior to implantation in inbred rats. After 2 to 4 weeks, the repair tissue consisted of hyaline articular cartilage with slight inflammatory cell infiltration in both groups; the immune response was somewhat more conspicuous in the allografts. However, inflammation resolved by 8 weeks and auto- and allografted repair tissues were almost identical after 6 months.

Freed et al.[18] cultured chondrocytes expanded by serial passage (P4) on polyglycolic acid (PGA) scaffolds for 3 to 4 weeks *in vitro* prior to implantation as allografts in rabbits. Compared to native rabbit articular cartilage, constructs contained 25% as much total collagen and 86% as much GAG per gram dry weight at the time of implantation. After 1 and 6 months, the histological scores of defects repaired with cell-PGA constructs did not differ significantly from those following implantation of PGA alone, except for qualitatively better surface smoothness, cell columnarization, and spatial uniformity of GAG in the defects grafted with cell-PGA constructs.

Grande et al.[19] cultured osteoprogenitor cells derived from skeletal muscle on PGA scaffolds for 2 to 3 weeks *in vitro* prior to implantation as allografts in rabbits. At the time of implantation, cells were attached to the scaffold but had not undergone chondrogenesis. After 3 months, defects repaired with cell-PGA constructs consisted of a cartilaginous surface region similar in thickness to the host cartilage and normal appearing subchondral bone, while implantation of PGA alone resulted in a patchy mixture of fibrous and hyaline cartilage.

Kawamura et al.[12] cultured chondrocytes in collagen gels for 2 weeks *in vitro* prior to implantation as allografts in rabbits. At the time of implantation, constructs appeared stiffer than uncultured cells in collagen gels and histologically resembled hyaline cartilage. After 6 months, the repair tissue still consisted of a thick plug of hyaline cartilage; i.e., the region at the base was neither vascularized nor replaced by bone. It was suggested that a mechanical mismatch between the thin layer of host cartilage and the thick plug of cartilaginous repair tissue, and the lack of regeneration of a proper subchondral bony base would contribute to long-term implant failure.

In Vitro Chondrogenesis

Buschmann et al.[20,21] showed that high cell density cultures of calf articular chondrocytes in agarose gels formed a mechanically functional cartilaginous matrix. After 7 weeks *in vitro*, construct compositions and mechanical properties (i.e., fractions of DNA and GAG, compressive modulus, streaming potential) reached values of about 25% those of native calf cartilage. Constructs responded to mechanical forces in a manner similar to that of native cartilage: static compression suppressed ECM synthesis by an amount that increased with increasing compression amplitude and culture time, while dynamic compression stimulated ECM synthesis by an amount that increased with ECM accumulation and culture time. The authors postulated that several mechanisms could be involved in mechanotransduction, including cell-ECM interactions and/or changes in interstitial fluid flow and streaming potential.

Hauselmann et al.[22] demonstrated the phenotypic stability of calf articular cartilage after prolonged (8 month) cultivation in alginate beads. The ECM formed by adult human chondrocytes cultured in gels for 30 days was similar to that of human articular cartilage and could be used to study PG turnover.[23] The ECM consisted of two compartments: a small amount of cell-associated matrix (corresponding to the pericellular and territorial ECM), and a larger amount of matrix further removed from the cells (corresponding to interterritorial ECM). Aggregated PGs in the cell-associated ECM turned over relatively quickly ($t_{1/2}$ of 29 days) as compared to those in the further-removed ECM ($t_{1/2} > 100$ days). These findings were attributed to the effects of proteolytic enzymes located at the cell membrane.

Freed et al.[24] characterized cartilaginous constructs based on calf articular or human rib chondrocytes and synthetic polymer scaffolds. Fibrous polyglycolic acid (PGA) meshes yielded constructs with higher cellularities and GAG production rates as compared to porous polylactic acid (PLLA) sponges; these findings were attributed to differences in polymer geometry (mesh vs. sponge, pore size distribution) and degradation (faster for PGA than PLLA). PGA scaffolds were subsequently characterized in detail and produced on a commercial scale.[25]

Grande et al.[26] showed that the choice of scaffold affected ECM synthesis rates, e.g., PGA and collagen scaffolds, respectively, enhanced GAG and protein synthesis rates of calf chondrocytes cultured in a perfused system. Sittinger et al.[27] observed PG and collagen deposition by human articular chondrocytes cultured on synthetic polyester meshes coated with poly-L-lysine or type II collagen and embedded in agarose gels. Dunkelman et al.[28] and Grande et al.[26] both reported that cell-polymer constructs were more likely to form cartilaginous ECM if cultured in perfused vessels rather than statically.

Carver and Heath[29,30] demonstrated that physiologicial levels of compression enhanced GAG deposition and improved the compressive moduli of engineered cartilage. In particular, constructs based on equine chondrocytes and PGA scaffolds were subjected to intermittent hydrostatic pressures of 500 and 1000 psi (3.4 and 6.9 MPa) in a semi-continuous perfusion system for 5 weeks. Structural and functional improvements were observed in constructs based on cells obtained from young but not adult horses. In a recent study, fetal human chondrocytes cultured at high density in serum-free medium formed 1.5 to 2.0 mm thick hyaline cartilage over 120 days whereas otherwise identical cultures containing serum could not be maintained for more than 30 days.[31]

Freed and Vunjak-Novakovic studied *in vitro* chondrogenesis using a variety of methods to seed and cultivate calf chondrocytes on polymer scaffolds as follows. Static seeding of scaffolds two or more mm thick resulted in bilaminar constructs with a fibrous upper region and a cartilaginous lower region.[32] In contrast, dynamic cell seeding in spinner flasks allowed relatively uniform cell seeding of scaffolds 2 to 5 mm thick at an essentially 100% yield.[33] An increase in the initial density of seeded cells resulted in comparable construct cellularities and collagen contents, but markedly higher GAG contents.[34]

Mixing during 3D culture markedly improved construct morphology and composition.[32,35] For example, 10 mm diameter × 5 mm thick scaffolds seeded and cultured in mixed flasks weighed twice as much as those seeded and cultured in mixed dishes, and contained about 2.5 times more of each GAG and total collagen.[35] However, constructs grown in mixed flasks formed outer capsules that were up to 300 μm thick and contained high concentrations of elongated cells and collagen and little GAG; this finding was attributed to the effects of turbulent flow conditions on cells at the construct surface.[35] In contrast, constructs cultured in rotating vessels had relatively uniform distributions of cells and ECM and were up to 5 mm thick after 6 weeks in culture.[36] With increasing culture time, construct ECM biosynthesis rates and the fractional loss of newly synthesized macromolecules into the culture medium both decreased[36] but construct GAG fractions and mechanical properties improved.[37] The collagen networks of constructs and native cartilage were similar with respect to fibril density and diameter and fractions of collagen types II, IX and X.[38]

Vunjak-Novakovic et al.[39] studied the relationships between construct compositions (fractions of water and ECM components) and mechanical properties in static and dynamic compression (equilibrium modulus, dynamic stiffness, hydraulic permeability, streaming potential) using three different culture environments: static flasks, mixed flasks, and rotating vessels. Constructs cultured in static and mixed flasks had lower concentrations of ECM and worse mechanical properties as compared to constructs cultured in rotating vessels. The structure-function relationships detected for chondrocyte-PGA constructs appeared consistent with those previously reported for chondrocytes cultured in agarose gels,[20] native calf cartilage,[40] and adult human cartilage.[41]

Martin et al.[42-44] demonstrated that bone marrow stromal cells (BMSC) expanded in monolayers, seeded onto scaffolds and cultured in mixed Petri dishes formed large, 3D cartilaginous tissues. The presence of a 3D scaffold was required, as demonstrated by the small size and noncartilaginous nature of control cell pellet cultures. The presence of fibroblast growth factor 2 (FGF) during 2D expansion promoted differentiation of BMSC during 3D cultivation. As compared to avian (embryonic chick) BMSC, mammalian (calf) BMSC required a more structurally stable 3D scaffold and the presence of additional biochemical signals.

23.3 Cell-Polymer-Bioreactor System

The literature reviewed in Section 23.2 above demonstrates the feasibility of using cell-based tissue engineering approaches to *in vivo* articular cartilage repair and *in vitro* studies of chondrogenesis. In the next section we will first describe the *in vitro* cell-polymer-bioreactor system and then use selected examples from our own work to illustrate its use in studies of the development and modulation of

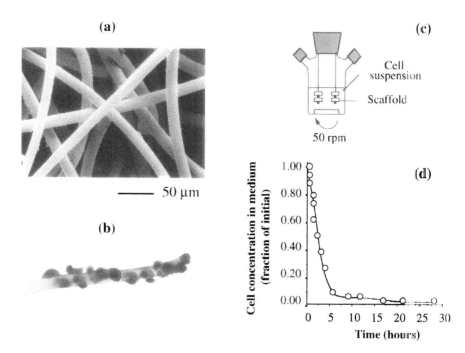

FIGURE 23.2   Cell seeding of polyglycolic acid (PGA) mesh. (a) PGA ultrastructure (scanning electron micrograph). (b) Chondrocytes attach to PGA fibers and maintain their spherical morphology (H&E stained histological section). (c) Dynamic cell seeding: magnetic stirring generates convective motion of cells into porous scaffolds that are fixed to needles embedded in the stopper of the flask. (d) Chondrocytes attached to PGA scaffolds with an effective yield of 100% over 24 h.

construct structure and function. The unifying hypothesis of our work is that isolated chondrocytes or precursor cells can form functional cartilage tissue *in vitro*, if cultured on a 3D structural template in an environment that provides the necessary biochemical and physical signals. Ideally, engineered cartilage should display the key structural features of native cartilage, be able to withstand physiologic loads, and be able to integrate with adjacent host tissues following *in vivo* implantation.

Experimental Methods

Cells: Cell types studied included articular chondrocytes and their precursors. *Chondrocytes* were obtained from the articular cartilage of 2 to 3 week old bovine calves[20,24] and used immediately after isolation. *Bone marrow stromal cells* (BMSC) were obtained from the marrow of 2 to 3 week old bovine calves[43] or 16 day embryonic chicks.[42]

   Scaffolds: Our best characterized scaffolds are made of *polyglycolic acid* (PGA) in form of 97% porous nonwoven meshes of 13 μm diameter fibers (Fig. 23.2a).[25] Other scaffolds that have been studied include *polylactic acid* (PLLA)[24] and *polylactic-co-glycolic acid* (PLGA) sponges.[45]

   Cell seeding: Polymer scaffolds (5 to 10 mm in diameter, 2 to 5 mm thick) were fixed in place and seeded with cells using well-mixed spinner flasks [33] (Fig. 23.2c).

   Bioreactor cultivation: Tissue culture systems under investigation are schematically presented in Fig. 23.3. Static and mixed *dishes* contained one construct per well in 6 to 7 ml medium; mixed dishes were placed on an orbital shaker at 75 rpm.[32] In *spinner flasks*, scaffolds were fixed to needles (8 to 12 per flask, in 100 to 120 cm³ medium), seeded with isolated cells under mixed conditions and cultured either statically or exposed to unidirectional turbulent flow using a non-suspended magnetic bar at 50-80 rpm.[35] *Rotating vessels* included the slow turning lateral vessel (STLV) and the high aspect ratio vessel (HARV), each of which was rotated around its central axis such that the constructs (8 to 12 per vessel, in 100 to

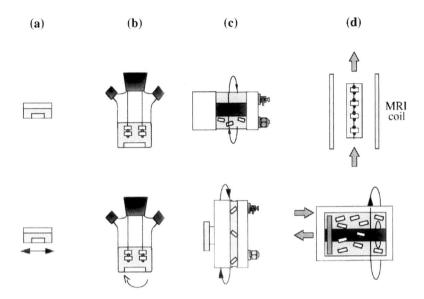

(a) **(b)** **(c)** **(d)**

FIGURE 23.3 Tissue culture bioreactors. (a) Static and orbitally mixed Petri dishes. (b) Static and magnetically stirred flasks. (c) Rotating vessels: the slow turning lateral vessel (above) and the high aspect ratio vessel (below). (d) Perfused chamber in which cultured constructs are monitored using magnetic resonance imaging (MRI, above); perfused rotating vessel (below).

120 cm³ medium) settled freely in a laminar flow field.[46,47] *Perfused vessels* included columns used to culture constructs and non-invasively monitor the progression of chondrogenesis using magnetic resonance imaging (MRI),[48] and a rotating perfused vessel developed by NASA for flight studies.[37] In all vessels, medium was exchanged batchwise (at a rate of ~3 cm³ per construct and day), and gas was exchanged continuously, by surface aeration or by diffusion through a silicone membrane.

Analytical techniques: Construct size and distributions of cells and tissue components were assessed by image analysis.[33,36] Constructs for histological assessment were fixed in neutral buffered formalin, embedded in paraffin, sectioned (5 to 8 μm thick), and stained with hematoxylin and eosin (H&E for cells), safranin-O (for GAG), and monoclonal antibodies (for collagen types I, II, IX, and X).[36,38,42] Ultrastructural analyses included scanning and transmission electron microscopy (SEM, TEM).[38] Biochemical compositions were measured following papain or protease-K digestion of lyophilized constructs.[24,25,36] Cell number was assessed by measuring the amount of DNA using Hoechst 33258 dye.[49] Sulfated GAG content was determined by dimethylmethylene blue dye binding.[50] Total collagen content was determined from hydroxyproline content after acid hydrolysis and reaction with *p*-dimethylamino-benzaldehyde and chloramine-T.[51] Type II collagen content was determined by inhibition ELISA.[36,38,52] The presence of other collagen types (e.g., I, IX, X) was demonstrated and semiquantitatively measured using SDS-PAGE and Western blots.[38] GAG distribution was determined by MRI.[48,53] Synthesis rates of GAG, total protein, and collagen were measured by incorporation and release of radiolabeled tracers.[36] Cell metabolism was assessed based on the ratio of lactate production and glucose consumption, and ammonia production rates.[54] Mechanical construct properties (e.g., compressive modulus, dynamic stiffness, hydraulic permeability, streaming potential) were measured in static and dynamic radially confined compression.[39,55]

Developmental Studies

As described above (Section 23.2, Table 23.1), articular cartilage repair has been enhanced following the transplantation of chondrocytes and osteochondral progenitor cells in conjunction with polymer scaffolds. However, identification of specific factors that influence *in vivo* regeneration and/or repair can be

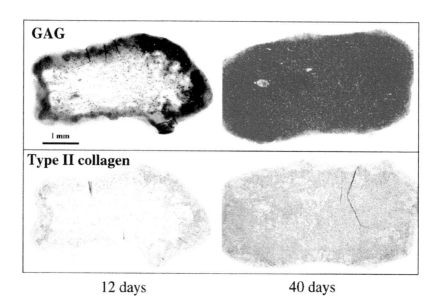

FIGURE 23.4   Temporo-spatial pattern of ECM deposition. Calf chondrocytes cultured on PGA scaffolds in rotating vessels. Chondrogenesis was initiated peripherally in 12 day constructs (left panels) and proceeded appositionally resulting in a continous cartilaginous ECM in 40 day constructs (right panels). Histological cross sections were stained with safranin-O for GAG (top panels) or with a monoclonal antibody to collagen type II (bottom panels).

difficult due to host systemic responses (e.g., neuro-endocrinological, immunological). Controlled *in vitro* studies carried out in the cell-polymer-bioreactor system can thus provide useful, complementary information regarding the process of cartilage matrix regeneration starting from isolated cells (herein referred to as developmental studies).

Chondrogenesis *in vivo* and *in vitro* is thought to be initiated by precursor cell aggregation.[56] Cartilaginous ECM is deposited, with concurrent increases in the amounts of GAG and collagen types II and IX, both in mesenchymal cells obtained from embryonic chick limbs[57] and in human limbs at various developmental stages.[58] ECM deposition starts at the center of the developing limb bud and spreads peripherally,[57] in conjunction with cellular conditioning of their microenvironment.[59]

In calf chondrocyte-PGA constructs, amounts of GAG and collagen type II also increased concomittantly[36] (Fig. 23.4). By culture day 12, cartilaginous tissue had formed at the construct periphery; by day 40, constructs were continuously cartilaginous matrix over their entire cross sections (6.7 mm diameter × 5 mm thick). Chondrogenesis was initiated peripherally and progressed both inward toward the construct center and outward from its surface; these findings could be correlated with construct cell distributions, as described below. The temporo-spatial patterns of GAG distribution could also be monitored in living constructs using MRI.[48] Constructs cultured 6 weeks contained an interconnected network of collagen fibers that resembled that of calf articular collagen with respect to overall organization and fiber diameter (Fig. 23.5A). Type II collagen represented more than 90% of the total collagen, as quantitated by an ELISA[36,38] and demonstrated qualitatively in Fig. 23.5B. Construct collagen type II was not susceptible to extraction with a chaotropic agent (guanidine hydrochloride, GuHCl), suggesting some degree of cross-linkage. However, construct collagen had only 30% as many pyridinium cross-links as native calf cartilage.[38]

Construct wet weight fractions of cartilaginous ECM increased, the amount of polymer decreased, and construct cellularity plateaued over 6 weeks of culture in rotating vessels[36] (Fig. 23.6). Over the same time interval, construct ECM synthesis rates decreased by approximately 40% and the fraction of newly synthesized macromolecules released into the culture medium decreased from about 25% of total at 4 days to less than 4%; the latter can be attributed in part to collagen network development.[36] The mass of the

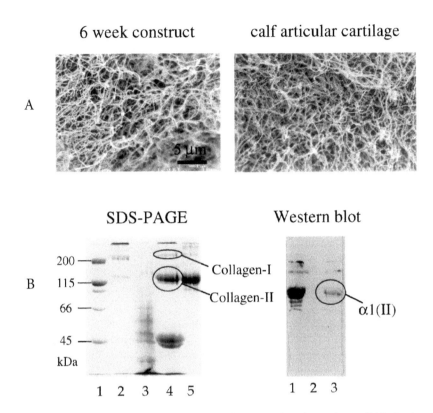

FIGURE 23.5   Collagen structure and type. Calf chondrocytes cultured on PGA scaffolds for 6 weeks in rotating vessels. (A) Scanning electron micrographs showed similar collagen network ultrastructures for constructs and native calf articular cartilage. (B) The presence of type II collagen in constructs was demonstrated using pepsin-digested constructs in conjunction with SDS-PAGE, and confirmed by Western blot (with a monoclonal antibody to αII). Lanes on SDS-PAGE: (1) molecular weight standards, (2) collagen type I, (3) GuHCl extract of construct, (4) pepsin extract of construct, (5) collagen type II; Lanes on Western blot: (1) collagen type II, (2) GuHCl extract of construct, (3) pepsin extract of construct.

PGA scaffold decreased to about 40% of initial over 6 weeks.[25] The time constant for scaffold degradation was of the same order of magnitude as the time constant of ECM deposition, a situation associated with enhanced tissue regeneration according to the hypothesis of isomorphous tissue replacement.[60]

Modulation of Cartilaginous Structure and Function

The structure and function of articular cartilage are determined, at least in part, by environmental factors.[61] It is likely that the same factors that affect *in vivo* cartilage development, maintenance, and remodeling also affect *in vitro* chondrogenesis. In the selected examples described below, we will describe the effects of (1) cell, scaffold, and biochemical factors and (2) cultivation conditions and time on the structure and function of engineered cartilage. In principle, *in vitro* cultivation of a cell-polymer construct prior to *in vivo* implantation can help localize cell delivery and promote device fixation and survival, while maintaining an ability for integration at the graft-host interface. In contrast, cells transplanted in the absence of a carrier vehicle tended to leak away from the defect site,[9] while cells implanted immediately after loading in/on biomaterials were more vulnerable to mechanical forces and metabolic changes experienced during fixation or following implantation.[12]

Cells, the Scaffold, and Biochemical Signals

Chondrogenesis depends on the cells themselves (e.g., type, *in vitro* expansion, density, spatial arrangement), the scaffold (e.g., material, structure, degradation rate), and the presence of biochemical factors

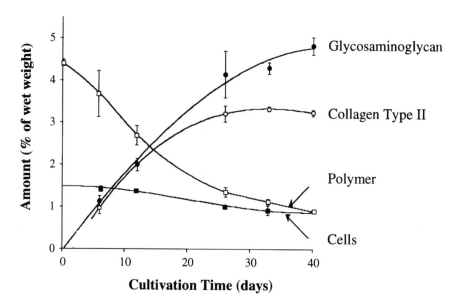

FIGURE 23.6   Tissue regeneration kinetics. Calf chondrocytes cultured on PGA scaffolds in rotating vessels. ECM components (GAG and collagen type II) accumulated, cellularity remained constant, and polymer mass decreased with increasing culture time. Data represent the average ± SD of three independent measurements.

(e.g., growth factors, hormones). The choice of cell type, which includes differentiated chondrocytes isolated from cartilage (articular or rib) and osteochondral progenitor cells isolated from bone marrow (herein referred to as bone marrow stromal cells, BMSC), can affect *in vitro* culture requirements (e.g., medium supplements) and *in vivo* construct function (e.g., integration potential). Polymer scaffolds vary with respect to surface properties (e.g., chemistry and wettability, which affect cell spreading and proliferation), geometry (e.g., dimensions, porosity, and pore size, which affect the spatial cell arrangement and the transmission of biochemical and mechanical signals), and physical properties (e.g., mechanical integrity and degradation rate, which determine whether the polymer can provide a structurally stable template for tissue regeneration).

Watt[61] suggested that a cell cultured *in vitro* will tend to retain its differentiated phenotype under conditions that resemble its natural *in vivo* environment. In the case of chondrocytes, phenotypic stability is enhanced by cultivation in alginate or agarose.[22,23,63] Moreover, chondrocytes dedifferentiated by serial passage in monolayers redifferentiated (i.e., reacquired a spherical shape, ceased dividing, and resumed the synthesis of GAG and collagen type II) when transferred into 3D cultures.[64,65] When cultured on 3D fibrous PGA scaffolds, chondrocytes retained their spherical shape and formed cartilaginous tissue.[25,66]

Chondrocytes cultured at high cell densities tended to express their differentiated phenotype.[63,67] It was hypothesized that the effective cross-talk between cells depends on the presence of homotypically differentiated cells in the immediate cell environment.[67] The term "community effect" was later coined by Gurdon[69] who suggested that the ability of a cell to respond to phenotypic induction is enhanced by, or even dependent on, other neighboring cells differentiating in the same way at the same time. A postulated underlying mechanism involves changes in gene transcription and translation caused by cell-cell/ECM interactions.[62,70,71]

In cell-polymer constructs, the density of cells initially seeded at the construct periphery was sufficient to initiate chondrogenesis in that region. In particular, corresponding temporo-spatial patterns of cartilaginous ECM deposition and cell distribution were observed (compare Figs. 23.4 and 23.7). The finding that cell densities were initially higher peripherally than centrally, which implies that cell seeding density and proliferation rate were relatively higher peripherally, can be attributed to enhanced rates of nutrient and gas transfer at the construct surface. Over the 6 week culture period, self-regulated cell proliferation

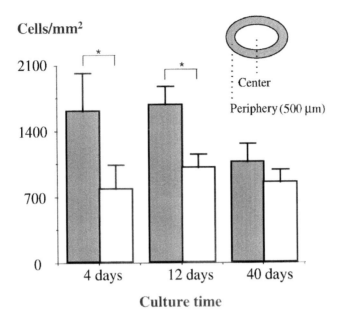

Cells/mm²

FIGURE 23.7   Temporo-spatial pattern of cell density. Calf chondrocytes cultured on PGA scaffolds in rotating vessels. Cell density was initially higher at the construct periphery (white bars) than at its center (shaded bars), while cell distribution in 40 day constructs was spatially uniform. Number of cells/mm² was assessed by image analysis of H&E stained histological sections (average ± SD of 24 independent measurements).

and ECM deposition resulted in constructs with physiological cellularities and spatially uniform distributions of components[36] (Figs. 23.4 and 23.7). Increases in the size, cellularity, and absolute amount of cartilaginous ECM were observed when chondrocyte-PGA constructs were cultured in medium supplemented with insulin-like growth factor I (IGF-I, 10-300 ng/ml) and serum (10%).[72]

In the case of osteochondral progenitor cells, Caplan et al.[10] suggested that principles of skeletal tissue engineering should be governed by the same motifs as embryonic development. BMSC differentiation is thought to be regulated by cell-to-cell contacts in an environment capable of activating the differentiation program.[73] *In vitro* (in BMSC aggregates), the induction of chondrogenesis depended on the presence of transforming growth factor-β1 (TGF-β) and dexamethasone.[74] *In vivo* (in rabbits), osteochondral repair recapitulated embryonic events and depended on the spatial arrangement and density of precursor cells and the presence of specific bioactive factors.[10]

In cell-polymer constructs, chondrocytic differentiation of BMSC depended both on scaffold-related factors and on exogenous biochemical signals.[42-44] Avian BMSC cultured in the absence of polymer scaffolds formed small bilaminar tissues in which the lower region contained GAG and upper region appeared undifferentiated (Fig. 23.8a). The same BMSC formed constructs consisting of a single tissue phase when cultured on PGA scaffolds in mixed Petri dishes (Fig. 23.8b), while BMSC expansion in the presence of FGF prior to culture on PGA scaffolds resulted in the most cartilaginous ECM (Fig. 23.8c). When FGF-expanded mammalian BMSC were cultured on nonwoven PGA mesh (Fig. 23.2a), constructs first contracted and then collapsed (Fig. 23.8d), while the same cells cultured on a scaffold consisting of a continuous polymer phase (polylactic-co-glycolic acid and polyethylene glycol (PLGA/PEG) sponge)[45] maintained their original dimensions (Fig. 23.8e). When FGF-expanded mammalian BMSC were cultured on PLGA/PEG scaffolds in mixed dishes, chondrogenesis was observed in media supplemented with transforming growth factor beta 1 (TGF-β), insulin, and dexamethasone (Fig. 23.8f) while osteogenesis was observed in media supplemented with betaglycerophosphate and dexamethasone (Fig. 23.8g). In the absence of these supplements, constructs consisted mainly of type I collagen and resembled loose connective tissue.

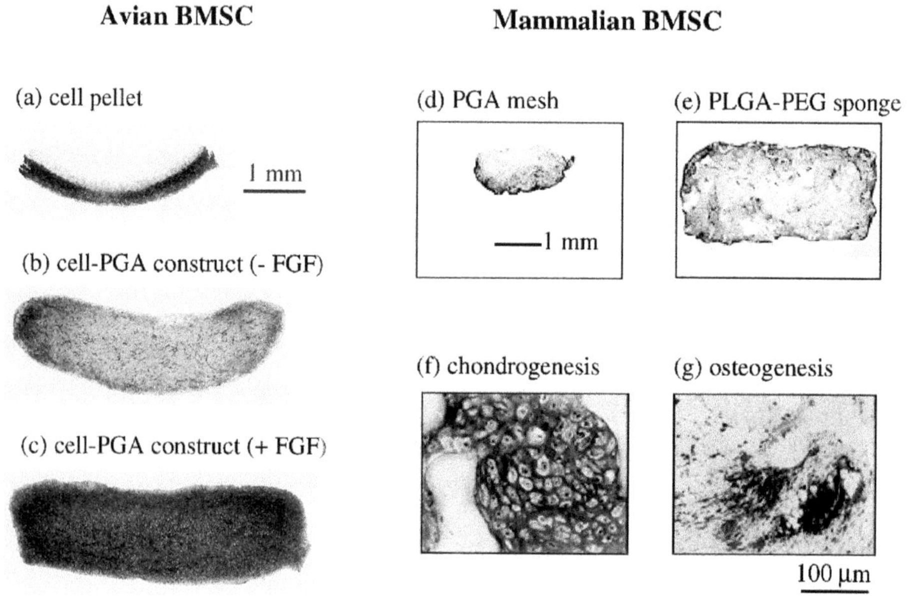

Avian BMSC   **Mammalian BMSC**

(a) cell pellet   (d) PGA mesh   (e) PLGA-PEG sponge

1 mm

——1 mm

(b) cell-PGA construct (- FGF)

(f) chondrogenesis   (g) osteogenesis

(c) cell-PGA construct (+ FGF)

100 µm

FIGURE 23.8 Chondrogenesis starting from bone marrow stromal cells (BMSC). (a–c) avian (chick embryo) BMSC cultured in media containing serum (10%) and ascorbic acid (50 µg/ml): (a) without polymer scaffolds (as cell pellets); (b) on PGA scaffolds, or (c) after expansion in the presence of FGF (1 ng/ml). (d–e) FGF-expanded mammalian (bovine calf) BMSC cultured on (d) PGA scaffolds (nonwoven meshes) or (e) PLGA/PEG scaffolds (sponges consisting of a continuous polymer phase). (f–g) FGF-expanded mammalian BMSC were cultured on PLGA/PEG sponges in media containing serum (10%), ascorbic acid (50 µg/ml) and either: (f) TGFβ (10 ng/ml), insulin (5 µg/ml), dexamethasone (100 mM), or (g) bGP (7 mM) and dexamethasone (10 mM).

Cultivation Conditions and Time

Tissue culture bioreactors permit the *in vitro* cultivation of larger, better organized engineered cartilage than can be grown in static Petri dishes.[47] Flow and mixing within bioreactors are expected to affect tissue formation in at least two ways: by enhancing *mass transfer* (e.g., of gases and nutrients) and by direct *physical stimulation* of the cells (e.g., by hydrodynamic forces).

The transport of chemical species lies at the heart of physiology and to a large extent determines tissue structure.[75,76] Cells communicate with each other by a combination of diffusion and convective flow, which are in turn driven by hydrodynamic, concentration, and osmotic gradients. *In vivo*, mass transfer to chondrocytes involves diffusion and convective transport by the fluid flow that accompanies tissue loading;[77] the presence of blood vessels in immature cartilage can further enhance mass transfer. *In vitro*, mixing-induced convection can enhance mass transport at construct surfaces. In contrast, mass transfer within constructs, which occurs by diffusion only, can become the limiting factor in the cultivation of a large construct with a dense ECM.[78] As compared to constructs grown statically, constructs grown in orbitally mixed Petri dishes and in mixed spinner flasks were larger and contained higher amounts of tissue components.[32,35] Cell metabolism in constructs cultured in mixed and static flasks were found to be aerobic and anaerobic, respectively, as assessed by lactate to glucose ratios and ammonia production rates.[54]

The form of a skeletal tissue represents a diagram of underlying forces transmitted across the ECM to the individual cells.[61] Mechanotransduction is thought to involve four steps: mechanocoupling, biochemical coupling, signal transmission, and effector cell response.[79] *In vivo*, load-bearing and immobilized articular cartilage respectively contained high and low GAG fractions.[80,81] *In vitro*, physiologic levels of dynamic compression increased the rates of GAG and protein synthesis in cartilage explants,[82,83] while static loading supressed GAG synthesis.[82,84] Physiological levels of dynamic compression also increased the GAG content and improved the mechanical properties of engineered cartilage.[29,30] The motion of

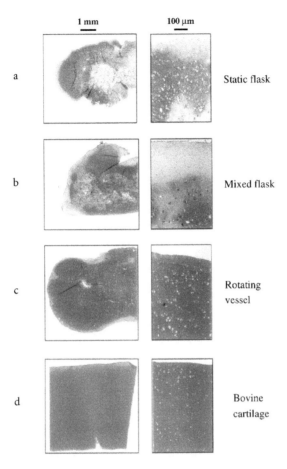

1 mm   100 µm

a — Static flask

b — Mixed flask

c — Rotating vessel

d — Bovine cartilage

FIGURE 23.9 Culture conditions affect construct morphology. Representative cross sections of 6 week constructs (calf chondrocytes/PGA) cultured in static flasks, mixed flasks, and rotating vessels are compared to fresh calf cartilage (low and high power H&E stained histological sections).

medium in roller bottles stimulated chondrocytes to form cartilaginous nodules,[85,86] and fluid shear enhanced PG size and synthesis rate in chondrocyte monolayers.[87] Turbulent mixing in spinner flasks induced the formation of a fibrous outer capsule at the construct surface, the thickness of which increased with both the mixing intensity and the duration of tissue cultivation.[35] This finding was attributed to direct effects of mechanical forces, i.e., cells exposed to external forces tend to flatten and activate stress-protection mechanisms in order to remain firmly attached to their substrate[88] and increase their stiffnesses by cytoskeletal rearrangements.[89]

The effects of culture conditions on the morphology, composition, and mechanical properties of chondrocyte-PGA constructs were studied over 6 weeks using three different bioreactors: static flasks, mixed flasks, and rotating vessels.[39] In static cultures, GAG accumulated mostly at the periphery, presumably due to diffusional constraints of mass transfer (Fig. 23.9a). In mixed flasks, turbulent shear caused the formation of a thick outer capsule with little or no GAG (Fig. 23.9b). Only in rotating vessels, were GAG fractions high and spatially uniform (Fig. 23.9c). Construct fractions of GAG (Fig. 23.10a) and total collagen (Fig. 23.10b) increased in the following order: static flasks, mixed flasks, rotating vessels, native cartilage.[39] Construct equilibrium moduli and hydraulic permeabilities (Figs. 23.10c,d) varied in a manner consistent with sample composition.[39] As compared to native calf cartilage, 6-week constructs cultured in rotating bioreactors had similar cellularities, 75% as much GAG and 40% as much total collagen per unit wet weight, but only 20% the compressive modulus and fivefold higher hydraulic

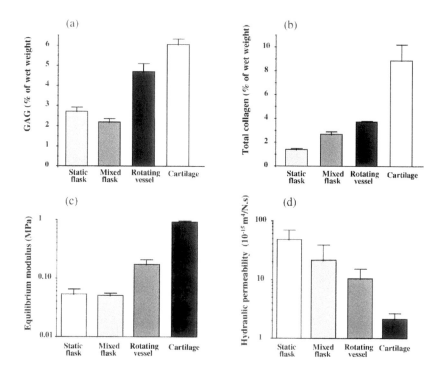

FIGURE 23.10   Culture conditions affect construct compositions and mechanical properties. Constructs (calf chondrocytes/PGA) cultured for 6 weeks bioreactors were compared with respect to: (a,b) wet weight fractions of GAG and total collagen, (c) equilibrium modulus, and (d) hydraulic permeability. As compared to static and mixed flasks, rotating vessels yielded constructs with the best properties, but these remained inferior to native calf cartilage. Data represent the average ± SD of three to six independent measurements.

permeability. The apparent lack of functional organization of ECM in constructs may be explained either by the use of immature cartilage (2 to 4 week old calves), or by the absence of specific factors in the *in vitro* culture environment which are normally present *in vivo*.

It is possible that the mechanisms by which the dynamic fluctuations in shear and pressure in rotating vessels enhanced chondrogenesis resembled those associated with dynamic loading *in vivo*. However, the acting hydrodynamic forces were different in nature and several orders of magnitude lower than those resulting from joint loading.[46,90,91] Studies of engineered cartilage subjected to physiological levels of dynamic compression[29,30] and shear should thus allow a more direct comparison of *in vitro* and *in vivo* tissue responses.

Chondrocytes can be phenotypically stable for prolonged periods of time in 3D cultures (e.g., for 8 months in alginate beads).[22] The effect of prolonged cultivation (7 months in rotating bioreactors) on the structure and function of chondrocyte-PGA constructs is shown in Fig. 23.11. As compared to native calf articular cartilage, 7 month constructs had comparable GAG fractions (Fig. 23.11a), 30% as much total collagen (Fig. 23.11b), comparable equilibrium moduli (Fig. 23.11c), and comparable hydraulic permeability (Fig. 23.11d). At 7 months, constructs were phenotypically stable (75% of the total construct collagen was type II) and consisted of metabolically active cells (component cells attached and spread in Petri dishes and were enzymatically active).[37]

A successful approach to cartilage tissue engineering must also provide the potential for constructs to integrate with the adjacent cartilage and subchondral bone. Most of the *in vivo* studies described in Section 23.2 addressed this issue. In general, the implantation of chondrocytes and BMSC without a cartilaginous ECM resulted in repair tissue that deteriorated with time *in vivo*,[9,11] while implantation of cartilaginous constructs integrated relatively poorly with adjacent host tissues.[10,12] *In vitro* systems can be used to study the effects of specific factors on construct integration in the absence of uncontrollable

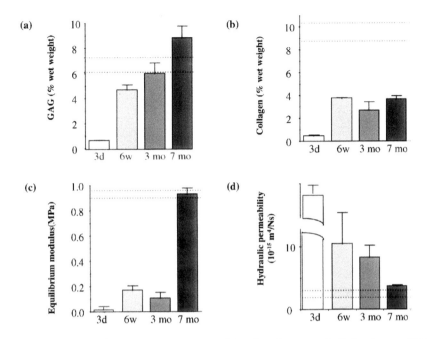

FIGURE 23.11 Culture time affects construct structure and function. Constructs (calf chondrocytes/PGA) cultured for 3 days (3 d), 6 weeks (6 w), 3 or 7 months (3 mo, 7 mo) in rotating vessels were compared with respect to: (a,b) wet weight fractions of GAG and total collagen, (c) equilibrium modulus, and (d) hydraulic permeability. All properties improved with culture time and approached values measured for native calf cartilage (normal ranges denoted by dotted lines). Data represent the average ± SD of 3 independent measurements.

variables intrinsic to *in vivo* studies. In one such study, constructs were cultured for various times, sutured into ring-shaped explants of native cartilage, and cultured for an additional period of time as composites.[92] The integration process involved cell migration into the construct-explant interface and the formation of a new tissue which was initially fibrous but became progressively cartilaginous with increasing culture time (Fig. 23.12a). Construct equilibrium modulus, which was negligible at the beginning of cultivation, increased to approximately 15% of native calf cartilage after 6 weeks (Fig. 23.11c). The adhesive strength at the construct-explant interface was approximately 65% higher for composites made with 6 day constructs, which consisted mainly of cells, as compared to composites made with 5 week constructs, which had a well-formed ECM (Fig. 23.12b).

23.4   Summary and Future Directions

Tissue engineering offers a cell-based approach to articular cartilage repair. In this chapter, we reviewed the state of the art of cartilage tissue engineering and focused on a cell-polymer-bioreactor system which can be used for controlled studies of chondrogenesis and the modulation of engineered cartilage by environmental factors.

A procedure in which autologous chondrocytes are obtained from an articular cartilage biopsy, expanded in culture, and transplanted in conjunction with a periosteal flap[3] is currently the only FDA-approved cell-based treatment for articular cartilage repair. However, *in vivo* studies in dogs had variable results and showed long-term degradation of the repair tissue.[8,9] The clinical study has been viewed with some skepticism[5,6] and long-term, prospective randomized clinical studies are needed to better evaluate the potential of this technique.

Alternatively, autologous BMSC have been isolated from bone marrow aspirates, expanded, and implantated in conjunction with various gels to repair osteochondral defects in experimental animals.[10,14] Following implanatation, the cells underwent a site-specific differentiation and formed a cartilaginous zone

(a) Integration: **(b) Adhesive strength (MPa)**

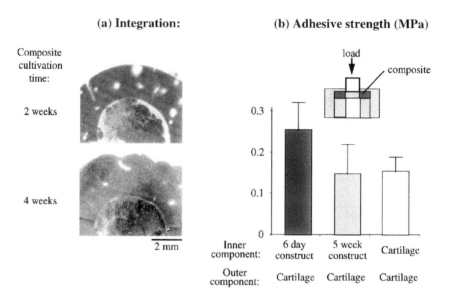

FIGURE 23.12   Culture time affects construct integration potential. (a) Composites made from 6 day constructs (calf chondrocytes/PGA) and cultured for an additional 2 or 4 weeks (upper or lower panel, respectively; safranin-O stained histological sections). (b) Adhesive strengths of composites cultured 4 weeks, including construct-cartilage composites made from 6 day or 5 week constructs and cartilage-cartilage composites (adhesion was estimated by fixing the outer ring in place and uniaxially loading the newly integrated central portion to failure as shown in the inset).

at the surface of the defect and a vascularized bony tissue at its base. In contrast to grafts based on mature chondrocytes, which failed to develop subchondral bone and to fully integrate with the host tissue, grafts based on precursor cells suffered from the progressive thinning of the cartilaginous surface zone.

A 3D scaffold permits the *in vitro* cultivation of cell-polymer constructs that can be readily manipulated, shaped, and fixed to the defect site.[18] As compared to such a pre-formed cartilaginous construct, cells injected under a periosteal flap or immobilized in a hydrated gel are more vulnerable to environmental factors and mechanical forces.[12] The selection of an appropriate scaffold depends in part on the starting cell type. For example, nonwoven fibrous PGA meshes supported chondrogenesis starting from chondrocytes[25] and avian BMSC,[42] while a scaffold with more structural stability appeared to be required for chondrogenesis starting from mammalian BMSC (Fig. 23.8).

Tissue constructs resembling native cartilage were engineered *in vitro* using isolated cells, 3D polymer scaffolds, and bioreactors (Figs. 23.4 through 23.6). Construct structure (histological, biochemical) and function (mechanical, metabolic) depended on cultivation conditions and duration.[39] The cell-polymer-bioreactor system can thus provide a basis for controlled *in vitro* studies of the effects of time and specific biochemical and physical factors on chondrogenesis (Figs. 23.7 through 23.11). Moreover, *in vitro* studies can be used to assess the potential of a cell-polymer construct to integrate with adjacent tissues (Fig. 23.12). Some of the current research needs include:

1. *Development of design criteria.* Specific construct design criteria (e.g., required cell metabolic activity, ECM composition, and mechanical properties) need to be established based on the results of further *in vitro* and *in vivo* experimentation and phenomenological modeling of cell and tissue responses to environmental signals.

2. *Selection of a cell source.* Autologous BMSC and mature chondrocytes are the most likely immediate candidates; allogeneic fetal chondrocytes represent an option for the future. Both BMSC and chondrocytes maintain their chondrogenic potential when expanded in the presence of FGF and then cultured on 3D scaffolds.[42,43] BMSC-based grafts recapitulate embryonic events of endochondral bone formation in response to local environmental factors[10] resulting in repair tissue

that is relatively well integrated but can undergo ossification, leading to progressive thinning at the articular surface.[11] On the other hand, chondrocyte-based grafts do not integrate as well[12] but consist of phenotypically stable cartilage with a mechanically functional ECM[37] that may promote survival in the presence of mechanical loading. Human fetal articular chondrocytes were recently demonstrated to regenerate hyaline cartilage when cultured at high densities in serum-free medium.[31] However, this approach has unresolved ethical issues.

3. *Selection of an appropriate scaffold for human chondrocytes and BMSC.* Ideally, a tissue engineering scaffold should meet all of the following criteria: (1) reproducible processing into complex, 3D shapes, (2) highly porous structure that permits a spatially uniform cell distribution during cell seeding and minimizes diffusional constraints during *in vitro* cultivation, (3) controlled degradation at a rate matching that of cellular deposition of ECM (to provide a stable template during *in vitro* chondrogenesis) followed by complete elimination of the foreign material (to maximize long-term *in vivo* biocompatibility).

4. *Development of methods for in vitro seeding and cultivation of human cells.* Ideally, a tissue culture bioreactor should provide: (1) a means to achieve efficient, spatially uniform cell distribution throughout a scaffold (e.g., dynamic seeding), (2) uniform concentrations of biochemical species in the bulk phase and their efficient transport to the construct surface (e.g., well-mixed culture conditions), (3) steady state conditions (e.g., automated control based on biosensors triggering appropriate changes in medium and gas supply rates), to more closely mimic the *in vivo* cellular environment, and (4) applied physical forces (e.g., hydrostatic pressure and shear, dynamic compression), to more closely mimic the *in vivo* tissue environment.

5. *Development of methods to promote graft survival, integration, and maturation.* Articular cartilage repair refers to healing that restores a damaged articular surface without actually replicating the complete structure and function of the tissue while articular cartilage regeneration refers to the formation of a new tissue that is indistinguishable from normal articular cartilage, including the zonal organization, composition, and mechanical properties.[2] Ideally, engineered cartilage should meet the criteria for regeneration, since any other repair tissue represents a mechanical discontinuity likely to cause long-term device failure.[10] Local pretreatment of the host tissues at the site of the defect (e.g., with proteolytic enzymes) may enhance graft integration.[10] Further *in vivo* studies are needed to evaluate whether implanted constructs develop characteristic architectural features of articular cartilage in conjunction with physiological loading.

This chapter describes technologies that can potentially lead to articular cartilage regeneration *in vitro* and *in vivo*. Representative studies are summarized in which cells (autologous or allogeneic chondrocytes or BMSC) were isolated, cultivated, and in some cases used to repair large full-thickness cartilage defects. Extension of these results to a human cell source and scale is expected to have a major clinical impact. At this time, tissue engineering studies are mainly observational. The increasing use of models to describe specific aspects of tissue formation (e.g., patterns of ECM deposition, structure-function correlations) is expected to help in the design of hypothesis-driven experiments and interpretation of their results.

Acknowledgments

This work was supported by the National Aeronautics and Space Association (Grant NAG9-836). The authors would like to thank R. Langer for general advice and I. Martin for reviewing the manuscript.

Defining Terms

Bioreactors: Tissue culture vessels mixed by magnetic stirring or rotation.

Bone marrow stromal cell (BMSC): A bone marrow-derived precursor cell with the potential to differentiate into various tissues including cartilage.

Chondrocyte: A cartilage cell.

Chondrogenesis: The process of cartilage formation.

Extracellular matrix (ECM): The biochemical components present in the extracellular space of a tissue, e.g., collagen type II and glycosoaminoglycan (GAG) in articular cartilage.

Polymer scaffold: A synthetic material designed for cell cultivation, characterized by its specific chemical composition and 3D structure.

Tissue construct: The tissue engineered *in vitro* using isolated cells, polymer scaffolds, and bioreactors.

References

1. Buckwalter, J.A., Mankin, H.J. Articular cartilage. Part I: tissue design and chondrocyte-matrix interactions. *J. Bone Joint Surg.* 79-A, 600, 1997a.
2. Buckwalter, J.A., Mankin, H.J. Articular cartilage repair and transplantation. *Arthrit. Rheum.* 41, 1331, 1998.
3. Brittberg, M., Lindahl, A., Nilsson, A., Ohlsson., C., Isaksson, O., Peterson, L. Treatment of deep cartilage defects in the knee with autologous chondrocyte transplantation. *NEJM* 331, 889, 1994.
4. Arnst, C., Carey, J. Biotech bodies. *Business Week,* July 27, 56, 1998.
5. Messner, K., Gillquist, J. Cartilage repair: a critical review. *Acta Orthop. Scand.* 67, 523, 1996.
6. Newman, A.P. Articular cartilage repair. *Am. J. Sports Med.* 26, 309, 1998.
7. Brittberg, M., Nilsson, A., Lindahl, A., Ohlsson, C., Peterson, L. Rabbit articular cartilage defects treated with autologous cultured chondrocytes. *Clin. Orthop. Rel. Res.* 326, 270, 1996.
8. Shortkroff, S., Barone, L., Hsu, H.P., Wrenn, C., Gagne, T., Chi, T., Breinan, H., Minas, T., Sledge, C.B., Tubo, R., Spector, M. Healing of chondral and osteochondral defects in a canine model: the role of cultured chondrocytes in regeneration of articular cartilage. *Biomaterials* 17, 147, 1996.
9. Breinan, H.A., Minas, T., Barone, L., Tubo, R., Hsu, H.P., Shortkroff, S., Nehrer, S., Sledge, C.B., Spector, M. Histological evaluation of the course of healing of canine articular cartilage defects treated with cultured autologous chondrocytes. *Tissue Eng.* 4, 101, 1998.
10. Caplan, A.I., Elyaderani, M., Mochizuki, Y., Wakitani, S., Goldberg, V.M. Principles of cartilage repair and regeneration. *Clin. Orthop. Rel. Res.* 342, 254, 1997.
11. Wakitani, S., Goto, T., Pineda, S.J., Young, R.G., Mansour, J.M., Caplan, A.I., Goldberg, V.M. Mesenchymal cell-based repair of large, full-thickness defects of articular cartilage. *J. Bone Joint Surg.* 76A, 579, 1994.
12. Kawamura, S., Wakitani, S., Kimura, T., Maeda, A., Caplan, A.I., Shino, K., Ochi, T. Articular cartilage repair-rabbit experiments with a collagen gel-biomatrix and chondrocytes cultured in it. *Acta Orthop. Scand.* 69, 56, 1998.
13. Butnariu-Ephrat, M., Robinson, D., Mendes, D.G., Halperin, N., Nevo, Z. Resurfacing of goat articular cartilage from chondrocytes derived from bone marrow. *Clin. Orthop. Rel. Res.* 330, 234, 1996.
14. Nevo, Z., Robinson, D., Horowitz, S., Hashroni, A., Yayon, A. The manipulated mesenchymal stem cells in regenerated skeletal tissues. *Cell Transpl.* 7, 63, 1998.
15. Chu, C., Coutts, R.D., Yoshioka, M., Harwood, F.L., Monosov, A.Z., Amiel, D. Articular cartilage repair using allogeneic perichondrocyte-seeded biodegradable porous polylactic acid (PLA): a tissue-engineering study. *J. Biomed. Mater. Res.* 29, 1147, 1995.
16. Chu, C., Dounchis, J.S., Yoshioka, M., Sah, R.L., Coutts, R.D., Amiel, D. Osteochondral repair using perichondrial cells: a 1 year study in rabbits. *Clin. Orthop. Rel. Res.* 340, 220, 1997.
17. Noguchi, T., Oka, M., Fujino, M., Neo, M., Yamamuro, T. Repair of osteochondral defects with grafts of cultured chondrocytes: comparison of allografts and isografts. *Clin. Orthop. Rel. Res.* 302, 251, 1994.
18. Freed, L.E., Grande, D.A., Emmanual, J., Marquis, J.C., Lingbin, Z., Langer, R. Joint resurfacing using allograft chondrocytes and synthetic biodegradable polymer scaffolds, *J. Biomed. Mater. Res.* 28, 891, 1994.
19. Grande, D.A., Southerland, S.S., Manji, R., Pate, D.W., Schwartz, R.E., Lucas, P.A. Repair of articular cartilage defects using mesenchymal stem cells. *Tissue Eng.* 1, 345, 1995.

20. Buschmann, M.D., Gluzband, Y.A., Grodzinsky, A.J., Kimura, J.H., Hunziker, E.B. Chondrocytes in agarose culture synthesize a mechanically functional extracellular matrix. *J. Orthop. Res.* 10, 745, 1992.

21. Buschmann, M.D., Gluzband, Y.A., Grodzinsky, A.J., Hunziker, E.B. Mechanical compression modulates matrix biosynthesis in chondrocyte/agarose culture. *J. Cell Sci.* 108, 1497, 1995.

22. Hauselmann, H.J., Fernandes, R.J., Mok, S.S., Schmid, T.M., Block, J.A., Aydelotte, M.B., Kuettner, K.E., Thonar, E.J.-M. Phenotypic stability of bovine articular chondrocytes after long-term culture in alginate beads. *J. Cell Sci.* 107, 17, 1994.

23. Haeuselmann, H.J., Masuda, K., Hunziker, E.B., Neidha, M., Mok, S.S., Michel, B.A., Thonar E.J.-M. Adult human chondrocytes cultured in alginate form a matrix similar to native human articular cartilage. *Am. J. Physiol.* 271, C742, 1996.

24. Freed, L.E., Marquis, J.C., Nohria, A., Mikos, A.G., Emmanual, J., Langer, R. Neocartilage formation *in vitro* and *in vivo* using cells cultured on synthetic biodegradable polymers. *J. Biomed. Mater. Res.* 27, 11, 1993.

25. Freed, L.E., Vunjak-Novakovic, G., Biron, R., Eagles, D., Lesnoy, D., Barlow, S., Langer, R. Biodegradable polymer scaffolds for tissue engineering. *Bio/Technology* 12, 689, 1994.

26. Grande, D.A., Halberstadt, C., Naughton, G., Schwartz, R., Manji, R. Evaluation of matrix scaffolds for tissue engineering of articular cartilage grafts. *J. Biomed. Mater. Res.* 34, 211, 1997.

27. Sittinger, M., Bujia, J., Minuth, W.W., Hammer, C., Burmester, G.R. Engineering of cartilage tissue using bioresorbable polymer carriers in perfusion culture. *Biomaterials*, 15, 451, 1994.

28. Dunkelman, N.S., Zimber, M.P., LeBaron, R.G., Pavelec, R., Kwan, M., Purchio, A.F. Cartilage production by rabbit articular chondrocytes on polyglycolic acid scaffolds in a closed bioreactor system. *Biotech. Bioeng.* 46, 299, 1995.

29. Carver, S.E., Heath, C.A. A semi-continuous perfusion system for delivering intermittent physiological pressure to regenerating cartilage. *Tissue Eng.* (in press) 1998.

30. Carver, S.E., Heath, C.A. Increasing extracellular matrix production in regenerating cartilage with intermittent physiological pressure. *Biotech. Bioeng.* (in press) 1998.

31. Adkisson, H.D., Maloney, W.J., Zhang, J., Hruska, K.A. Scaffold-independent neocartilage formation: a novel approach to cartilage engineering. *Trans. Orthop. Res. Soc.* 23, 803, 1998.

32. Freed, L.E., Marquis, J.C., Vunjak-Novakovic, G., Emmanual, J., Langer, R. Composition of cell-polymer cartilage implants, *Biotech. Bioeng.* 43, 605, 1994.

33. Vunjak-Novakovic, G., Obradovic, B., Bursac, P., Martin, I., Langer, R., Freed, L.E. Dynamic seeding of polymer scaffolds for cartilage tissue engineering. *Biotechnol. Prog.* 14, 193, 1998.

34. Freed, L.E., Vunjak-Novakovic, G., Marquis, J.C., Langer, R. Kinetics of chondrocyte growth in cell-polymer implants, *Biotech. Bioeng.* 43, 597, 1994.

35. Vunjak-Novakovic, G., Freed, L.E., Biron, R.J., Langer, R. Effects of mixing on the composition and morphology of tissue engineered cartilage, *J. A.I.Ch.E.* 42, 850, 1996.

36. Freed, L.E., Hollander, A.P., Martin, I., Barry, J., Langer, R., Vunjak-Novakovic, G. Chondrogenesis in a cell-polymer-bioreactor system. *Exp. Cell Res.* 240, 58, 1998.

37. Freed, L.E., Langer, R., Martin, I., Pellis, N., Vunjak-Novakovic, G., Tissue engineering of cartilage in space, *PNAS* 94, 13885, 1997.

38. Riesle, J., Hollander, A.P., Langer, R., Freed, L.E., Vunjak-Novakovic, G. Collagen in tissue engineered cartilage: types, structure and crosslinks. *J. Cell. Biochem.* 71, 313, 1998.

39. Vunjak-Novakovic, G., Martin, I., Obradovic, B., Treppo, S, Grodzinsky, A.J., Langer, R., Freed, L. Bioreactor cultivation conditions modulate the composition and mechanical properties of tissue engineered cartilage. *J. Orthop. Res.* (in press) 1998.

40. Sah, R.L., Trippel, S.B., Grodzinsky, A.J. Differential effects of serum, insulin-like growth factor-I, and fibroblast growth factor-2 on the maintenance of cartilage physical properties during long-term culture. *J. Orthop. Res.* 14, 44, 1996.

41. Armstrong, C.G., Mow, V.C. Variations in the intrinsic mechanical properties of human articular cartilage with age, degeneration, and water content. *J. Bone Joint Surg.* 44A, 88, 1982.

42. Martin, I., Padera, R.F., Vunjak-Novakovic, G., Freed, L.E. *In vitro* differentiation of chick embryo bone marrow stromal cells into cartilaginous and bone-like tissues. *J. Orthop. Res.* 16, 181, 1998.

43. Martin, I., Shastri, V.P., Langer, R., Vunjak-Novakovic, G., Freed, L.E. Engineering autologous cartilaginous implants. BMES Annual Fall Meeting, *Ann. Biomed. Eng.* 26, S-139, 1998.

44. Martin, I., Shastri, V.P., Padera, R.F., Langer, R., Vunjak-Novakovic, G., Freed, L.E. Bone marrow stromal cell differentiation on porous polymer scaffolds. *Trans. Orthop. Res. Soc.* 24, 57, 1999.

45. Shastri, V.P., Martin, I., Langer, R. A versatile approach to produce 3-D polymeric cellular solids. *4th US-Japan Symposium on Drug Delivery Systems*, 1, 36, 1997.

46. Freed, L.E., Vunjak-Novakovic, G. Cultivation of cell-polymer constructs in simulated microgravity. *Biotechnol. Bioeng.* 46, 306, 1995.

47. Freed, L.E., Vunjak-Novakovic, G. Tissue culture bioreactors: chondrogenesis as a model system, In *Principles of Tissue Engineering*, R.P. Lanza, R. Langer, and W.L. Chick, (eds.), Landes & Springer, 1997, chap. 11.

48. Williams, S.N.O., Burstein, D., Gray, M.L., Langer, R., Freed, L.E., Vunjak-Novakovic, G. MRI measurements of fixed charge density as a measure of glycosaminoglycan content and distribution in tissue engineered cartilage. *Trans. Orthop. Res. Soc.* 23, 203, 1998.

49. Kim, Y.J., Sah, R.L., Doong, J.Y.H. et al. Fluorometric assay of DNA in cartilage explants using Hoechst 33258. *Anal. Biochem.* 174, 168, 1988.

50. Farndale, R.W., Buttler, D.J., Barrett, A.J. Improved quantitation and discrimination of sulphated glycosaminoglycans by the use of dimethylmethylene blue. *Biochim. Biophys. Acta* 883, 173, 1986.

51. Woessner, J.F. The determination of hydroxyproline in tissue and protein samples containing small proportions of this amino acid. *Arch. Biochem. Biophys.* 93, 440, 1961.

52. Hollander, A.P., Heathfield, T.F., Webber, C., Iwata, Y., Bourne, R., Rorabeck, C., Poole, R.A. Increased damage to type II collagen in osteoarthritic articular cartilage detected by a new immunoassay. *J. Clin. Invest.* 93, 1722, 1994.

53. Bashir, A., Gray, M.L., Burstein, D. Gd-DTPA2 as a measure of cartilage degradation. *Magn. Res. Med.* 36, 665, 1996.

54. Obradovic, B., Freed, L.E., Langer, R., Vunjak-Novakovic, G. Bioreactor studies of natural and engineered cartilage metabolism. *Fall meeting of the AIChE*, Los Angeles, November, 1997.

55. Frank, E.H., Grodzinsky, A.J. Cartilage electromechanics: II. A continuum model of cartilage electrokinetics and correlation with experiments. *J. Biomech.* 20, 629, 1987.

56. Tachetti, C., Tavella, S., Dozin, B., Quarto, R., Robino, G., and Cancedda, R. Cell condensation in chondrogenic differentiation. *Exp. Cell Res.* 200, 26, 1992.

57. Kulyk, W.M., Coelho, C.N.D., Kosher, R.A. Type IX collagen gene expression during limb cartilage differentiation. *Matrix* 11, 282, 1991.

58. Treilleux, I., Mallein-Gerin, F., le Guellec, D., Herbage, D. Localization of the expression of type I, II, III collagen and aggrecan core protein genes in developing human articular cartilage. *Matrix* 12, 221, 1992.

59. Gerstenfeld, L.C., Landis, W.J. Gene expression and extracellular matrix ultrastructure of a mineralizing chondrocyte cell culture system. *J. Cell Biol.* 112, 501, 1991.

60. Yannas, I.V. *In vivo* synthesis of tissues and organs, In *Principles of Tissue Engineering*, R.P. Lanza, R. Langer, and W. Chick, eds., Academic Press & Landes, Austin, 1997, chap. 12.

61. Thompson, D.W. *On Growth and Form*. Cambridge University Press, New York, 1977.

62. Watt, F. The extracellular matrix and cell shape. *TIBS* 11, 482, 1986.

63. Bruckner, P., Hoerler, I., Mendler, M., Houze, Y., Winterhalter, K.H., Eiach-Bender, S.G., Spycher, M.A. Induction and prevention of chondrocyte hypertrophy in culture *J. Cell Biol.* 109, 2537, 1989.

64. Benya, P.D., Shaffer, J.D. Dedifferentiated chondrocytes reexpress the differentiated collagen phenotype when cultured in agarose gels. *Cell* 30, 215, 1982.

65. Bonaventure, J., Kadhom, N., Cohen-Solal, L., Ng, K.H., Bourguignon, J., Lasselin, C., Freisinger, P. Reexpression of cartilage-specific genes by dedifferentiated human articular chondrocytes cultured in alginate beads. *Exp. Cell Res.* 212, 97, 1994.

66. Vacanti, C., Langer, R., Schloo, B., Vacanti, J.P. Synthetic biodegradable polymers seeded with chondrocytes provide a template for new cartilage formation *in vivo*. *Plast. Reconstr. Surg.* 88, 753, 1991.

67. Watt, F. Effect of seeding density on stability of the differentiated phenotype of pig articular chondrocytes. *J. Cell Sci.* 89, 373, 1988.

68. Abbot, J., Holtzer, H. The loss of phenotypic traits by differentiated cells. *J. Cell Biol.* 28, 473, 1966.

69. Gurdon, J.B. A community effect in animal development. *Nature* 336, 772, 1988.

70. Brockes, J.P. Amphibian limb regeneration: rebuilding a complex structure. *Science* 276, 81, 1997.

71. Zanetti, N.C., Solursh, M. Effect of cell shape on cartilage differentiation, In *Cell Shape: Determinants, Regulation and Regulatory Role*. Academic Press, New York, 1989, chap. 10.

72. Blunk, T., Sieminski, A.L., Nahir, M., Freed, L.E., Vunjak-Novakovic, G., Langer, R. Insulin-like growth factor-I (IGF-I) improves tissue engineering of cartilage *in vitro*. *Proc. Keystone Symp. on Bone and Collagen: Growth and Differentiation*, 1997. Paper 19.

73. Osdoby, P., Caplan, A.I. Scanning electron microscopic investigation of *in vitro* osteogenesis. *Calcif. Tissue Int.* 30, 45, 1980.

74. Johnstone, B., Hering, T.M., Caplan, A.I., Goldberg, V.M., Yoo, J.U. *In vitro* chondrogenesis of bone marrow-derived mesenchymal progenitor cells. *Exp. Cell Res.* 238, 265, 1998.

75. Grodzinsky, A.J., Kamm, R.D., Lauffenburger, D.A. Quantitative aspects of tissue engineering: basic issues in kinetics, transport and mechanics, In *Principles of Tissue Engineering*, R.P.Lanza, R. Langer, and W. Chick, eds., Academic Press & Landes, Austin, 1997, chap. 14.

76. Lightfoot, E.N. The roles of mass transfer in tissue function, In *The Biomedical Engineering Handbook*, J.D. Bronzino, ed., CRC Press, Boca Raton, FL, 1995, chap. 111.

77. O'Hara, B.P., Urban, J.P.G., Maroudas, A. Influence of cyclic loading on the nutrition of articular cartilage. *Ann. Rheum. Dis.* 49, 536, 1990.

78. Bursac, P.M., Freed, L.E., Biron, R.J., Vunjak-Novakovic, G. Mass transfer studies of tissue engineered cartilage. *Tissue Eng.* 2, 141, 1996.

79. Dunkan, R.L., Turner, C.H. Mechanotransduction and the functional response of bone to mechanical strain. *Calc. Tissue Int.* 57, 344, 1995.

80. Slowman, S.D., Brandt, K.D. Composition and glycosaminoglycan metabolism of articular cartilage from habitually loaded and habitually unloaded sites. *Arthrit. Rheum.* 29, 88, 1986.

81. Kiviranta, I., Jurvelin, J., Tammi, M., Saamanen, A.-M., Helminen, H.J. Weight-bearing controls glycosaminoglycan concentration and articular cartilage thickness in the knee joints of young beagle dogs. *Arthritis Rheum.* 3, 801, 1987.

82. Sah, R.L.-Y., Kim, Y.J., Doong, J.Y.H., Grodzinsky, A.J., Plaas, A.H., Sandy, J.D. Biosynythetic response of cartilage explants to dynamic compression. *J. Orthop. Res.* 7, 619, 1989.

83. Parkinnen, J.J., Ikonen, J., Lammi, M.J., Laakkonen, J., Tammi, M., Helminen, H.J. Effect of cyclic hydrostatic pressure on proteoglycan synthesis in cultured chondrocytes and articular cartilage explants. *Arch. Biochem. Biophys.* 300, 458, 1993.

84. Schneidermann, R., Keret, D., Maroudas, A. Effects of mechanical and osmotic pressure on the rate of glycosaminoglycan synthesis in the human adult femoral head cartilage: an *in vitro* study. *J. Orthop. Res.* 4, 393, 1986.

85. Kuettner, K.E., Pauli, B.U., Gall, G., Memoli, V.A., Schenk, R. Synthesis of cartilage matrix by mammalian chondrocytes *in vitro*. Isolation, culture characteristics, and morphology. *J. Cell Biol.* 93, 743, 1982.

86. Kuettner, K.E., Memoli, V.A., Pauli, B.U., Wrobel, N.C., Thonar, E.J.-M.A., Daniel, J.C. Synthesis of cartilage matrix by mammalian chondrocytes *in vitro*— maintenance of collagen and proteoglycan. *J. Cell Biol.* 93, 751, 1982.

87. Smith, R.L., Donlon, B.S., Gupta, M.K., Mohtai, M., Das, P., Carter, D.R., Cooke, J., Gibbons, G., Hutchinson, N., Schurman, D.J. Effect of fluid-induced shear on articular chondrocyte morphology and metabolism *in vitro*. *J. Orthop. Res.* 13, 824, 1995.

88. Franke, R.P., Grafe, M., Schnittler, H., Seiffge, D., Mittermayer, C. Induction of human vascular endothelial stress fibers by fluid shear stress. *Nature* 307, 648, 1984.

89. Wang, N., Ingber, D.E. Control of cytoskeletal mechanics by extracellular matrix, cell shape and mechanical tension. *Biophys. J.* 66, 2181, 1994.

90. Berthiaume, F., Frangos, J. Effects of flow on anchorage-dependent mammalian cells-secreted products, In *Physical Forces and the Mammalian Cell*, J. Frangos, ed., Academic Press, San Diego, 1993, chap. 5.

91. Buckwalter, J.A., Mankin, H.J. Articular cartilage, part II: degeneration and osteoarthrosis, repair, regeneration, and transplantation. *J. Bone Joint Surg.* 79A, 612, 1997.

92. Obradovic, B., Martin, I., Padera, R.F., Treppo, S., Freed, L.E., Vunjak-Novakovic, G. Integration of engineered cartilage into natural cartilage, *Annual Meeting of the AIChE*, Miami, Nov. 1998.

Further Information

Buckwalter, J.A., Ehrlich, M.G., Sandell, L.J., Trippel, S.B. (eds.). *Skeletal Growth and Development: Clinical Issues and Basic Science Advances*, American Academy of Orthopaedic Surgeons, 1998.

Buckwalter, J.A., Mankin, H.J. Articular cartilage repair and transplantation. *Arthrit. Rheum.* 41, 1331, 1998.

Caplan, A.I., Elyaderani, M., Mochizuki, Y., Wakitani, S., Goldberg, V.M. Principles of cartilage repair and regeneration. *Clin. Orthop. Rel. Res.* 342, 254, 1997.

Comper, W.D. (ed). *Extracellular Matrix: Molecular Components and Interactions*, Hardwood Academic Publishers, the Netherlands, 1996.

Newman, A.P. Articular cartilage repair. *Am. J. Sports Med.* 26, 309, 1998.

24

Tissue Engineering of the Kidney

H. David Humes

University of Michigan

Tissue engineering is one of the most intriguing and exciting areas in biotechnology due to its requirements for state-of-the-art techniques from both biologic and engineering disciplines. This field is on the threshold of the development of an array of products and devices comprised of cell components, biologic compounds, and synthetic materials to replace physiologic function of diseased tissues and organs.

Successful tissue and organ constructs depend on a thorough understanding and creative application of molecular, cellular, and organ biology and the principles of chemical, mechanical, and material engineering to produce appropriate structure-function relationships to restore, maintain, or improve tissue or organ function. This approach depends on the most advanced scientific methodologies, including stem cell culture, gene transfer, growth factors, and biomaterial technologies.

The kidney was the first solid organ whose function was approximated by a machine and a synthetic device. In fact, renal substitution therapy with hemodialysis or chronic ambulatory peritoneal dialysis (CAPD) has been the only successful long-term *ex vivo* organ substitution therapy to date [1]. The kidney was also the first organ to be successfully transplanted from a donor individual to an autologous recipient patient. However, the lack of widespread availability of suitable transplantable organs has kept kidney transplantation from becoming a practical solution to most cases of chronic renal failure.

Although long-term chronic renal replacement therapy with either hemodialysis or CAPD has dramatically changed the prognosis of renal failure, it is not complete replacement therapy, since it only provides filtration function (usually on an intermittent basis) and does not replace the homeostatic, regulatory, metabolic, and endocrine functions of the kidney. Because of the nonphysiologic manner in which dialysis performs or does not perform the most critical renal functions, patients with ESRD on dialysis continue to have major medical, social, and economic problems [2]. Accordingly, dialysis should be considered as renal substitution rather than renal replacement therapy.

Tissue engineering of a biohybrid kidney comprised of both biologic and synthetic components will most likely have substantial benefits for the patient by increasing life expectancy, increasing mobility and flexibility, increasing quality of life with large savings in time, less risk of infection, and reduced costs. This approach could also be considered a cure rather than a treatment for patients.

24.1 Fundamentals of Kidney Function

The kidneys are solid organs located behind the peritoneum in the posterior abdomen and are critical to body homeostasis because of their excretory, regulatory, metabolic, and endocrinologic functions. The excretory function is initiated by filtration of blood at the glomerulus, which is an enlargement of the proximal end of the tubule incorporating a vascular tuft. The structure of the glomerulus is designed to provide efficient ultrafiltration of blood to remove toxic waste from the circulation yet retain important circulating components, such as albumin. The regulatory function of the kidney, especially with regard to fluid and electrolyte homeostasis, is provided by the tubular segments attached to the glomerulus.

The ultrafiltrate emanating from the glomerulus courses along the kidney tubule, which resorbs fluid and solutes to finely regulate their excretion in various amounts in the final urine. The kidney tubules are segmented, with each segment possessing differing transport characteristics for processing the glomerular ultrafiltrate efficiently and effectively to regulate urine formation. The segments of the tubule begin with the proximal convoluted and straight tubules, where most salt and water are resorbed. This segment leads into the thin and thick segments of Henle's loop, which are critical to the countercurrent system for urinary concentration and dilution of water. The distal tubule is next and is important for potassium excretion. The final segment is the collecting duct, which provides the final regulation of sodium, hydrogen, and water excretion. The functional unit of the kidney is therefore composed of the filtering unit (the glomerulus) and the regulatory unit (the tubule). Together they form the basic component of the kidney, the nephron. In addition to these excretory and regulatory functions, the kidney is an important endocrine organ. Erythropoietin, active forms of vitamin D, renin, angiotensin, prostaglandins, leukotrienes, and kallikrein-kinins are some of the endocrinologic compounds produced by the kidney.

In order to achieve its homeostatic function for salt and water balance in the individual, the kidney has a complex architectural pattern (Fig. 24.1). This complex organization is most evident in the exquisitely regulated structure-function interrelationships between the renal tubules and vascular structures to coordinate the countercurrent multiplication and exchange processes to control water balance with urinary concentration and dilution [3]. This complex structure is the result of a long evolutionary process in which animals adapted to many changing environmental conditions. Although well suited for maintaining volume homeostasis, the mammalian kidney is an inefficient organ for solute and water excretion. In humans, approximately 180 liters of fluid are filtered into the tubules daily, but approximately 178 liters must be reabsorbed into the systemic circulation. Because of the importance of maintaining volume homeostasis in an individual to prevent volume depletion, shock, and death, multiple redundant physiologic systems exist within the body to maintain volume homeostasis. No such redundancy, however, exists to replace renal excretory function of soluble metabolic toxic by-products of metabolic activity. Accordingly, chronic renal disease becomes a clinical disorder due to loss of renal excretory function and buildup within the body of metabolic toxins which require elimination by the kidneys. Because of the efficiency inherent in the kidneys as an excretory organ, life can be sustained with only 5–10% of normal renal excretory function. With the recognition that the complexity of renal architectural organization is driven by homeostatic rather than excretory function and that renal excretory function is the key physiologic process which must be maintained or replaced to treat clinical renal failure, the approach to a tissue engineering construct becomes easier to entertain, especially since only a fraction of normal renal excretory function is required to maintain life.

For elimination of solutes and water from the body, the kidney utilizes simple fundamental physical principles which govern fluid movement (Fig. 24.2). The kidney's goal in excretory function is to transfer solutes and water from the systemic circulation into tubule conduits in order to eliminate toxic by-products from the body in a volume of only several liters. Solute and fluid removal from the systemic circulation is the major task of the renal filtering apparatus, the glomerulus. The force responsible for this filtration process is the hydraulic pressure generated within the system circulation due to myocardial contraction and blood vessel contractile tone. Most of the filtered fluid and solutes must be selectively reabsorbed by the renal tubule as the initial filtrate courses along the renal tubules. The reabsorptive process depends upon osmotic forces generated by active solute transport by the renal epithelial cell and the colloid oncotic pressure within the peritubular capillary (Fig. 24.2). The approach of a tissue-engineering construct for renal replacement is to mimic these natural physical forces to duplicate filtration and reabsorption processes to attain adequate excretory function lost in renal disorders.

Glomerular Ultrafiltration

The process of urine formation begins within the capillary bed of the glomerulus [4]. The glomerular capillary wall has evolved into a structure with the property to separate as much as one-third of the plasma entering the glomerulus into a solution of a nearly ideal ultrafitrate. The high rate of ultrafiltration across the glomerular capillary is a result of hydraulic pressure generated by the pumping action of the heart and the vascular tone of the preglomerular and postglomerular vessels as well as the high hydraulic permeability of the glomerular capillary walls. This hydraulic pressure as well as the hydraulic permeability of the glomerular capillary bed is at least two times and two orders of magnitude higher, respectively, than most other capillary networks within the body [5]. Despite this high rate of water and solute flux across the glomerular capillary wall, this same structure retards the filtration of important circulating macromolecules, especially albumin, so that all but the lower-molecular-weight plasma proteins are restricted in their passage across the filtration barrier.

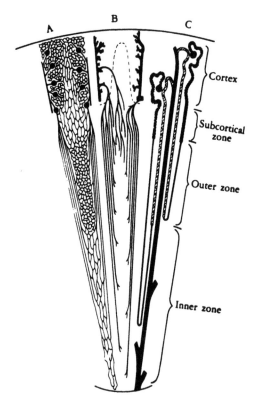

FIGURE 24.1 Representation of the complex morphologic architecture of a section of a mammalian kidney in which these components are schematized separately: (A) arterial and capillary blood vessels; (B) venous drainage; (C) two nephrons with their glomeruli and tubule segments (From Kriz, W. and Lever, A.F. [3]. With permission.)

A variety of experimental studies and model systems have been employed to characterize the sieving properties of the glomerulus. Hydrodynamic models of solute transport through pores have been successfully used to describe the size selective barrier function of this capillary network to macromolecules [6]. This pore model, in its simplest form, assumes the capillary wall to contain cylindrical pores of identical size and that macromolecules are spherical particles. Based upon the steric hindrances that macromolecules encounter in the passage through small pores, whether by diffusion or by convection (bulk flow of fluid), definition of the glomerular capillary barrier can be a fluid-filled cylindrical pore (Fig. 24.3). This modeling characterizes the glomerular capillary barrier as a membrane with uniform pores of 50 Å radius [7]. This pore size predicts that molecules with radii smaller than 14 Å appear in the filtrate in the same concentration as in plasma water. Since there is no restriction to filtration, fractional clearance of this size molecule is equal to one. The filtration of molecules of increasing size decreases progressively, so that the fractional clearance of macromolecules the size of serum albumin (36 Å) is low.

The glomerular barrier, however, does not restrict molecular transfer across the capillary wall only on the basis of size (Fig. 24.4). This realization is based upon the observation that the filtration of the circulating protein, albumin, is restricted to a much greater extent than would be predicted from size alone. The realization that albumin is a polyanion at physiologic pH suggests that molecular charge, in addition to molecular size, is another important determination of filtration of macromolecules [8]. The

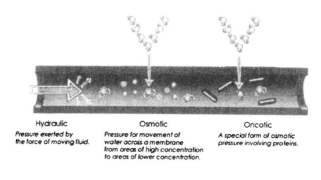

Hydraulic	Osmotic	Oncotic
Pressure exerted by the force of moving fluid.	*Pressure for movement of water across a membrane from areas of high concentration to areas of lower concentration.*	*A special form of osmotic pressure involving proteins.*

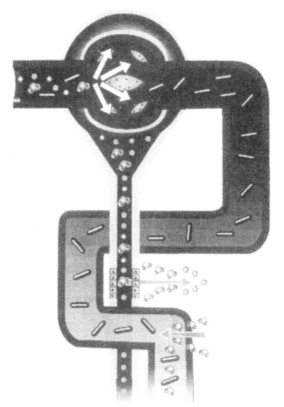

FIGURE 24.2   Physical forces which govern fluid transfer within the kidney.

greater restriction to the filtration of circulating polyanions, including albumin, is due to the electrostatic hindrance by fixed negatively charged components of the glomerular capillary barrier. These fixed negative charges, as might be expected, simultaneously enhance the filtration of circulating polycations.

Thus, the formation of glomerular ultrafiltrate, the initial step in urine formation, depends upon the pressure and flows within the glomerular capillary bed and the intrinsic permselectivity of the glomerular capillary wall. The permselective barrier excludes circulating macromolecules from filtration based upon size as well as net molecular charge, so that for any given size, negatively charged macromolecules are restricted from filtration to a greater extent than neutral molecules.

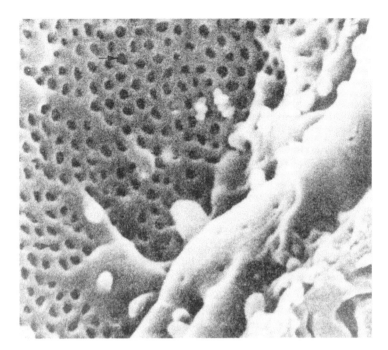

FIGURE 24.3 Scanning electron micrograph of the glomerular capillary wall demonstrating the fenestrae (pores) of the endothelium within the glomerulus (mag × 50,400). (Reprinted with permission from Schrier RW, Gottschalk CW. 1988. Diseases of the Kidney, p 12, Boston, Little, Brown.)

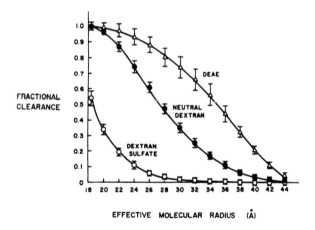

FIGURE 24.4 Fractional clearances of negatively charged (sulfate) dextrans, neutral dextrans, and positively charged (DEAE) dextrans of varying molecular size. These data demonstrate that the glomerular capillary wall behaves as both a size-selective and charge-selective barrier [8].

Tubule Reabsorption

Normal human kidneys form approximately 100 ml of filtrate every minute. Since daily urinary volume is roughly 2 l more than 98% of the glomerular ultrafiltrate must be reabsorbed by the renal tubule. The bulk of the reabsorption, 50–65%, occurs along the proximal tubule. Similar to glomerular filtration, fluid movement across the renal proximal tubule cell is governed by physical forces. Unlike the fluid transfer across the glomerular capillary wall, however, tubular fluid flux is principally driven by osmotic and oncotic pressures rather than hydraulic pressure (Fig. 24.2). Renal proximal tubule fluid reabsorption is based upon active Na^+ transport, requiring the energy-dependent Na^+K^+ ATPase located along the basolateral membrane of the renal tubule cell to promote a small degree of luminal hypotonicity [9]. This small degree of osmotic difference (2–3 mOsm/kgH$_2$O) across the renal tubule is sufficient to drive isotonic fluid reabsorption due to the very high diffusive water permeability of the renal tubule cell membrane. Once across the renal proximal tubule cell, the transported fluid is taken up by the peritubular capillary bed due to the favorable oncotic pressure gradient. This high oncotic pressure within the peritubular capillary is the result of the high rate of protein-free filtrate formed in the proximate glomerular capillary bed [10]. As can be appreciated, the kidney has evolved two separate capillary networks to control bulk fluid flow from various fluid compartments of the body. The glomerular capillary network has evolved an efficient structure to function as a highly efficient filter to allow water and small solutes, such as urea and sodium, to cross the glomerular capillary wall while retaining necessary macromolecules, such as albumin. This fluid transfer is driven by high hydraulic pressures within the glomerular capillary network generated by the high blood flow rates to the kidney and a finely regulated vascular system. The permselectivity of the filter is governed by an effective pore size to discriminate macromolecular sieving based upon both size and net molecular charge. The high postglomerular vascular resistance and the protein-free glomerular filtrate results, respectively, in low hydraulic pressure and high oncotic pressure within the peritubular capillary system which follows directly in series from the glomerular capillary network. The balance of physical forces within the peritubular capillaries, therefore, greatly favors the uptake of fluid back into the systemic circulation. The addition of a renal epithelial monolayer with high rates of active Na^+ transport and high hydraulic permeability assists further in the high rate of salt and water reabsorption along the proximal tubule. Thus, an elegant system has evolved in the nephron to filter and reabsorb large amounts of fluid in bulk to attain high rates of metabolic product excretion while maintaining regulatory salt and water balance.

Endocrine

As an endocrine organ, the kidney has been well recognized as critical in the production of erythropoietin, a growth factor for red blood cell production, and vitamin D, a compound important in calcium metabolism, along with, but not limited to, prostaglandins, kinins, and renin. For the purposes of this chapter, this discussion will be limited to erythropoietin production as an example of a potential formulation of a tissue-engineering construct to replace this lost endocrine function in chronic end-stage renal disease.

More than 40 years ago erythropoietin was shown to be the hormone that regulates erythropoiesis, or red blood cell production, in the bone marrow [11]. In adults, erythropoietin is produced primarily (greater than 90%) by specialized interstitial cells in the kidney [12]. Although the liver also synthesizes erythropoietin, the quantity is not adequate (less than 10%) to maintain adequate red cell production in the body [13]. The production of erythropoietin by the kidney is regulated by a classic endocrinologic feedback loop system. As blood flows through the kidney, the erythropoietin-producing cells are in an ideal location to sense oxygen delivery to tissues by red cells in the bloodstream, since they are located adjacent to peritubular capillaries in the renal interstitium.

As demonstrated in Fig. 24.5, erythropoietin production is inversely related to oxygen delivery to the renal interstitial cells. With hypoxemia or decline in red blood cell mass, a decline in oxygen delivery occurs to these specialized cells, and increased erythropoietin production develops. Upon return to normal oxygen delivery with normoxia and red blood cell mass, the enhanced production of erythropoietin is suppressed, closing the classic feedback loop. Of importance, the regulation of erythropoietin in the kidney cells depends upon transcriptional control, not upon secretory control, as seen with insulin [14]. The precise molecular mechanism of the oxygen sensor for tissue oxygen availability has not been delineated but appears to depend on a heme protein.

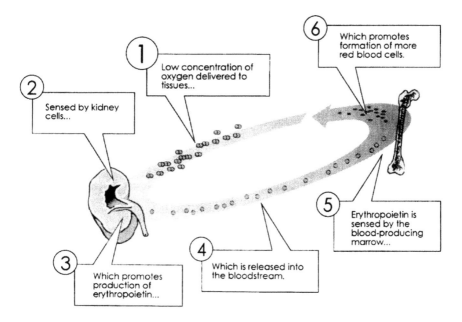

FIGURE 24.5 Endocrinologic back loop which regulates erythropoietin production by the kidney.

Once erythropoietin is released, it circulates in the bloodstream to the bone marrow, where it signals the marrow to produce red blood cells. In this regard, all blood cells, both white and red cells, originate from a subset of bone marrow cells, called *multipotent stem cells*. These stem cells develop during embryonic development and are maintained through adulthood via self-regulation. Under appropriate stimulation, stem cells proliferate and produce committed, more highly differentiated progenitor cells which are then destined to a specific differentiated line of blood cells, including neutrophils, lymphocytes, platelets, and red cells. Specifically, erythropoietin binds to receptors on the outer membrane of committed erythroid progenitor cells, stimulating the terminal steps in erythroid differentiation. Nearly 200 years ago, it was first recognized that anemia is a complication of chronic renal failure. Ordinarily an exponential increase in serum erythropoietin levels is observed when hemoglobin level in patients declines below 10 g/dl. In the clinical state of renal disease, however, the normal increase in erythropoietin in response to anemia is impaired [14]. Although the oxygen delivery (or hemoglobin) to erythropoietin feedback loop is still intact, the response is dramatically diminished. In patients with end-stage renal disease (ESRD), the hematocrit levels are directly correlated to circulating erythropoietin levels. In fact, ERSD patients with bilateral nephrectomies have the lowest hematocrits and lowest rates of erythropoiesis, demonstrating that even the small amount of erythropoietin produced by the end-stage kidney is important. Thus, the loss of renal function due to chronic disease results in an endocrine deficiency of a hormone normally produced by the kidney and results in a clinical problem that complicates the loss of renal excretory function.

24.2 Tissue-Engineering Formulation Based upon Fundamentals

In designing an implantable bioartificial kidney for renal replacement function, essential functions of kidney tissue must be utilized to direct the design of the tissue-engineering project. The critical elements of renal function must be replaced, including the excretory, regulatory (reabsorptive), and endocrinologic functions. The functioning excretory unit of the kidney, as detailed previously, is composed of the filtering unit, the glomerulus, and the regulatory or reabsorptive unit, the tubule. Therefore, a bioartificial kidney requires two main units, the glomerulus and the tubule, to replace renal excretory function.

Bioartificial Glomerulus: The Filter

The potential for a bioartificial glomerulus has been achieved with the use of polysulfone fibers *ex vivo* with maintenance of ultrafiltration in humans for several weeks with a single device [15, 16]. The availability of hollow fibers with high hydraulic permeability has been an important advancement in biomaterials for replacement function of glomerular ultrafiltration. Conventional hemodialysis for ESRD has used membranes in which solute removal is driven by a concentration gradient of the solute across the membranes and is, therefore, predominantly a diffusive process. Another type of solute transfer also occurs across the dialysis membrane via a process of ultrafiltration of water and solutes across the membrane. This convective transport is independent of the concentration gradient and depends predominantly on the hydraulic pressure gradient across the membrane. Both diffusive and convective processes occur during traditional hemodialysis, but diffusion is the main route of solute movement.

The development of synthetic membranes with high hydraulic permeability and solute retention properties in convenient hollow fiber form has promoted ERSD therapy based upon convective homofiltration rather than diffusive hemodialysis [17, 18]. Removal of uremic toxins, predominantly by the convective process, has several distinct advantages, because it imitates the glomerular process of toxin removal with increased clearance of higher-molecular-weight solutes and removal of all solutes (up to a molecular weight cutoff) at the same rate. The comparison of the differences between diffusive and convective transport across a semipermeable membrane is detailed in Fig. 24.6. This figure demonstrates the relationship between molecular size and clearance by diffusion and convection. As seen, the clearance of a molecule by diffusion is negatively correlated with the size of the molecule. In contrast, clearance of a substance by convection is independent of size up to a certain molecular weight. The bulk movement of water carries passable solutes along with it in approximately the same concentration as in the fluid.

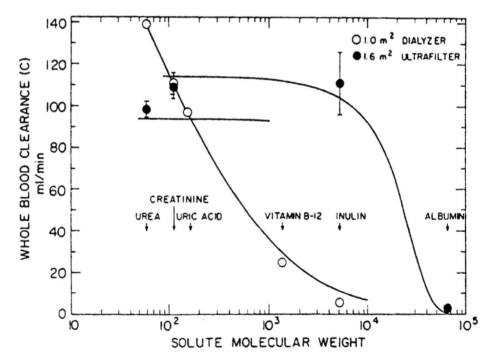

FIGURE 24.6 Relationship between solute molecular size and clearance by diffusion (open circles) and convection (closed circles). Left curve shows solute clearance for a 1.0 m² dialyzer with no ultrafiltration where solute clearance is diffusion. Right curve shows clearance for a 1.6 m² ultrafilter where solute clearance is by convection. Smaller molecules are better cleared by diffusion, larger molecules by convection. Normal kidneys clear solutes in a pattern similar to convective transport. (Adapted from Henderson, L.W. et al., 1975 [18].)

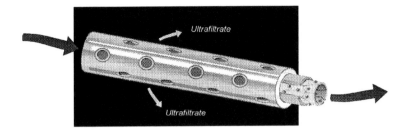

FIGURE 24.7 Conceptual schematization of bioartificial glomerulus.

Development of an implantable device which mimics glomerular filtration will thus depend upon convective transport. This physiologic function has been achieved clinically with the use of polymeric hollow fibers *ex vivo*. Major limitations to the currently available technology for long-term replacement of filtration function include bleeding associated with required anticoagulation, diminution of filtration rate due to protein deposition in the membrane over time or thrombotic occlusion, and large amounts of fluid replacement required to replace the ultrafiltrate formed from the filtering unit. The use of endothelial-cell-seeded conduits along filtration surfaces may provide improved long-term hemocompatibility and hemofiltaration *in vivo* [19–21], as schematized in Fig. 24.7.

In this regard, endothelial cell seeding of small-caliber vascular prosthesis has been shown experimentally to reduce long-term platelet deposition, thrombus formation, and loss of graft patency [21]. Recent results in humans have demonstrated success in autologous endothelial cell seeding in small-caliber grafts after growth of these cells along the graft lumen *ex vivo* to achieve a confluent monolayer prior to implantation. Long-term persistent endothelialization and patency of the implanted graft has been reported [19]. A potential rate-limiting step in endothelial-cell-lined hollow fibers of small caliber is thrombotic occlusion, which limits the functional patency of this filtration unit. In this regard, gene transfer into seeded endothelial cells for constitutive expression of anticoagulant factors can be envisioned to minimize clot formation in these small-caliber hollow fibers. Since gene transfer for *in vivo* protein production has been clearly achieved with endothelial cells [22, 23], gene transfer into endothelial cells for the production of an anticoagulant protein is clearly conceivable.

For differentiated endothelial cell morphology and function, an important role for various components of the extracellular matrix (ECM) has been demonstrated [24, 25]. The ECM has been clearly shown to dictate phenotype and gene expression of endothelial cells, thereby modulating morphogenesis and growth. Various components of ECM, including collagen by type I, collagen type IV, laminin, and fibronectin, have been shown to affect endothelial cell adherence, growth, and differentiation. Of importance, ECM produced by MDCK cells, a permanent renal epithelial cell line, has the ability to induce capillary endothelial cells to produce fenestrations [25, 26]. Endothelial cell fenestrations are large openings which act as channels or pores for convective transport though the endothelial monolayer and are important in the high hydraulic permeability and sieving characteristics of glomerular capillaries. Thus, the ECM component on which the endothelial cells attach and grow may be critical in the functional characteristics of the lining monolayer.

Bioartificial Tubule: The Reabsorber

As detailed above, the efficiency of reabsorption, even though dependent upon natural physical forces governing fluid movement across biologic as well as synthetic membranes, requires specialized epithelial cells to perform vectorial solute transport. Critical to the advancement of this tubule construct, as well as for the tissue-engineering field in general, is the need for the isolation and growth *in vitro* of specific cells, referred to as *stem progenitor cells*, from adult tissues.

Stem or Progenitor Cells

These cells are those that possess stem-cell-like characteristics with a high capacity for self-renewal under defined conditions into specialized cells to develop correct structure and functional components of a physiologic organ system [27–29]. Stem cells have been extensively studied in three adult mammalian tissues: the hematopoietic system, the epidermis, and the intestinal epithelium. Recent work has also suggested that stem cells may also reside in the adult nervous system [30]. Little insight into possible renal tubule stem cells had been developed until recent data demonstrating methodology to isolate and grow renal proximal tubule stem or progenitor cells from adult mammalian kidneys [31, 32]. This series of studies was promoted by the clinical and experimental observations suggesting that renal proximal tubule progenitor cells must exist, because they have the ability to regenerate after severe neophrotoxic or ischemic injury to form a fully functional and differentiated epithelium [33, 34]. Whether proximal tubule progenitor cells are pluripotent, possessing the ability to differentiate into cells of other segments (such as loop of Henle, distal convoluted tubule) as in embryonic kidney development, is at present unclear; the clinical state of acute tubular necrosis certainly supports the idea that proximal tubule progenitor cells have the ability to replicate and differentiate into proximal tubule cells with functionally and morphologically differentiated phenotypes.

In this regard, recent data have demonstrated, using renal proximal tubule cells in primary culture, that the growth factors transforming growth factor-β1 (TGF-β1) and the epidermal growth factor (EGF), along with the retinoid, retinoic acid, promoted tubulogenesis in renal proximal tubule progenitor cells in tissue culture [31]. These observations defined a coordinated interplay between growth factors and retinoids to induce pattern formation and morphogenesis. This finding is one of the first definitions of inductive factors which may be important in the organogenesis of a mammalian organ. In addition, using immunofluorescence microscopy, retinoic acid induced laminin A- and B$_1$-chain production in these cells and purified soluble laminin completely substituted for retinoic acid in kidney tubulogenesis. These results clearly demonstrate the manner in which retinoic acid, as a morphogen, can promote pattern formation and differentiation by regulating the production of an extracellular matrix molecule.

Further work has demonstrated, in fact, that a population of cells resides in the adult mammalian kidney which have retained the capacity to proliferate and morphogenically differentiate into tubule structures *in vitro* [32]. These experiments have identified non-serum-containing growth conditions, which select for proximal tubule cells with a high capacity for self-renewal and an ability to differentiate phenotypically, collectively and individually, into proximal tubule structures in collagen gels. Regarding the high capacity for self-renewal, genetic marking of the cells with a recombinant retrovirus containing the *lacZ* gene and dilution analysis demonstrated that *in vitro* tubulogenesis often arose from clonal expansion of a single genetically tagged progenitor cell. These results suggest that a population of proximal tubule cells exists within the adult kidney in a relatively dormant, slowly replicative state, but with a rapid potential to proliferate, differentiate, and pattern-form to regenerate the lining proximal tubule epithelium of the kidney following severe ischemic or toxic injury.

Bioartificial Tubule Formulation

The bioartificial renal tubule is now clearly feasible when conceived as a combination of living cells supported on polymeric substrata [35]. A bioartificial tubule uses epithelial progenitor cells cultured on water and solute-permeable membranes seeded with various biomatrix materials so that expression of differentiated vectorial transport and metabolic and endocrine function is attained (Figs. 24.8 and 24.9). With appropriate membranes and biomatrices, immunoprotection of cultured progenitor cells can be achieved concurrent with long-term functional performance as long as conditions support tubule cell viability [35, 36]. The technical feasibility of an implantable epithelial cell system derived from cells grown as confluent monolayers along the luminal surface of polymeric hollow fibers has been achieved [35]. These previously constructed devices, however, have used permanent renal cell lines which do not have differentiated transport function. The ability to purify and grow renal proximal tubule progenitor cells with the ability to differentiate morphogenically may provide a capability for replacement renal tubule function.

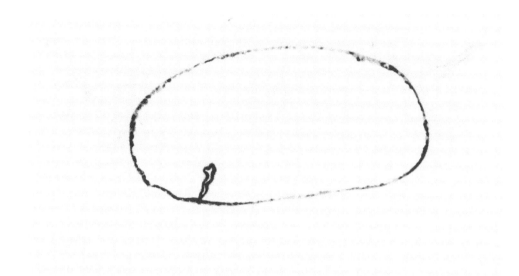

FIGURE 24.8 Light micrograph of an H&E section (100×) of hollow fiber lined with collagen type IV and confluent monolayer of human renal tubule epithelial cells along the inner component of the fiber. In this fixation process, the hollow fiber is clear with the outer contour of the hollow fiber identified by the irregular line (disregard artifact in lower left quadrant).

A bioartificial proximal tubule satisfies a major requirement of reabsorbing a large volume of filtrate to maintain salt and water balance within the body. The need for additional tubule equivalents to replace another nephronal segment function, such as the loop of Henle, to perform more refined homeostatic elements of the kidney, including urine concentration or dilution, may not be necessary. Patients with moderate renal insufficiency lose the ability to finely regulate salt and water homeostasis—because they are unable to concentrate or dilute—yet are able to maintain reasonable fluid and electrolyte homeostasis due to redundant physiologic compensation via other mechanisms. Thus, a bioartificial proximal tubule, which reabsorbs iso-osmotically the majority of the filtrate, may be sufficient to replace required tubular function to sustain fluid electrolyte balance in a patient with end-stage renal disease.

Bioartificial Kidney

The development of a bioartificial filtration device and a bioartificial tubule processing unit would lead to the possibility of an implantable bioartificial kidney, consisting of the filtration device followed in series by the tubule unit (Fig. 24.10). The filtrate formed by this device will flow directly into the tubule unit. The tubule unit should maintain viability, because metabolic substrates and low-molecular-weight growth factors are delivered to the tubule cells from the ultrafiltration unit. Furthermore, immunoprotection of the cells grown within the hollow fiber is achievable due to the impenetrance of immunologically competent cells through the hollow fiber. Rejection of transplanted cells will, therefore, not occur. This arrangement thereby allows the filtrate to enter the internal compartments of the hollow fiber network, which are lined with confluent monolayers of renal tubule cells for regulated transport function.

This device could be used either extracoporeally or implanted within a patient. In this regard, the specific implant site for a bioartificial kidney will depend upon the final configuration of both the bioartificial filtration and tubule device. As currently conceived, the endothelial-line bioartificial filtration hollow fibers can be placed into an arteriovenous circuit using the common iliac artery and vein, similar to the surgical connection for a renal transplant. The filtrate is connected in series to a bioartificial proximal tubule, which is embedded into the peritoneal membrane, so that reabsorbate will be transported into the peritoneal cavity and reabsorbed into the systemic circulation. The processed filtrate

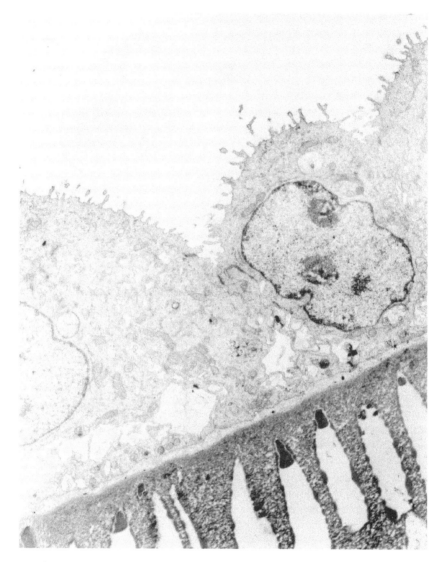

FIGURE 24.9 Electron micrograph of a single hollow fiber lined with extracellular matrix and a confluent mono-layer (see Fig. 24.8) of renal tubule cells along the inner component of the fiber. As displayed, the differentiated phenotype of renal tubule cells on the hollow fiber prelined with matrix is apparent. The well-developed microvilli and apical tight junctions can be appreciated (14,000×).

exiting the tubule unit is then connected via tubing to the proximate ureter for drainage and urine excretion via the recipient's own urinary collecting system.

Although an implantable form of this therapy is in the conceptual phase of development, a functioning extracorporeal bioartificial renal tubule has been developed. The technical feasibility of an epithelial cell system derived from cells grown as confluent monolayers along the luminal surface of polymeric hollow fibers has been recently achieved [38]. Because of its anatomic and physiologic similarities with humans and the relative simplicity with which it can be bred in large numbers, the pig is currently considered the best source of organs for both human xenotransplantation and immuno-isolated cell therapy devices [39–41]. Yorkshire breed pig renal tubule progenitor cells have been expanded and cultured on semi-permeable hollow fiber membranes seeded with various biomatrix materials, so that expression of differentiated vectorial transport, metabolic, and endocrine function has been attained [38, 42, 43]. This

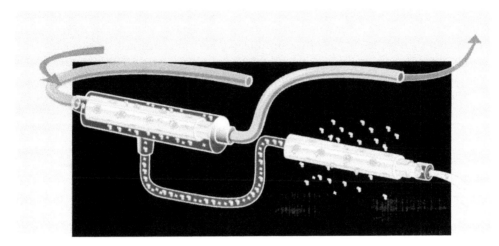

FIGURE 24.10   Conceptual schematization of an implantable tissue engineered bioartificial kidney with an endo-thelial-cell-lined hemofilter in series with a proximal tubule-cell-lined reabsorber.

bioartificial renal tubule has been evaluated in uremic and non-uremic large animals [44]. A customized extracorporeal circuit using standard arterial venous blood tubing with a dialysis machine has been developed which delivers the post-filtered blood through the extracapillary space and the ultrafiltrate through the liminal space of the bioartificial tubule. Experiments have confirmed the functional metabolic performance and active tubule transport properties of the bioartificial renal tubule using this extracorporeal circuit [44]. Proximal tubule cells derive embryonically from mesodermal progenitors closely related to bone marrow precursor cells and have retained many elements of immunologically competent cells, including the ability for antigen presentation and production of a variety of immunologically active cytokines [45]. Since the kidney participates in this complex and dynamic network of pro- and anti-inflammatory cytokines, cell replacement therapy with an extracorporeal bioartificial renal tubule assist device may play a critical role in the future treatment of renal failure.

Bioartificial Endocrine Gland

The Erythropoietin Generator

Because specialized cells are programmed to carry out specific biologic tasks, cell therapy may deliver several key proteins in a coordinated cascade to promote a biologic or physiologic process. Targeted delivery of a specific deficient protein, hormone, or neurotransmitter may be achieved with site-specific implantation of cells which can produce this deficient compound after being encapsulated in special polymeric membranes. The membranes allow cell nutrients into the encapsulated space to maintain cell viability and allow cellular metabolic wastes to exit along with the desired protein, hormone, or neurotransmitter while shielding the cells from the host's destructive immune response. This strategy is being employed, for example, to deliver dopamine produced by bovine adrenal cells to the substantia nigra where a deficiency of this neurotransmitter at this site leads to Parkinson's disease [46].

Regulated and homeostatic drug dosing may also be achieved with cell therapy. For hormonal therapy, such as insulin for diabetes mellitus, appropriate insulin levels within the body are only crudely attained with a once-a-day or twice-a-day dosing. Any hormone-producing cell has a highly evolved biologic sensing system to monitor the ambient environment and respond with graded production and release of the hormone to regulate the sensed level of the moiety which is regulated. The circulating level of a protein or a hormone may be regulated at several levels: at the gene level by transcriptional mechanisms, at the protein level by translational processes, or at the secretory level by cellular processes. The complexity of regulation increases several-fold, as control progresses from transcriptional to translational to excretory processes. Accordingly, a more refined differentiated cell phenotype is required to maintain a regulated secretory process compared to a transcriptional process. The lack of success of encapsulation of insulin-producing cells is due to the fact that the cells are unable to maintain a viable, highly differentiated state to sense ambient glucose levels and release performed insulin in a regulated, differentiated secretory pathway. In contrast, since erythropoietin production is regulated by transcriptional mechanisms, the ability to identify and perhaps grow cells from adult mammalian kidneys with the ability to regulate erythropoietin production in response to oxygen delivery may allow the design of an implantable cell therapy device to sense circulating oxygen levels and regulate erythropoeitin production based upon a biologic sensing mechanism. Recently, genetically engineered polymer encapsulated myoblasts have been shown to continuously deliver human and mouse erythropoietin in mice [47].

24.3 Clinical and Economic Implications

Although long-term chronic renal replacement therapy with either hemodialysis or CAPD has dramatically changed the prognosis of renal failure, it is not complete replacement therapy, since it only provides filtration function (usually on an intermittent basis) and does not replace the excretory, regulatory, and endocrine functions of the kidney. Because of the nonphysiologic manner in which dialysis performs or does not perform the most critical renal functions, patients with ESRD on dialysis continue to have major medical, social, and economic problems. Renal transplant addresses some of these issues, but immunologic barriers and organ shortages keep this approach from being ideal for a large number of ESRD patients.

Although dialysis or transplantation therapies can prolong the life of a patient with ESRD disease, it is still a serious medical condition, with ESRD patients having only one-fifth the life expectancy of a normal age-matched control group. ESRD patients also experience significantly greater morbidity. Patients with ESRD have five times the hospitalization rate, nearly twice the disability rate, and five times the unemployment rate of age-matched non-ESRD individuals [2]. Accordingly, this new technology based upon the proposed bioengineering prototypes would most likely have substantial benefits to the patient by increasing life expectancy, increasing mobility and flexibility, increasing quality of life with large savings in time, less risk of infection, and reduced costs.

Besides the personal costs to the patient and family, care of chronic kidney failure is monetarily expensive on a per-capita basis in comparison to most forms of medical care [1, 2]. The 1989 estimated Medicare payment (federal only) per ESRD patient during the entire year averaged $30,900. The patient and private insurance obligations were an addition $6900 per patient. The total cost of a patient per year with end-stage renal disease, therefore, is approximately $40,000. In 1988 the expected life span after beginning dialysis for an ESRD patient was approximately 4 years; therefore, the total cost per patient of ESRD during his or her lifetime was approximately $160,000 in 1988.

The total cost in direct medical payments for ESRD, by both public and private payers, increased from $6 billion in 1989 to over $14 billion in 1996 [48]. These estimates do not include a number of indirect cost items, since they do not include patient travel costs and lost labor production. The number of patients receiving chronic dialytic therapy in the U.S. is at present over 250,000 with a current growth rate at 8 to 10% per year. It is conceivable that in the not too distant future, tissue engineering technology could supplant current treatments for ESRD. Although it is difficult to estimate the value of a technology, on a purely economic basis there may be an opportunity for major cost savings with this technology.

24.4 Summary

Three technologies will most likely dominate medical therapeutics in the next century. One is "cell therapy"—the implantation of living cells to produce a natural substance in short supply from the patient's own cells due to injury and destruction from various clinical disorders. Erythropoietin cell therapy is an example of this approach to replace a critical hormone deficiency in end-stage renal disease. A second therapy is tissue engineering, wherein cells are cultured to replace masses of cells that normally function in a coordinated manner. Growing a functional glomerular filter and tubule reabsorber from a combination of cells, biomaterials, and synthetic polymers to replace renal excretory and regulatory functions is an example of this formulation. Over the last few years, an extracorporeal bioartificial renal tubule has become a reality, demonstrating physiologic and biochemical regulatory function in large animal studies. Finally, a third technology that will dominate future therapeutics is gene therapy, in which genes are transferred into living cells either to deliver a gene product to a cell in which it is missing or to produce a foreign gene product by a cell to promote a new function. The use of genes which encode for anticoagulant proteins as a means to deliver in a targeted and local fashion an anticoagulant to maintain hemocompatibility of a tissue engineered hemofilter is an example of the application of this third technology.

The kidney was the first organ whose function was substituted by an artificial device. The kidney was also the first organ to be successfully transplanted. The ability to replace renal function with these revolutionary technologies in the past was due to the fact that renal excretory function is based upon natural physical forces which govern solute and fluid movement from the body compartment to the external environment. The need for coordinated mechanical or electrical activities for renal substitution was not required. Accordingly, the kidney may well be the first organ to be available as a tissue-engineered implantable device as a fully functional replacement part for the human body.

References

1. Iglehart JK. 1993. The American Health Care System: The End Stage Renal Disease Program. N Engl J Med 328:366.
2. Excerpts from United States Renal Data System 1991 Annual Data Report. Prevalence and cost of ESRD therapy. Am J Kidney Dis 18(5)(supp)2:21.
3. Kriz W, Lever AF. 1969. Renal countercurrent mechanisms: Structure and function. Am Heart J 78:101.
4. Brenner BM, Humes HD. 1977. Mechanisms of glomerular ultra-filtration. N Engl J Med 297:148.
5. Landis EM, Pappenheimer JR. Exchange of substances through the capillary walls. In WF Hamilton, P Dow (eds), Handbook of Physiology: Circulation, sec 2, vol 2, p 961, Washington, DC, American Physiological Society.
6. Anderson JL, Quinn JA. 1974. Restricted transport in small pores. A model for steric exclusion and hindered particle motion. Biophys J 14:130.
7. Chang RLS, Robertson CR, Deen WM, et al. 1975. Permselectivity of the glomerular capillary wall to macromolecules: I. Theoretical considerations. Biophys J 15:861.
8. Brenner BM, Hostetter TH, Humes HD. 1978. Molecular basis of proteinuria of glomerular origin. N Engl J Med 298:826.
9. Andreoli TE, Schafer JA. 1978. Volume absorption in the pars recta: III. Luminal hypotonic-sodium reabsorption. Circ Res 52:491.
10. Knox FG, Mertz JI, Burnett JC, et al. 1983. Role of hydrostatic and oncotic pressures in renal sodium reabsorption. Circ Res 52:491.
11. Jacobson LO, Goldwasser E, Fried W, et al. 1957. Role of kidney in erythropoiesis. Nature 179:633.
12. Maxwell PH, Osmond MK, Pugh CW, et al. 1993. Identification of the renal erythropoietin-producing cells using transgenic mice. Kidney Int 441:1149.
13. Fried W. 1972. The liver as a source of extrarenal erythropoietin production. Blood 49:671.
14. Jelkmann W. 1992. Erythropoietin: Structure, control of production, and function. Physiol Rev 72(2):449.
15. Golper TA. 1986. Continuous arteriorvenous hemofiltration in acute renal failure. Am J Kidney Dis 6:373.
16. Kramer P, Wigger W, Rieger J, et al. 1977. Arterior-venous hemofiltration: A new and simple method for treatment of overhydrated patients resistant to diuretics. Klin Wochenschr 55:1121.
17. Colton CK, Henderson LW, Ford CA, et al. 1975. Kinetics of hemodiafiltration. In vitro transport characteristics of a hollow-fiber blood ultrafilter. J Lab Clin Med 85:355.

18. Henderson LW, Colton CK, Ford CA. 1975. Kinetics of hemodiafiltration: II. Clinical characterization of a new blood cleansing modality. J Lab Clin Med 85:372.

19. Kadletz M, Magometschnigg H, Minar E, et al. 1992. Implantation of in vitro endothelialized polytetrafluoroethylene grafts in human beings. J Thorac Cardiovasc Surg 104:736.

20. Schnider PA, Hanson SR, Price TM, et al. 1988. Durability of confluent endothelial cell monolayers of small-caliber vascular prostheses in vitro. Surgery 103:456.

21. Shepard AD, Eldrup-Jorgensen J, Keough EM, et al. 1986. Endothelial cell seeding of small caliber synthetic grafts in the baboon. Surgery 99:318.

22. Zweibel JA, Freeman SM, Kantoff PW, et al. 1989. High-level recombinant gene expression in rabbit endothelial cells transduced by retroviral vectors. Science 243:220.

23. Wilson JM, Birinyi LK, Salomon RN, et al. 1989. Implantation of vascular grafts lined with genetically modified endothelial cells. Science 244:1344.

24. Carey DJ. 1991. Control of growth and differentiation of vascular cells by extacellular matrix proteins. Annu Rev Physiol 53:161.

25. Carley WW, Milici AJ, Madri JA. 1988. Extracellular matrix specificity for the differentiation of capillary endothelial cells. Exp Cell Res 178:426.

26. Milici AJ, Furie MB, Carley WW. 1985. The formation of fenestrations and channels by capillary endothelium in vitro. Proc Natl Acad Sci USA 82:6181.

27. Garlick JA, Katz AB, Fenjves ES, et al. 1991. Retrovirus-mediated transduction of cultured epidermal keratinocytes. J Invest Dermatol 97:824.

28. Hall PA, Watt FM. 1989. Stem cells: The generation and maintenance of cellular diversity. Development 106:619.

29. Potten CS, Lieffler M. 1990. Stem cells; lessons for and from the crypt. Development 110:1001.

30. Reynolds BA, Weiss S. 1992. Generation of neurons and astrocytes from isolated cells of the adult mammalian central nervous system. Science 255:1707.

31. Humes HD, Cieslinski DA. 1992. Interaction between growth factors and retinoic acid in the induction of kidney tubulogenesis. Exp Cell Res 201:8.

32. Humes HD, Krauss JC, Cieslinski DA, et al. Tubulogenesis from isolated single cells of adult mammalian kidney: Clonal analysis with a recombinant retrovirus (submitted).

33. Coimbra T, Cieslinski DA, Humes HD. 1990. Exogenous epidermal growth factor enhances renal repair in mercuric chloride-induced acute renal failure. Am J Physiol 259:F 483.

34. Humes HD, Cieslinski DA, Coimbra T, et al. 1989. Epidermal growth factor enhances renal tubule cell regeneration and repair and accelerates the recovery of renal function in postischemic acute renal failure. J Clin Invest 84:1757.

35. Ip TK, Aebischer P. 1989. Renal epithelial-cell-controlled solute transport across permeable membranes as the foundation for a bioartificial kidney. Artif Organs 13:58.

36. Aebischer P, Wahlberg L, Tresco PA, et al. 1991. Macroencapsulation of dopamine-secreting cells by coextrusion with an organic polymer solution. Biomaterials 12:50.

37. Tai IT, Sun AM. 1993. Microencapsulation of recombinant cells: A new delivery system for gene therapy. FASEB J 7:1061.

38. McKay SM, Funke AJ, Buffington DA, Humes HD. 1998. Tissue engineering of a bioartificial renal tubule. ASAIO J 44:179–183.

39. Cozzi E, White D. 1995. The generation of transgenic pigs as potential organ donors for humans. Nat Med 1:965–966.

40. Cooper DKC, Ye Y, Rolf JLL, Zuhdi N. 1991. The pig as potential organ donor for man. In Cooper DKC, Kemp E, Reemtsma K, White DJG (eds), Xeno-Transplantation. Springer, Berlin. pp 481–500.

41. Calne RY. 1970. Organ transplantation between widely disparate species. Transplant Proc 2:550–553.

42. Humes HD, Cieslinski DA. 1992. Interaction between growth factors and retinoic acid in the induction of kidney tubulogenesis. Exp Cell Res 201:8–15.

43. Humes HD, Krauss JC, Cieslinski DA, Funke AJ. 1996. Tubulogenesis from isolated single cells of adult mammalian kidney: clonal analysis with a recombinant retrovirus. Am J Physiol Renal 271(40):F42–F49.

44. Weitzel WF, Browning A, Buffington DA, Funke AJ, Gupte A, MacKay S, Humes HD. Analysis of a renal proximal tubule assist device (RAD) during CVVH on uremic dogs, J Am Soc of Nephrol Abstract, 31st Annual Meeting, (In press).

45. Ong ACM, Fine LG. 1994. Tubular-derived growth factors and cytokines in the pathogenesis of tubulointerstitial fibrosis: Implications for human renal disease progression. Am J Kidney Dis 23:205–209.

46. Aebischer P, Tresco PA, Winn SR, et al. Long-term cross-species brain transplantation of a polymer-encapsulated dopamine-secreting cell line. Exp Neurol 111:269.

47. Relulier E, Schneider BL, Deglon N, Beuzard Y, Aebischer P. 1998. Continuous delivery of human and mouse erythropoietin in mice by genetically engineered polymer encapsulated myoblasts. Gene Ther 5:1014–1022.

48. Excerpts from the United States Renal Data System 1998 Annual Data Report. The economic cost of ESRD and Medicare spending for alternative modalities of treatment. J Kidney Dis 32(2)(supp)1:S118.

Index

9 780367 446758